Nursing Assistant Care

Susan Alvare
Diana Dugan, RN
Jetta Fuzy, RN, MS

Hartman Publishing, Inc.
hartmanonline.com

Credits

MANAGING EDITOR
Susan Alvare

COVER AND INTERIOR DESIGNER
Kirsten Browne

ILLUSTRATOR/PAGE LAYOUT
Thaddeus Castillo

PROOFREADERS
Kristin Calderon
Celia McIntire

PHOTOGRAPHY
Art Clifton/Dick Ruddy/Susana Marks

SALES/MARKETING
Debbie Rinker/Caroyl Scott/Cheryl Garcia/Kendra Robertson

CUSTOMER SERVICE
Fran Desmond/Tom Noble/Angela Storey/Kim Williams

Copyright Information

8529 Indian School Road, NE
Albuquerque, New Mexico 87112
(505) 291-1274
web: www.**hartman**online.com
e-mail: orders@**hartman**online.com

ISBN-13 978-1-888343-80-9 (paperback)
ISBN-10 1-888343-80-X

ISBN-13 978-1-888343-83-0 (hardcover)
ISBN-10 1-888343-83-4

NOTICE TO READERS
Though the guidelines and procedures contained in this text are based on consultations with healthcare professionals, they should not be considered absolute recommendations. The instructor and readers should follow employer, local, state, and federal guidelines concerning healthcare practices. These guidelines change, and it is the reader's responsibility to be aware of these changes and of the policies and procedures of her or his healthcare facility.

The publisher, author, editors, and reviewers cannot accept any responsibility for errors or omissions or for any consequences from application of the information in this book and make no warranty, expressed or implied, with respect to the contents of the book. The Publisher does not warrant or guarantee any of the products described herein or perform any analysis in connection with any of the product information contained herein.

GENDER USAGE
This textbook utilizes the pronouns he, his, she, and hers interchangeably to denote care team members and residents.

PRINTED IN CANADA

Special Thanks

Sincere thanks to all of our knowledgeable and insightful reviewers:

Kathryn L. Stockton, RN, BSN

Linda S. Stricklin, RN, BSN, MSHP

Leona M. Howell, MS, BSN

Karla Jones, RN, MS

Steven O. Ross, RNC

Lois Moore, RN, MS, MPH

Margaret Pearson, CEO

Anne Snyder, COO

Table of Contents

Chapter 5
Quality Infection Control

Chapter 6
Safety and Body Mechanics

Chapter 7
Emergency Care and Disaster Preparation

Chapter 8
Human Needs and Human Development

Chapter 9
The Healthy Human Body

Chapter 10
Moving, Lifting, and Positioning

Chapter 11
Admitting, Transferring, and Discharging

Chapter 12
The Resident's Unit

Chapter 13
Personal Care Skills

Chapter 14
Urinary Elimination

Chapter 15
Bowel Elimination

Chapter 16
Nutrition and Hydration

Chapter 19
Confusion, Dementia, and Alzheimer's Disease

Chapter 20
Mental Health and Mental Illness

Chapter 21
Rehabilitation and Restorative Care

Chapter 22
Subacute Care

Table of Procedures

Using this Textbook

This book will help you master what you need to know to provide excellent care to residents with very different needs. It will also teach you to take care of yourself and your career.

Understanding how the book is organized will help you make the most of this resource.

We have assigned each chapter its own colored tab. Each colored tab contains the chapter number and title, and you'll see them on the side of every page.

6 Safety and Body Mechanics

1. Explain HIPAA and list ways to protect residents' privacy

Everything in this book, the student workbook, and your instructor's teaching material is organized around learning objectives. A learning objective is a very specific piece of knowledge or a very specific skill. After reading the text, if you can DO what the learning objective says, you know you have mastered the material.

---

key terms

You'll find **bold** key terms throughout the text. These terms are defined in the text and again in the glossary at the back of this book.

Washing hands

All care procedures are highlighted by the same black bar for easy recognition.

---

g O&R

Guidelines and observing and reporting are colored for easy reference.

This icon helps you find important information about abuse and neglect and how to recognize and prevent both. Ways to support and promote Residents' Rights are also included.

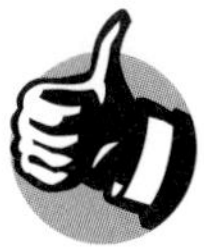

These icons call out interesting and educational tidbits that you can use inside and outside of work.

Chapter Review

Chapter-ending questions test your knowledge of the information found in the chapter. If you have trouble answering a question, you can return to the text and reread the material.

Chapter 1
Understanding Long-Term Care

1. Compare long-term care to other healthcare settings

Welcome to the world of health care. Health care is found in many different places. Nursing assistants work in many of these settings. In each, similar tasks will be done. However, each setting is also unique.

This textbook will focus on settings that provide long-term care. **Long-term care** (LTC) is for people who need 24-hour care. It assists those with ongoing conditions. Other terms for long-term care facilities are:

- nursing homes
- nursing facilities
- skilled nursing facilities
- extended care facilities

The people who live in these facilities may be disabled and/or elderly. They may come from hospitals or other facilities. Some will have a terminal illness. **Terminal** means the person is expected to die from the illness. Some people come to nursing homes for conditions that need care for six months or longer. Other people come for short stays. Some people recover. They may return to their homes or to assisted living facilities.

Most conditions seen in nursing homes are **chronic**. This means they last a long period of time, even a lifetime. Chronic conditions include physical disabilities, heart disease, stroke, and dementia. (You will learn more about these disorders and diseases in chapter 18.) In a nursing home, you will form relationships with residents for longer than in other healthcare settings.

While people live in this type of facility, it is their home. This is why the people who live there are called **residents** (Fig. 1-1). It will be a resident's home until he or she returns home, moves to another place, or dies.

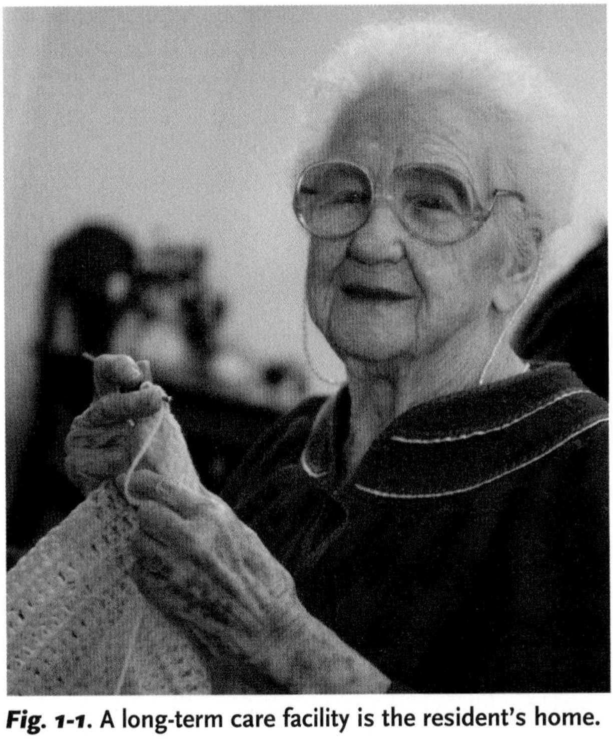

Fig. 1-1. **A long-term care facility is the resident's home.**

Other types of healthcare settings are:

Acute care is given in hospitals and ambulatory surgical centers. It is for people who have an immediate illness. People are admitted for short stays for surgery or diseases. Acute care is 24-hour skilled care for temporary, but serious, illnesses or injuries (Fig. 1-2). **Skilled care** is medically necessary care given by a skilled nurse or therapist. This care is available 24 hours a day. It is ordered by a doctor, and involves a treatment plan.

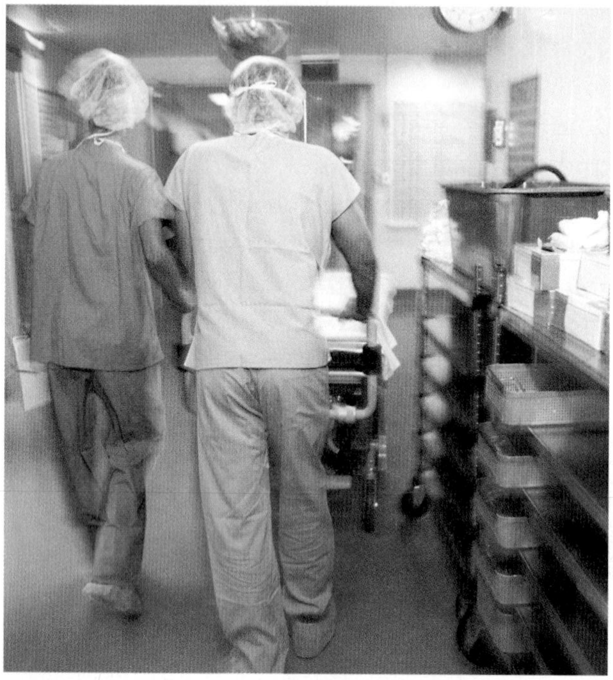

Fig. 1-2. **Acute care is performed in hospitals.**

Subacute care can be given in a hospital or in a nursing home. The residents need more care and observation than some long-term care facilities can give. The cost is usually less than a hospital but more than long-term care. You will learn about subacute care in chapter 22.

Outpatient care is usually given for less than 24-hours. It is for people who have had treatments or surgery that need short-term skilled care.

Rehabilitation is care given by a specialist. Physical, occupational, and speech therapists restore or improve function after an illness or injury.

In **assisted living**, residents need some help with daily care, such as showers, meals, and dressing. They may also need help with medications. Staff give whatever daily care the resident needs. Residents who live in assisted living facilities are generally more independent. They do not usually need skilled care.

Assisted living facilities allow independent living in a home-like environment. An assisted living facility may be attached to a long-term care facility. It may also stand alone.

Home health care takes place in a person's home (Fig. 1-3). In some ways, working as a home health aide is similar to working as a nursing assistant. Almost all care in this textbook applies to home health aides. Most of the personal care and basic nursing procedures are the same. Home health aides may also clean, shop for groceries, do laundry, and cook.

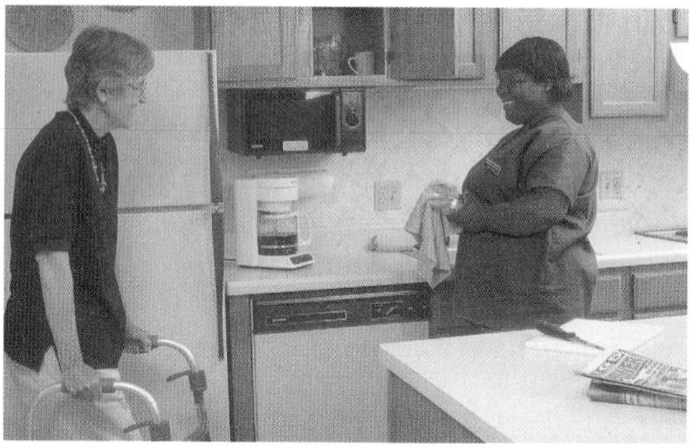

Fig. 1-3. **Home care is performed in a person's home.**

Home health aides may have more contact with the family. They also will work more independently, although a supervisor monitors their work. The advantage of home health care is that clients do not have to leave home. They may have lived there for many years. Staying at home may be comforting.

Adult daycare is given at a facility during daytime work hours. Generally, adult daycare cares for people who need some help but are not seriously ill or disabled. Adult daycare centers give different levels of care.

Adult daycare can also provide a break for spouses, family members, and friends. A center may be a part of another facility, or it may stand alone. The daily fee is usually much less than the cost of a long-term care facility.

Hospice care is for people who have six months or less to live. A doctor decides this. Hospice workers give physical and emotional care and comfort. They also support families. Hospice care can take place in facilities or in homes.

Residents' **diagnoses**, or medical conditions, will vary. The stages of illnesses or diseases affect how sick people are and how much care they will need. The job of nursing assistants will also vary. This is due to the person's different symptoms, abilities, and needs.

This textbook focuses on care for residents living in long-term care settings. Acute care facilities will not be covered. Subacute care will be covered in some depth later in the textbook.

2. Describe a typical long-term care facility

A long-term care facility may give only skilled nursing care. It may offer assisted living, dementia care, or even subacute care. Some facilities offer specialized care. Others care for all types of residents. The typical long-term care facility offers personal care for all residents and focused care for residents with special needs. When specialized care is offered, the employees must have special training. Residents with similar needs may be placed in units together.

For-profit companies or nonprofit organizations can own facilities.

3. Explain Medicare and Medicaid

The Centers for Medicare & Medicaid Services (CMS), was formerly known as the Health Care Finance Administration (HCFA). It is a federal agency within the U.S. Department of Health and Human Services. CMS runs two national healthcare programs, Medicare and Medicaid. They both help pay for health care and health insurance for millions of Americans. CMS has many other responsibilities as well.

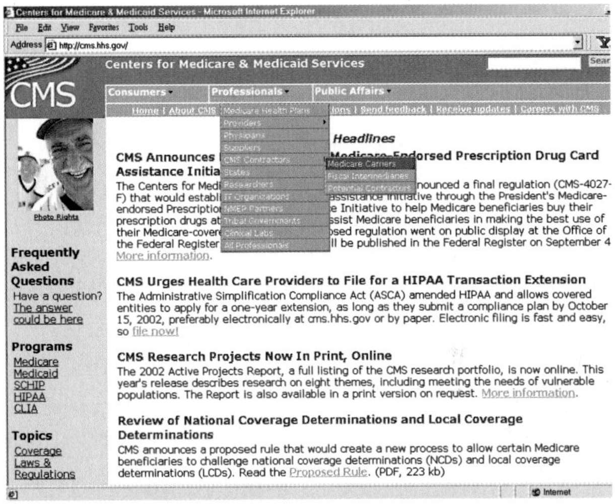

Fig. 1-4. **The CMS web site.**

Medicare is a health insurance program for people who are 65 or older. It also covers people younger than 65 who are disabled or ill and cannot work.

Medicare has two parts: Hospital Insurance (Part A), and Medical Insurance (Part B). Part A helps pay for care from a hospital, skilled nursing facility, home health agency, or hospice. Part B helps pay for physician services and other medical services and equipment. Medicare covers a percentage of healthcare costs. Medicare will only pay for care it determines to be medically necessary.

Medicaid is a medical assistance program for low-income people. It is funded by both the federal government and each state. Eligibility is determined by income and special circumstances. People must qualify for this program.

Medicare and Medicaid pay long-term care facilities a fixed amount for services. This is based on the resident's need upon admission.

4. Describe the long-term care survey process

Inspections are done to make sure long-term care facilities (and home health agencies) follow state and federal regulations. Inspections are done every nine to 15 months by the state agency that licenses facilities. These inspections are called **surveys**. They may be done more often if a facility has been cited. To **cite** means to find a problem through a survey. Inspections may be done less often if the facility has a good record. Inspection teams include a variety of trained healthcare professionals.

Surveyors study how well staff care for its residents. They focus on how residents' nutritional, physical, psychosocial, and spiritual needs are met. They do this by interviewing residents and family. They observe staff's interactions with residents and care given. They review resident charts. They observe meals. Surveys are one reason the "paperwork" part of a nursing assistant's job is so important. You will learn more about this throughout the textbook.

If a facility is cited for not following a federal regulation, surveyors use federal tags (F-tags) to note these problems.

When surveyors are in your facility, try not to be nervous. Give the same great care you do every day. Answer any questions to the best of your ability. If you do not know the answer, be honest. Never guess. Tell the surveyor that you do not know the answer but will find out as quickly as possible. Then do just that. Do not offer any information unless asked.

5. Explain policies and procedures

All facilities must have manuals outlining policies and procedures. A **policy** is a course of action to be followed. A very basic policy is that healthcare information must remain confidential. A **procedure** is a method, or way, of doing something. A facility will have a procedure for reporting information about residents. The procedure explains what form to complete, when and how often to fill it out, and to whom it is given. You will be told where to find a list of policies and procedures that all staff are expected to follow.

Common policies at long-term care facilities include:

- All resident information must stay confidential.
- The plan of care must always be followed.
- Nursing assistants should not do tasks not included in the job description.
- Nursing assistants must report important events or changes in residents to a nurse.
- Personal problems must not be discussed with the resident or the resident's family.
- Nursing assistants should not take money or gifts from residents or their families (Fig. 1-5).
- Nursing assistants must be on time for work. They must be dependable.

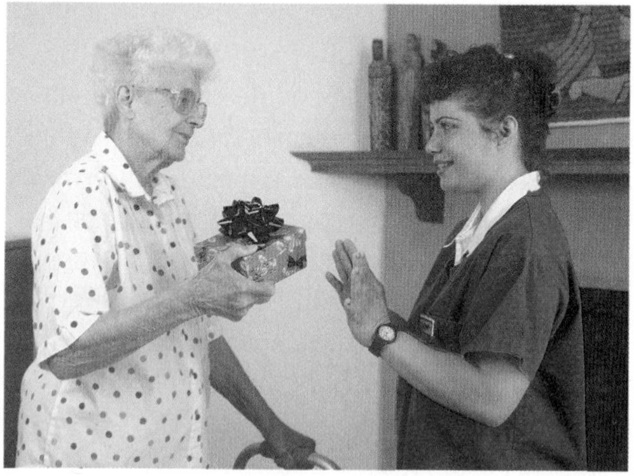

Fig. 1-5. **Nursing assistants should not accept money or gifts from residents or their families because it could lead to conflict.**

Everyone needs a reminder on how to do a task from time to time. Do not hesitate to look at the procedure manual to review steps. Nursing assistants who ask questions when they are unsure give safer resident care. Always ask if you have questions.

Your employer will have policies and procedures for every resident care situation. Written procedures may seem long and complicated, but each step is important. Become familiar with your facility's policies and procedures.

6. Describe residents who live in long-term care facilities

There are some general statements that can be made about residents in nursing homes. However, more important than understanding the entire population is understanding the individuals for whom you will care. Make sure you know how to care for residents based on their needs, illnesses, and preferences.

According to the National Center for Health Statistics, almost 91 percent of long-term care residents in the U.S. are over age 65. Only nine percent are younger than 65. Almost 72 percent of residents are female (Fig. 1-6). More than 85 percent are Caucasian. This is a much larger percentage than the U.S. population as a whole. About one-third of residents come from a private residence. Over 50 percent come from a hospital or other facility.

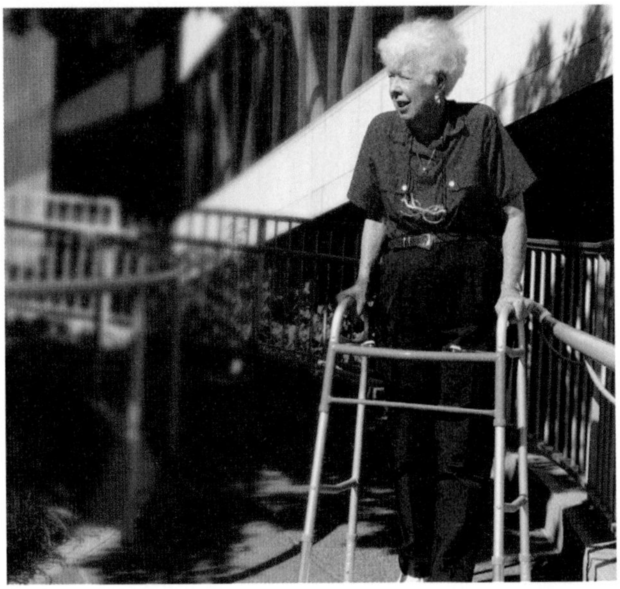

***Fig. 1-6.* Women make up a higher percentage of nursing home residents.**

The length of stay of almost one-half of residents is six months or more. The **length of stay** is the number of days a person stays in a healthcare facility. These residents need enough help with their activities of daily living that 24-hour care is needed. Often, they did not have caregivers available to give enough care for them to live in the community. The groups with the longest average stay are the mentally retarded and developmentally disabled. They are often younger than 65. You will learn more about these groups in chapter 18.

The other half of residents stay for less than six months. This group generally falls into two categories. The first is residents admitted for terminal care. They will die in the facility. The second category is residents admitted for rehabilitation or illness. They will recover and return to the community. As you can imagine, care of these residents may be very different.

Various studies place the number of nursing home residents with dementia between 50 and 90 percent. **Dementia** is defined as a serious loss of mental abilities. These include thinking, remembering, reasoning, and communicating. Dementia and other mental disorders are major causes of nursing home admissions. Many residents are admitted with other disorders. However, the disorders are often not the reason for admission. It is most often the lack of ability to care for oneself and lack of a support system that leads people into a facility.

A support system is vital in allowing the elderly to live outside a facility. For every elderly person in a long-term care facility, at least two with the same disorders and disabilities live in the community.

You may see this lack of outside support among your residents. It is one reason you will care for the "whole person," instead of only the illness or disease. Residents have many needs besides bathing, eating and drinking, and toileting. These needs will go unmet if staff do not work to meet them.

Chapter Review

1. Which of these statements about long-term care is true?
   a. Long-term care is for people who need 24-hour care and assistance for conditions that are long-term.
   b. Long-term care is for people who have chronic conditions.
   c. Long-term care is for people who have terminal illnesses.
   d. All of the above
2. What are some ways that working as a home health aide is different than working as a nursing assistant in long-term care?
   a. Home health aides do not have to bathe residents.
   b. Home health aides do not have supervision.
   c. Home health aides may have to clean the home and cook meals.
   d. Home health aides do not have to shop for groceries.
3. What types of services may a long-term care facility give?
4. Briefly describe what the Medicare and Medicaid programs do.
5. List three ways that surveyors decide how well a facility cares for its residents.
6. Define policies and procedures. List four examples of facility policies.
7. Almost 91 percent of residents in nursing homes are over what age?
8. Who makes up the majority of nursing home residents—men or women?

Chapter 2
The Nursing Assistant and The Care Team

1. Explain the nursing assistant's role

Nursing assistants can have many different titles. "Nurse aide," "unlicensed assistive personnel," and "certified nursing assistant" are some. This book will use the term "nursing assistant."

A nursing assistant (NA) does delegated or assigned nursing tasks. These include taking residents' temperature and blood pressure. **Delegation** means transferring authority to a person to for a specific task. A nursing assistant also gives personal care, such as bathing residents and helping them with hair care.

Other nursing assistant duties are:

- feeding residents
- helping residents with toileting and elimination needs
- helping residents to move safely around the facility
- keeping residents' living areas neat and clean
- encouraging residents to eat and drink (Fig. 2-1)
- caring for supplies and equipment
- helping dress residents
- making beds
- giving backrubs
- helping residents with mouth care

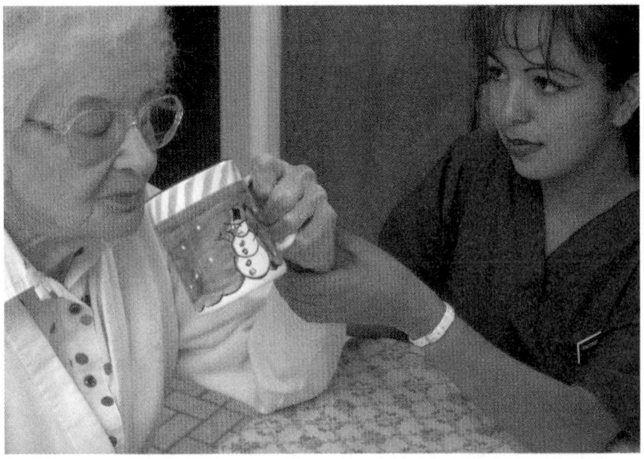

Fig. 2-1. **Encouraging residents to drink often will be an important part of your job.**

Nursing assistants are not allowed to give medications. Nurses are responsible for this. Some states allow nursing assistants to work with medications after receiving special training.

Nursing assistants spend more time with residents than other team members do. They are the "eyes and ears" of the team. Observing changes in a resident's condition and reporting them is a very important role. You will also write down important information about the resident (Fig. 2-2). This is called **charting**.

Nursing assistants are part of a team of health professionals. Everyone, including residents, works together to meet goals. Goals include helping residents to recover from illnesses or to do as much as they can for themselves.

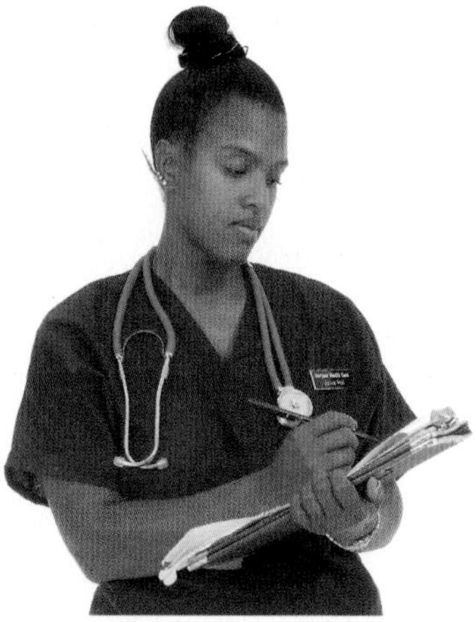

Fig. 2-2. **Writing down what you observe is an important duty you will have.**

Organizing Your Work

It is important to organize and prioritize your work every day. Do you use sticky notes to remind yourself to do things at home? Many nursing assistants and other team members use a similar method at work. A small notebook can make the difference between feeling organized and feeling overwhelmed.

2. Explain professionalism and list examples of professional behavior

Professional means dealing with work or a job. The opposite of professional is **personal**. It refers to your life outside your job. This includes your family, friends, and home life. **Professionalism** is behaving properly on the job. It includes how you dress, the words you use, and what you talk about. It also means being on time, completing tasks, and reporting to the nurse. Professionalism is also following the care plan, making careful observations, and always reporting accurately. Following policies and procedures is an important part of professionalism.

Residents, coworkers, and supervisors respect employees who are professional. Professionalism helps you keep your job. It also helps you earn promotions and raises.

A professional relationship with a resident includes:

- keeping a positive attitude
- being clean and neatly dressed and groomed
- doing only the assigned tasks you are trained to do
- keeping all residents' information confidential
- being polite and cheerful, even if you are not in a good mood (Fig. 2-3)
- not discussing your personal problems
- not using profanity, even if a resident does
- listening to the resident

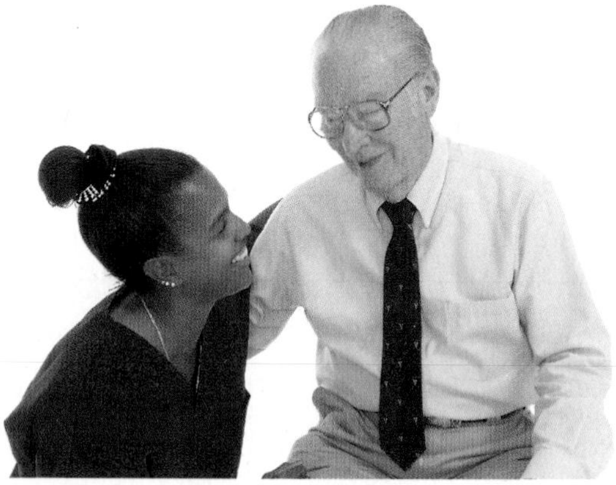

Fig. 2-3. **Being polite and cheerful with residents is something that will be expected of you.**

- calling a resident "Mr.," "Mrs.," "Ms.,", or "Miss," or by the name he or she prefers
- never giving or accepting gifts
- always explaining the care you will give before giving it
- following practices, such as handwashing, to protect yourself and residents

A professional relationship with an employer includes:

- completing tasks efficiently
- always following all policies and procedures
- always documenting and reporting carefully and correctly

- communicating problems with residents or tasks
- reporting anything that keeps you from completing tasks
- asking questions when you do not know or understand something
- taking directions or criticism without getting upset
- always being on time
- telling your employer if you cannot report for work
- following the chain of command
- participating in education programs
- being a positive role model

The best nursing assistants have these qualities:

Compassion. Being **compassionate** is being caring, concerned, considerate, empathetic, and understanding. **Empathy** means entering into the feelings of others. Compassionate people understand others' problems. They care about them. Compassionate people are also sympathetic. **Sympathy** means sharing in the feelings and difficulties of others.

Honesty. An honest person tells the truth and can be trusted. Residents must be able to trust those who care for them. The care team depends on your honesty in planning care. Employers count on truthful records of your care and observations.

Tact. **Tact** is the ability to understand what is proper and appropriate when dealing with others. It is the ability to speak and act without offending others.

Conscientiousness. People who are **conscientious** always try to do their best. They are always alert, observant, accurate, and responsible. Conscientious care means making correct observations and reports, following assignments, and taking responsibility for actions (Fig. 2-4). For example, taking accurate measurements of vital signs, such as temperature or pulse, is important. The care team will make decisions from your measurements. Without conscientious care, a resident's health and well-being are in danger.

Dependability. Nursing assistants must make and keep commitments. You must get to work on time. You must skillfully do tasks, avoid too many absences, and help your peers when they need it.

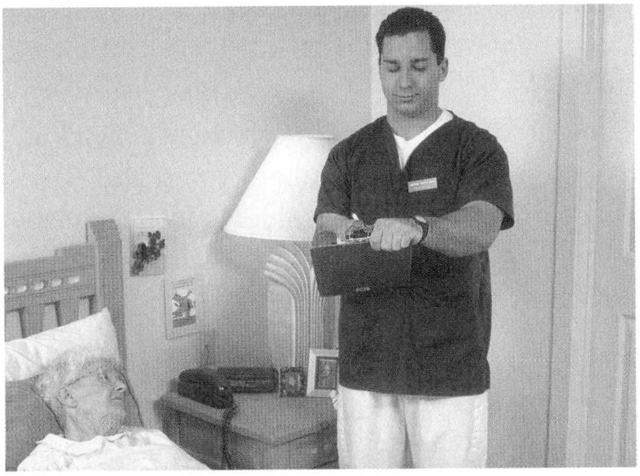

Fig. 2-4. **Nursing assistants must be conscientious in documenting observations and procedures.**

Respect. Being respectful means valuing other people's individuality. This includes their age, religion, culture, feelings, and beliefs. People who are respectful treat others politely and kindly. You should care about people's self-esteem. Do not do or say things that will harm it. You must not disrespect others by gossiping. Respect the culture and practices of each person.

Lack of prejudice. You will work with different people from many backgrounds. Give each resident quality care regardless of age, gender, sexual orientation, religion, race, ethnicity, or condition.

Tolerance. You may not like or agree with things that your residents or their families do or have done. However, your job is to care for each resident as assigned, not to judge him or her. Put aside your opinions. See each resident as an individual who needs your care.

NAs: In demand in 1945

Nursing assistants have been in demand for many years. This list of unfilled positions in hospitals appeared late in 1945:

- *Registered Nurses 65,000*
- *Non-nursing personnel 90,000*
- *Nurses' Aides 90,000*
- *Untrained volunteers 45,000*

3. Describe good personal grooming habits

Good grooming makes you feel great. And, it makes others feel good about you (Fig. 2-5). Grooming affects how residents feel about the care you give. Good grooming habits nursing assistants should follow are:

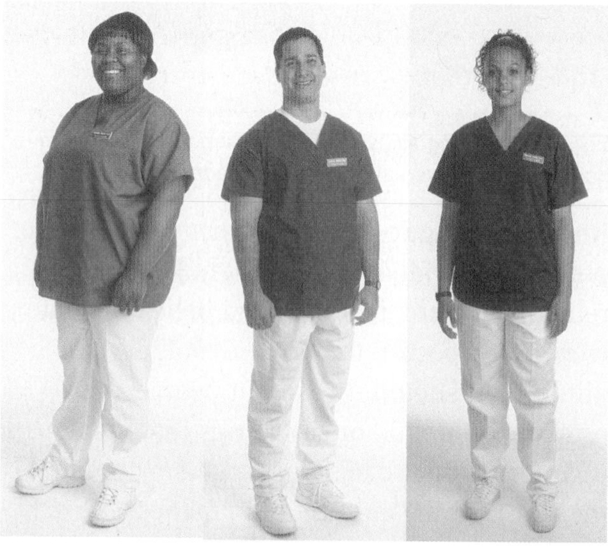

Fig. 2-5. **Good grooming includes being clean and neatly dressed. Keep long hair tied back, and apply makeup lightly.**

- Bathe or shower daily. Use deodorant or anti-perspirant. Use little or no perfume or cologne. Some residents may dislike or be allergic to scents.
- Brush your teeth often. Use mouthwash when needed.
- Keep your hair clean and neatly brushed or combed. Tie long hair back in a bun or ponytail. Long hair that is not tied back can block your vision. It may even fall into residents' faces as you give them care. Men should keep facial hair short and neat.
- Dress neatly. Keep your uniform washed and ironed. Do not wear clothes that are too tight or too baggy, torn or stained, or too revealing (short skirts, low-cut blouses, see-through fabrics).
- Do not wear jewelry that is large or gets in the way. If you wear rings or bracelets, remove them while working. Rings and bracelets house bacteria. This causes disease. Sharp edges can scratch or tear a resident's fragile skin. Residents can pull on earrings, causing injury. The main exception to this rule is to wear a simple, waterproof watch. You will use it to take a resident's pulse and respirations and record events.
- Wear comfortable, clean, and quality shoes. Change the laces if they are stained or soiled. Keep shoes clean (Fig. 2-6).

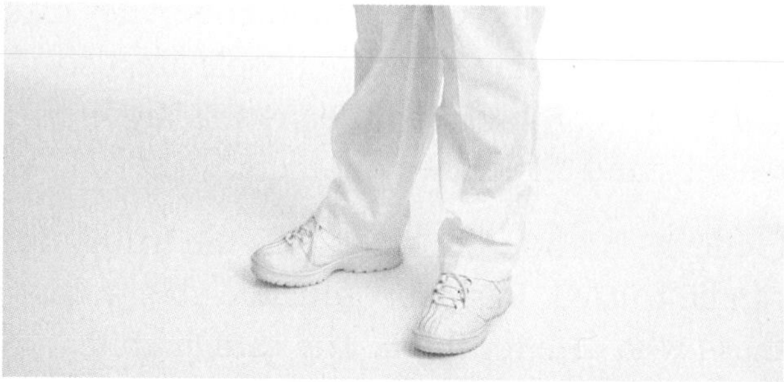

Fig. 2-6. **Wear clean, proper shoes for the job.**

- Keep fingernails short and clean. Long nails can tear a resident's skin. Do not wear false nails. False nails hide bacteria no matter how well you wash your hands.
- Wear little or no makeup. If you wear it, apply it lightly.

Kill the scent.

Wearing colognes and perfumes when you know a resident does not like scents or has allergies may be considered abuse. You must try to meet the needs of residents in every way. That means respecting their individual problems. Put their comfort first.

4. Identify the role of each member of the care team

Residents have different needs and problems. This means that people with different kinds of education and experience help care for them (Fig. 2-7). This group is the **care team**. Members of the care team include:

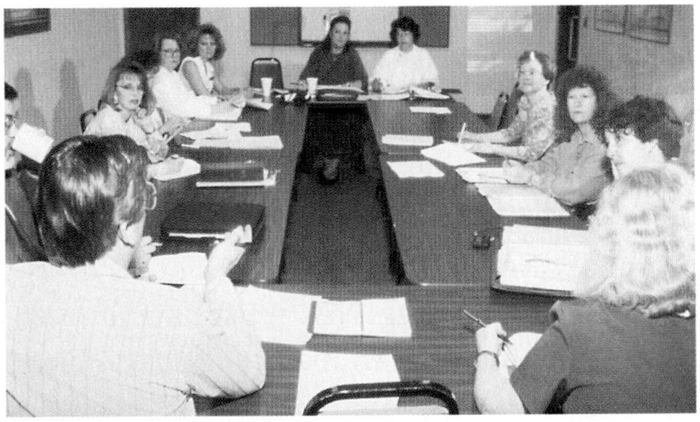

Fig. 2-7. **The care team is made up of many different people.**

Registered Nurse (RN). A **registered nurse** is a licensed professional. He or she has completed two to four years of education. RNs have diplomas or college degrees. They have passed a licensing exam run by the state board of nursing. Registered nurses may have other degrees or education in specialty areas.

The nurse assesses residents' status, monitors progress, and provides skilled nursing care. The nurse gives treatments, including drug therapies, as prescribed by a doctor. The nurse also assigns tasks and supervises your daily care of residents.

Licensed Practical Nurse (LPN) or Licensed Vocational Nurse (LVN). A **licensed practical nurse** or **licensed vocational nurse** is a licensed professional. He or she has completed one to two years of education. A LPN/LVN passes medications and gives treatments. LPNs may also supervise your daily care of residents.

Physician or Doctor (MD or DO). A doctor diagnoses disease or disability and prescribes treatment. Doctors attend four-year medical schools after receiving a bachelor's degree. Many doctors also take specialized training programs after medical school (Fig. 2-8).

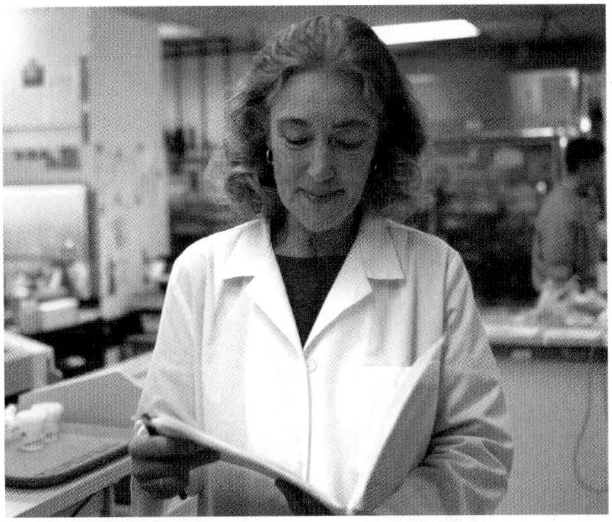

Fig. 2-8. **Doctors diagnose disease and prescribe treatment.**

Physical Therapist (PT). The **physical therapist** gives therapy in the form of heat, cold, massage, ultrasound, electricity, and exercise to people with muscle, bone, and joint problems. Goals of physical therapy are improving blood circulation, healing, regaining mobility, and easing pain. For example, a PT helps a person to safely use a walker, cane or wheelchair (Fig. 2-9).

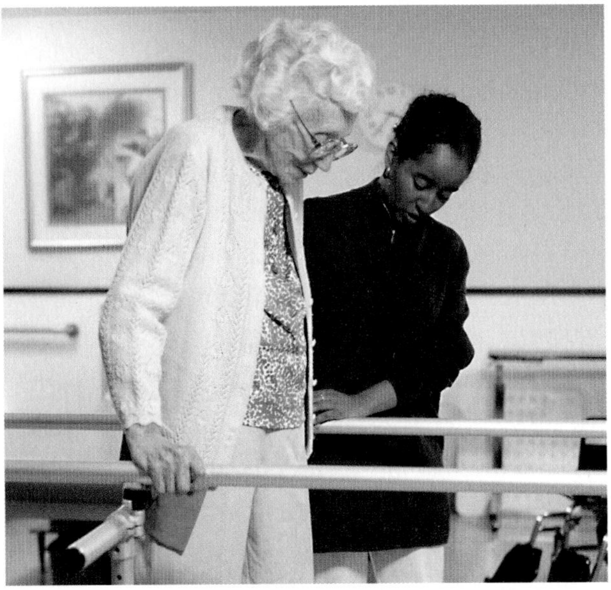

Fig. 2-9. **A physical therapist will help restore specific abilities.**

Occupational Therapist (OT). An **occupational therapist** helps residents learn to compensate for disabilities. An OT helps residents be able to do **activities of daily living** (ADLs). ADLs are personal daily care tasks. They include bathing, dressing, caring for teeth and hair, toileting, and eating and drinking. This often involves equipment called **assistive** or **adaptive devices** (Fig. 2-10). (See chapter 21 for more information.) For example, an OT can teach a person to use a special fork to feed himself. The OT observes a resident's needs and plans a treatment program.

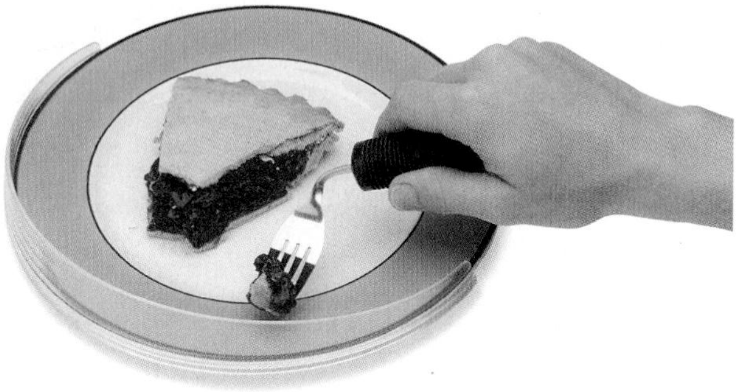

Fig. 2-10. **An occupational therapist will help residents learn to use adaptive devices, such as this one for eating. (Photo courtesy of North Coast Medical, Inc. 800-821-9319.)**

Speech Language Pathologist (SLP). A **speech language pathologist**, or **speech therapist**, helps with speech and swallowing problems. An SLP makes a plan of care to meet short- and long-term recovery goals. An SLP teaches exercises to help the resident improve or overcome speech problems. For example, after a stroke, a person may not be able to talk. An SLP may use a picture board to help the person communicate thirst or pain. An SLP also evaluates a person's ability to swallow food and drink.

Registered Dietitian (RDT). A **registered dietitian** or **nutritionist** creates diets for residents with special needs. Special diets can improve health and help manage illness.

Medical Social Worker. A **medical social worker** helps with social needs. For example, a medical social worker helps residents find compatible roommates. He or she also helps with support services. These include obtaining clothing and personal items if the family is not involved or does not visit often. A medical social worker may book appointments and transportation.

Activities Director. The **activities director** plans activities, such as bingo or special performances. This helps residents socialize and stay physically and mentally active.

Nursing Assistant (NA) or Certified Nursing Assistant (CNA). The **nursing assistant** (NA) does delegated or assigned tasks, such as taking a resident's temperature. NAs also give personal care, such as bathing residents and helping with toileting. NAs must have at least 75 hours of training. In many states, training exceeds 100 hours.

Resident and Resident's Family. The resident is an important member of the care team. The resident has the right to make decisions about his or her own care. The resident helps plan care and makes choices. The team revolves around the resident and his or her condition, treatment, and progress. Without the resident, there is no care team.

The resident's family may also be involved in these decisions. The family is a great source of information. They know the resident's personal preferences, history, diet, rituals, and routines.

5. Explain the chain of command and scope of practice

As a nursing assistant, you will follow instructions given by a nurse. The nurse acts on the doctor's instructions. This is called the **chain of command**. It describes the line of authority in the facility.

The chain of command coordinates care to provide the best care for residents. It also protects you and your employer from liability. **Liability** is a legal term. It means a person can be held responsible for harming someone else. Example: Something you did for a resident harmed him. However, what you did was assigned to you. It was done according to policy and procedure. Then, you may not be liable, or responsible, for hurting the resident. If you do something not assigned to you and it harms a resident, you could be held responsible. That is why it is important to follow instructions and know the chain of command (Fig. 2-11).

Everyone must know what they can and cannot do. This is so that you do not harm a resident or involve yourself or your employer in a lawsuit. Some states certify that a nursing assistant is qualified to work. However, nursing assistants are not licensed healthcare providers. Everything in your job is assigned to you by a licensed healthcare professional.

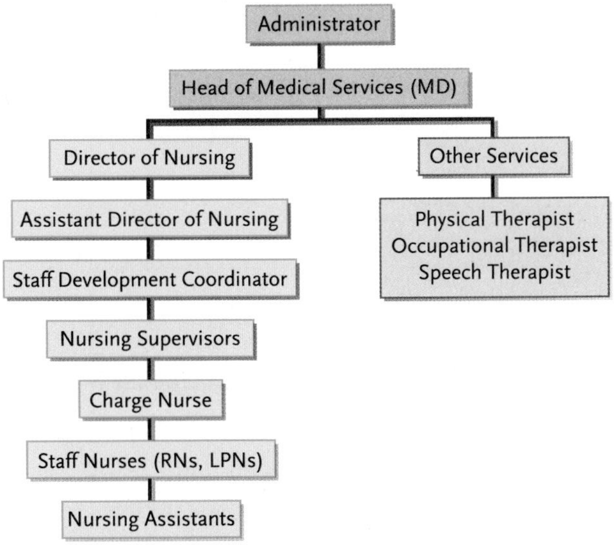

Fig. 2-11. **The chain of command describes the line of authority in a facility.**

You work under the authority of another person's license. That is why these professionals will show great interest in what you do and how you do it.

Every state grants the right to do various jobs in health care through licensure. Examples include nursing, medicine, or physical therapy. All members of the care team work under each profession's "scope of practice." A **scope of practice** defines the things you are allowed to do and how to do them correctly.

Never call yourself a nurse.

Do not identify yourself as a nurse. A nurse has had more training and has different responsibilities. So never use the term "nurse" lightly. Always identify yourself as a nursing assistant.

6. Define "care plan" and explain its purpose

A care plan is created for each resident. A **care plan** is written and developed by the nurse. It helps the resident achieve his or her goals. The resident assists with developing the care plan. The care plan outlines the steps and tasks the care team, including the NA, must perform (Fig. 2-12).

The care plan is a guide. It helps the resident reach and maintain the best level of health possible. Activities not listed on the care plan should not be done without permission from a nurse. The care plan must be followed very carefully.

In this text you will read how important it is to make observations and report them to the nurse. Sometimes even simple observations are very important. The information you collect and the changes you observe are both important in deciding how the care plan needs to change.

7. Describe the nursing process

To communicate with other care team members, nurses use the **nursing process**. This is an organized method used by nurses to determine the nursing care for residents. The process has five steps:

- **assessment**: getting information from many sources, such as medical history and a physical assessment, and reviewing it

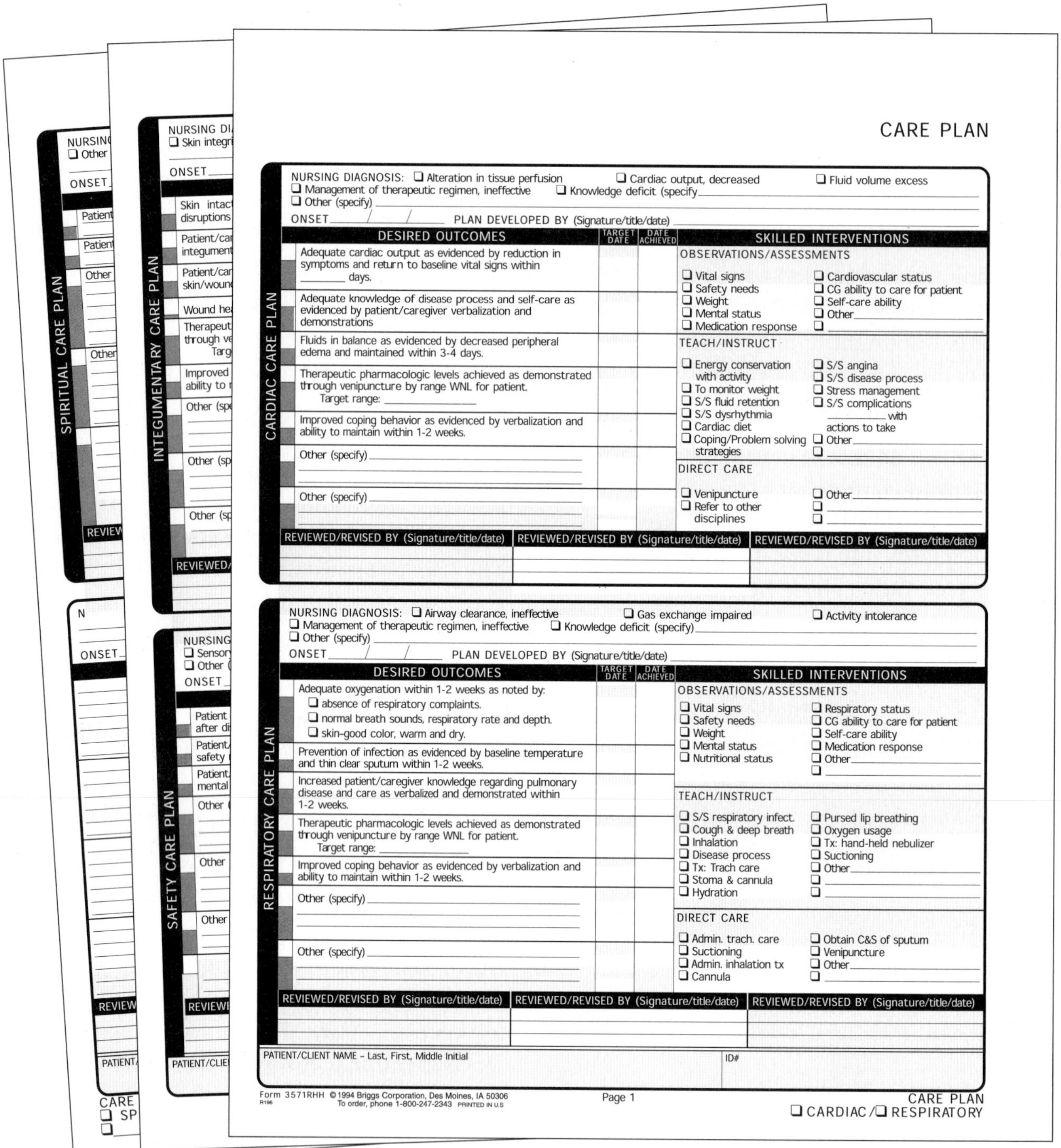
CARE PLAN

CARDIAC CARE PLAN

NURSING DIAGNOSIS: ❑ Alteration in tissue perfusion ❑ Cardiac output, decreased ❑ Fluid volume excess
❑ Management of therapeutic regimen, ineffective ❑ Knowledge deficit (specify
❑ Other (specify)
ONSET ___/___/___ PLAN DEVELOPED BY (Signature/title/date)

DESIRED OUTCOMES	TARGET DATE	DATE ACHIEVED
Adequate cardiac output as evidenced by reduction in symptoms and return to baseline vital signs within ______ days.		
Adequate knowledge of disease process and self-care as evidenced by patient/caregiver verbalization and demonstrations		
Fluids in balance as evidenced by decreased peripheral edema and maintained within 3-4 days.		
Therapeutic pharmacologic levels achieved as demonstrated through venipuncture by range WNL for patient. Target range: ______		
Improved coping behavior as evidenced by verbalization and ability to maintain within 1-2 weeks.		
Other (specify)		
Other (specify)		

SKILLED INTERVENTIONS

OBSERVATIONS/ASSESSMENTS
❑ Vital signs ❑ Cardiovascular status
❑ Safety needs ❑ CG ability to care for patient
❑ Weight ❑ Self-care ability
❑ Mental status ❑ Other
❑ Medication response ❑

TEACH/INSTRUCT
❑ Energy conservation with activity ❑ S/S angina
❑ To monitor weight ❑ S/S disease process
❑ S/S fluid retention ❑ Stress management
❑ S/S dysrhythmia ❑ S/S complications ______ with actions to take
❑ Cardiac diet
❑ Coping/Problem solving strategies ❑ Other
❑

DIRECT CARE
❑ Venipuncture ❑ Other
❑ Refer to other disciplines ❑
❑

REVIEWED/REVISED BY (Signature/title/date) | REVIEWED/REVISED BY (Signature/title/date) | REVIEWED/REVISED BY (Signature/title/date)

RESPIRATORY CARE PLAN

NURSING DIAGNOSIS: ❑ Airway clearance, ineffective ❑ Gas exchange impaired ❑ Activity intolerance
❑ Management of therapeutic regimen, ineffective ❑ Knowledge deficit (specify)
❑ Other (specify)
ONSET ___/___/___ PLAN DEVELOPED BY (Signature/title/date)

DESIRED OUTCOMES	TARGET DATE	DATE ACHIEVED
Adequate oxygenation within 1-2 weeks as noted by: ❑ absence of respiratory complaints. ❑ normal breath sounds, respiratory rate and depth. ❑ skin-good color, warm and dry.		
Prevention of infection as evidenced by baseline temperature and thin clear sputum within 1-2 weeks.		
Increased patient/caregiver knowledge regarding pulmonary disease and care as verbalized and demonstrated within 1-2 weeks.		
Therapeutic pharmacologic levels achieved as demonstrated through venipuncture by range WNL for patient. Target range: ______		
Improved coping behavior as evidenced by verbalization and ability to maintain within 1-2 weeks.		
Other (specify)		
Other (specify)		

SKILLED INTERVENTIONS

OBSERVATIONS/ASSESSMENTS
❑ Vital signs ❑ Respiratory status
❑ Safety needs ❑ CG ability to care for patient
❑ Weight ❑ Self-care ability
❑ Mental status ❑ Medication response
❑ Nutritional status ❑ Other
❑

TEACH/INSTRUCT
❑ S/S respiratory infect. ❑ Pursed lip breathing
❑ Cough & deep breath ❑ Oxygen usage
❑ Inhalation ❑ Tx: hand-held nebulizer
❑ Disease process ❑ Suctioning
❑ Tx: Trach care ❑ Other
❑ Stoma & cannula ❑
❑ Hydration ❑

DIRECT CARE
❑ Admin. trach. care ❑ Obtain C&S of sputum
❑ Suctioning ❑ Venipuncture
❑ Admin. inhalation tx ❑ Other
❑ Cannula ❑

REVIEWED/REVISED BY (Signature/title/date) | REVIEWED/REVISED BY (Signature/title/date) | REVIEWED/REVISED BY (Signature/title/date)

PATIENT/CLIENT NAME – Last, First, Middle Initial | ID#

Form 3571RHH ©1994 Briggs Corporation, Des Moines, IA 50306 R196 To order, phone 1-800-247-2343 PRINTED IN U.S. Page 1 CARE PLAN ❑ CARDIAC /❑ RESPIRATORY

Fig. 2-12. **A sample resident care plan. (Reprinted with permission of Briggs Corporation, 800-247-2343.)**

- **nursing diagnosis**: the identification of health problems after looking at all the resident's needs; done to make a care plan
- **planning**: setting goals and creating a care plan to meet the resident's needs
- **implementation**: putting the care plan into action; giving care
- **evaluation**: a careful examination to see if the goals were met

The goal of the nursing process is to meet the resident's nursing needs. Good communication between all care team members and the resident is vital. It helps ensure the success of the nursing process.

This process constantly changes as new information is collected. Nursing assistants are an important part of this process. You will be observing and reporting on your residents. Your accurate observations are an important part of the nursing process.

8. Describe "The Five Rights of Delegation"

While care planning, nurses decide which tasks to delegate. Everything you do in your job is delegated to you by a licensed healthcare professional. Licensed nurses are accountable for care. This includes all delegated tasks. The National Council of State Boards of Nursing identified "The Five Rights of Delegation." This can be used as a mental checklist to help nurses in the decision-making process.

"The Five Rights of Delegation" are the "Right Task," "Right Circumstance," "Right Person," "Right Direction/Communication," and "Right Supervision/Evaluation." Before delegating tasks, nurses may consider these questions:

- Is there a match between the resident's needs and the NA's skills, abilities, and experience?
- What is the level of resident stability?
- Is the NA the right person to do the job?
- Can the nurse give appropriate direction and communication?
- Is the nurse available to give the supervision, support and help that the NA needs?

There are questions you may want to ask yourself before accepting a task. Consider these questions:

- Do I have all the information I need to do this job? Are there questions I should ask?
- Do I believe that I can do this task? Do I have the necessary skills?
- Do I have the needed supplies, equipment and other support?
- Do I know who my supervisor is, and how to reach him/her?
- Do we both understand who is doing what?

Never be afraid to ask for help. Always ask if you need any more information or are unsure about something. If you feel that you do not have the skills for a task, talk to the nurse.

Chapter Review

1. List six examples of duties that NAs perform.
2. What is one duty that NAs do not usually perform?
3. Describe professionalism. List five examples of professional behavior with a resident.
4. List seven examples of professional behavior with an employer.
5. What personal qualities will make you a good NA?
6. What is one reason why an NA should keep her long hair tied back?
7. Why is it not a good idea for an NA to wear jewelry while working?
8. Choose three members of the care team. Describe the roles they play.
9. Name one reason why the chain of command is important.
10. Why are observing and reporting even simple observations about a resident important?
11. List five steps in the nursing process.
12. List the "Five Rights of Delegation."
13. What should an NA do if he feels he does not have the skills necessary to do a task?

Chapter 3
Legal and Ethical Issues

1. Define the terms "law" and "ethics"

There are many important legal and ethical issues in resident care. **Ethics** is the knowledge of right and wrong. An ethical person has a sense of duty toward others. He or she always tries to do what is right. For example, an NA politely asks another NA to stop gossiping about coworkers.

Ethics tell us what we *should* do. Laws tell us what we *must* do. Laws are usually based on ethics. **Laws** are rules set by the government to protect people and help them live peacefully together. For example, stealing a resident's personal possession is against the law. When people break the law, they may be punished. They may have to pay a fine or spend time in prison.

2. List examples of legal and ethical behavior

Ethics and laws protect those receiving care. They guide those giving care (Fig. 3-1). Professional and ethical behavior in healthcare is vital to the safety and well-being of residents. NAs and other team members follow a code of ethics. They must also know the laws that apply to their jobs.

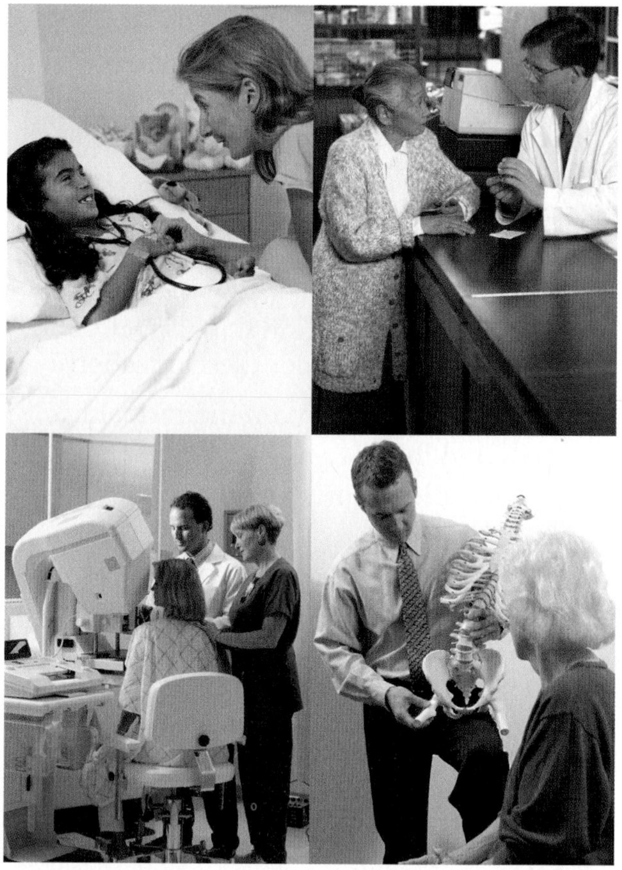

Fig. 3-1. **Behaving ethically and following the law applies to all healthcare providers.**

GUIDELINES
Legal and Ethical Behavior

- Be honest at all times. Stealing from a resident and lying about care you gave are examples of dishonesty. Communicate honestly with all team members.

- Protect residents' privacy. Do not discuss their cases except with other members of the care team. Keeping resident information confidential is one of the Residents' Rights. They are covered later in this chapter. All team members must keep resident information confidential.
- Keep staff information confidential. You should not share information about your coworkers at home or anywhere else.
- Report abuse or suspected abuse of a resident. You will learn more about abuse later in this chapter.
- Follow the care plan and your assignments. If you make a mistake, report it promptly. This helps prevent any further problems. Reporting mistakes promotes the safety and well-being of all residents.
- Do not do any task outside your scope of practice.
- Report all resident observations and incidents to the nurse.
- Document accurately and promptly.
- Follow rules on safety and infection control. You will learn more about these rules in chapters 5 and 6.
- Do not accept gifts or tips.
- Do not get personally or sexually involved with residents or family members.

3. Describe a nursing assistant's code of ethics

Many places have adopted a formal code of ethics. This helps their employees deal with issues of right and wrong. Codes of ethics differ. All revolve around the idea that a resident is a valuable person who deserves ethical care. A sample code of ethics for nursing assistants is shown below:

1. I will strive to provide and maintain the highest quality of care for my residents. I will fully recognize and follow all of the Residents' Rights.
2. I will communicate well, serve on committees, and read all material as provided and required by my employer. I will attend educational in-services, and join organizations relevant to nursing assistant care.
3. I will show a positive attitude toward my residents, staff, family members, and other visitors.
4. I will always provide privacy for my residents. I will maintain confidentiality of resident, staff, and visitor information.
5. I will be trustworthy and honest in all dealings with residents, staff, and visitors.
6. I will strive to preserve resident safety. I will promptly report mistakes I make, along with anything that I deem dangerous, to the right person(s).
7. I will have empathy for my residents, the staff, and all visitors, giving support and encouragement whenever needed.
8. I will respect all people, without regard to age, sex, ethnicity, religion, economic situation, sexual orientation, or diagnosis.
9. I will strive to have the utmost patience with all people at my facility.

4. Explain the Omnibus Budget Reconciliation Act (OBRA)

Due to reports of poor care and abuse in nursing homes, the U.S. government passed the **Omnibus Budget Reconciliation Act (OBRA)** in 1987. It has been updated several times.

OBRA set minimum standards for nursing assistant training. NAs must complete at least 75 hours of training. NAs must also pass a competency evaluation (testing program) before they can be employed. They must attend regular in-service education to keep skills updated. OBRA requires that states keep a current list of nursing assistants in a state registry.

OBRA increases minimum staff requirements. It specifies the minimum services that nursing homes must provide.

Another important part of OBRA is the resident assessment requirements. OBRA requires complete assessments on every resident. The assessment forms are the same for every facility.

A resident assessment system was developed in 1990. It is revised periodically. It is called the **Minimum Data Set (MDS)**. The MDS is a detailed form with guidelines for assessing residents. It also details what to do if resident problems are identified (Fig. 3-2). Facilities must complete the MDS for each resident within 14 days of admission and again each year. In addition, the MDS for each resident must be reviewed every three months. A new MDS must be done when there is any major change in the resident's condition.

OBRA made major changes in the survey process. You first learned about the survey process in chapter 1. The results from surveys are available to the public and posted in the facility.

OBRA also identified important rights for residents in nursing homes. You will learn more about them in the next learning objective.

What is the State Board of Nursing and reciprocity?

In your state, this agency might have a different name. However, the responsibilities will be similar. Many state boards of nursing are in charge of the licensing of nurses and the testing or certification of nursing assistants. This agency may handle other issues relating to NAs. Find out who is in charge of the NA registry in your state. Know the telephone number and address.

When you complete an approved NA course and pass an exam, you may be eligible for certification. Keep proof of certification in a safe place. When you move to another state, your NA certification may transfer to the new state. This is called reciprocity. Contact the agency in that state that handles nursing assistant issues. Find out if you qualify for reciprocity. Gather any important paperwork from your original state before you leave. Obtaining a new certificate in your new state is your responsibility.

5. Explain Residents' Rights

Residents' Rights relate to how residents must be treated while living in a facility. They are an ethical code of conduct for healthcare workers. You need to be familiar with Residents' Rights. Residents' Rights are very detailed. They include:

Quality of life: Residents have the right to the best care available. Dignity, choice, and independence are important parts of quality of life.

Services and activities to maintain a high level of wellness: Residents must have the correct care. Their care should keep them as healthy as possible every day. Health should not decline as a direct result of the facility's care.

The right to be fully informed about rights and services: Residents must be told what care and services are available. They must be told the charges for each service. Legal rights must be explained in a language they can understand. This includes being given a written copy of their rights. They have the right to be notified in advance of any change of room or roommate. They have the right to communicate with someone who speaks their language. They have the right to assistance for any sensory impairment. Blindness is one sensory impairment.

Numeric Identifier________________________________

MINIMUM DATA SET (MDS) – *VERSION 2.0*

FOR NURSING HOME RESIDENT ASSESSMENT AND CARE SCREENING

BASIC ASSESSMENT TRACKING FORM

SECTION AA. IDENTIFICATION INFORMATION

1.	RESIDENT NAME ⊛	(Exactly as appears on Medicare Card) a. (First) b. (Middle Initial) c. (Last) d. (Jr./Sr.)
2.	GENDER ⊛	1. Male 2. Female
3.	BIRTHDATE ⊛	*(Complete all four digits)* Month – Day – Year
4.	RACE/⊛ ETHNICITY	1. American Indian/Alaskan Native 2. Asian/Pacific Islander 3. Black, not of Hispanic origin 4. Hispanic 5. White, not of Hispanic origin
5.	SOCIAL⊛ SECURITY AND ⊛ MEDICARE NUMBERS [C in 1st box if non Med. no.]	a. Social Security Number b. Medicare number (or comparable railroad insurance number)
6.	FACILITY PROVIDER NO. ⊛	a. State No. *(Facility Medicaid Provider number)* *(Facility Medicare Provider number)* b. Federal No.
7.	MEDICAID NO. *["+" if pending, "N" if not a Medicaid recipient]* ⊛	*(Resident Medicaid number)*
8.	REASONS FOR ASSESS-MENT *Use 8a if NOT Medicare covered, leave 8b blank. Use 8a & b if Medicare covered.*	[Note–Other codes do not apply to this form] a. Primary reason for assessment 1. Admission assessment (required by day 14) - may be 2. Annual assessment 3. Significant change in status assessment - may be 4. Significant correction of prior full assessment - may be 5. Quarterly review assessment 10. Significant correction of prior quarterly assessment 0. *NONE OF ABOVE* **b.** ***Codes for assessments required for Medicare PPS or the State*** *1. Medicare 5 day assessment* *2. Medicare 30 day assessment* *3. Medicare 60 day assessment* *4. Medicare 90 day assessment* *5. Medicare readmission/return assessment* *6. Other state required assessment* *7. Medicare 14 day assessment* *8. Other Medicare required assessment*

9. Signatures of Persons who Completed a Portion of the Accompanying Assessment or Tracking Form

I certify that the accompanying information accurately reflects resident assessment or tracking information for this resident and that I collected or coordinated collection of this information on the dates specified. To the best of my knowledge, this information was collected in accordance with applicable Medicare and Medicaid requirements. I understand that this information is used as a basis for ensuring that residents receive appropriate and quality care, and as a basis for payment from federal funds. I further understand that payment of such federal funds and continued participation in the government-funded health care programs is conditioned on the accuracy and truthfulness of this information, and that I may be personally subject to or may subject my organization to substantial criminal, civil, and/or administrative penalties for submitting false information. I also certify that I am authorized to submit this information by this facility on its behalf.

Signature and Title	Sections	Date
a.		
b.		
c.		
d.		
e.		
f.		
g.		
h.		
i.		
j.		
k.		
l.		

GENERAL INSTRUCTIONS

Complete this information for submission with all full and quarterly assessments (Admission, Annual, Significant Change, State or Medicare required assessments, or Quarterly Reviews, etc.).

MDS RUG III CASE MIX GROUPS

- RU = Rehabilitation Ultra High
- RV = Rehabilitation Very High
- RH = Rehabilitation High
- RM = Rehabilitation Medium
- RL = Rehabilitation Low
- SE = Extensive Services
- SS = Special Care
- CC, CB, CA = Clinically Complex

⊛ = Key items for computerized resident tracking

☐ = When box blank, must enter number or letter

[a.] = When letter in box, check if condition applies

Code "–" if information unavailable or unknown

◆ = Quality Indicator/ Quality Measure

■ = **Related to the Top 26 RUG III Case Mix Classifications**

☐ = **Related to the Lower RUG III Case Mix Classifications**

QM LEGEND: Chronic Care & Post-Acute

Percent of short stay residents who had moderate to severe pain
Percent of short stay residents with delirium
Percent of short stay residents with pressure sores
Percent of residents whose need for help with daily activities has increased
Percent of residents who have moderate to severe pain
Percent of residents who were physically restrained
Percent of high-risk residents who have pressure sores
Percent of low-risk residents who have pressure sores
Percent of residents with a urinary tract infection
Percent of residents who spent most of their time in bed or in a chair
Percent of residents who have become more depressed or anxious
Percent of low-risk residents who lose control of their bowels or bladder
Percent of residents who have/had a catheter inserted and left in their bladder
Percent of residents whose ability to move about in and around their room got worse

TRIGGER LEGEND

1 - Delirium
2 - Cognitive Loss/Dementia
3 - Visual Function
4 - Communication
5A - ADL-Rehabilitation
5B - ADL-Maintenance
6 - Urinary Incontinence and Indwelling Catheter
7 - Psychosocial Well-Being
8 - Mood State
9 - Behavioral Symptoms
10A - Activities (Revise)
10B - Activities (Review)
11 - Falls
12 - Nutritional Status
13 - Feeding Tubes
14 - Dehydration/Fluid Maintenance
15 - Dental Care
16 - Pressure Ulcers
17 - Psychotropic Drug Use
17* - For this to trigger, O4a, b, or c must = 1-7
18 - Physical Restraints

QI LEGEND

1 Incidence new fractures
2 Prevalence of falls
3 Prevalence of behavioral symptoms affecting others
4 Prevalence of symptoms of depression
5 Prevalence of depression w/o antidepressants
6 9+ medications
7 Incidence of cognitive impairment
8 Prevalence of bladder or bowel incontinence
9 Prevalence of occasional bladder or bowel incontinence w/o plan
10 Prevalence of indwelling catheter
11 Prevalence of fecal impaction*
12 Prevalence of UTI
13 Prevalence of weight loss
14 Prevalence of tube feeding
15 Prevalence of dehydration*
16 Prevalence of bedfast residents
17 Incidence of decline in late loss ADLs
18 Incidence of decline in ROM
19 Prevalence of antipsychotic use in absence of psychotic conditions
20 Prevalence of antianxiety/hypnotic use
21 Prevalence of hypnotic use > 2x/wk
22 Prevalence of daily restraints
23 Prevalence of little or no activity
24 Prevalence of stage 1-4 pressure ulcers*

*SENTINEL HEALTH EVENT

For additional information on MDS required schedule and documentation to justify skilled care, see page 8.

MDS 2.0 September 2000

1 of 9

Fig. 3-2. **A sample MDS form. (Reprinted with permission of the Briggs Corporation, 800-247-2343.)**

The right to participate in their own care: Residents have the right to participate in planning their treatment, care, and discharge. Residents have the right to refuse medication, treatment, and restraints. They have the right to be told of changes in their condition. They have the right to review their medical record.

Informed consent is a concept that goes along with this. A person has the legal and ethical right to direct what happens to his or her body. Doctors also have an ethical duty to involve the person in his or her health care. **Informed consent** is the process in which a person, with the help of a doctor, makes informed decisions about his or her health care.

The right to make independent choices: Residents have the right to make choices about their doctors, care, and treatments. They can make personal decisions. These include what to wear and how to spend their time. They can join in community activities, both inside and outside the nursing home.

The right to privacy and confidentiality: Residents can expect privacy with care given. Their medical and personal information cannot be shared with anyone but the healthcare team. Residents have the right to private, unrestricted communication with anyone they choose (Fig. 3-3).

The right to dignity, respect, and freedom: Residents must be respected and treated with dignity by caregivers. They cannot be abused in any way. You will learn more about abuse in the next learning objective.

The right to security of possessions: Residents' personal possessions must be safe at all times. They cannot be taken or used by anyone without a resident's permission. Residents have the right to manage their own finances. If the nursing home handles residents' financial affairs, it must be done properly.

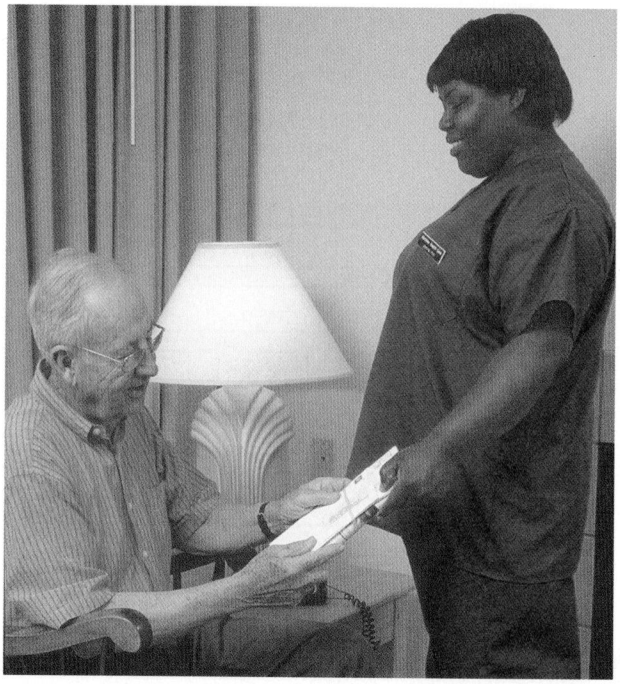

Fig. 3-3. **Residents have the right to private communication with anyone. Do not open residents' mail.**

Rights during transfers and discharges: Location changes must be made safely and with the resident's knowledge and consent. Residents have the right to stay in a facility unless a transfer or discharge is needed.

The right to complain: Residents have the right to complain without fear of punishment. Nursing homes must quickly try to resolve complaints.

The right to visits: Residents have the right to visits from family, doctors, groups, and others (Fig. 3-4).

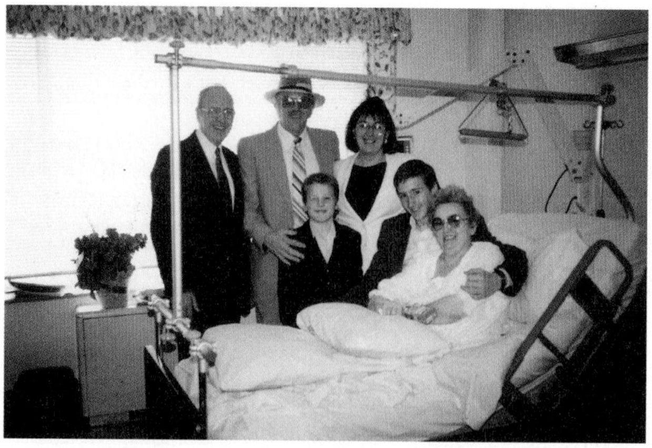

Fig. 3-4. **Residents have the right to visitors.**

Residents' Council

A Residents' Council is a group of residents who meet regularly to discuss issues related to the nursing home. This Council gives residents a voice in facility operations. Topics of discussion may include facility policies, decisions regarding activities, concerns, and problems. The Residents' Council offers residents a chance to provide suggestions on improving the quality of care. Council executives are elected by residents. Family members are invited to attend meetings with or on behalf of residents. Staff may participate in this process when invited by Council members.

6. Define and list signs of abuse and neglect

Abuse is purposely causing physical, mental, or emotional pain or injury to someone in your care. Some examples are:

- An NA pushes a resident when she does not move fast enough in the hall.
- An NA loudly announces that a resident wet the bed last night in front of other residents and visitors.

Neglect is harming the person in your care physically, mentally, or emotionally by failing to give needed care. For example, a nursing assistant leaves the side rail down on a resident's bed. The resident has a doctor's order for side rails. The resident falls out of bed. She breaks her hip.

To put it more simply: Abuse is something you DO; neglect is something you DO NOT DO.

There are different types of abuse, including:

- Physical abuse
- Sexual abuse
- Psychological abuse
- Financial abuse
- Domestic violence
- Workplace violence
- Involuntary seclusion
- Sexual harassment
- Substance abuse

Physical abuse is any treatment, intentional or not, that causes harm to a person's body. This includes slapping, bruising, cutting, burning, physically restraining, pushing, shoving, or even rough handling.

Sexual abuse is forcing a person to perform or participate in sexual acts.

Psychological or **mental abuse** is emotionally harming a person by threatening, scaring, humiliating, intimidating, isolating, insulting, or treating him or her as a child. It includes verbal abuse. **Verbal abuse** is oral or written words, pictures, or gestures that threaten, embarrass, or insult a resident.

Financial abuse is stealing, taking advantage of, or improperly using the money, property, or other assets of another.

Domestic violence is abuse by spouses, intimate partners, or family members. It can be physical, sexual, or emotional. The victim can be a woman, man, elderly person, or a child.

Workplace violence is abuse of staff by residents or other staff members. It can be verbal, physical, or sexual. This includes improper touching and discussion about sexual subjects.

Involuntary seclusion is confinement or separation from others in a certain area. It is done without consent or against one's will.

Sexual harassment is any unwelcome sexual advance or behavior that creates an intimidating, hostile or offensive working environment. Requests for sexual favors, unwanted touching, and other acts of a sexual nature are examples of sexual harassment.

Substance abuse is the use of legal or illegal drugs, cigarettes, or alcohol in a way that harms oneself or others. You will learn more about this in chapter 20.

Reporting abuse is the law. If you see or suspect that a caregiver, family member, or a resident is abusing a person, report it at once to the charge nurse. If action is not taken, keep reporting up the chain of command. Do this until action is taken.

If no appropriate action is taken at the facility level, call the state abuse hotline. Usually this is an anonymous call. If no abuse hotline exists in your area, contact the proper state agency.

OBSERVING AND REPORTING

Abuse and Neglect

These are "suspicious" injuries. They should be reported:

- poisoning or traumatic injury
- teeth marks
- belt buckle or strap marks
- old and new bruises, contusions and welts
- fractures, dislocation
- burns of unusual shape and in unusual locations; cigarette burns
- scalding burns
- scratches and puncture wounds
- scalp tenderness and patches of missing hair
- swelling in the face, broken teeth, nasal discharge

Signs that could indicate abuse include:

- yelling obscenities
- fear, apprehension, fear of being alone
- poor self-control
- constant pain
- threatening to hurt others
- withdrawal or apathy (Fig. 3-5)

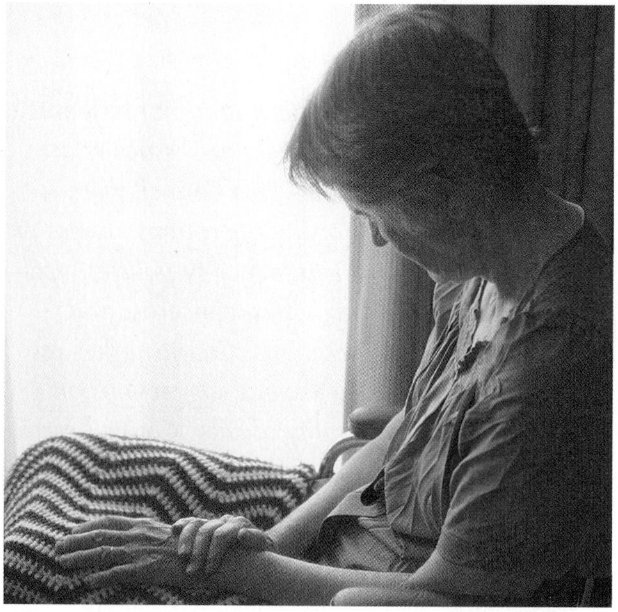

Fig. 3-5. **Withdrawal is an important change to report.**

- alcohol or drug abuse
- agitation or anxiety, signs of stress
- low self-esteem
- mood changes, confusion, disorientation
- private conversations are not allowed, or the family member/caregiver is present during all conversations

Signs that could indicate neglect include:

- pressure sores
- body not clean
- body lice
- unanswered call lights
- soiled bedding or incontinence briefs not being changed
- poorly-fitting clothing
- refusal of care
- unmet needs relating to hearing aids, glasses, etc.
- weight loss
- poor appetite
- dehydration
- uneaten food
- fresh water or beverages not being passed each shift

If you suspect abuse or neglect, you are legally required to report it. If residents want to make a complaint of abuse, you must help them in every way. This includes telling them of the process and their rights.

Never retaliate against (punish) residents complaining of abuse. If you see someone being cruel or abusive to a resident who made a complaint, you must report it. All care team members are responsible for residents' safety.

They are all your residents.

All of the residents in your area or unit are your residents. Even though you may be assigned a number of residents, you must still respond to any resident in need. Never say, "He/she is not my resident."

7. List examples of behavior supporting and promoting Residents' Rights

Protect your residents' rights in these ways:

- Never abuse a resident physically, psychologically, or sexually.
- Watch for and report any signs of abuse or neglect.
- Call the resident by the name he or she prefers.
- Involve residents in your plans.
- Always explain a procedure to a resident before starting it.
- Respect a resident's refusal of care. Report the refusal to the nurse at once.
- Tell the nurse if a resident has questions about the goals of care or the care plan.
- Be truthful when documenting care.
- Do not talk or gossip about a resident.
- Knock. Ask for permission before entering a resident's room. (Fig. 3-6).
- Do not accept gifts or money.
- Do not open a resident's mail or look through his things.

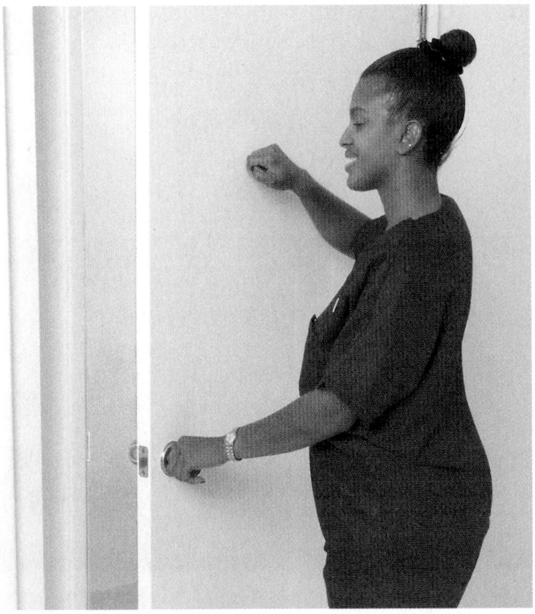

Fig. 3-6. **Always respect your residents' privacy. Knock before entering their rooms, even if the door is open.**

- Respect residents' personal possessions.
- Report observations about a resident's condition or care.
- Help resolve disputes by reporting them to the nurse.

8. Identify the ombudsman's role

An **ombudsman** is assigned by law as the legal advocate for residents. The ombudsman visits and listens to residents. He or she decides what action to take if there is a problem. An ombudsman can help resolve conflicts and settle disputes. They provide an ongoing presence in nursing homes. They monitor care and conditions.

An ombudsman typically:

- advocates for Residents' Rights and quality care
- educates consumers and care providers
- investigates and resolves complaints
- appears in court and/or in legal hearings
- works with investigators from the police, adult protective services, and health departments to resolve complaints (Fig. 3-7)
- gives information to the public

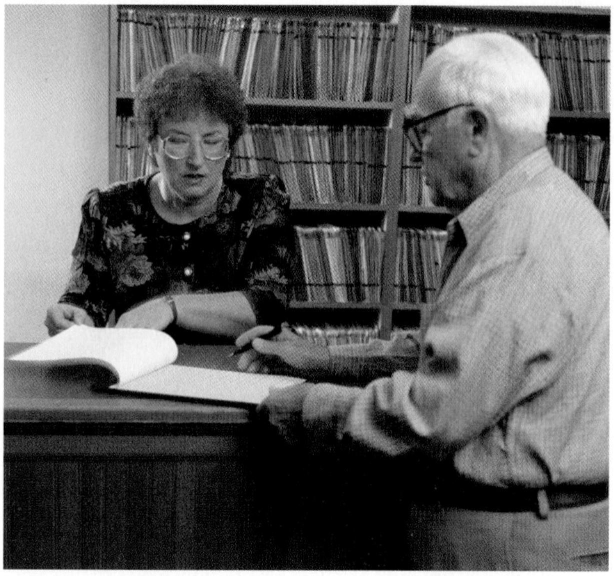

Fig. 3-7. **An ombudsman is a legal advocate for residents. He or she visits the facility and listens to residents. He or she also works with other agencies to resolve complaints.**

9. Explain HIPAA and list ways to protect residents' privacy

To respect confidentiality means to keep private things private. You will learn confidential (private) information about your residents. You may learn about health, finances, and relationships. Ethically and legally, you must protect this information. You should not tell anyone except members of the care team **anything** about your residents.

Congress passed the Health Insurance Portability and Accountability Act (HIPAA) in 1996. It was refined and revised in 2001 and again in 2002. One reason for this law is to keep health information private and secure. All healthcare organizations must take special steps to protect health information. They and their employees can be fined and/or imprisoned if they break rules to protect patient privacy. This applies to all healthcare providers. This includes doctors, nurses, nursing assistants, and all care team members.

Under this law, health information must be kept private. It is called **protected health information (PHI)**. PHI includes the patient's name, address, telephone number, social security number, e-mail address, and medical record number. Only those who must have information for care or to process records should know this information (Fig. 3-8). They must protect the information. It must not become known or used by anyone else. It must be kept confidential.

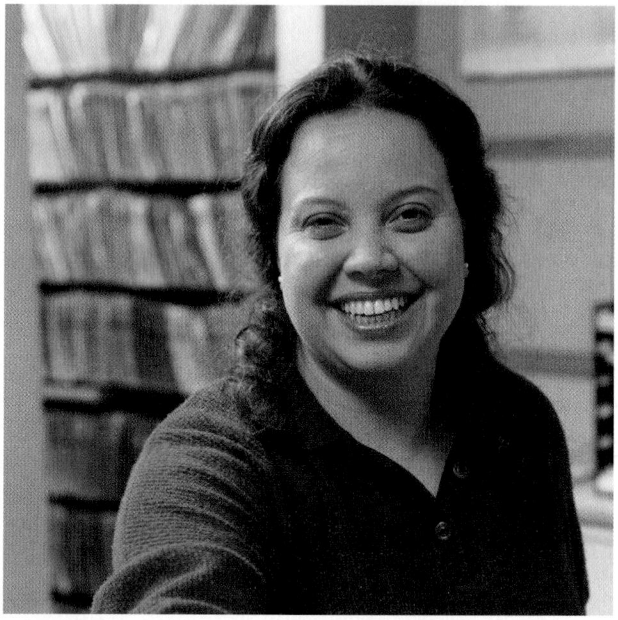

Fig. 3-8. **Special care must be taken to keep medical records confidential. Only people who give care or process records should have access to this information.**

NAs cannot give out any resident information to anyone not directly involved in the resident's care. For example, if a neighbor asks you how a resident is doing, reply, "I'm sorry, but I cannot share that information. It's confidential." That is the correct response to anyone who does not have a legal reason to know about the resident.

Other ways to protect residents' privacy are:

- Make sure you are in a private area when you listen to or read your messages.
- Know with whom you are speaking on the phone. If you are not sure, get a name and number. Call back after you get approval.
- When talking to a care team member on the phone, do not use cellular phones. They can be scanned.

- Do not talk about residents in public (Fig. 3-9). Public areas include elevators, grocery stores, lounges, waiting rooms, parking garages, schools, restaurants, etc.

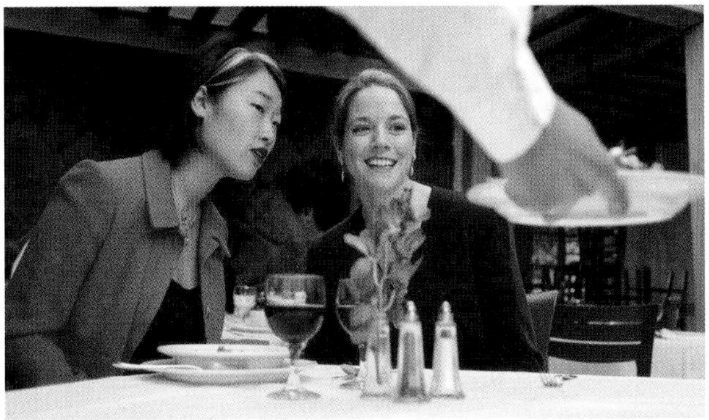

Fig. 3-9. **Do not discuss any information about residents in public places, such as grocery stores or restaurants. Only discuss residents' information with the care team.**

- Use confidential rooms for reports to other care team members.
- If you see a resident's family member or a former resident in public, be careful with your greeting. He or she may not want others to know about the family member or that he or she has been a resident.
- Do not bring family or friends to the facility to meet residents.
- Make sure nobody can see health or personal information on your computer screen.
- Log off when you are not on your computer.
- Do not give confidential information in e-mails. You do not know who has access to them.
- Make sure fax numbers are correct before faxing information. Use a cover sheet with a confidentiality statement.
- Do not leave documents where others may see them.
- Store and file documents according to your facility's policy.
- If you find documents with a resident's information, give them to the nurse.

All healthcare workers must follow HIPAA regulations no matter where they are or what they are doing. There are serious penalties for violating these rules. Penalties differ depending upon the violation. They can include:

- Fines ranging from $100 to $250,000
- Prison sentences of up to ten years

Confidentiality is a legal and ethical obligation. It is part of respecting your residents and their rights. Discussing a resident's care or personal affairs with anyone other than members of the care team violates the law.

10. Explain The Patient Self-Determination Act (PSDA)

The Patient Self-Determination Act (PSDA) encourages all people to make decisions about advance directives. **Advance directives** allow people to choose what medical care they wish to have if they cannot make those decisions themselves (Fig. 3-10). Advance directives can also name someone to make decisions for a person if that person becomes ill or disabled. Living Wills and Durable Power of Attorney for Health Care are examples of advance directives.

A **Living Will** states the medical care a person wants, or does not want, in case he or she becomes unable to make those decisions him- or herself. It is called a "Living Will" because it takes effect while the person is still living. It may also be called a "directive to physicians," "health care declaration," or "medical directive."

A **Durable Power of Attorney for Health Care** is a signed, dated, and witnessed paper that appoints someone else to make the medical decisions for a person in the event he or she becomes unable to do so. This can include instructions about medical treatment the person wants to avoid.

A **do-not-resuscitate** (**DNR**) order is another

Form 3128/2P
BRIGGS, Des Moines, IA 50306 (800) 247-2343
PRINTED IN U.S.A.

ACKNOWLEDGEMENT OF RECEIPT

ADVANCE DIRECTIVES/MEDICAL TREATMENT DECISIONS

This is to acknowledge that I have been informed in writing in a language that I understand of my rights and all rules and regulations to make decisions concerning medical care, including the right to accept or refuse medical or surgical treatment and the right to formulate and to issue Advance Directives to be followed should I become incapacitated.

❑ **I have chosen to formulate and issue the following Advance Directives.**
I understand it is my responsibility to provide to the facility copies of all pertinent documentation which verify those advance directives specified below for placement in my medical record.

DATE ISSUED		DATE ISSUED	
________	❑ Living Will		❑ Medication Restrictions
________	❑ Do Not Resuscitate	________	Type(s) ________
________	❑ Do Not Hospitalize		❑ Other Treatment Restrictions
________	❑ Organ Donation	________	Type(s) ________
________	❑ Autopsy Request		❑ Other Advance Directives
	❑ Feeding Restrictions	________	Type ________
________	Type(s) ________	________	Type ________

❑ **I do not choose to formulate or issue any Advance Directives at this time.**
I want efforts made to prolong my life and I want life-sustaining treatment to be provided.

ACKNOWLEDGEMENT SIGNATURES

Resident/Patient/Client X ____________________ Date ________

Legal Representative ____________________ Date ________

If Legal Representative Signed, Complete the Following:

Print Name	Relationship to Resident/Patient/Client	Type of Legal Appointment

Witness ____________________ Date ________

Witness ____________________ Date ________
(Second Witness Signature Required if Acknowledged by Resident/Patient/Client "Mark".)

If Resident/Patient/Client Unable to Sign Name, State Medical Reason:

____

____

Physician Signature ____________________ Date ________

WHITE - Medical Record **PINK - Resident/Patient/Client**

NAME–Last	First	Middle	Attending Physician	Med. Rec. No.

Form 3128/2P © 1991 Briggs Corporation, Des Moines, IA 50306 (800) 247-2343 PRINTED IN U.S.A.
(12-91)

ACKNOWLEDGEMENT OF RECEIPT
Advance Directives/Medical Treatment Decisions

Fig. 3-10. **A sample advance directive form. (Reprinted with permission of the Briggs Corporation, 800-247-2343.)**

tool that helps medical providers honor wishes about care. A DNR order tells medical professionals not to perform CPR. CPR (cardiopulmonary resuscitation) refers to medical procedures to restart the heart and breathing during heart failure. You will learn more about CPR in chapter 7. A DNR means that medical personnel will not attempt emergency CPR if breathing or the heartbeat stops. In general, DNR (do-not-resuscitate) orders are appropriate for those in the final stages of a terminal illness or who suffer from a serious condition.

The PSDA requires all healthcare agencies receiving Medicare and Medicaid money to give adults, during admission or enrollment, information about their rights relating to advance directives.

These rights include:

- The right to participate in and direct healthcare decisions
- The right to accept or refuse treatment
- The right to prepare an advance directive
- Information on policies that govern these rights

The act prohibits discriminating against a patient who does not have an advance directive. The PSDA requires documentation of patient information and ongoing community education on advance directives.

Living Wills and Wills

*A Living Will is not the same thing as a will. A **will** is a legal declaration of how a person wishes his or her possessions to be disposed of after death. If a resident tells you he or she wants to prepare a will, notify the nurse.*

Chapter Review

1. What is the difference between ethics and laws?
2. List five examples of legal and ethical behavior for an NA.
3. What do codes of ethics all revolve around?
4. What is the minimum number of hours of training that NAs must complete?
5. Describe three parts of OBRA.
6. What is the purpose of Residents' Rights?
7. If you see or suspect abuse, what is your responsibility?
8. All of these statements about Residents' Rights are true EXCEPT:
   a. Residents cannot refuse medication.
   b. Residents have the right to refuse treatment.
   c. Residents have the right to be free from restraints.
   d. Residents can choose what to wear for the day.
9. You see an NA slap a resident with dementia on the hand because she is refusing to let the NA bathe her. What kind of abuse is this?
   a. Physical abuse
   b. Psychological abuse
   c. Neglect
   d. Domestic violence
10. Which of these is NOT an example of abuse or neglect?
    a. A nursing assistant helps a resident to make a complaint.
    b. An NA steals a resident's money.
    c. An NA leaves a resident in a soiled bed.
    d. An NA threatens to hit a resident.
11. Pick three of the examples of behavior promoting residents' rights in learning objective 7. Describe how it supports or promotes specific rights found in Residents' Rights.

12. What does an ombudsman do?
13. What are some examples of a person's protected health information (PHI)?
14. To whom is an NA allowed to give information about a resident?
15. To what members of the healthcare team is HIPAA applicable?
16. Do HIPAA's guidelines apply if an NA is shopping at the grocery store?
17. List three rights relating to advance directives that the PSDA requires be given to a resident at the time of admission.

Chapter 4
Communication and Cultural Diversity

1. Define "communication"

Communication is the exchange of information with others. It is a process of sending and receiving messages. People communicate with signs and symbols, such as words, drawings, and pictures. They also communicate with behavior.

The simplest form of communication is between two people (Fig. 4-1). The person who communicates first is the "sender" who sends a message. The person who receives the message is called the "receiver." Receiver and sender constantly switch roles as they communicate.

The third step is giving feedback. The receiver repeats the message or responds to it. This lets the sender know the message was received and understood. Feedback is especially important when working with the elderly. Take time to make sure residents understand messages.

All three steps must occur before the process is complete. During a conversation, this three-step process occurs over and over.

Effective communication is a vital part of your job. Nursing assistants must communicate with supervisors, the care team, residents, and family members. A resident's health depends on how well you communicate your observations and concerns to the nurse. You must also be able to communicate clearly and respectfully in stressful or confusing situations.

2. Explain verbal and nonverbal communication

Communication is either verbal or nonverbal. **Verbal communication** uses words or sounds, spoken or written. Oral reports are an example of verbal communication. **Nonverbal communication** is communicating without using words. Examples are shaking your head or shrugging your shoulders. Nonverbal communication includes how a person says something. You might say, "I'll be right there, Mrs. Gonzales." This communicates that you are ready and willing to help. But saying the same phrase in a different tone can sound angry, "I'll *be* right *there*, Mrs. Gonzales!"

Body language is another form of nonverbal communication. Movements, facial expressions, and posture can show different attitudes or emotions. Just as with speaking, you send messages with body language. Other people receive and interpret them. For example, slouching in a chair and sitting erect send two different messages (Fig. 4-2). Slouching says that you are bored, tired, or hostile. Sitting up straight shows interest.

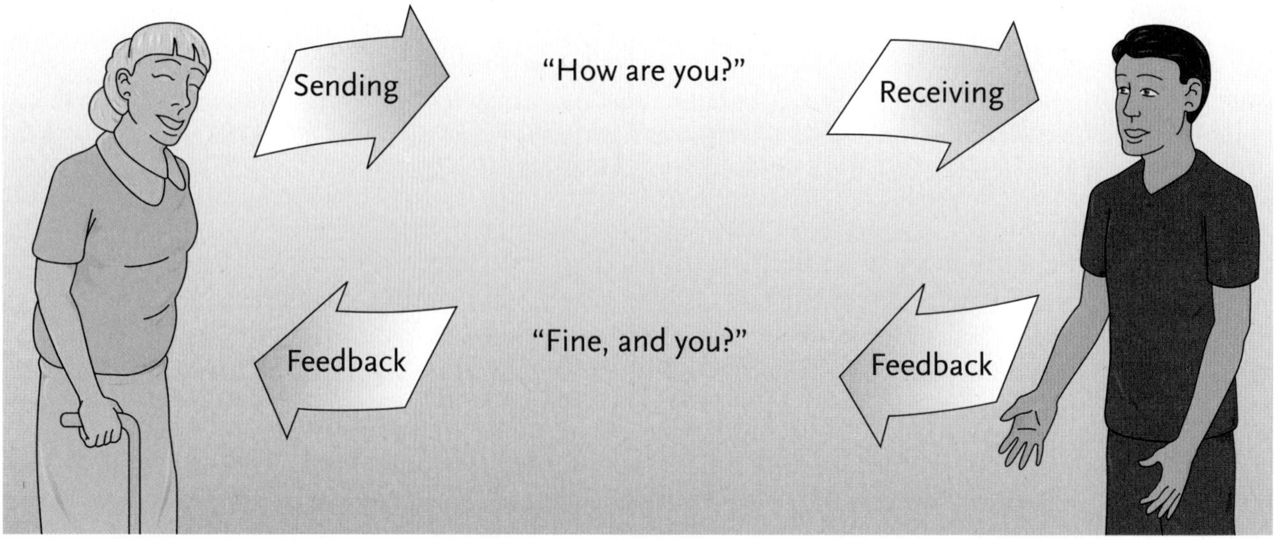

Fig. 4-1. **The communication process consists of sending a message, receiving it, and giving feedback.**

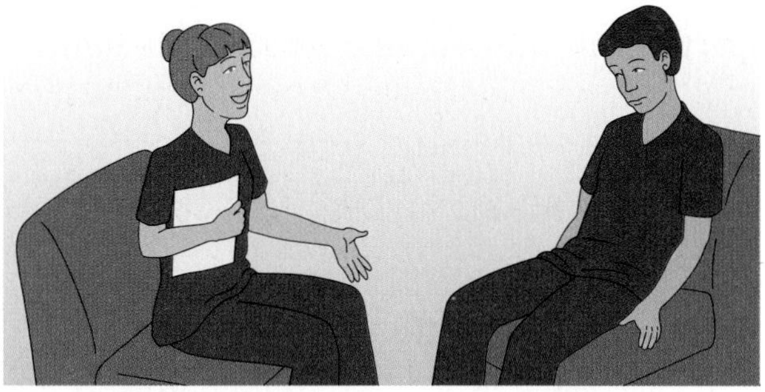

Fig. 4-2. **Body language often speaks as plainly as words. Which of these people seems more interested in their conversation?**

Here are some examples of positive and negative nonverbal communication:

Positive nonverbal communication

- smiling in a friendly way
- leaning forward to listen
- with consent, putting your hand over a resident's hand while listening to her

Negative nonverbal communication

- rolling your eyes or crossing your arms
- tapping your foot
- pointing at someone while speaking

3. Describe ways different cultures communicate

Cultural diversity has to do with the variety of people who live and work together in the world. Positive responses to cultural diversity include acceptance and knowledge, not **bias**, or prejudice. A **culture** is a system of behaviors people learn from the people they live and grow up with. Each culture may have different lifestyles, religions, customs, and behaviors.

Nonverbal communication may depend on personality or background. Some people are more animated when they speak. They use lots of gestures and facial expressions. Others are quiet or calm, regardless of their moods. Depending on their cultural background, people may motion with their hands when they talk. They may stand close to the person they are talking to, or touch the other person.

People from some cultural groups stand further apart when talking than those from other groups. When one person moves closer, the other person may view it as a threat. Be sensitive to your residents' needs. Let them decide how close they want to be to you.

The use of touch and eye contact also varies with culture and personality (Fig. 4-3). For some people, touch is welcome. It expresses caring and warmth. For others, it seems threatening or harassing. In the United States, we speak of "looking someone straight in the eye" or speaking "eye to eye." We see eye contact as a sign of honesty. In some cultures, looking someone in the eye is disrespectful.

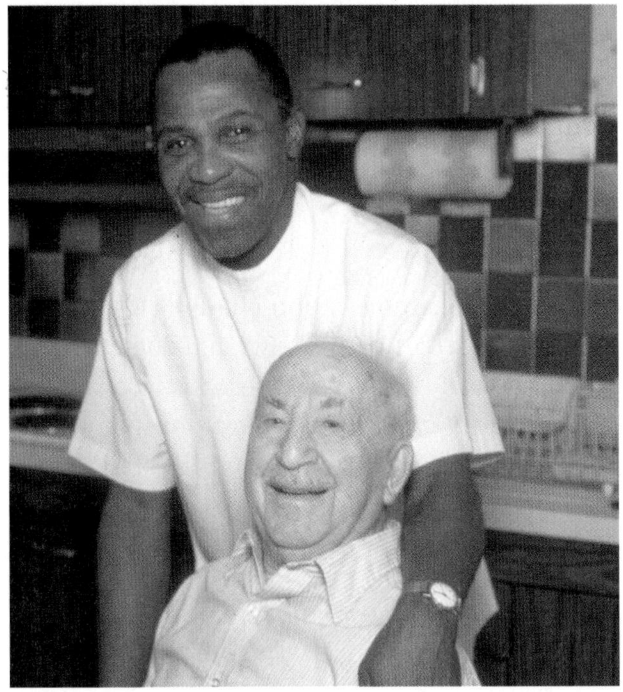

Fig. 4-3. **How a person perceives touch may depend on his or her background.**

Learning each resident's behavior can be a challenge. However, it is an important part of communication. It is especially vital in a multicultural society (a society made up of many cultures), like the United States. Be aware of all the messages you send and receive. As you listen and observe, you will better understand your residents' needs and feelings.

STOP ***Ask, acknowledge, and accept.***

Focus on compassionate, respectful, and sensitive care. Treat your residents as they wish to be treated, not how you want to treat them. Your culture and experiences shape your thinking. Others come from different cultures and experiences. They have shaped the way they think. Something you may want or need from others may be different from what your resident wants or needs. Ask questions. Find out what is appropriate. Never try to make residents change their beliefs in any way.

4. Identify barriers to communication

Communication can be blocked or disrupted (Fig. 4-4). These are some barriers and ways to avoid them:

Resident does not hear you, does not hear correctly, or does not understand. Face the resident. Speak more slowly than you do with family and friends. Speak clearly. Use a low, pleasant voice. Do not whisper or mumble. Use a pleasant, professional tone. If the resident wears a hearing aid, check that it is on and works properly.

Resident is hard to understand. Be patient. Take time to listen. Ask the resident to repeat

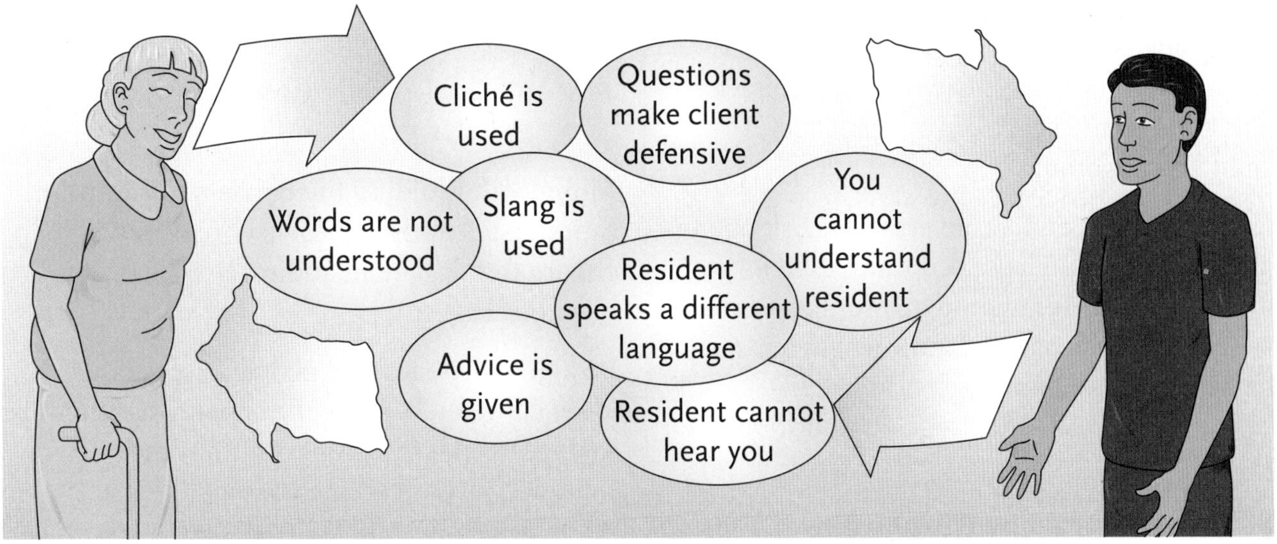

Fig. 4-4. **Barriers to communication.**

or explain. State the message in your own words to make sure you have understood.

Message uses words receiver does not understand. Do not use medical terms with residents. Use simple, everyday words. Ask what a word means if you are not sure.

Do not use slang words. Do not curse. Slang can confuse the message. Avoid slang. It is unprofessional. It may not be understood. Never curse or use profanity, even if the resident does.

Avoid clichés. Clichés are phrases that are used repeatedly. They do not really mean anything. For example, "Everything will be fine" is a cliché. Instead, listen to what your resident is really saying. Respond with a meaningful message. If a resident is afraid of having a bath, say "I understand that it seems scary to you. What can I do to make you more comfortable?" Do not say, "Oh, it'll be over before you know it."

Asking "why" makes the resident defensive. Avoid asking "why" when a resident speaks. "Why" questions make people feel defensive. For example, a resident may say she does not want to go for a walk. If you ask "why not?" you may get an angry response. Instead, ask, "Are you too tired to take a walk? Is there something else you want to do?" Your resident may then be willing to discuss the issue.

Giving advice is inappropriate. Do not offer your opinion or advice. Giving medical advice is not within the scope of your practice. It could be dangerous.

Yes/no answers end a conversation. Ask open-ended questions. They need more than a "yes" or "no" answer. Yes and no answers end conversation. If you want to know what your resident likes to eat, do not ask "Do you like vegetables?" Try "Which vegetables do you like best?"

Resident speaks a different language. If a resident speaks a different language than you, speak slowly and clearly. Keep your messages short and simple. Be alert for words the resident understands. Also be alert for signs the resident is only pretending to understand you. You may need to use pictures or gestures to communicate. Ask the resident's family, friends, or other staff members who speak the resident's language for help. Be patient and calm.

Nonverbal communication changes the message. Be aware of your body language and gestures. Look for nonverbal messages from residents and clarify them. For example, "Mr. Feldman, you say you're feeling fine but you seem to be in pain. Can I help?"

STOP ***Speak so they can understand.***

Abuse comes in many forms. When you care for residents, always use a language they can understand or find an interpreter (someone who speaks their language). Do not speak with other staff in a different language in front of residents.

You can also try to learn a few words in residents' native languages. This can be done by working with an interpreter or with residents' family members or friends. Flash cards and books can also help. Speaking a few words in residents' native languages may be very comforting to them.

5. List ways to make communication accurate and complete

Along with avoiding the barriers to communication listed earlier, these techniques will help ensure that you send and receive clear, complete messages:

Be a good listener. Let people express their ideas completely. Concentrate on what they are saying. Do not interrupt. Do not finish their sentences even if you know what they are going to say. Restate the message in your own words to make sure you have understood.

Give feedback as you listen. Active listening is focusing on the person sending the message and giving feedback. Feedback might be an acknowledgment, a question, or repeating the sender's message. Offer general but leading responses, such as "Oh?" or "Go on," or "Hmm." By doing this you are actively listening, giving feedback, and encouraging the sender to expand the message.

Bring up topics of concern. If you know of a topic that might concern a resident, raise it in a general, non-threatening way. This lets the resident to decide whether to discuss it. For example, if you see that your resident is unusually quiet, you could say, "Mrs. Jones, you seem so quiet today."

Let some pauses happen. Use silence for a few moments at a time. This allows the resident to gather thoughts and compose messages.

Tune in to other cultures. Learn words and phrases of your resident's culture. This shows that you respect the culture and are interested in what the resident has to say. It will help you understand your residents more fully. Be careful about using new words and terms. Some may have a different meaning than you think. The important thing is to understand words and expressions when others use them. Do not be judgmental. Accept people who are different from you.

Accept a resident's religion. Religious differences also affect communication. Religion can be very important in people's lives, particularly when they are ill or dying. Respect residents' religious beliefs and practices, especially if they are different from yours. Never question your residents' beliefs. Do not discuss your beliefs with them.

Understand the importance of touch. Softly patting residents' hands or shoulders or holding their hands may communicate caring. Some people's backgrounds may make them less comfortable being touched. Ask permission. Be sensitive to your residents' feelings. You must touch residents in order to do your job. However, recognize that some residents feel more comfortable when there is little physical contact. Learn about your residents. Adjust care to their needs.

Ask for more. When residents report symptoms, events, or feelings, have them repeat what they have said. Ask them for more information.

Make sure communication aids are clean and in good working order. These include hearing aids, glasses, dentures, and wrist or hand braces. Tell the nurse if they do not work properly or are dirty or damaged (Fig. 4-5).

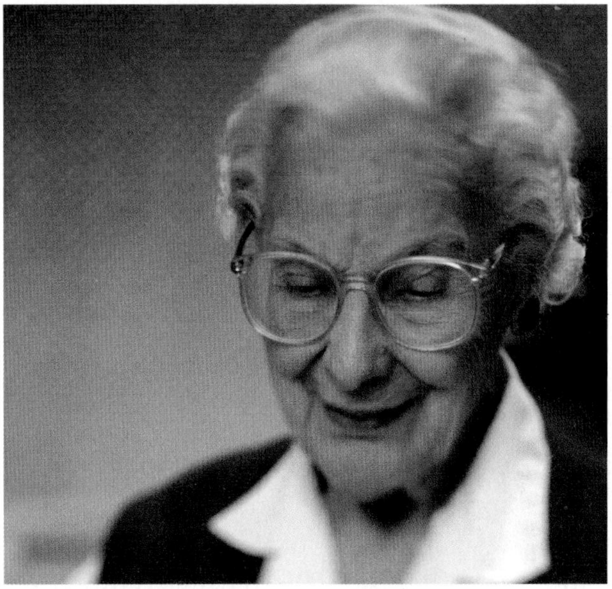

Fig. 4-5. **Glasses must be clean and in good condition. Tell the nurse if you think communication aids are not clean or not working properly.**

Communicating with Residents

When communicating with your residents, remember:

Always greet the resident by his or her preferred name.

Identify yourself.

Focus on the proper topic to be discussed.

Face the resident while speaking. Avoid talking into space.

Talk with the resident while giving care.

Listen and respond when the resident speaks. Praise the resident. Smile often.

Encourage the resident to interact with you and others.

Be courteous.

Tell the resident when you are leaving the room.

Call residents by the names they prefer. *Never use disrespectful terms such as "sweetie" or "honey."*

6. Explain how to develop effective interpersonal relationships

Having good relationships with residents, their family members, and the care team will help you to give excellent care. Develop warm professional relationships with residents based on trust. Good communication will help you get to know them. It will also help them learn to trust you. The following can help you communicate well and develop good relationships:

Avoid changing the subject when your resident is speaking. This is true even if the subject makes you feel uncomfortable or helpless. A resident might say, "I'm having so much pain today." Do not try to avoid the topic. This tells the resident that you are not interested in him or what he is talking about.

Do not ignore a request. Ignoring a request is considered neglect. Honor it if you can. Explain why any requests cannot be fulfilled. Always report such requests to the nurse.

Do not talk down to an elderly or disabled person. Talk to your residents and their families as you would talk to any person. Adjust if someone is visually or hearing-impaired. Guidelines for visually and hearing-impaired residents are found later in the chapter.

Sit near the person. This shows you find what he or she is saying important and worth your time.

Lean forward in your chair when someone is speaking to you. This communicates interest. Pay attention to your nonverbal communication. If you fold your arms, you send the negative message that you wish to distance yourself from the speaker.

Talk directly to the person whom you are assisting. Do not talk to other staff while helping residents (Fig. 4-6). Avoid gossip. Do not criticize other staff members.

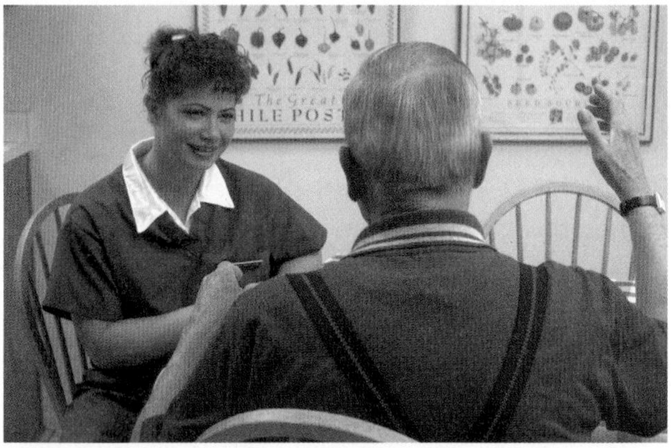

Figure 4-6. **When helping residents, do not talk to other staff. Do not talk over residents' heads. Look and speak directly to the person you are helping.**

Approach the person who is talking. Even if you are in another area of the room, approach the person. This tells the person you are interested in what he or she has to say.

Put yourself in other people's shoes. Try to understand what they are going through. This is called empathy. Ask yourself how you would feel if you were bedbound or needed help to go to the bathroom. Do not tell residents you know how they feel. You do not know this. Do say things like, "I can imagine this must be hard for you."

Show residents' families and friends that you have time for them, too. Communicate with them. Do not discuss a resident's care with friends or family members. Listen if they want to talk. Be respectful and nice. Give privacy for visits. Do not interfere with private family business. If you see any abusive behavior towards a resident, report it immediately to the nurse.

Families are great sources of information for residents' personal preferences, history, diet, habits, and routines. Ask them questions.

7. Explain the difference between facts and opinions

A fact is something that is definitely true. For example, "Mr. Ford has lost four pounds this month." You can back up this fact with evidence: weighing Mr. Ford and comparing his current weight to his weight last month. An opinion is something believed to be true, but is not definitely true. "I think Mr. Ford looks thinner," is an opinion. It might be true, but you cannot back it up with evidence. It is important to separate facts from opinions. This will make you a better communicator. Use facts to communicate more effectively.

When communicating with members of the healthcare team, separate facts and opinions. For example, "Mr. Morgan is acting like he had a stroke," is an opinion. It could very well be wrong. Instead, report the facts: "Mr. Morgan has lost strength on his right side and his speech is slurred." When you report your opinion, begin it with "I think...." Then it is clear that you are giving your opinion and not a fact you have observed.

8. Explain objective and subjective information and describe how to observe and report accurately

When making a report, you must get the right information before documenting it. Facts, not opinions, are most useful to the nurse and the care team. Two kinds of factual information are needed in your reporting. **Objective information** is based on what you see, hear, touch, or smell. Objective information is collected by using the senses. **Subjective information** is something you cannot or did not observe. It is based on something the resident reported to you that may or may not be true. An example of objective information is, "Mr. McClain is holding his head and rubbing his temples." A subjective report might be, "Mr. McClain says he has a headache." The nurse needs factual information in order to determine care and treatment. Both objective and subjective reports are valuable.

Make sure what you observe and what the resident reports to you are clearly noted. For example, "Ms. S reports pain in left shoulder." You are not expected to make diagnoses based on what you observe. Your observations, however, can alert staff to possible problems. To report accurately, observe accurately. To observe accurately, use as many senses as possible to gather information (Fig. 4-7).

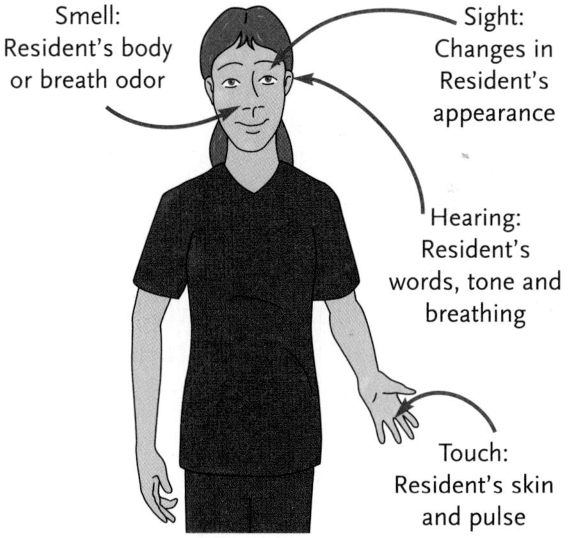

Fig. 4-7. **Reporting what you observe means using more than one sense.**

Sight. Look for changes in appearance. This includes rashes, redness, paleness, swelling, discharge, weakness, sunken eyes, posture or gait (walking) changes.

Hearing. Listen to what the resident tells you about his condition, family, or needs. Is he speaking clearly and making sense? Does he show emotions, such as anger, frustration, or sadness? Is breathing normal? Does he wheeze, gasp, or cough? Is the area calm and quiet enough for him to rest as needed?

Touch. Does the skin feel hot or cool, moist or dry? Is the pulse rate regular?

Smell. Do you notice odor from the resident's body? Odors could suggest poor bathing, infections, or incontinence. **Incontinence** is the inability to control the bladder or bowels. Breath odor could suggest use of alcohol or tobacco, indigestion, or poor oral care.

Using all your senses will help you make the most complete report of a resident's situation.

9. Describe basic medical terminology and abbreviations

In your training, you will learn medical terms for specific conditions. For example, the medical term for a resident whose skin is pale or blue is **cyanotic**.

Medical terms are made up of word parts. These parts are roots, prefixes, and suffixes. A root is the part of a word that gives it meaning. A prefix comes at the front of the word. It works with a word root to make a new term. A suffix is found at the end of a word. A suffix by itself does not form a full word. When you add a prefix or a root, the suffix turns it into a working medical term.

Here are some examples:

- The root "scope" means an instrument to look inside. The prefix "oto" means ear. An otoscope is an instrument used to examine the ear.
- The prefix "brady" means slow. The root "cardia" means heart. "Bradycardia" is slow heart rate or pulse.
- The suffix "meter" means measuring instrument. The prefix "thermo" means heat. A thermometer is an instrument that measures temperature.

Your instructor has more examples of roots, prefixes, and suffixes.

When speaking with residents and their families, use simple, non-medical terms. When you speak with the care team, medical terms will help you give more complete information.

Abbreviations are a way to communicate more efficiently. For example, the abbreviation "p.r.n." means "as necessary." "BP" means "blood pressure." Learn the standard medical abbreviations your facility uses. Use them to report information briefly and accurately. You may need to know these abbreviations to read assignments or care plans.

A list of abbreviations is found at the end of this textbook. Check with your facility to see if there are terms you must know.

10. Explain how to give and receive an accurate report of a resident's status

Nursing assistants must make brief, accurate oral and written reports to residents and staff. Good communication is needed to collect information about residents. These skills will help you get information from residents and their families to pass to the care team. This information may be written or given in oral reports shift to shift. Remember that all resident information is confidential. Only share information with members of the care team.

Your careful observations are important to the health and well-being of all residents. Deciding what to report immediately to the nurse involves critical thinking. For the nursing assistant, critical thinking is making good observations to get help for a potential problem. Signs and symptoms that should be reported will be discussed in this book. In addition, anything that endangers your resident should be reported immediately, including:

- falls
- chest pain

- severe headache
- trouble breathing
- abnormal pulse, respiration, or blood pressure
- change in mental status
- sudden weakness or loss of mobility
- high fever
- loss of consciousness
- change in level of consciousness
- bleeding
- change in condition
- bruises, abrasions, or other signs of abuse (chapter 3)

For an oral report, write notes so you do not forget important details. Following an oral report, document when, why, about what, and to whom an oral report was given. Use your notes to write these reports. Do not rely on memory.

Sometimes the nurse or another member of the care team will give you a brief oral report on a resident. Listen carefully. Take notes (Fig. 4-8). Ask about anything you do not understand. At the end of the report, restate what you have been told to make sure you understand it.

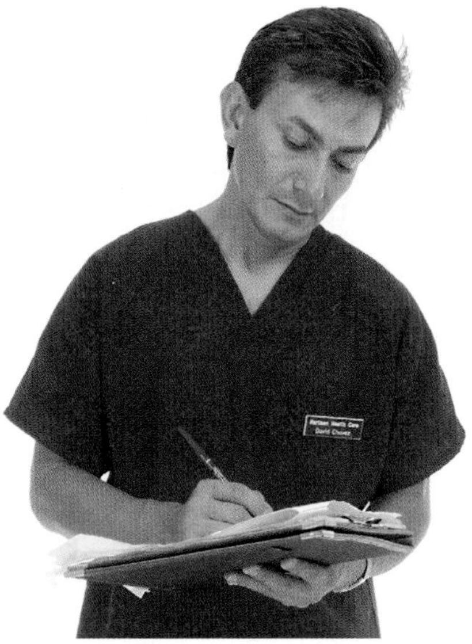

Figure 4-8. **Take notes so you can remember facts and report accurately.**

Some facilities use a method of reporting called "rounds." Staff members move from room-to-room and discuss each resident and the care plan. You may be involved in rounds at your facility. If you are, listen closely. Take notes. Offer valuable information gathered about residents to staff.

11. Explain documentation and describe related terms and forms

NAs spend more time with residents than other members of the care team. You may notice things about your residents that nurses or doctors do not know. You will not diagnose or decide treatment. However, you will have valuable information about residents. This will help in care planning. Documenting accurately is key to care planning. A thorough written record shows your observations to others. It helps you remember details about each resident.

You will see many residents during the day. You cannot remember everything about them. Documentation gives you an up-to-date record of each resident's care. You must learn to document accurately. Always observe and record carefully. Follow your facility's policies and procedures. Because documentation is so important, do not put it off.

A medical chart (record) is the legal record of a resident's care. What is written in the chart is considered in court to be what actually happened. The information found in the chart includes:

- Admission forms
- Resident's history and results of physical examinations
- Care plans
- Doctor's orders
- Doctor's progress notes
- Nursing assessments
- Nurse's notes

- Flow sheets
- Graphic record
- Intake and output record
- Consent forms
- Lab and test results
- Surgery reports
- Advance directives

If your facility allows you to chart in a medical record, remember: there are legal aspects to your documentation. Careful charting is important for these reasons:

1. It is the only way to guarantee clear and complete communication among all the members of the care team.

2. It is a legal record of every resident's treatment. Medical charts are used in court as evidence.

3. Documentation protects you and your employer from liability by proving what you did.

4. Documentation gives an up-to-date record of the status and care of each resident.

GUIDELINES

Careful Documentation

- Write your notes immediately after the care is given. This helps you to remember important details. Always wait to document until after you have completed care. Never record any care before it is done.
- Think about what you want to say before writing. This will help you be as brief and as clear as possible.
- Write facts, not opinions.
- Write neatly. Use black ink.
- If you make a mistake, draw one line through it. Write the correct word or words. Put your initials and the date. Never erase what you have written. Never use correction fluid (Fig. 4-9).
- Sign your full name and title. Write the correct date.

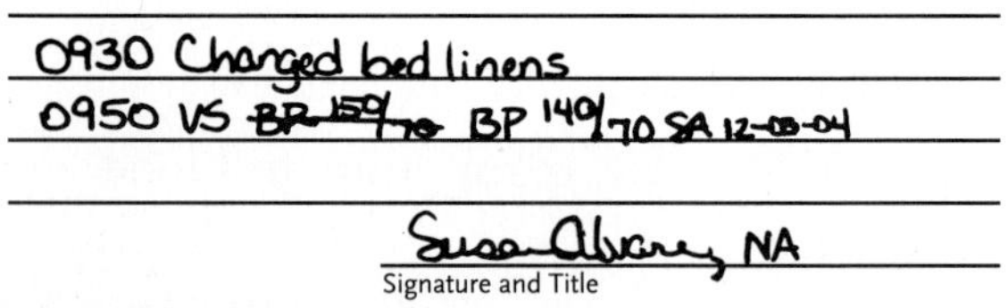

Fig. 4-9. **Corrected notes.**

- Document as specified in the care plan. Some facilities have a "check-off" sheet for documenting care. It is also called an ADL (activities of daily living) or flow sheet (Fig. 4-10). You will learn more about ADLs in chapters 8 and 13.

Computers

Some facilities use computers to document information. Computers record and store information. It can be retrieved when it is needed. This is faster and more accurate than writing information by hand. If your facility uses computers for documentation, you will be trained to use them.

HIPAA privacy guidelines apply to computer use. Make sure nobody can see private and protected health or personal information on your computer screen. Do not share confidential information with anyone except the care team.

24-Hour Clock (Military Time)

Facilities may use the 24-hour clock, or military time, to document information. Figure 4-11 shows the 24-hour clock and the corresponding military time. Examples of the way the numbers are written are:

Example #1: Regular to Military

11:00 a.m. = 1100 (eleven-hundred hours)

Example #2: Military to Regular

1115 = 11:15 a.m.

To change the hours between 1:00 p.m. to 11:59 p.m. to military time, add 12 to the regular time. For example, to change 4:00 p.m. to military time, add 4 + 12. The answer is 1600 hours.

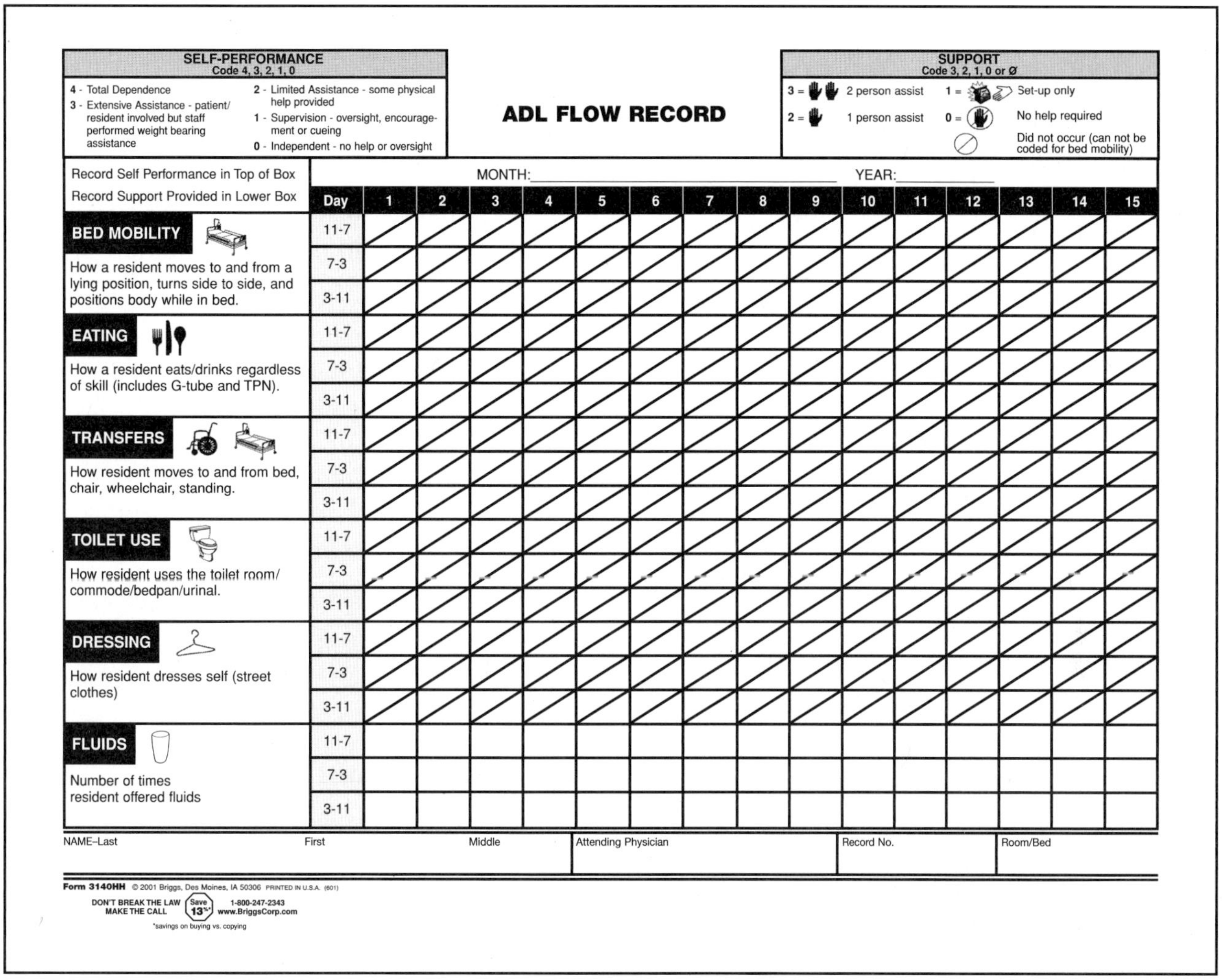

SELF-PERFORMANCE
Code 4, 3, 2, 1, 0

4 - Total Dependence
3 - Extensive Assistance - patient/resident involved but staff performed weight bearing assistance
2 - Limited Assistance - some physical help provided
1 - Supervision - oversight, encouragement or cueing
0 - Independent - no help or oversight

ADL FLOW RECORD

SUPPORT
Code 3, 2, 1, 0 or Ø

3 = 2 person assist
2 = 1 person assist
1 = Set-up only
0 = No help required
Ø Did not occur (can not be coded for bed mobility)

MONTH:______ YEAR:______

Record Self Performance in Top of Box / Record Support Provided in Lower Box	Day	1	2	3	4	5	6	7	8	9	10	11	12	13	14	15
BED MOBILITY. How a resident moves to and from a lying position, turns side to side, and positions body while in bed.	11-7															
	7-3															
	3-11															
EATING. How a resident eats/drinks regardless of skill (includes G-tube and TPN).	11-7															
	7-3															
	3-11															
TRANSFERS. How resident moves to and from bed, chair, wheelchair, standing.	11-7															
	7-3															
	3-11															
TOILET USE. How resident uses the toilet room/commode/bedpan/urinal.	11-7															
	7-3															
	3-11															
DRESSING. How resident dresses self (street clothes)	11-7															
	7-3															
	3-11															
FLUIDS. Number of times resident offered fluids	11-7															
	7-3															
	3-11															

NAME–Last First Middle | Attending Physician | Record No. | Room/Bed

Form 3140HH © 2001 Briggs, Des Moines, IA 50306 PRINTED IN U.S.A. (601)
DON'T BREAK THE LAW MAKE THE CALL Save 13%* 1-800-247-2343 www.BriggsCorp.com
*savings on buying vs. copying

Fig. 4-10. **Some facilities use ADL or flow sheets. (Reprinted with permission of Briggs Corporation, 800-247-2343.)**

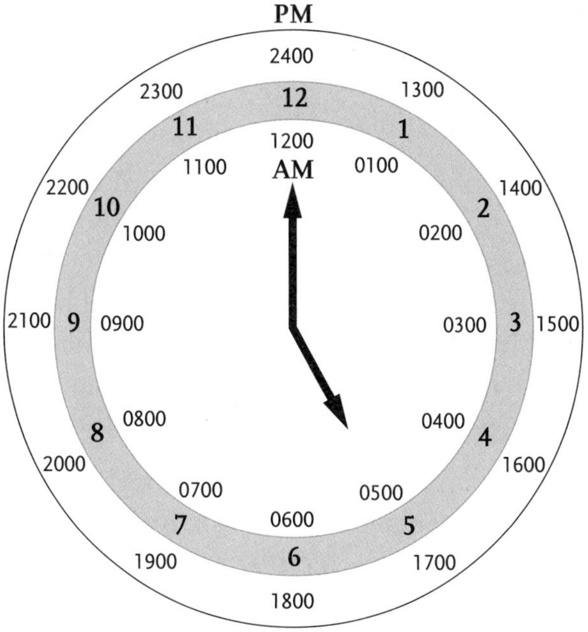

Fig. 4-11. **Divisions in the 24-hour clock.**

To change from military time to regular time, subtract 12. For example, to change 2200 hours to standard time, subtract 12 from 22. The answer is 10:00 p.m.

Minimum Data Set (MDS) manual

You first learned about the MDS manual in chapter 3. It is an assessment tool to give facilities a structured, standardized approach to care. The MDS manual offers a detailed guide to help nurses complete assessments accurately. The reporting you do on changes in your residents may "trigger" a needed assessment. Always report changes you notice to the nurse. They may be a sign of an illness or problem. By reporting them promptly, a new MDS assessment can be done if needed.

Kardex

Some facilities use a Kardex filing system. The Kardex is a type of card file that keeps resident information organized and easy to find. Information found in a Kardex includes the resident's care plan, diagnoses, special needs, and equipment used. It is usually kept at the nurse's station.

12. Describe incident reporting and recording

An **incident** is an accident or unexpected event during the course of care. It is not part of the normal routine in a facility. An error in care, such as feeding a resident from the wrong meal tray, is an incident. A fall or injury to a resident, employee, or visitor is another type of incident. An accusation from a resident or family member against staff is another example of an incident. Employee injuries also require reporting.

Reporting and documenting incidents is done to protect everyone involved. This includes the resident, your employer, and you. If you are required to document incidents at your facility, complete the report as soon as possible. Give it to the charge nurse. This is important so that you do not forget any details.

State and federal guidelines require incidents to be recorded in an incident report (Fig. 4-12). Report an incident to the nurse as soon as possible. The information in an incident report is confidential.

If a resident falls, and you did not see it, do not write "Mr. G fell." Instead write "found Mr. G on the floor," or "Mr. G states that he fell." For your protection, write a brief and accurate description of the events as they happened. Never place any blame or liability within the incident report.

Incident reports help show areas where changes can be made to avoid repeating the same incident. The following are guidelines for completing an incident report:

GUIDELINES

Incident Reporting

- Tell what happened. State the time, and the mental and physical condition of the resident.
- Tell how the person tolerated the incident (what was his reaction).
- State the facts. Do not give opinions.
- Do not write on the medical record about anything in the incident report (incident reports are confidential).
- Describe the action taken to give care.
- Include suggestions for change.

Incident Reports

Do not let anyone try to talk you out of filling out an incident report. It is important to have these reports on file. Complete it the same day the incident occurs. You may want to keep a copy of the incident report for yourself. This will protect you should the report be lost by the facility.

13. Discuss the nursing assistant's role in care planning and at care conferences

Nursing assistants have an important role in care planning. Care plans are prepared from the observations of staff caring for the resident. At care planning meetings, do not be afraid to speak up. Share your observations. If you are not sure what is important to say, talk to a nurse before the meeting to find out.

Care plans may be written at a special care conference. This is a meeting to share and gather information. Members of the care team may attend. At the conference, you will add your observations to help the nurses prepare the care plans.

Form 875/2 (if 2 part set) or
Form 875/3 (if 3 part set)

BRIGGS, Des Moines, IA 50306 (800) 247-2343

Printed in U.S.A.

INCIDENT REPORT

"An incident is any happening which is not consistent with the routine operation of the hospital or the routine care of a particular patient. It may be an accident or a situation which might result in an accident."

PERSON INVOLVED	(Last Name) (First Name) (Middle Initial) Mr. ❑: Mrs. ❑: Child ❑: Male ❑: Female ❑: Age ______		
PATIENT ❑	Room No.	State Cause for Hospitalization	
	Patient's Condition Before Incident Normal ❑: Senile ❑: Disoriented ❑: Sedated ❑: Other		
	Were Bed Rails Present? Yes ❑: No ❑: Up ❑: Down ❑: Ordered ❑:	Was Height of Bed Adjustable? Yes ❑: No ❑: Up ❑: Down ❑:	
EMPLOYEE ❑	Department	Job Title	
VISITOR ❑	Home Address	Home Phone	
OTHER ❑	Occupation	Reason for Presence at the Hospital	
Exact Location of Incident		Date of Incident	Time of Incident ❑ A.M. ❑ P.M.

Property Involved ❑: Equipment Involved ❑: Describe

Description of Incident by Person Involved

Describe Exactly What Happened: Why It Happened: What Causes Were. If an injury, State Part of Body Injured. If Property or Equipment Damaged, Describe Damage.

Name, Address & Phone No. of Witness(es)

Was It Necessary to Notify Physician? Yes ❑ No ❑	Time of Notification ______ a.m./p.m.	Time Responded ______ a.m./p.m.
Was Person Involved Seen by a Physician? Yes ❑ No ❑	Time Seen ❑ A.M. ❑ P.M.	Where
Physician's Name		T.______ P.______ R.______ B.P.______

Statement of Physician:

Date of Report	Title & Signature of Person Preparing Report

Additional Comments:

Form 875 BRIGGS, Des Moines, IA 50306 (800) 247-2343
PRINTED IN U.S.A.

INCIDENT REPORT

Fig. 4-12. **A sample incident report. (Reprinted with permission of Briggs Corporation, 800-247-2343.)**

Residents, family, and friends may attend the care conference. Members of the community, such as ombudsmen, share helpful information too.

14. Demonstrate effective communication on the telephone

At times, you may answer the telephone at your facility. General rules for speaking on the phone are:

- Be cheerful when greeting a caller. Say, "Good morning," "Good afternoon," or "Good evening."
- Identify your facility: "Lincolnwood Facility."
- Identify yourself and your position: "Nancy Jones, Nursing Assistant."
- Listen closely to the caller's request. Write down messages. Ask for correct spelling of names.
- Get a telephone number, if needed.
- Say "Thank you," and "Goodbye."

Do not give out any information about staff or residents over the phone. All resident and staff information is confidential. It must not be given over the telephone. Refer this type of phone call to a supervisor.

You may place a caller on hold if you need to get someone to take the call. Ask the caller if she can hold first.

Follow your facility's policy on personal phone calls. Some places ban the use of personal cell phones and pagers.

15. Explain the resident call system

Residents signal staff by using a facility call system. "Signal light" or "call light" are other names for this system. It allows residents to call for assistance when needed. Think of this system as a resident's lifeline. A lifeline can literally save a life. Always respond to call lights promptly. Do this even if the person is not your assigned resident. Never ignore a call light. Always leave call lights within reach of residents when leaving their rooms.

16. List guidelines for communicating with residents with special needs

Some residents need special communication techniques. This includes residents with:

- hearing or visual impairments
- stroke
- angry or combative behavior
- inappropriate behavior
- dementia *
- mental illness *

* Information on residents with dementia, such as Alzheimer's disease, is in chapter 19. Guidelines for communicating with residents who are mentally ill are in chapter 20.

Hearing Impairment

An **impairment** is a loss of function or ability. It can be a partial or complete loss. Those who are hearing-impaired or deaf may have lost their hearing gradually. They may have been born without the ability to hear. Hearing loss may affect how well residents can express their needs.

GUIDELINES
Hearing Impairment

- If the resident has a hearing aid and does not seem to be hearing well, make sure he or she is wearing it and that it is working properly (Fig. 4-13).
- Reduce or remove noise, such as TVs, radios, and loud speech. Close doors if needed.
- Get residents' attention before speaking. Do not startle them by approaching from behind. Walk in front or touch them lightly on the arm to show you are near.

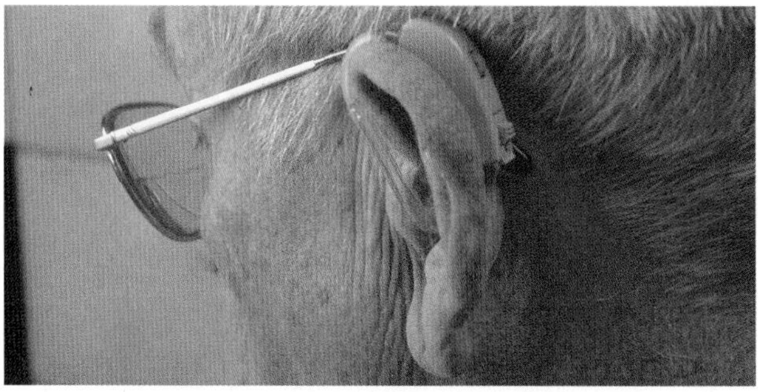

Fig. 4-13. **This is one type of hearing aid. Hearing aids must be turned on to work properly.**

- Speak clearly, slowly, and in good lighting. Directly face the person (Fig. 4-14). The light should be on your face, rather than on the resident's. Ask if he or she can hear what you are saying.

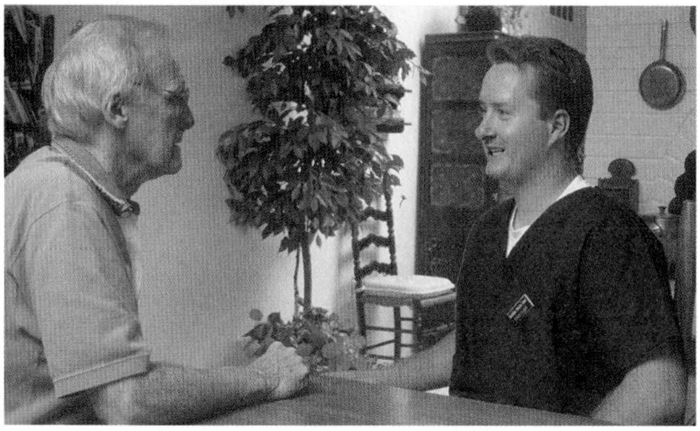

Fig. 4-14. **Speak face-to-face in good light.**

- Do not shout. Do not mouth the words in an exaggerated way.
- Lower the pitch of your voice.
- Do not chew gum or eat while speaking.
- Keep hands away from your face while talking.
- Know which ear hears better. Speak to and stand on that side.
- Use short sentences and simple words. Avoid sudden topic changes.
- Repeat what you have said using different words, when needed. Some hearing-impaired people want you to repeat exactly what you said. This is because they miss only a few words.
- Use picture cards or a notepad as needed.
- Hearing impaired residents may hear less when tired or ill. This is true of everyone.
- A hearing decline can be a normal aspect of aging. Be matter-of-fact about this. Show your understanding. Be supportive.

Vision Impairment

Vision impairment can affect people of all ages. It can exist at birth or develop gradually. It can occur in one eye or both. It may be the result of injury, illness, or aging.

GUIDELINES

Vision Impairment

- If the person has glasses, make sure they are clean and that he or she wears them. Also, make sure that they are in good condition and fit well.
- Identify yourself when you enter the room. Do not touch the resident until you have said your name. Explain what you would like to do.
- Always tell the resident what you are doing while caring for him.
- Talk directly to the resident. Do not talk to another person.
- Provide good lighting at all times.
- When you enter a new room with the resident, orient him or her to the area.
- Use the face of an imaginary clock as a guide to explain the position of objects in front of resident (Fig. 4-15).
- Do not move personal items or furniture without the resident's knowledge and permission.
- Offer large-print newspapers, magazines, and books.
- Use large clocks, clocks that chime, and radios to help keep track of time.
- Get books on tape and other aids from the local library or support organizations.

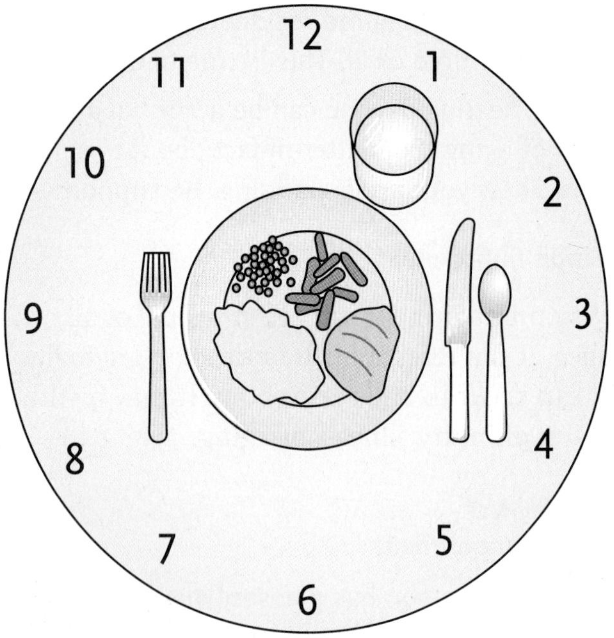

Fig. 4-15. **Use the face of an imaginary clock to explain the position of objects.**

- Put everything back where it was found.
- Encourage the use of other senses, such as hearing, touch, and smell.
- If the resident has a guide dog, do not play with or distract it.
- Tell resident when you are leaving the room.

Stroke

The medical term for a stroke is a cerebral vascular accident (CVA). CVA, or **stroke**, occurs when a clot or a ruptured blood vessel suddenly cuts off the blood supply to the brain (Fig. 4-16). Without blood, part of the brain gets no oxygen. This causes brain cells to die. Brain tissue is further damaged by leaking blood, clots, and swelling. These cause pressure on surrounding healthy tissue. You will learn more about caring for someone who has had a stroke in chapter 18.

Strokes can be mild or severe. Afterward, a resident may experience any of these effects:

- weakness on one side of the body, called **hemiparesis**

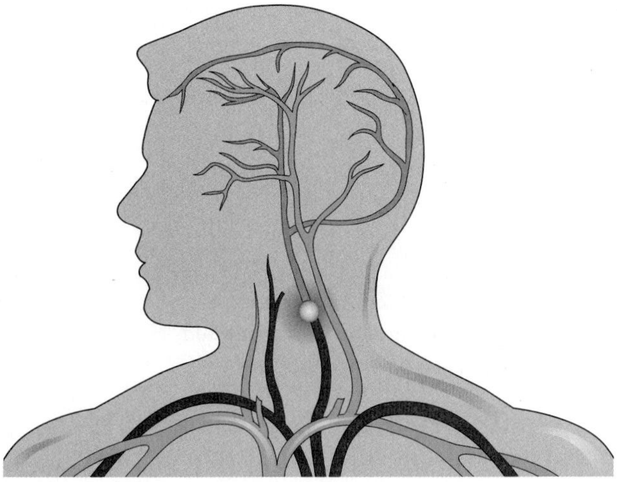

Fig. 4-16. **A stroke is caused when the blood supply to the brain is cut off suddenly by a clot or ruptured blood vessel.**

- paralysis on one side of the body, called **hemiplegia**
- tendency to ignore a weak or paralyzed side of the body
- trouble speaking or inability to speak, called **aphasia**
- inability to express needs through speech or written words, called **expressive aphasia**
- trouble understanding spoken or written words
- loss of sensations, such as temperature or touch
- loss of bowel or bladder control
- confusion
- laughing or crying without reason, or inappropriately, called **emotional lability**
- poor judgment
- memory loss
- loss of thinking and learning abilities
- trouble swallowing, called **dysphagia**

GUIDELINES
Communication and Stroke

Depending on the severity of the stroke and speech loss or confusion, these tips may help:

- Keep questions and directions simple. Give directions one step at a time.
- Phrase questions so they can be answered with a "yes" or "no." For example, when helping a resident with eating, ask, "Would you like to start with a drink of milk?"
- Agree on signals, such as shaking or nodding the head or raising a hand or finger for "yes" or "no."
- Use a pencil and paper if a resident can write. A thick handle or tape around it may help the resident hold it more easily.
- Never call the weaker side the "bad side," or talk about the "bad" leg or arm. Use the term "weaker" or "involved" to refer to the side with paralysis or weakness.
- Use pictures, gestures, or pointing. Use communication boards or special cards to aid communication (Fig. 4-17).
- Keep the call signal within reach of residents. They can let you know when you are needed.

STOP *Never talk about residents as if they were not there. Just because they cannot speak does not mean they cannot hear. Treat all residents with respect.*

Combative Behavior

Residents may display **combative**, meaning violent or hostile, behavior. Such behavior includes hitting, pushing, kicking, or verbal attacks. It may result from disease affecting the brain. It may also be due to frustration. It may just be part of someone's personality. In general, combative behavior is not a reaction to you. Try not to take it personally.

Always report and document combative behavior. Even if you are not upset, the care team needs to be aware of it. Use these guidelines when dealing with combative behavior:

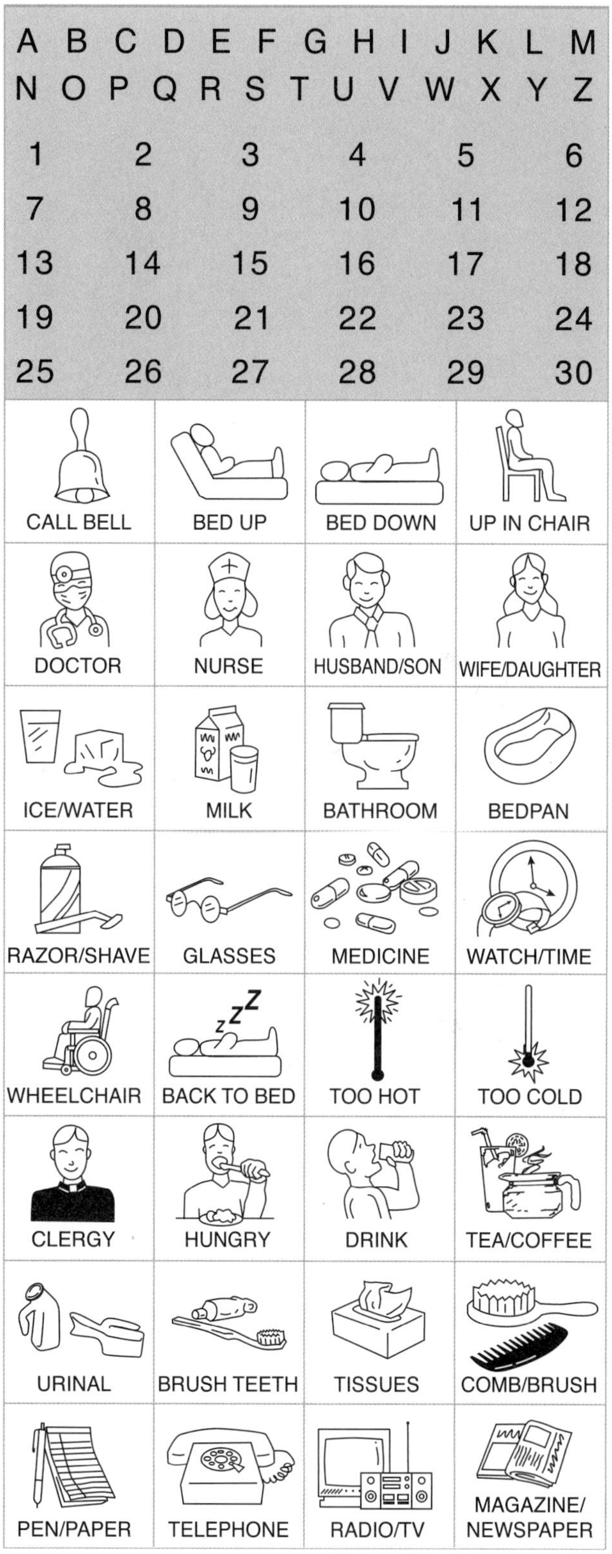

Fig. 4-17. **A sample communication board.**

GUIDELINES
Combative Behavior

- Block physical blows or step out of the way. Never hit back (Fig. 4-18).

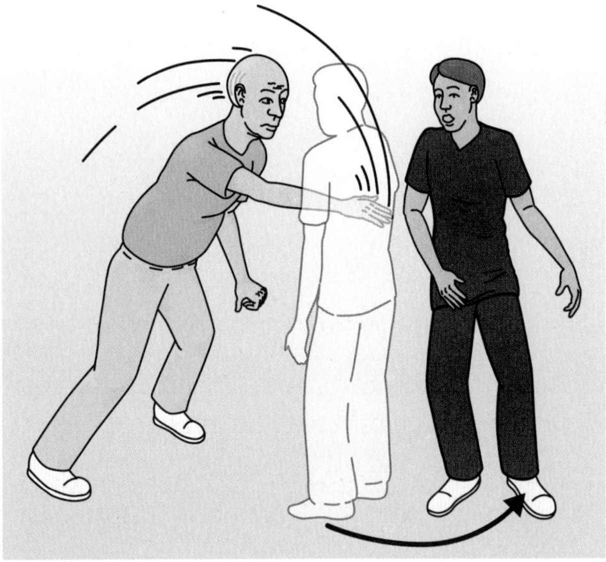

Fig. 4-18. **Step out of the way of a combative resident, but never hit back.**

- Stay at a safe distance.
- Stay calm. Lower the tone of your voice.
- Be flexible and patient.
- Stay neutral.
- Do not respond to verbal attacks. Do not argue. Do not accuse the resident of wrongdoing.
- Do not use gestures that could frighten or startle the resident.
- Be reassuring and supportive.
- Consider what provoked the resident. Leave the resident alone if you can safely do so. Get help to take the resident to a quieter place.

Anger

Anger is a natural emotion. Residents and their families may express it. There are many causes of anger. Some are disease, fear, pain, and loneliness. Some residents may be angry due to their loss of independence. Anger may just be a part of someone's personality. Some people get angry more easily than others.

Anger is expressed in different ways. Some are shouting, yelling, threatening, throwing things, and pacing. Others express anger by withdrawing, being silent, or sulking.

Always report angry behavior to the nurse. Use these guidelines when dealing with angry residents:

GUIDELINES

Angry Behavior

- Stay calm.
- Do not respond to verbal attacks. Do not argue.
- Empathize with the resident. Try to understand what he or she is feeling.
- Try to find out what caused the resident's anger. Using silence may help the resident explain.
- Treat the resident with dignity and respect. Explain what you are going to do and when you will do it.
- Answer call lights promptly.
- Stay at a safe distance if the resident becomes combative.

Assertive vs. Aggressive Behavior

A resident is behaving assertively when he or she expresses thoughts, feelings, and beliefs in a direct and honest way. Being assertive involves respect for a resident's own needs and feelings and for those of other people.

A resident is behaving aggressively when he or she expresses thoughts, feelings, and beliefs in ways that humiliate, disgrace, or overpower the other person. Little or no respect is shown for the needs or feelings of others.

Inappropriate Behavior

Some residents will show inappropriate behavior. This includes sexual advances and comments. Sexual advances include any sexual words, comments, or behavior that makes you feel uncomfortable. Report this behavior to the nurse immediately.

Inappropriate behavior also includes residents removing their clothes or touching themselves in public. Illness, dementia, confusion, and medication may cause this behavior.

If you encounter any embarrassing situation, be matter-of-fact. Do not over-react. This may actually reinforce the behavior. Try to distract the person. If that does not work, gently direct the resident to a private area. Notify the nurse.

Confused residents may have problems that mimic inappropriate sexual behavior. They may have an uncomfortable rash, clothes that are too tight, too hot, or too scratchy, or the need to go to the bathroom. Consider and watch for these problems.

When residents act inappropriately, report it, even if you think it was harmless.

STOP ***Never hit a resident.***

Unfortunately, it is not uncommon to read or hear about physical abuse of the elderly by caregivers. These caregivers may be family, friends, or care team members. Often, physical abuse is due to stressful situations causing the caregiver to lash out quickly. You can never hit a resident, NO MATTER WHAT. Even if a resident strikes you first, you may not strike back. If you feel that your reactions are out of control, seek help.

Chapter Review

1. Write out a short sample conversation you might have with a resident. Use the three basic steps of communication.
2. Which of these is an example of nonverbal communication?
   a. Telling a joke
   b. Laughing at a joke
3. Nonverbal communication that may be affected by cultural background includes:
   a. Making hand motions while talking
   b. Making eye contact
   c. Standing far away from another person
   d. All of the above
4. What does the word "culture" mean?
5. What are two things an NA can do if a resident speaks a different language?
6. How can an NA show a resident that she is listening and encourage him to give more information?
7. What can silence or pauses help a resident do?
8. Why should an NA sit near a resident who has started a conversation?
9. For each statement, decide whether it is a fact or an opinion. Write "F" for fact and "O" for opinion.

   _____ Mr. Moore looked terrible today.

   _____ Mr. Gaston had a fever of 100.7.

   _____ Ms. Martino needs to make some friends.

   _____ Ms. Martino has not had a visitor since last week.
10. For each of these, decide whether it is an objective or subjective observation. Write "O" for objective and "S" for subjective.

    _____ Resident seems depressed.

    _____ Red skin on resident's hip.

    _____ Resident is running a fever.

    _____ Resident has noisy breathing.

    _____ Resident says he is nauseous.
11. What does the abbreviation "ROM" stand for?

12. What does the abbreviation "NPO" stand for?
13. List ten signs and symptoms that should be reported immediately to the nurse.
14. Describe four reasons why careful documentation is important.
15. List four guidelines for documentation.
16. Convert 10:00 p.m. to military time.
17. What is an incident at a facility?
18. List four guidelines for incident reporting.
19. What is the purpose of care conferences?
20. Give an example of a proper greeting when answering the phone.
21. What is the purpose of the resident call light or call system?
22. When a resident has a hearing impairment, on whose face should the light be shining while communicating—the resident's or the NA's?
23. How can an NA explain the position of objects in front of a visually impaired resident?
24. How should questions be phrased to a resident who has had a stroke?
25. How should an NA refer to the weaker side of a resident who has had a stroke?
26. What should an NA always do after a resident behaves inappropriately?

Chapter 5
Quality Infection Control

1. Define "infection control" and related terms

Infection control is the set of methods used to control and prevent the spread of disease. It is the responsibility of all members of the care team. Know your facility's infection control policies and procedures. They help protect you, residents, and others from disease.

A **microorganism** is a tiny living thing. It is not visible to the eye without a microscope. Microorganisms are always present in the environment. **Infections** occur when harmful microorganisms, called **pathogens**, enter the body. For infections to develop, pathogens must invade and grow within the human body.

There are two main types of infections, systemic and localized. A **systemic infection** occurs when pathogens enter the bloodstream and move throughout the body. It causes general symptoms such as fever, chills, or mental confusion. A **localized infection** is limited to a specific part of the body. It has local symptoms. Its symptoms are near the site of infection. For example, if a wound becomes infected, the area around it may become red, hot, and painful.

Another type of infection is a nosocomial infection. A **nosocomial infection**, or hospital-acquired infection (HAI), is an infection acquired in a hospital or other healthcare facility.

Asepsis means no pathogens are present. It refers to the clean conditions you want to create in your facility. In health care, an object can only be called "**clean**" if it has not been contaminated with pathogens. An object that is "**dirty**" has been contaminated with pathogens.

Preventing the spread of infection is important. To know how to do this, you must first know how it is spread.

2. Describe the chain of infection

The **chain of infection** describes how disease is transmitted from one being to another (Fig. 5-1). Definitions and examples of the six links in the chain of infection are:

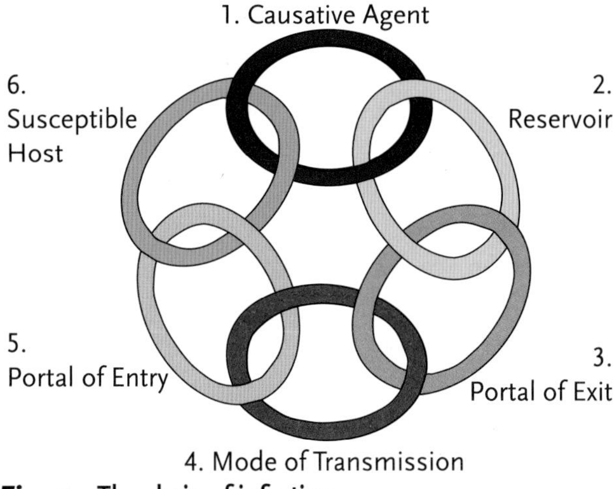

***Fig. 5-1.* The chain of infection.**

Link 1: The causative agent is a pathogen or microorganism that causes disease. Normal flora are the microorganisms that live in and on the body. They do not cause harm. When they enter a different part of the body, they may cause an infection. Causative agents include bacteria, viruses, fungi, and protozoa.

Link 2: A reservoir is where the pathogen lives and grows. It can be a person, animal, plant, soil or substance. Microorganisms grow best in warm, dark, and moist places where food is present. Some microorganisms need oxygen to survive. Others do not. Reservoirs include the lungs, blood, and large intestine.

Link 3: The portal of exit is any opening on an infected person allowing pathogens to leave. These include the nose, mouth, eyes, or a cut in the skin (Fig. 5-2).

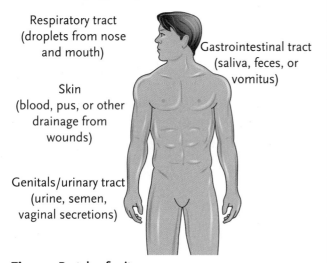

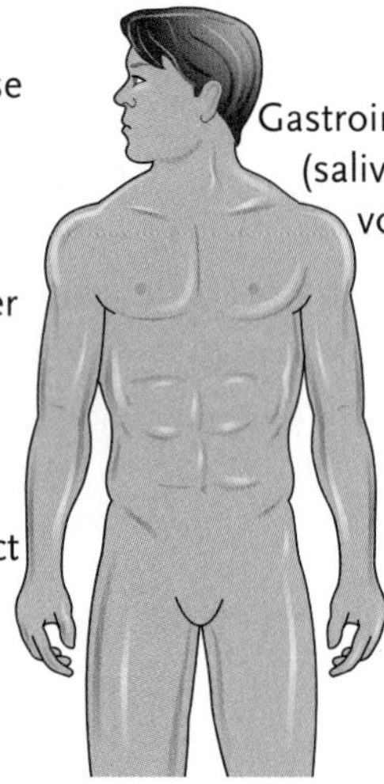

Fig. 5-2. **Portals of exit.**

Link 4: The mode of transmission describes how the pathogen travels from one person to another. Transmission can happen through the air. It can also occur through direct or indirect contact. **Direct contact** happens by touching the infected person or his or her secretions. **Indirect contact** results from touching something contaminated by the infected person, such as a tissue or clothes.

Link 5: The portal of entry is any body opening on an uninfected person that lets pathogens enter. This includes the nose, mouth, eyes, other mucous membranes, a cut in the skin, or dry/cracked skin (Fig. 5-3). **Mucous membranes** include the linings of the mouth, nose, eyes, rectum, or genitals.

Link 6: A susceptible host is an uninfected person who could get sick. This includes all healthcare workers and anyone in their care who is not already infected.

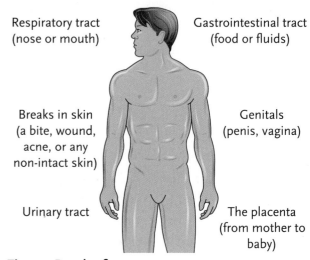

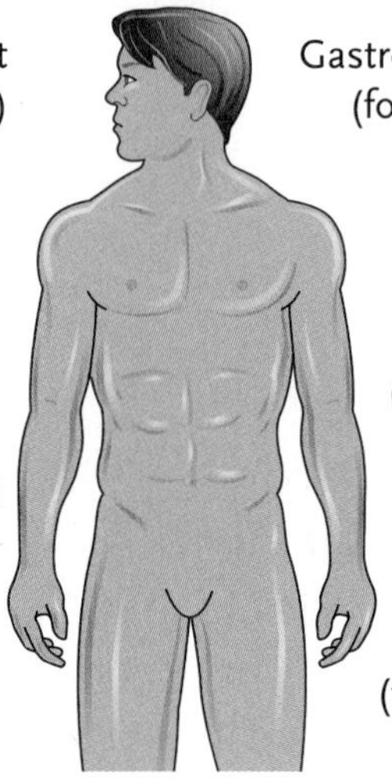

Fig. 5-3. **Portals of entry.**

If one of the links in the chain of infection is broken, then the spread of infection stops. Infection control practices help stop pathogens from traveling (Link 4), and getting on your hands, nose, eyes, mouth, skin, etc. (Link 5). You can also reduce your chances of getting sick (Link 6) by having immunizations for diseases such as hepatitis B and influenza.

Transmission of most **infectious**, or contagious, diseases can be prevented by always taking a few precautions. Washing your hands is the most important way to stop the spread of infection. All caregivers should wash their hands often.

3. Explain why the elderly are at a higher risk for infection and identify symptoms of an infection

The elderly are at a higher risk for infection. This is due, in part, to weakened immune systems as a result of aging. Weakened immune systems can also result from chronic illnesses.

Other physical changes of aging may also contribute to infections in the elderly. These include decreased circulation and slow wound healing.

Older adults are at risk for malnutrition. This adds to an increased risk of infection. Someone who is **malnourished** is not getting proper nutrition. It is a serious condition (see chapter 16). Also, the elderly may have limited mobility, which is another risk factor. Lack of mobility increases the risk of pressure sores and skin infections.

The elderly are hospitalized more often than younger people. This makes them more likely to get nosocomial infections. Difficulty swallowing and incontinence increase the risk of respiratory and urinary tract infections. Some medications increase the chance of infection. Feeding tubes and other types of tubes, such as catheters (chapter 14), increase the risk of infection.

Infection is more dangerous for the elderly. Even a simple cold can turn into a life-threatening illness, such as pneumonia. It also may take longer for older people to recover from an infection or illness. This is why preventing infection is so important. You play an important role in preventing infection.

You will need to recognize signs and symptoms of infections so that you can report them to the nurse.

OBSERVING AND REPORTING
Localized and Systemic Infections

Signs and symptoms of a localized infection are:

- redness
- swelling
- pain
- heat
- **drainage** (fluid from a wound or a cavity)

Signs and symptoms of a systemic infection are:

- fever
- chills
- headache
- change in other vital signs
- nausea, vomiting, and diarrhea
- mental confusion

If you notice any of these symptoms, tell the nurse immediately.

4. Describe the Centers for Disease Control and Prevention (CDC) and explain Standard Precautions

The **Centers for Disease Control and Prevention (CDC)** is a federal government agency that issues guidelines to protect and improve health. It promotes public health and safety through education. The CDC tries to control and prevent disease. In 1996, the CDC recommended a new infection control system to reduce the risk of contracting infectious diseases. In 2004, the CDC proposed some changes to this system.

There are two levels of precautions within the infection control system. They are Standard Precautions and Transmission-Based, or Isolation, Precautions. To **isolate** means to keep something separate, or by itself. In the 2004 proposed guidelines the CDC suggests that the term "Expanded Precautions" be used instead of "Transmission-Based Precautions."

Following **Standard Precautions** means treating all blood, body fluids, non-intact skin (like abrasions, pimples, or open sores), and mucous membranes (lining of mouth, nose, eyes, rectum, or genitals) as if they were infected. This is the only safe way of doing your job. You cannot tell by looking at your residents or their charts if they have a contagious disease such as HIV, hepatitis, or influenza.

Under Standard Precautions, "body fluids" include saliva, sputum (mucus coughed up), urine, feces, semen, vaginal secretions, and pus or other wound drainage. It does not include sweat.

Standard Precautions and Transmission-Based Precautions are a way to stop the spread of infection. They interrupt the mode of transmission. In other words, these guidelines do not stop an infected person from giving off pathogens. However, by following these guidelines you help stop those pathogens from infecting you or those in your care.

1. Practice Standard Precautions with every single person in your care.
2. Transmission-Based Precautions vary based on how an infection is transmitted. When indicated, they are used in addition to the Standard Precautions. You will learn more about them in learning objective 9.

GUIDELINES

Standard Precautions

- **Wear gloves** if you may come into contact with: blood; body fluids or secretions; broken skin (abrasions, acne, cuts, stitches or staples); or mucous membranes (linings of the mouth, nose, eyes, vagina, rectum, and penis). Such situations include mouth care, bathroom assistance, perineal care, helping with a bedpan or urinal, cleaning up spills, cleaning basins, urinals, bedpans, and other containers that have held body fluids; and disposing of wastes.
- **Wash your hands** before putting on gloves. Wash them immediately after removing your gloves. Be careful not to touch clean objects with your used gloves.
- **Remove gloves** immediately when finished with a procedure.
- **Immediately wash all skin surfaces that have been contaminated** with blood and body fluids.
- **Wear a disposable gown** if you may come into contact with blood or body fluids.
- **Wear a mask and protective goggles** if you may come into contact with splashing or spraying blood or body fluids.
- **Wear gloves and use caution when handling razor blades, needles, and other sharps. Sharps** are needles or other sharp objects. Discard them carefully in a puncture-resistant biohazard container.
- **Never attempt to cap needles or sharps.** Dispose of them in an approved container. (Fig. 5-4).

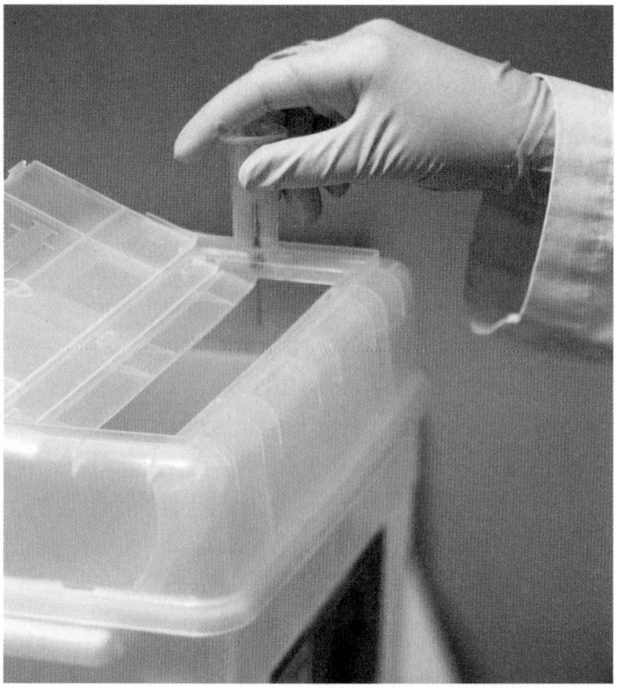

Fig. 5-4. **One type of biohazardous waste container.**

- **Avoid nicks and cuts** when shaving residents.
- **Carefully bag all contaminated supplies.** Dispose of them according to your facility's policy.
- **Clearly label body fluids** that are saved for a specimen with the resident's name and a biohazard label. Keep them in a container with a lid.
- **Dispose of contaminated wastes** according to your facility's policy.

Again, Standard Precautions should ALWAYS be practiced on those in your care regardless of their infection status. You cannot tell by how someone looks or acts, or even by reading his chart, if he carries a bloodborne disease. If you practice Standard Precautions, you greatly reduce the risk of getting disease from those in your care. You will also keep one resident's infection from harming another.

You will learn more about following Standard Precautions in the next several learning objectives.

5. Explain the term "hand hygiene" and identify when to wash hands

In your work you will use your hands constantly. Microorganisms are on everything you touch. Washing your hands is the single most important thing you can do to prevent the spread of disease (Fig. 5-5).

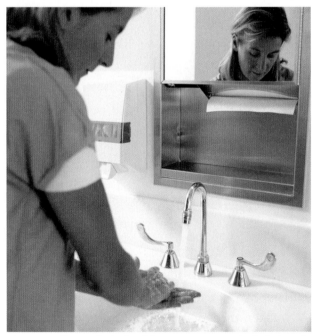

Fig. 5-5. **All people in health care must wash their hands often. Washing your hands is the most important thing you can do to prevent the spread of disease.**

The CDC has defined **hand hygiene** as handwashing with either plain or antiseptic soap and water and using alcohol-based hand rubs. Alcohol-based hand rubs include gels, rinses, and foams. They do not require the use of water.

Alcohol-based hand rubs have proven effective in reducing bacteria on the skin. However, they are not a substitute for proper handwashing. Always use soap and water for visibly soiled hands. It is important to wash your hands often. Once they are clean, alcohol-based products can be used in addition to handwashing. Use hand lotion to prevent dry, cracked skin.

If you wear rings, consider removing them while working. Rings may increase the risk of contamination. Keep fingernails short and clean. Do not wear false nails. False nails increase the risk of contamination.

You should wash your hands:

- when you get to work
- before and after touching meal trays and/or handling food
- before and after feeding residents
- before, between, and after all contact with residents
- after contact with any body fluids
- after handling contaminated items
- before putting on gloves and after removing gloves
- before getting clean linen
- after touching garbage or trash
- after picking up anything from the floor
- after using the bathroom
- after blowing your nose or coughing or sneezing into your hand
- before and after you eat
- after smoking
- after touching areas on your body, such as your mouth, face, eyes, hair, ears, or nose
- before and after applying makeup
- before leaving the facility

Wash hands before resident care.

As you move between residents' rooms, always wash your hands. Taking care of residents means you will get many microorganisms on your hands. Wash your hands before giving care. It will help prevent the spread of disease.

Washing hands

Equipment: soap, paper towels

1. Turn on water at sink.
2. Angle your arms down. Hold your hands lower than your elbows. Wet your hands and wrists thoroughly (Fig. 5-6).

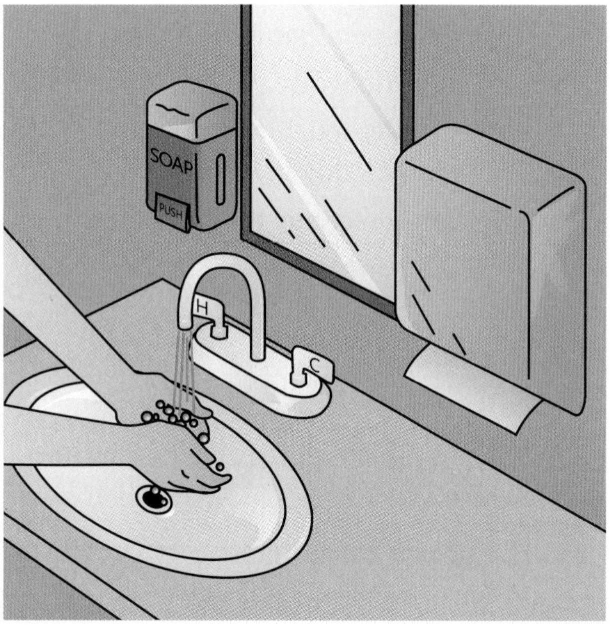

Fig. 5-6.

3. Apply skin cleanser or soap to your hands.
4. Lather all surfaces of your fingers and hands, including your wrists (Fig. 5-7). Use friction for at least 10 seconds.
5. Clean your nails by rubbing them in palm of other hand.
6. Rinse all surfaces of your hands and wrists. Run water down from wrists to fingertips.
7. Use a clean, dry paper towel to dry all surfaces of your hands, wrists, and fingers.

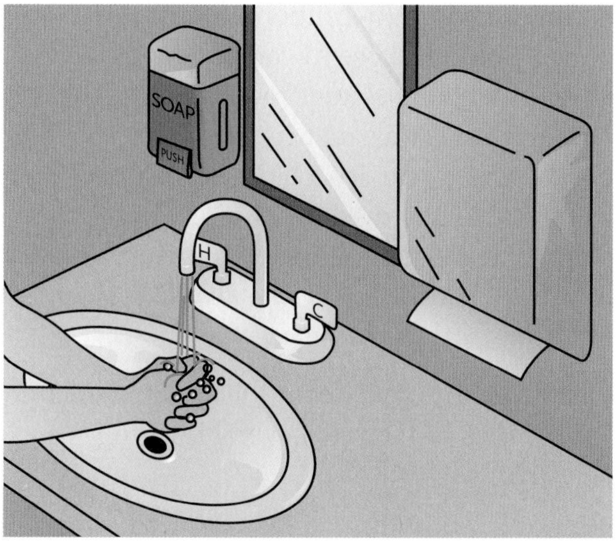

Fig. 5-7.

8. Use a clean, dry paper towel or clean, dry area of paper towel to turn off the faucet (Fig. 5-8). Do not contaminate your hands by touching the surface of the sink or faucet.

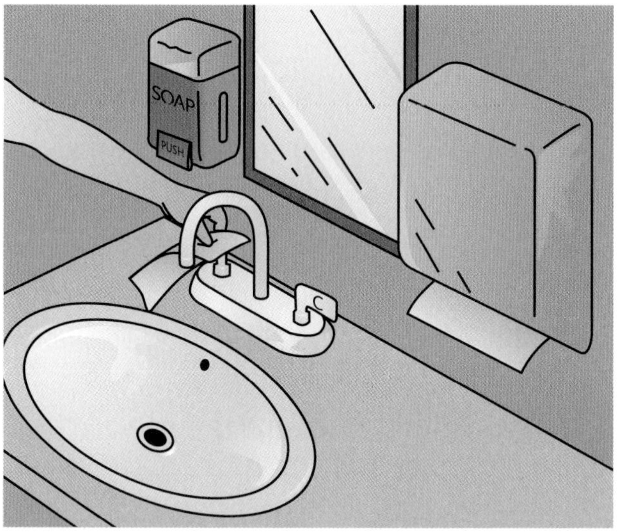

Fig. 5-8.

9. Dispose of used paper towel(s) in wastebasket immediately after shutting off faucet.

6. Discuss the use of personal protective equipment (PPE) in facilities

Personal protective equipment (PPE) is a **barrier** (a block or obstacle) between a person and disease. PPE helps protect you from potentially infectious material. Your employer is responsible for giving you the appropriate PPE to wear. PPE includes gloves, gowns, masks, goggles, and face shields.

Gloves protect the hands. Gowns protect the skin and/or clothing. Masks protect the mouth and nose. Goggles protect the eyes. Face shields protect the entire face—the mouth, nose, and eyes.

Gloves

You must wear gloves when there is a chance of contact with body fluids, open wounds, or mucous membranes. Mucous membranes are the membranes that line body cavities, such as the mouth or nose. Your facility will have policies and procedures on when to wear gloves. Learn and follow them. Always wear gloves for these tasks:

- any time you might touch blood or any body fluid, including vomitus, urine, feces, or saliva
- doing or helping with mouth care or care of any mucous membrane
- doing or helping with perineal care (care of the genitals and anal area)
- performing personal care on a resident whose skin is broken by abrasions, cuts, rash, acne, pimples, or boils
- helping with personal care when you have open sores or cuts on your hands
- shaving a resident
- disposing of soiled bed linens, gowns, dressings, and pads

Clean, non-sterile gloves are generally adequate. They may be vinyl, latex, or nitrile. Some people are allergic to latex. If you are, let the nurse know. Alternative gloves will be provided. Tell the nurse if you have dry, cracked, or broken skin. Gloves should fit your hands comfortably. They should not be too loose or too tight.

If you have cuts or sores on your hands, first cover these areas with bandages or gauze. Then put on gloves. Disposable gloves are worn only once. They may not be washed or disinfected for reuse. Change gloves right before contact with mucous membranes or broken skin, or if gloves are soiled, torn, or damaged. Wash your hands before putting on fresh gloves.

Putting on gloves

1. Wash your hands.
2. If you are right-handed, slide one glove on your left hand (reverse if left-handed).
3. With gloved hand, slide the other hand into the second glove.
4. Interlace fingers. Smooth out folds and create a comfortable fit.
5. Carefully look for tears, holes, or discolored spots. Replace the glove if needed.
6. If wearing a gown, pull the cuff of the gloves over the sleeve of gown (Fig. 5-9).

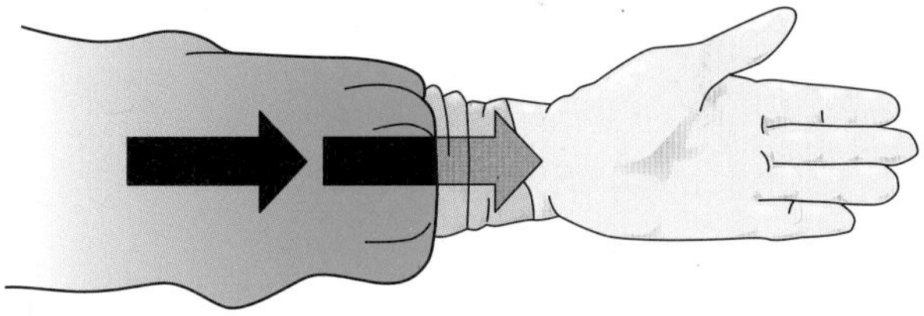

Fig. 5-9.

Remove gloves promptly after use and before caring for another resident. Wash your hands. Remove your gloves before touching noncontaminated items or surfaces. You are wearing gloves to protect your skin from contamination. After giving care, your gloves are contaminated. If you open a door with the gloved hand, the doorknob is contaminated. Later, when you open the door with an ungloved hand, you will be infected. It is a common mistake to contaminate the room around you. Do not do this. Before touching surfaces, remove gloves. Wash your hands. Put on new gloves if needed.

Taking off gloves

1. Touch only the outside of one glove. Pull the first glove off by pulling down from the cuff (Fig. 5-10).

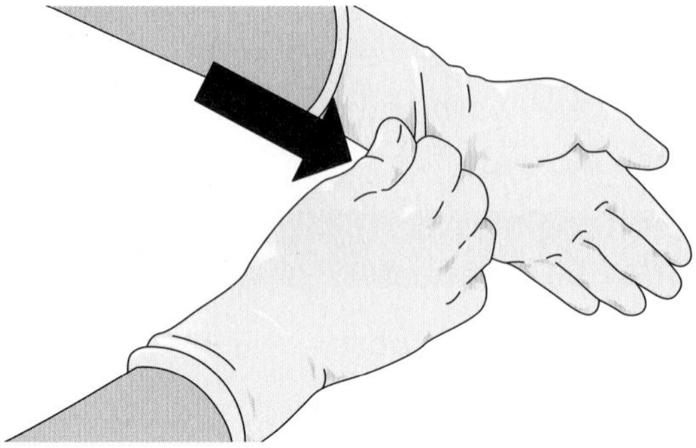

Fig. 5-10.

2. As the glove comes off, it should be turned inside out.
3. With the fingertips of your gloved hand, hold the glove you just removed. With your ungloved hand, reach two fingers inside the remaining glove. Be careful not to touch any part of the outside of glove (Fig. 5-11).

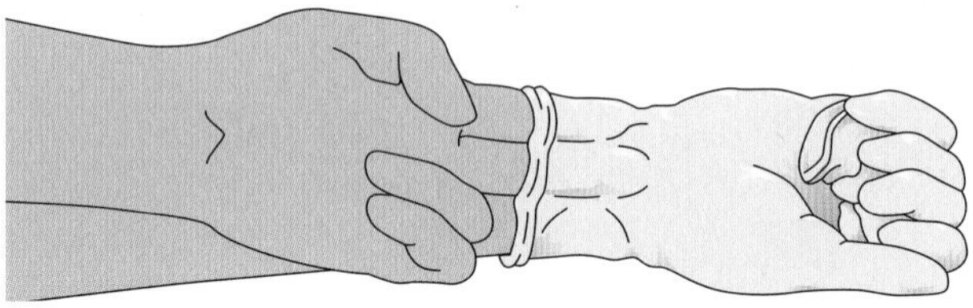

Fig. 5-11.

4. Pull down, turning this glove inside out and over the first glove as you remove it.
5. You should now be holding one glove from its clean inner side. The other glove should be inside it.
6. Drop both gloves into the proper container.
7. Wash your hands.

The guidelines for wearing other PPE are the same as for gloves. Wear PPE if there is a chance of contact with body fluids, mucous membranes, or open wounds. Gowns, masks, goggles, and face shields are worn when splashing or spraying of body fluids or blood could occur.

Gowns

Clean, non-sterile gowns protect your exposed skin. They also prevent soiling of your clothing. Gowns should fully cover your torso. They should fit comfortably over your body, and have long sleeves that fit snugly at the wrist. When finished with a procedure, remove the gown as soon as possible. Wash your hands.

Putting on a gown

1. Wash your hands.
2. Open the gown. Hold out in front of you and allow it to open. Do not shake it. Slip your arms into the sleeves. Pull gown on (Fig. 5-12).

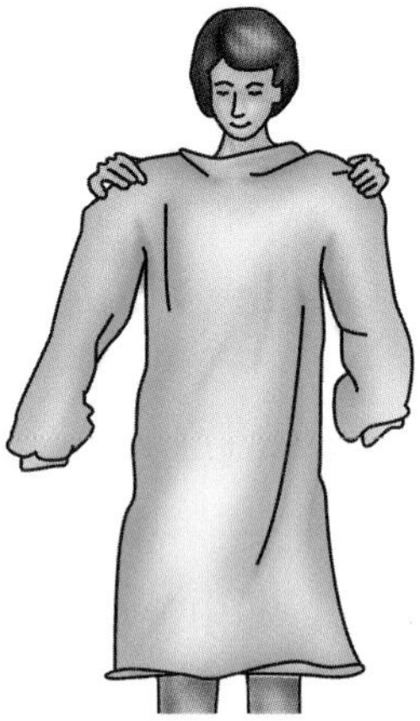

Fig. 5-12.

3. Tie the neck ties into a bow so they can be easily untied later.
4. Reach behind you. Pull the gown until it completely covers your clothing. Tie the back ties (Fig. 5-13).

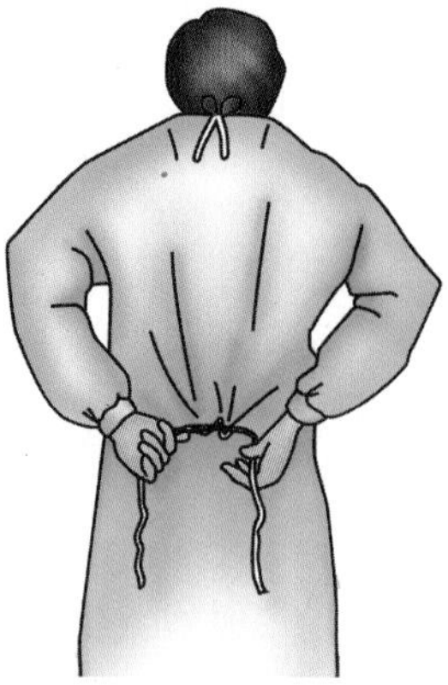

Fig. 5-13.

5. Use gowns only once and then discard or remove. When removing a gown, roll it dirty side in and away from the body. If gown is wet or soiled, remove it. Check clothing. Put on a new gown.
6. Put on your gloves after putting on gown.

Masks and Goggles

Masks should also be worn when caring for residents with respiratory illnesses. You will learn more about special masks and respiratory illnesses later in the chapter. Masks should fully cover your nose and mouth and prevent fluid penetration. Masks should fit snugly over the nose and mouth. Always change your mask between residents.

Goggles provide protection for your eyes. Eyeglasses alone do not provide proper eye protection. Goggles should fit snugly over and around your eyes or eyeglasses.

Putting on a mask and goggles

1. Wash your hands.
2. Pick up the mask by top strings or elastic strap. Do not touch mask where it touches your face.
3. Adjust the mask over your nose and mouth. Tie top strings, then bottom strings. Masks must always be dry or they must be replaced. Never wear a mask hanging from only the bottom ties (Fig. 5-14).

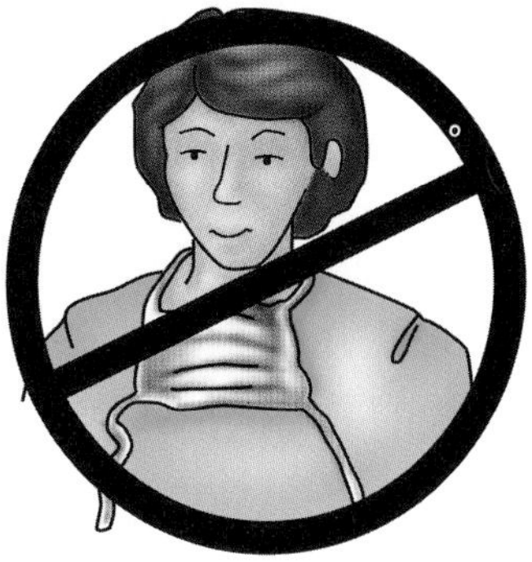

Fig. 5-14.

4. Put on the goggles.
5. Put on your gloves after putting on mask and goggles.

Face Shields

When additional skin protection is needed, a face shield can be used as a substitute to wearing a mask or goggles. Follow your facility's policies. The face shield should cover your forehead and go below the chin. It wraps around the sides of your face.

PPE Summary

Your employer will give you PPE as needed. It is your responsibility to know where it is kept and how to use it.

When applying PPE, remember this order:

1. Apply mask and goggles.
2. Apply gown.
3. Apply gloves last.

When removing PPE, remember this order:

1. Remove gloves.
2. Remove gown.
3. Remove mask and goggles.

7. List guidelines for handling equipment and linen

Facilities will have separate areas for clean and dirty items, such as equipment, linen, and supplies. They are normally called the "clean" and the "dirty," or "contaminated," utility rooms. Before entering a clean utility room, wash your hands. This helps keep the equipment in this room clean.

The contaminated or dirty utility room is usually separate from the clean utility room. It is used to store equipment that is not needed by the resident. Supplies in this room are not "clean," such as trash bags. Wash your hands before leaving this room so that you do not transfer pathogens to other areas in the facility. A sink is usually in this room. After washing your hands, do not touch anything in the room. If you do, you must wash your hands again. Know the location of clean and dirty utility rooms and what is stored in each.

Measures like sterilization and disinfection decrease the spread of pathogens and disease. **Sterilization** means all microorganisms are destroyed, not just pathogens. An autoclave is usually used to sterilize equipment. It creates steam or a gas that kills all microorganisms. **Disinfection** means that only pathogens are destroyed. However, disinfection does not kill all pathogens.

GUIDELINES

Handling Equipment, Linen, and Clothing

- Handle all equipment in a way that prevents
  - skin/mucous membrane contact
  - contamination of your clothing
  - transfer of disease to other residents or areas
- Do not use "re-usable" equipment again until it has been properly cleaned and reprocessed. Dispose of all "single-use" equipment properly.
- Clean and disinfect
  - all environmental surfaces
  - beds, bedrails, all bedside equipment (Fig. 5-15)
  - all frequently touched surfaces (such as doorknobs)

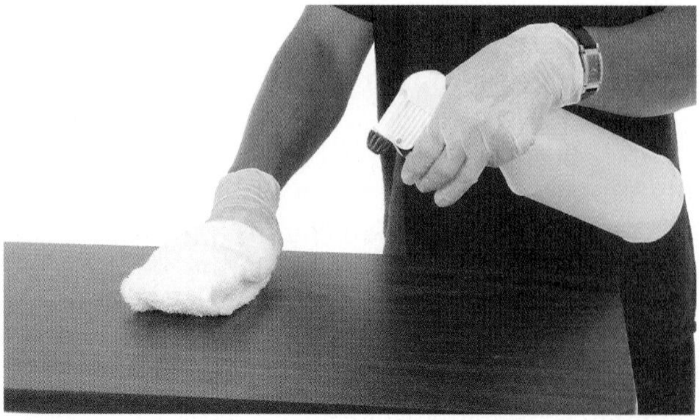

Fig. 5-15. **Use a solution of bleach and water to disinfect surfaces.**

- Handle, transport, and process soiled linens and clothing in a way that prevents
  - skin and mucous membrane exposure
  - contamination of clothing (hold linen and clothing away from uniform) (Fig. 5-16)
  - transfer of disease to other residents and areas (do not shake linen or clothes; fold or roll linen so that the dirtiest area is inside)

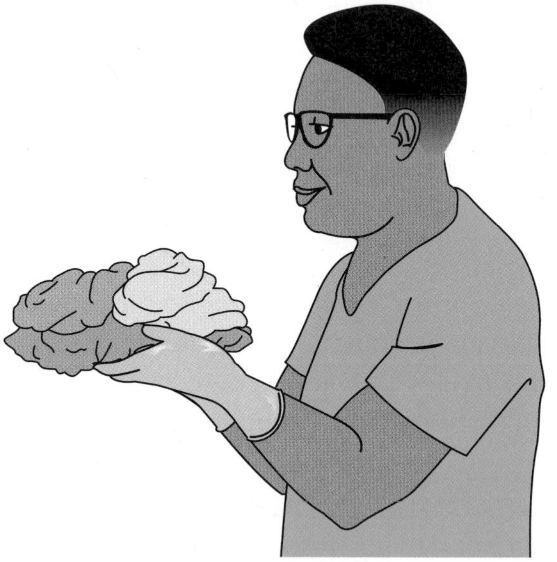

Fig. 5-16. **Hold dirty linen away from your uniform.**

You will learn more about cleaning equipment and supplies in chapter 12.

8. Explain how to handle spills

Spills can pose a serious risk of infection. Nursing homes will have cleaning solutions for spills. Clean spills using proper equipment and procedures.

GUIDELINES

Cleaning Spills Involving Blood, Body Fluids, or Glass

- Apply gloves before starting. In some cases, industrial-strength gloves are best.
- Clean up spills immediately with the proper cleaning solution.
- Do not pick up any pieces of broken glass, no matter how large, with your hands. Use a dustpan and broom or other tools.

- Waste containing broken glass, blood, or body fluids should be properly bagged. Put it in a trash bag and close it. Then put the first bag in a second, clean trash bag and close it. This is called **double-bagging**. Waste containing blood or body fluids may need to be placed in a special biohazard container. Follow facility policy.

9. Explain Transmission-Based Precautions

In 1996, the CDC set forth a second level of precautions beyond the Standard Precautions. These guidelines were for persons who are infected or may be infected with diseases. They were known as Transmission-Based, or Isolation, Precautions. If approved, the new name for these precautions will be "Expanded Precautions."

There are three categories of Transmission-Based Precautions:

- Airborne Precautions
- Droplet Precautions
- Contact Precautions

The category used depends on the disease and how it spreads. They may also be used in combination for diseases that have multiple routes of transmission.

Airborne Precautions

Airborne Precautions are used for diseases that are transmitted through the air after being expelled (Fig. 5-17). The pathogens are so small that they can attach to moisture in the air. They remain floating for some time. For certain care you will be required to wear N95 or HEPA respirators to avoid infection. Airborne diseases include tuberculosis, measles, and chicken pox. Tuberculosis (TB) is a disease that is transferred through moisture in the air. It can travel a long distance. TB can be fatal if not treated. More information on TB is found later in this chapter.

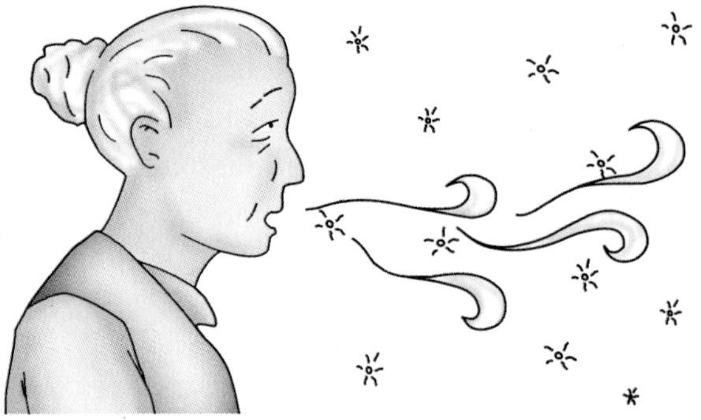

Fig. 5-17. **Airborne diseases stay suspended in the air.**

Droplet Precautions

Droplet Precautions are used when the disease-causing microorganism does not remain in the air. They usually travel only short distances after being expelled. Droplets normally do not travel more than three feet. Droplets can be created by coughing, sneezing, talking, laughing, or suctioning (Fig. 5-18). Droplet Precautions include wearing a face mask during care and restricting visits from uninfected people. Residents should wear masks when being moved from room to room. Cover your nose and mouth with a tissue when you sneeze or cough. Ask residents, family, and others to do the same.

If you sneeze on your hands, wash them promptly. An example of a droplet disease is the mumps.

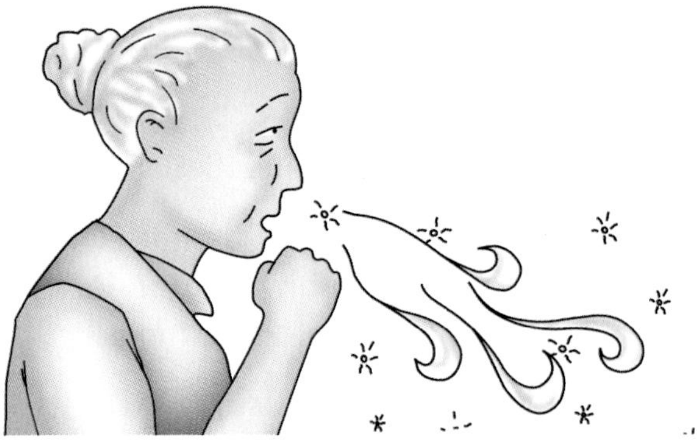

Fig. 5-18. **Droplet Precautions are followed when the disease causing microorganism does not remain in the air.**

Contact Precautions

Contact Precautions are used when the resident is at risk of transmitting a microorganism by touching an infected object or person (Fig. 5-19). Examples include bacteria that could infect an open skin wound or infection. Lice, scabies (a skin disease that causes itching), and conjunctivitis (pink eye) are also examples. Transmission can occur during transfers or bathing.

Contact Precautions include PPE and resident isolation. They require washing hands with antimicrobial soap. They also require not touching contaminated surfaces with ungloved hands or uninfected surfaces with contaminated gloves.

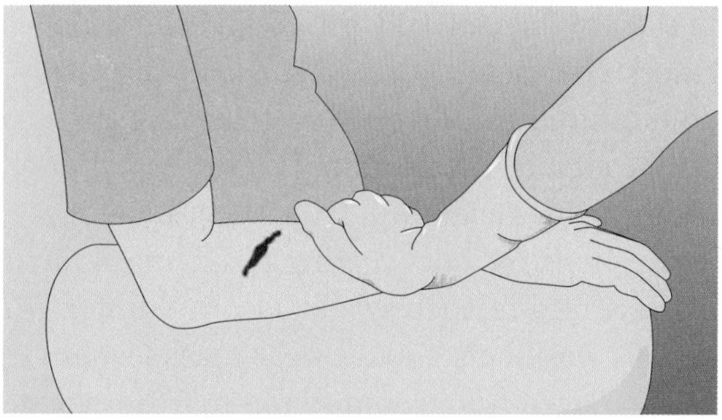

Fig. 5-19. **Contact Precautions are used when the person is at risk of transmitting or getting a microorganism from touching an infected object or person.**

Transmission-Based Precautions Summary

Staff often refer to residents who need Transmission-Based Precautions as being in "isolation." A sign should be on the door indicating "isolation" or alerting people to see the nurse before entering.

Two important points to remember are:

1. When they are indicated, Transmission-Based Precautions are always used IN ADDITION to Standard Precautions.

2. The resident must be reassured that it is the disease, not the person, that is being isolated. Talk with your resident. Explain why these steps are being taken.

Residents in isolation units experience big changes. They cannot move about freely. They are isolated or separated from everyone. Empathize with them. How might you feel if you were in isolation? Contact with residents in isolation should be as frequent as possible. This gives them a connection to the outside world. Place the call light within the resident's reach when leaving the isolation room.

10. Define "bloodborne pathogens" and describe two major bloodborne diseases

Bloodborne pathogens are microorganisms found in human blood. They can cause infection and disease in humans. They may also be in body fluids, draining wounds, and mucous membranes. Bloodborne diseases are transmitted by infected blood entering your bloodstream, or if infected semen or vaginal secretions contact your mucous membranes. Mucous membranes include the linings of the vagina, penis, rectum, nose, and mouth. You can be infected with a bloodborne disease through sexual contact with someone with that disease. It is not necessary to have sexual intercourse to transmit disease. Other kinds of sexual activity can cause infection. Using a needle to inject drugs and sharing needles can also transmit bloodborne diseases. In addition, infected mothers may transmit bloodborne diseases to their babies in the womb or at birth.

In health care, contact with infectious blood or body fluids is the most common way to get a bloodborne disease. Infections can be spread through accidental contact with contaminated blood or body fluids, needles or other sharp objects, or contaminated supplies or equipment. This chapter explains work practices, such as handwashing, Standard Precautions, isolation, and PPE, to prevent transmission of bloodborne diseases. Employers are required by law to help prevent exposure to bloodborne pathogens. You will read more about that law in the next learning objective.

You can safely touch, hug, and talk with residents who have a bloodborne disease

(Fig. 5-20). They need the same thoughtful, personal attention you give to all your residents. They should not be treated or cared for differently in any way.

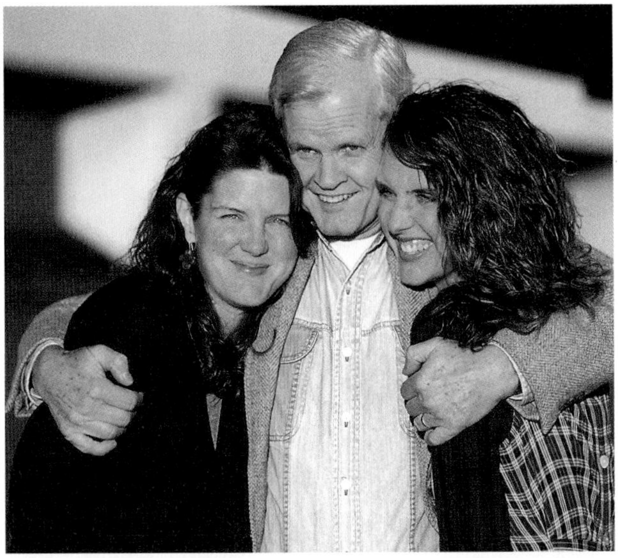

Fig. 5-20. **Hugs and touches cannot spread a bloodborne disease.**

The major bloodborne diseases in the United States are acquired immune deficiency syndrome (AIDS) and hepatitis. HIV is the virus that causes AIDS. **HIV** stands for human immunodeficiency virus. HIV weakens the immune system so that people cannot effectively fight infections. Some of these people will develop **AIDS** as a result of their HIV infection. People with AIDS lose all ability to fight infection. They can die from illnesses that a healthy body could fight. You will learn more about HIV and AIDS in chapter 18.

Hepatitis is inflammation of the liver caused by infection. Liver function can be permanently damaged by hepatitis. It can lead to other chronic, life-long illnesses. Several different viruses can cause hepatitis. The most common types of hepatitis are A, B, and C. Hepatitis B and C are bloodborne diseases. They can cause death. Many more people have hepatitis B (HBV) than HIV. The risk of getting hepatitis is greater than the risk of acquiring HIV. HBV is a serious threat to healthcare workers.

HBV can cause short-term illness that leads to:

- loss of appetite
- diarrhea and vomiting
- tiredness
- jaundice (yellow skin or eyes)
- pain in muscles, joints, and stomach

It can also cause long-term illness that leads to:

- liver damage (cirrhosis)
- liver cancer
- death

Your employer must offer you a free vaccine to protect you from hepatitis B. The HBV vaccine can prevent hepatitis B. Prevention is the best option for dealing with this disease. Take the vaccine when it is offered. It is the best protection against HBV. There is no vaccine for hepatitis C.

11. Explain OSHA's Bloodborne Pathogen Standard

The Occupational Safety and Health Administration (OSHA) is a federal government agency. It makes rules to protect workers from hazards on the job. OSHA has set standards for special procedures to follow in facilities. One of these is the Bloodborne Pathogens Standard. This law requires that healthcare facilities protect employees from bloodborne health hazards.

By law, employers must follow these rules to reduce the risk of acquiring infectious diseases. The Standard also guides employers and employees through the steps to follow if exposed to infectious material. Significant exposures include:

- Exposure by injection; a needle stick
- Mucous membrane contact
- Cut from an object containing a potentially infectious body fluid (includes human bites)

- Non-intact skin (OSHA includes acne as non-intact skin)

Guidelines employers must follow include:

- Employers must give in-service training on the risks of bloodborne pathogens and updates on any new safety standards.
- Employers must have an exposure control plan should an employee be accidentally exposed to infectious waste. It identifies the step-by-step method of what to do if exposed to infectious material. It also includes specific work practices that must be followed. All employees must be trained on it and know where to find it.
- Employers must give all employees, visitors, and residents proper personal protective equipment (PPE) to wear when needed (Fig. 5-21).
- Employers must place biohazard containers in each resident's room and in other areas in the facility to dispose of equipment and supplies contaminated with infectious waste. Biohazard containers are hard, leak-proof containers. They are clearly labeled.
- Employers must provide a free hepatitis B vaccine to all employees after hire.

If any potential exposures occur, you will need to fill out an incident report or a special exposure report form. Your employer will help you find out if you have been infected and take steps to keep you from becoming sick. To protect your health and that of others, report any potential exposures right away. Steps will also be taken to help keep similar incidents from occurring again. Your facility may require tests and other measures to keep you healthy.

In 2001, OSHA revised the Bloodborne Pathogens Standard. The revisions address the need for employers to select safer needle devices and to involve employees in choosing these devices. The updated standard also requires employers to keep a log of injuries from contaminated sharps.

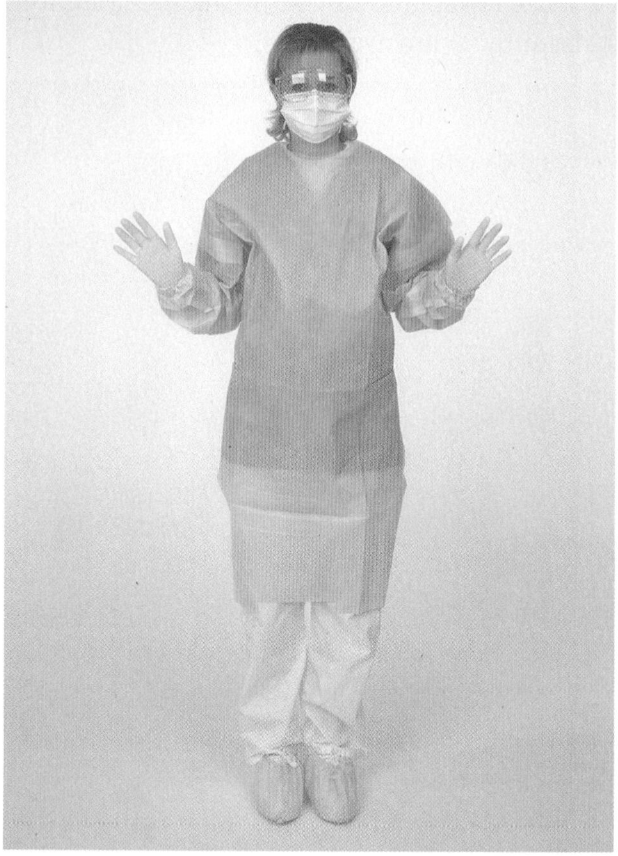

Fig. 5-21. **Using PPE is an important way to reduce the spread of infection.**

12. Define "tuberculosis" and list infection control guidelines

Tuberculosis, or TB, is an airborne disease. It is carried on mucous droplets suspended in the air. When a person infected with TB talks, coughs, breathes, or sings, he or she may release mucous droplets carrying it. TB usually infects the lungs. It causes coughing, trouble breathing, fever, and fatigue. If left untreated, TB can cause death.

There are two types of TB. **TB infection**, also called latent TB, and **TB disease**, also called active TB. Someone with TB infection carries the disease but does not show symptoms and cannot infect others. A person with active TB, or TB disease, shows symptoms of the disease and can spread TB to others. TB infection can progress to TB disease. The signs and symptoms of TB include:

- fatigue
- loss of appetite
- weight loss
- slight fever and chills
- night sweats
- prolonged coughing
- coughing up blood
- chest pain
- shortness of breath
- trouble breathing

Tuberculosis is more likely to be spread in small, confined, or poorly ventilated places. It is more likely to develop in those whose immune systems are weakened by illness, malnutrition, alcoholism or drug abuse. People with cancer or HIV/AIDS are more susceptible to developing TB disease when exposed. This is due to their weakened immune systems.

GUIDELINES
Tuberculosis

- Follow Standard Precautions and Airborne Precautions.
- Wear a mask and gown during resident care. Special masks, such as N95, high efficiency particulate air (HEPA), or other masks, may be needed (Fig. 5-22). They filter out very small particles, such as the germs that cause TB. You must be fit-tested for these special masks. You will also be trained on how to use the masks.

a. b.

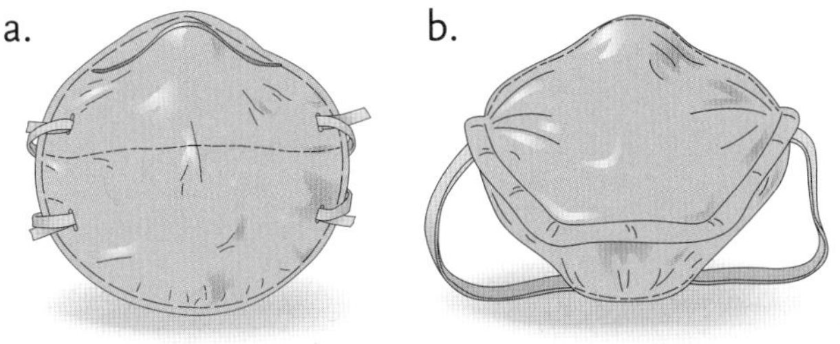

Fig. 5-22. **a) an N-95 respirator mask and b) a PFR-95 respirator mask.**

- Use special care when handling sputum or phlegm. **Phlegm** is thick mucus from the respiratory passage.
- Ensure good ventilation in the resident's room.
- Resident may be placed in a negative air pressure room. This is a room in which the flow of air is controlled. Airborne particles are not trapped in the room. Air flows into the room from outside. The air is changed often. The air is exhausted directly outside or forced through filters to remove particles. The door should always stay closed. The room should be identified as an "Acid-Fast Bacillus (AFB)" isolation room. When entering an AFB room, do not open or close the door quickly. This pulls contaminated room air into the hallway.
- Follow isolation procedures for airborne diseases if directed.
- Help the resident remember to take all medication prescribed. Failure to take all medication is a major factor in the spread of TB. **Multi-drug resistant TB** (MDR-TB) can develop when people with TB disease do not take all the prescribed medication. **Resistant** means drugs no longer work to kill the specific germs. When the full course of medication is not taken, the "strongest" bacilli are left. These are less likely to be killed by medication. If the TB bacilli develop a resistance to the drugs that treat TB, fighting the disease becomes more difficult.

13. Define the terms "MRSA" and "VRE"

Multidrug-resistant organisms (MDROs) are microorganisms, mostly bacteria, that are resistant to one or more antimicrobial agents. An **antimicrobial** agent destroys or resists pathogens. MDROs are increasing. This is a serious problem. Two commons types of MDROs are MRSA and VRE.

MRSA is methicillin-resistant *Staphylococcus aureus. Staphylococcus aureus* is a common type of bacteria that can cause illness. Methicillin is a powerful antibiotic drug. MRSA is an antibiotic-resistant infection often acquired in hospitals and other facilities.

MRSA can spread among those having close contact with infected people. It is almost always spread by direct physical contact, not through the air. If a person has MRSA on his skin, especially on the hands, and touches someone, he may spread MRSA. Spread also occurs through indirect contact by touching objects, such as sheets or clothes, contaminated by a person with MRSA.

You can prevent MRSA by practicing good hygiene. Handwashing, using soap and warm water, is the single most important way to control MRSA. Keep cuts and abrasions clean. Cover them with a proper bandage until healed. Avoid contact with other people's wounds or material contaminated by wounds.

VRE is vancomycin-resistant enterococcus. Enterococcus is a bacterium that lives in the digestive and genital tracts. They do not cause problems in healthy people. Vancomycin is a powerful antibiotic. It is often the antibiotic of last resort. It is generally limited to use against bacteria that are resistant to other antibiotics. Vancomycin-resistant enterococcus is a mutant strain of enterococcus. It originally developed in people who were exposed to the antibiotic.

VRE is dangerous. It cannot be controlled with antibiotics. It causes life-threatening infections in those with weak immune systems—the very young, the very old, and the very ill.

VRE is spread through direct and indirect contact. Once it establishes itself, it is very hard to get rid of. Preventing VRE is much easier. Help prevent its spread by washing your hands often. Wear PPE as directed. Disinfect items according to facility policy.

Chapter Review

1. What does "infection control" mean?
2. How does infection occur?
3. What is the chain of infection?
4. What is indirect contact? What is direct contact?
5. Why is infection more dangerous for elderly people?
6. List four signs of a localized infection and four signs of a systemic infection.
7. Under Standard Precautions, what does the phrase "body fluids" include?
8. On whom should Standard Precautions be practiced?
9. Under Standard Precautions, when should you wear gloves?
10. Define "mucous membranes."
11. What is the most important thing you can do to prevent the spread of disease?
12. What is hand hygiene?
13. List ten situations that require you to wash your hands.
14. How many times can disposable gloves be worn?
15. List two situations in which you should wear a mask.
16. In what order should PPE be applied? In what order should it be removed?
17. Describe the difference between "clean" and "dirty" in health care.
18. How should soiled linen be carried?

19. Describe three guidelines for cleaning spills.
20. What are Transmission-Based Precautions? List the three categories of Transmission-Based Precautions.
21. How are bloodborne diseases transmitted?
22. What is the most common way to be infected with a bloodborne disease in the healthcare setting?
23. What does HIV do to the immune system?
24. What is hepatitis?
25. List four guidelines employers must follow under the Bloodborne Pathogen Standard.
26. TB is more likely to develop in which people?
27. In what kind of setting is TB most likely to spread?
28. What is one of the best ways you can prevent the spread of MRSA and VRE?

Chapter 6
Safety and Body Mechanics

1. List common accidents in facilities and describe prevention guidelines

All staff members, including you, are responsible for safety. Elderly people have more safety concerns due to dementia, illness, disability, and diminished senses. Prevention is the key to safety.

There are many accidents and injuries that may occur, including:

- falls
- burns
- poisoning
- choking
- cuts
- not identifying a resident before performing care or serving food

Falls

Most accidents in a facility are falls. Falls can be caused by an unsafe environment or by loss of abilities. The consequences of falls can range from minor bruises to fractures and life-threatening injuries. Older people are often more seriously injured by falls, as their bones are more fragile. Hip fractures are one of the most common types of fractures from falls. Hip fractures cause the greatest number of deaths. They can lead to severe health problems. Be alert to the risk of falls.

Things that raise the risk of falls include:

- clutter
- throw rugs
- exposed electrical cords
- slippery or wet floors
- uneven floors or stairs
- poor lighting
- call lights that are out of reach or not promptly answered

Personal conditions that raise the risk of falls include medications, loss of vision, walking or balance problems, weakness, paralysis, and disorientation. **Disorientation** is confusion about person, place, or time.

To guard against falls:

- Clear all walkways of clutter, throw rugs, and cords.
- Use non-skid mats or carpeting where needed.
- Have residents wear non-skid shoes. Make sure their shoelaces are tied.
- Have residents wear clothing that fits properly, e.g. not too long.
- Keep frequently-used personal items close to residents, including call lights (Fig. 6-1).

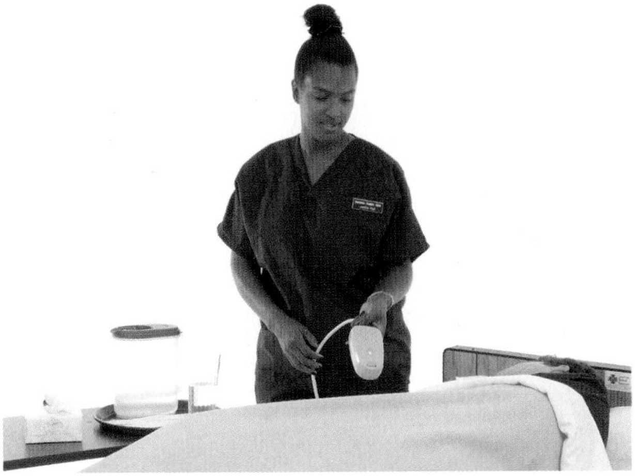

Fig. 6-1. **Keep call lights near residents so they can call you when needed.**

- Answer call lights promptly.
- Immediately clean up spills.
- Report loose hand rails immediately.
- Mark uneven flooring or stairs with colored tape to indicate a hazard.
- Improve lighting where needed.
- Lock wheelchairs before helping residents into or out of them (Fig. 6-2).

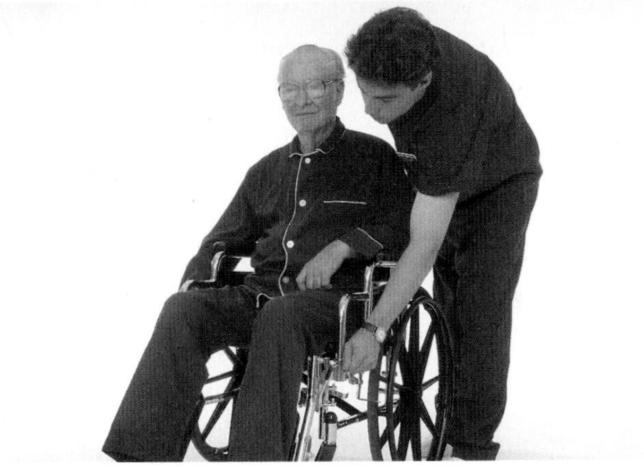

Fig. 6-2. **Always lock a wheelchair before a resident gets into or out of it.**

- Lock bed wheels before helping a resident into and out of bed or when giving care (Fig. 6-3).
- Return beds to their lowest position when you have finished with care.
- If side rails are ordered, check before leaving the room to make sure they are all raised.

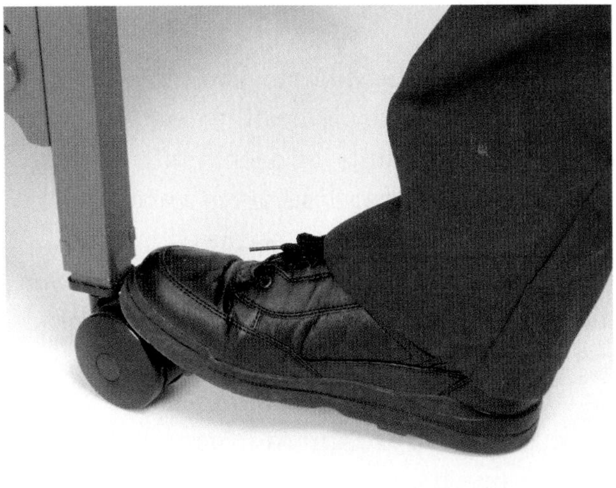

Fig. 6-3. **Always lock the bed wheels before helping a resident into or out of bed, and before giving care.**

- Get help when moving a resident. Do not assume you can do it alone. When in doubt, ask for help. Keep residents' canes or walkers handy.
- Offer trips to the bathroom often. Respond to residents' requests promptly (Fig. 6-4).
- Leave furniture in the same place as you found it.
- Know residents who are at risk for falls and give help.
- If a resident starts to fall, be in a good position to help support him or her. Never try to catch a falling resident. Use your body to slide him or her to the floor. If you try to reverse a fall, you may hurt yourself and/or the resident.

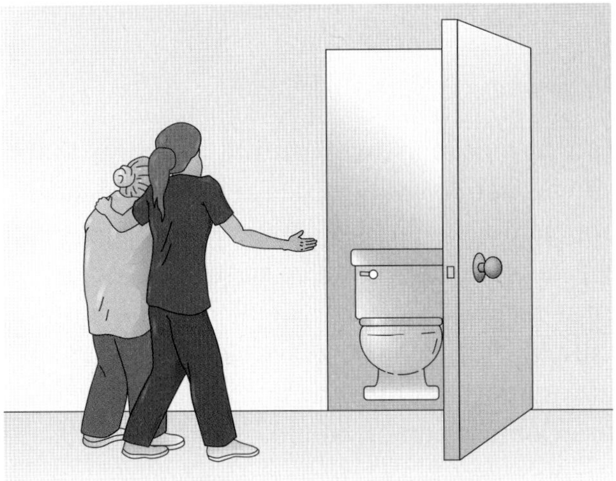

Fig. 6-4. **Offer trips to the bathroom often.**

Burns/Scalds

Burns can be caused by stoves and appliances, hot water or liquids, or heating devices. Small children, older adults, or people with loss of sensation due to paralysis are at greatest risk of burns. **Scalds** are burns caused by hot liquids. It takes five seconds or less for a serious burn to occur when the temperature of liquid is 140°F. Coffee, tea, and other hot drinks are usually served at 160°F to 180°F. These temperatures can cause almost instant burns that require surgery.

Follow these guidelines to guard against burns and scalds:

- Always check water temperature with a water thermometer or on your wrist before using.
- Report frayed electrical cords or unsafe-looking appliances immediately. Do not use them.
- Let residents know you are about to pour or set down a hot liquid.
- Pour hot drinks away from residents.
- Keep hot drinks and liquids away from edges of tables. Put a lid on them.
- Make sure residents are sitting down before serving hot drinks.
- If plate warmers or other equipment that produces heat are used, monitor them carefully.

Poisoning

Facilities have many harmful substances that should not be swallowed. These include cleaners, paints, medicines, toiletries, and glues. These products should be stored or locked away from confused residents or those with limited vision. Do not leave cleaning products in residents' rooms. The number for the Poison Control Center should be posted by all telephones.

Choking

Choking can occur when eating, drinking or taking medication. People who are weak, ill, or unconscious can choke on their own saliva. To guard against choking, residents should eat sitting as upright as they can (Fig. 6-5). Residents with swallowing problems may have special diets with liquids thickened to the consistency of honey or syrup. Thickened liquids are easier to swallow. You will learn more about helping with feeding and thickened liquids in chapter 16.

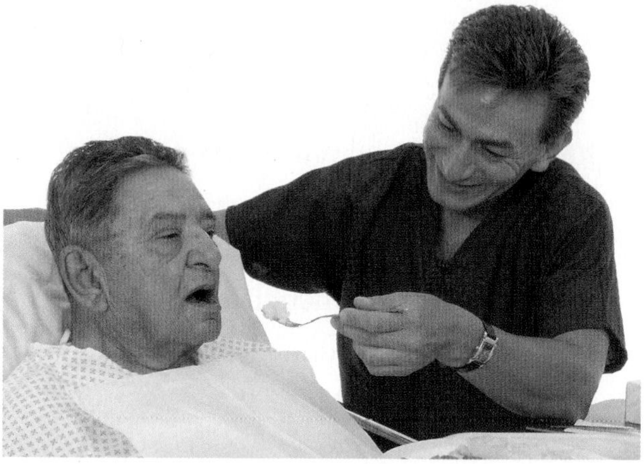

Fig. 6-5. **Residents should be sitting up straight while eating. Do not rush a resident who is eating.**

Cuts/Scrapes

Cuts and scrapes can happen quickly. Cuts often occur in the bathroom. Put sharp objects, such as razors, away after use. When moving a resident in a wheelchair, make sure that the resident's arms and legs are inside the chair. Be careful not to bump into walls or doorways. Push wheelchairs forward. Do not pull them behind you. If moving between floors, turn the chair around before entering the elevator, so the resident is facing forward. When approaching doors, move slowly.

Resident Identification

Residents must always be identified. Not identifying residents before giving care or serving food can cause serious problems, even death.

Facilities have different methods of identification. Some have ID bracelets. Some have pictures to identify residents. Identify each resident before starting any procedure or giving any care (Fig. 6-6). Always identify residents before placing meal trays or helping with feeding. Check the diet card against the resident's identification. Call the resident by name.

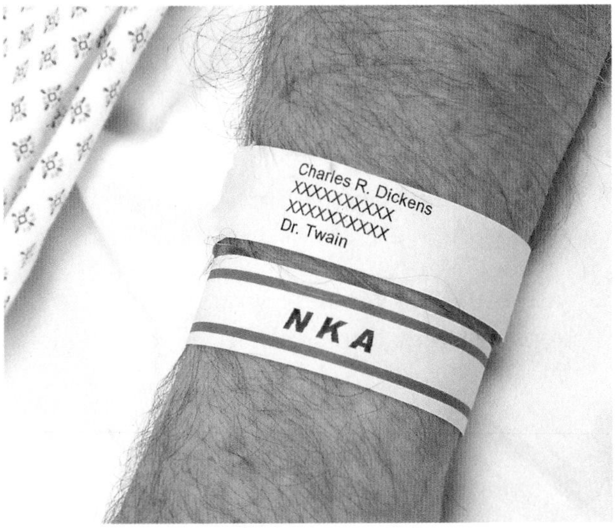

Fig. 6-6. **Identify all residents before giving care. The abbreviation "NKA" means "no known allergies".**

Help make your workplace safer. Report unsafe conditions before accidents occur. As you work, watch for safety hazards. Other general safety guidelines are:

- Do not run in halls, on stairs, or in the dining room.
- Keep paths clear and free of clutter.
- Wipe up spilled liquids right away.
- Discard trash properly.
- Follow instructions. Ask about anything you do not understand.
- Report injuries immediately.

Show up!

Assignments are based on the number of residents and the number of staff members available on that shift. It is important to work every day you are scheduled. Missing a day without good reason can compromise the safety of residents and staff. Staff may have too many residents to care for. If you must be absent, call your facility early to tell them. This lets your supervisor start trying to replace you sooner.

2. List safety guidelines for oxygen use

Residents with breathing problems may receive oxygen. It is more concentrated than what is in the air. Oxygen is prescribed by a doctor. NAs never stop, adjust, or administer oxygen. Oxygen may be piped into a resident's room through a central system. It may be in tanks or produced by an oxygen concentrator. An **oxygen concentrator** changes air in the room into air with more oxygen.

Oxygen is a very dangerous fire hazard because it makes other things burn. Oxygen itself does not burn. It merely supports combustion. **Combustion** means the process of burning. Working around oxygen requires special safety precautions.

GUIDELINES

Working Safely Around Oxygen Equipment

- Remove all fire hazards from the room or area. Fire hazards include electric razors, hair dryers, or other electrical appliances (Fig. 6-7). They also include flammable liquids. **Flammable** means easily ignited and capable of burning quickly. Examples of flammable liquids are alcohol and nail polish remover.
- Tell the nurse of fire hazards residents do not want removed.
- Post "No Smoking" and "Oxygen in Use" signs. Never allow smoking where oxygen is used or stored.
- Never allow candles, lit matches, or other open flames around oxygen.
- Learn how to turn oxygen off in case of fire if facility allows this. Never adjust the oxygen level.

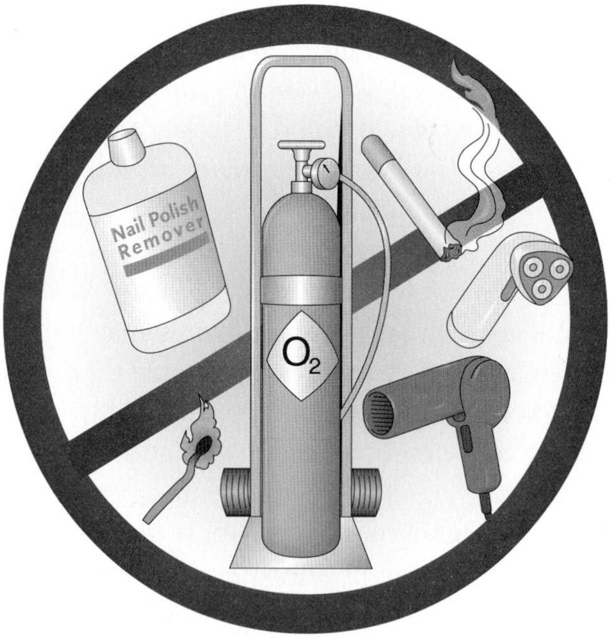

Fig. 6-7. **Examples of fire hazards.**

- Report if the nasal cannula or face mask causes irritation. Check behind ears for irritation from tubing (Fig. 6-8).

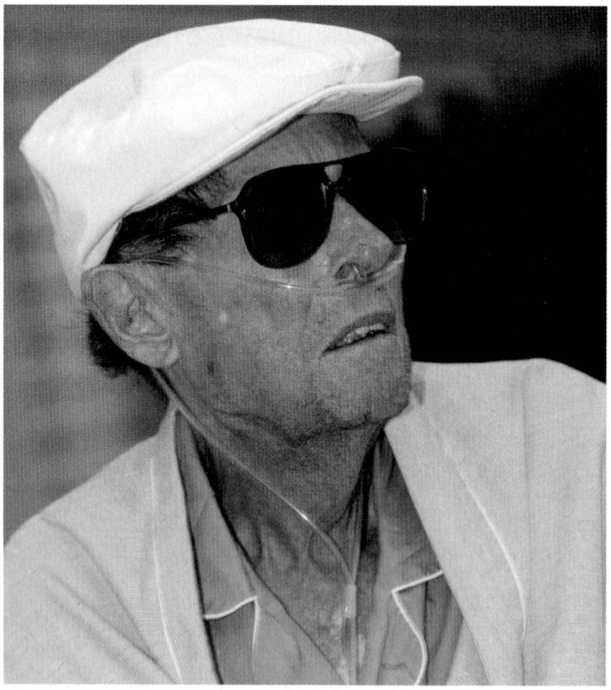

Fig. 6-8. **A resident with a nasal cannula.**

3. Explain the Material Safety Data Sheet (MSDS)

The Occupational Safety and Health Administration (OSHA - see chapter 5) is responsible for the safety of employees at work. OSHA requires that all dangerous chemicals have a **Material Safety Data Sheet** (MSDS). This sheet details the chemical ingredients, chemical dangers, emergency response actions to be taken, and safe handling procedures for the product (Fig. 6-9 on next page). Some facilities use a toll-free number to access MSDS information. MSDSs must be accessible in work areas for all employees. Important information about the MSDS includes:

1. Your employer must have an MSDS for every chemical used.
2. Your employer must provide easy access to the MSDS.
3. You must know where your MSDSs are kept and how to read them. If you do not know how, ask for help.

Emergency Eye Wash

An eye splash means spraying a substance into the eyes. If an eye splash occurs, follow facility policy on steps to take. Many facilities have eye wash stations. If one is available, follow directions at the station. To use an emergency eye wash bottle, flip the cup lid open. Open eyelid with your thumb and index finger. Press cup against your eye and squeeze the bottle repeatedly. Report the incident to the nurse as soon as possible.

4. Define the term "restraint" and give reasons why restraints were used

A **restraint** is a physical or chemical way to restrict voluntary movement or behavior. Common physical restraints are the vest restraint, belt restraint, wrist/ankle restraint, and the mitt restraint. Physical restraints are also called postural supports or protective devices. Side rails and special chairs, such as geriatric chairs, are also physical restraints (Figs. 6-10 and 6-11).

Material Safety Data Sheet
May be used to comply with OSHA's Hazard Communication Standard, 29 CFR 1910 1200. Standard must be consulted for specific requirements.

U.S. Department of Labor
Occupational Safety and Health Administration
(Non-Mandatory Form)
Form Approved
OMB No. 1218-0072

IDENTITY *(as Used on Label and List)*	*Note: Blank spaces are not permitted. If any item is not applicable or no information is available, the space must be marked to indicate that.*

Section I

Manufacturer's name	Emergency Telephone Number
Address *(Number, Street, City, State and ZIP Code)*	Telephone Number for Information
	Date Prepared
	Signature of Preparer *(optional)*

Section II—Hazardous Ingredients/Identity Information

Hazardous Components (Specific Chemical Identity, Common Name(s))	OSHA PEL	ACGIH TLV	Other Limits Recommended	% (optional)

Section III—Physical/Chemical Characteristics

Boiling Point		Specific Gravity ($H_20 = 1$)	
Vapor Pressure (mm Hg)		Melting Point	
Vapor Density (AIR = 1)		Evaporation Rate (Butyl Acetate = 1)	
Solubility in Water			
Appearance and Odor			

Section IV—Fire and Explosion Hazard Data

Flash Point (Method Used)	Flammable Limits	LEL	UEL
Extinguishing Media			
Special Fire Fighting Procedures			
Unusual Fire and Explosion Hazards			

OSHA 174 Sept. 1985

Fig. 6-9. A Material Safety Data Sheet.

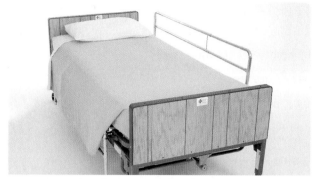

Fig. 6-10. **Side rails are considered restraints. They restrict movement.**

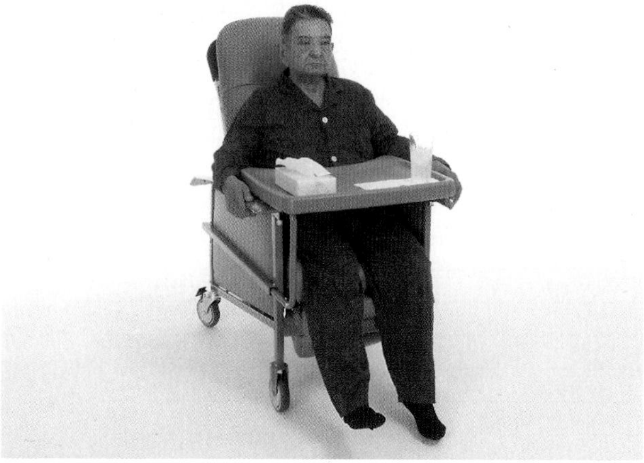

Fig. 6-11. **When the tray table is attached, a geriatric chair, or geri-chair, is a restraint.**

Chemical restraints are medications to control a person's behavior. In the past, restraints were commonly ordered for these reasons:

- To keep a person from hurting self or others
- To keep a person from pulling out tubing that is needed for treatment
- To keep a person with dementia or who is confused from wandering
- To prevent falls

Restraint usage was abused by caregivers. The abuse led to new restrictions and laws on their use. Today, the use of both physical and chemical restraints in facilities has greatly decreased.

Generally, restraints are only used as a last resort. **Restraints can never be used without a doctor's order.** It is against the law for staff to use restraints for convenience or discipline.

5. List physical and psychological problems associated with restraints

There are many problems with restraints. Some of the negative effects of restraint use are:

- reduced blood circulation
- stress on the heart
- incontinence
- constipation
- weakened muscles and bones
- loss of bone mass
- muscle atrophy (weakening or wasting of the muscle)
- pressure sores
- risk of suffocation
- pneumonia
- less activity, causing poor appetite and malnutrition
- sleep disorders
- loss of dignity
- loss of independence
- increased agitation
- increased depression and/or withdrawal
- poor self-esteem

Restraints have also caused severe injury and even death.

6. Define the terms "restraint-free" and "restraint alternatives" and list examples of restraint alternatives

Laws allow the use of restraints only when absolutely necessary for the safety of the person, others around that person, and staff. State and federal agencies encourage facilities to take steps toward a restraint-free environment.

Restraint-free care means that restraints are not used for any reason. They are usually not kept by the facility. To reach this goal, many nursing homes use creative ideas called **re-**

straint alternatives. A restraint alternative is any intervention used in place of a restraint or that reduces the need for a restraint.

Many scientific studies show that the use of restraints is no longer needed. People tend to respond better to the use of creative ways to reduce tension, pulling at tubes, wandering, and boredom.

Examples of restraint alternatives are:

- Improve safety measures to prevent accidents and falls. Improve lighting.
- Use postural devices to support and protect residents' bodies.
- Make sure call light is within reach. Answer call lights promptly.
- Ambulate the person when he or she is restless. Add exercise into the care plan. Provide activities for those who wander at night.
- Encourage activities and independence. Escort the person to social activities. Increase visits and social interaction.
- Give frequent help with toileting. Help with cleaning immediately after an episode of incontinence.
- Offer food or drink. Offer reading materials.
- Distract or redirect interest. Give the person a repetitive task.
- Decrease the noise level. Listen to soothing music. Use massage or relaxation techniques.
- Assess medication. Reduce pain by scheduling medications. Report pain to the nurse.
- Offer one-on-one time with a caregiver. Provide familiar caregivers. Increase the number of caregivers with family and volunteers.
- Use a team approach to meeting the person's needs. Offer training to teach gentle approaches to difficult people.

There are also several types of pads, belts, special chairs, and alarms that can be used instead of restraints (Fig. 6-12).

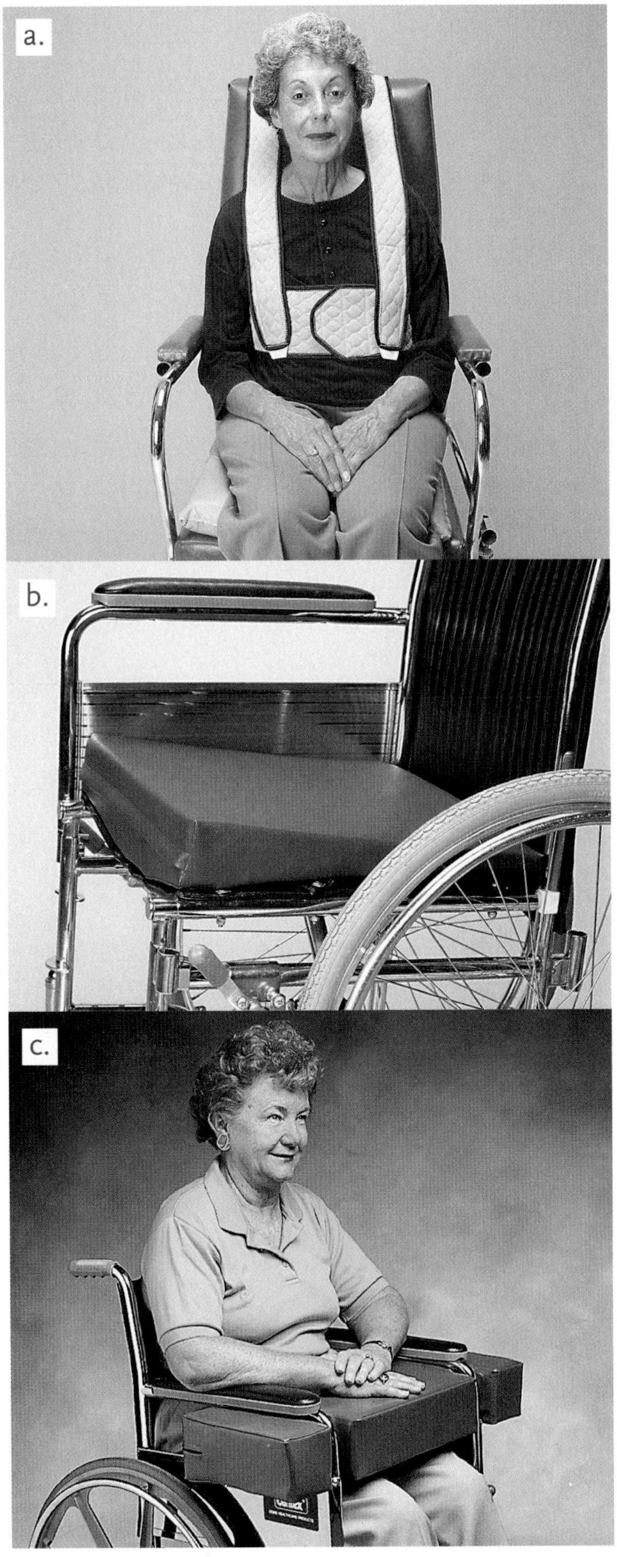

Fig. 6-12. **a) A Posey Torso Support, b) A Posey Deluxe Wedge Cushion, c) A lap-top cushion. (Photos courtesy of North Coast Medical, Inc., www.ncmedical.com, 800-821-9319.)**

Music soothes.

Some people use music to relax. Some like classical, others like reggae, country, R&B, jazz, or rock and roll. When new residents are admitted, ask them the type of music they like. It might help staff choose soothing music. Music may help calm residents.

7. Describe guidelines for applying a restraint and what must be done if a restraint is ordered

Do not use a restraint unless the nurse has told you to do so and you have been trained in its proper use. If you are asked to apply a restraint, follow these guidelines:

GUIDELINES

Applying Restraints

- Know your state's laws and facility rules regarding applying restraints. Make sure there is an order for a restraint before applying one.
- Follow the manufacturer's instructions when applying restraints.
- Use the correct size and style of restraint. Ask the nurse for help if needed.
- Always use a slip knot. A **slip knot** is a quick-release knot used to tie restraints so that they can be removed quickly when needed.
- Never tie the restraint to side rails. Only tie the restraint to the movable part of a bed frame.
- Check to make sure the restraint is not too tight. Place an open hand flat between the resident and the restraint. This helps to ensure that the device fits properly and is comfortable.
- If using a vest or belt style of restraint, apply the restraint over clothing. Be careful not to catch the resident's breasts or skin in the restraint. The criss-cross in a vest restraint must be placed on the front of the body.
- Place the call light within the resident's reach. Residents with mitt restraints will not be able to press the call light. Because of this, they must be checked every five minutes.
- Document the following when restraints are used:

  Type of restraint and time applied

  Each time of removal

  Care given when released

  Any circulation, skin, or other problems

A restrained resident must be monitored constantly. The resident must be checked at least every 15 minutes. At least every two hours the following must be done:

- Release the restraint for at least 15 minutes.
- Offer help with toileting. Check for episodes of incontinence. Give care.
- Offer fluids.
- Check the skin for irritation. Report any red, blue, or discolored areas to the nurse immediately.
- Check for swelling of the body part.
- Reposition the resident.
- Ambulate the resident if he or she is able.

8. Explain the principles of body mechanics

Back strain or injury is one of the greatest risks nursing assistants face. Prevention is very important. In this text you will learn correct procedures for helping with transfers, positioning, and ambulation. These procedures will include instructions for proper body mechanics.

Body mechanics is the way the parts of the body work together when you move. Good body mechanics help save energy and prevent injury. Good body mechanics help you push, pull, and lift objects or people who cannot fully support or move their own bodies. Basic principles of body mechanics will help keep you and residents safe.

Alignment: Alignment is based on the word "line." When you stand up straight, a vertical line could be drawn through the center of your body and your center of gravity (Fig. 6-13). When the line is straight, the body is in alignment. Whether standing, sitting or lying down, try to have your body in alignment. This means that the two sides of the body are mirror images of each other, with body parts lined up naturally. Maintain correct body alignment when lifting or carrying an object by keeping it close to your body. Point your feet and body in the direction you are moving. Avoid twisting at the waist.

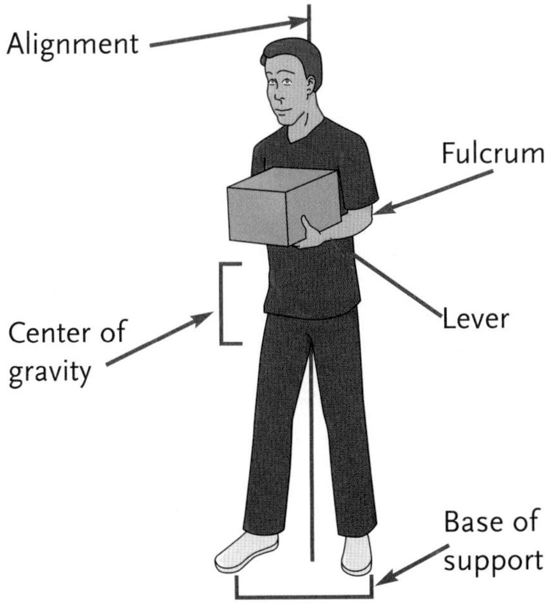

Fig. 6-13. **Proper body alignment is important when standing and sitting.**

Base of support: The base of support is the foundation of an object. The feet are the body's base of support. Standing with your legs shoulder-width apart gives a greater base of support. You will be more stable than someone standing with his or her feet together.

Fulcrum and lever: A **lever** moves an object by resting on a base of support, called a fulcrum. Think of a seesaw. The flat board you sit on is the lever. The triangular base the board rests on is the fulcrum. When two children sit on opposite sides of the seesaw, they easily move each other up and down. This is because the fulcrum and lever are doing the work.

If you think of your body as a set of fulcrums and levers, you can find ways to lift without working as hard. Think of your arm as a lever. The elbow is the fulcrum. When you lift something, rest it against your forearm. This will shorten the lever and make the item easier to lift than it would be if you were holding it in your hands.

Center of gravity: The center of gravity in your body is the point where the most weight is concentrated (Fig. 6-14). This point will depend on the position of the body. When you stand, your weight is centered in your pelvis. A low center of gravity gives a more stable base of support. Bending your knees when lifting lowers your pelvis. It lowers your center of gravity. This gives you more stability. It makes you less likely to fall or strain your muscles.

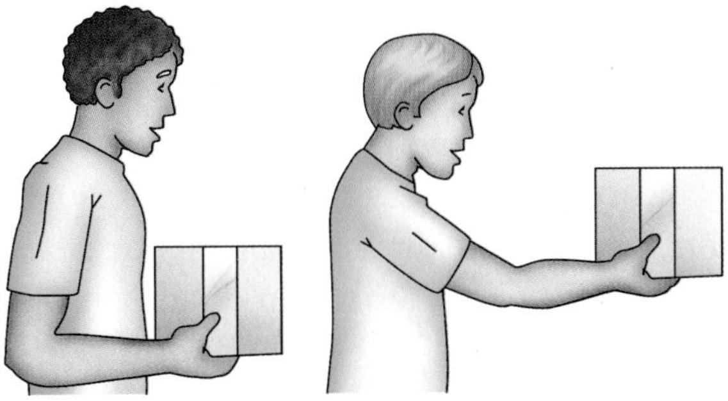

Fig. 6-14. **Holding things close to you moves weight toward your center of gravity. In this illustration, who is more likely to strain his back muscles?**

9. Apply principles of body mechanics to daily activities

By applying the principles of body mechanics to your daily activities, you can avoid injury and use less energy. Some examples of good body mechanics include:

Lifting a heavy object from the floor. Spread your feet shoulder-width apart. Bend your knees. Using the strong, large muscles in your thighs, upper arms, and shoulders, lift the object. Pull it close to your body, level with your pelvis. By doing this, you keep the object close to your center of gravity and base of support. When you stand up, push with your strong hip and thigh muscles. Raise your body and the object together (Fig. 6-15).

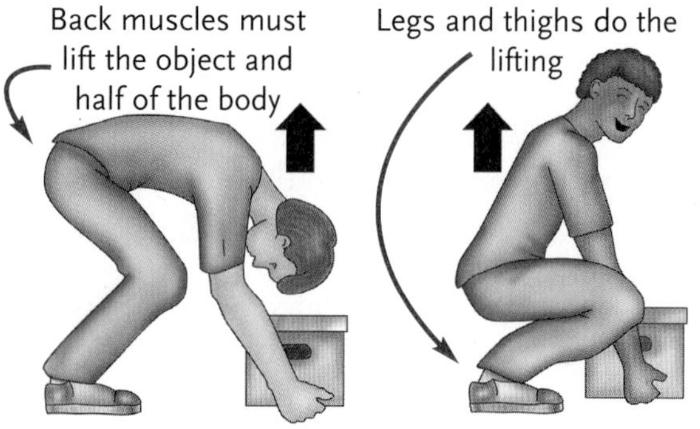

Fig. 6-15. **In this illustration, which person is lifting correctly?**

Do not twist when you are moving an object. Always face the object or person you are moving. Pivot your feet instead of twisting at the waist.

Helping a resident sit up, stand up, or walk. Whenever you support a resident's weight, assume a good stance. Place your feet twelve inches, or hip-width apart. Put one foot in front of the other, with your knees bent. Your upper body should stay upright and in alignment. If a resident starts to fall, do not try to "catch" him or her. Assist him or her to the floor. (Fig. 6-16).

Bend your knees to lower yourself, rather than bending from the waist. When a task requires bending, use a good stance. This lets you to use the big muscles in your legs and hips rather than the smaller muscles in your back.

If you are making an adjustable bed, adjust the height to a safe working level, usually waist high. If you are making a regular bed, lean or kneel to support yourself at working level. Avoid bending at the waist.

In addition, keep these tips in mind:

- Use both arms and hands to lift, pull, push, or carry objects.
- Hold objects close to you when you are lifting or carrying them.

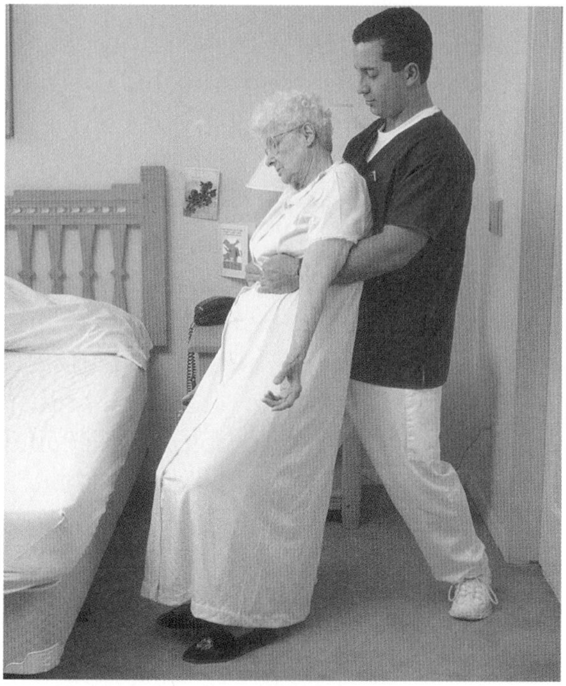

Fig. 6-16. **Maintaining a wide base of support and low center of gravity will enable you to help a falling resident.**

- Push, slide, or pull objects rather than lifting them.
- Avoid bending and reaching as much as possible. Move or position furniture so that you do not have to bend or reach.
- Get help when possible for lifting or helping residents.
- When moving a resident, let him know what you will do so he can help if possible. Count to three. Lift or move on three so everyone moves together.

Report to the nurse any task you feel that you cannot safely do. Never try to lift an object or a resident that you feel you cannot handle.

Bend your knees for ease.

When preparing to move or position a resident, always bend your knees. Be able to feel the bed with your knees before you begin the procedure. If you cannot feel the bed, stop and bend your knees. If you do not bend your knees properly, you could seriously hurt your back.

10. Identify major causes of fire and list fire safety guidelines

For a fire to occur, it must have these three things:

- Heat: makes the flame
- Fuel: object that burns
- Oxygen: gas that will keep the fire burning

There are many potential causes of a fire in facilities, including:

- smoking
- frayed or damaged electrical cords
- electrical equipment in need of repair
- space heaters
- overloaded electrical plugs
- oxygen use
- careless cooking
- flammable liquids or rags with oils on them
- stacks of newspapers or other clutter

Most facilities have a fire safety plan. All workers need to know this plan. Fire and disaster drills help you learn what to do in an emergency. The nurse will explain your facility's guidelines. Get residents to safety first. A fast, calm and confident response by the staff saves lives.

GUIDELINES

Reducing Fire Hazards and Responding to Fires

- Never leave smokers unattended. If residents smoke, make sure they are in the proper area for smoking. Be sure that cigarettes are extinguished. Empty ashtrays often. Before emptying ashtrays, make sure there are no hot ashes or hot matches in ashtray.
- Report frayed or damaged electrical cords immediately. Report electrical equipment in need of repair immediately.
- Fire alarms and exit doors should not be blocked. If they are, report this to the nurse.
- Every facility will have a fire extinguisher (Fig. 6-17). The PASS acronym will help you understand how to use it:

  Pull the pin.

  Aim at the base of fire when spraying.

  Squeeze the handle.

  Sweep back and forth at the base of the fire.

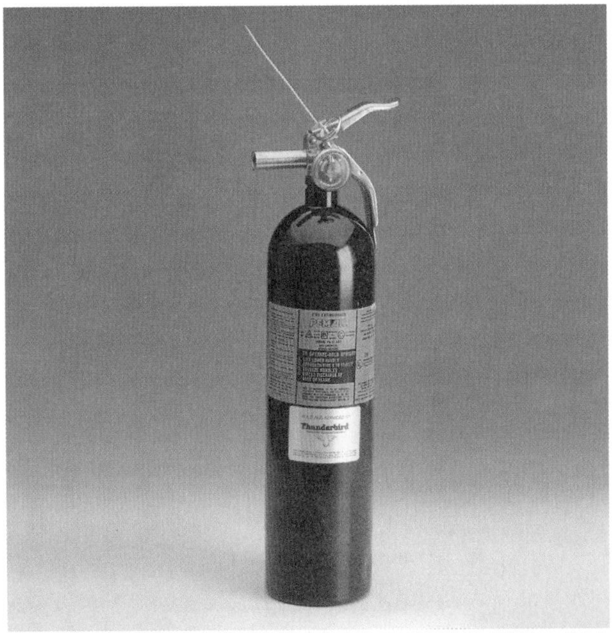

Fig. 6-17. **Know where the extinguisher is stored in your facility and how to use it.**

- In case of fire, the RACE acronym is a good rule to follow:

  Remove residents from danger.

  Activate 911.

  Contain fire if possible.

  Extinguish, or fire department will extinguish.

Follow these guidelines for helping residents exit the building safely:

- Know the facility's fire evacuation plan.
- Know which residents need one-on-one help or assistive devices.
- Stay calm.
- Remove anything blocking a window or door that could be used as a fire exit.
- If a door is closed, check for heat coming from it before opening it.
- If clothing catches fire, do not run. Stop, drop to the ground, and roll to extinguish flames.
- Stay low in a room to escape a fire.
- Use a covering over the face to reduce smoke inhalation.
- Never get into an elevator during a fire.
- Call for emergency help.

Chapter Review

1. What are the majority of accidents in facilities?
2. List eleven guidelines to prevent falls.
3. Describe five ways to guard against burns/scalds.
4. In what position should residents eat to avoid choking?
5. What should you always do before giving care or serving meal trays?
6. What are some examples of fire hazards that must be removed around oxygen?
7. What is the purpose of the MSDS?
8. Why are restraints no longer often used?
9. List ten problems with restraint use.
10. Define the terms "restraint-free" and "restraint alternatives."
11. List four things that must be done if a restraint is ordered.
12. What is body mechanics?
13. Where is the point where most weight is concentrated?

True or False. Mark each statement with a "T" for true or an "F" for false.

14. _____ By using the principles of good body mechanics at work, you can avoid injury and save energy.
15. _____ To lift a heavy object from the floor, place your feet together and keep your knees straight.
16. _____ The muscles of the thighs, upper arms, and shoulders are not as strong as the muscles in the back.
17. _____ A wide base of support and a low center of gravity means the feet are apart and the knees are bent.
18. _____ When moving an object, pivot your feet instead of twisting at the waist.
19. _____ It is a good idea to hold an object away from your body.
20. _____ Never try to catch a falling resident.
21. Name three things you can do at work to use good body mechanics.
22. List seven guidelines for reducing fire hazards and responding to fires.

Chapter 7
Emergency Care and Disaster Preparation

1. Demonstrate how to recognize and respond to medical emergencies

Medical emergencies may be caused by accidents or sudden illnesses. This chapter discusses what to do in a medical emergency. Heart attacks, strokes, diabetic emergencies, choking, automobile accidents, and gunshot wounds are all medical emergencies. Severe falls, burns, and cuts can also be emergencies.

In an emergency, try to remain calm, act quickly, and communicate clearly. Knowing these steps will help:

Assess the situation. Try to find out what has happened. Make sure you are not in danger. Note the time.

Assess the victim. Ask the hurt or ill person what has happened. If the person cannot respond, he may be unconscious. Being **conscious** means being mentally alert and having awareness of surroundings, sensations, and thoughts. Determine whether the person is conscious. Tap the person and ask if he is all right. Speak loudly. Use the person's name if you know it. If there is no response, assume the person is unconscious. This is an emergency. Call for help right away or send someone else to call.

If a person is conscious and able to speak, then he is breathing and has a pulse. Talk with the person about what happened. Check the person for injury. Look for these things:

- severe bleeding
- changes in consciousness
- irregular breathing
- unusual color or feel to the skin
- swollen places on the body
- medical alert tags
- anything the resident says is painful

If any of these exist, you may need medical help. Always get help before doing anything else.

If the hurt or ill person is conscious, he may be frightened. Listen to the person. Tell him what is being done to help him. Be calm and confident. Tell him that he is being taken care of.

After the emergency, you will need to document it in your notes. Complete an incident report. Try to remember as many details as you can. Remember, only report the facts. If you think a resident had a heart attack, write the signs and symptoms you observed. Record the actions you took. Knowing what information you will have to document will help you remember the important facts. For instance, it is especially important to remember the time at which a resident becomes unconscious.

Reporting Emergencies

If a resident needs emergency help, the nurse may ask you to call emergency services. Know the procedure for dialing an outside line. If you need to call emergency medical services, dial 911. When calling, give this information:

- the phone number and address of the emergency, directions or landmarks, and the location in the building
- the resident's condition, including any medical background you know
- your name and position
- details of any first aid being given

The dispatcher you speak with may need other information or may want to give you other instructions. Do not hang up the phone until the dispatcher hangs up or tells you to hang up.

Emergency Codes

Facilities often use codes to inform staff of emergencies without alarming residents and visitors. For example, "Code Red" usually means fire. "Code Blue" usually means cardiac arrest. Know the codes for your facility. Do not panic when you hear codes announced. Respond calmly to codes.

2. Demonstrate knowledge of first aid procedures

First aid is care given in an emergency before trained medical professionals can take over. **Cardiopulmonary resuscitation** (**CPR**) refers to medical procedures used when a person's heart or lungs have stopped working. CPR is used until medical help arrives. Quick action is necessary. CPR must be started immediately. Brain damage may occur within four to six minutes after the heartbeat and breathing stop. The person can die within ten minutes.

Only properly trained people should perform CPR. Your employer will probably arrange for you to be trained in CPR. If not, ask about American Heart Association or Red Cross CPR training. You may also contact one of these agencies yourself. CPR is an important skill to learn. If you are not trained, do not attempt to perform CPR. Performing CPR incorrectly can further injure a person.

Starting CPR

Know your facility's policies on whether you can initiate CPR if you have been trained. Some facilities do not allow nursing assistants to begin CPR without direction of the nurse. This is due, in part, to residents' Advance Directives. Some residents have made the decision that they do not want CPR. Notify the nurse immediately if an emergency occurs.

This textbook is not a CPR course. The following is a brief review for people who have had CPR training. It is a procedure to use on adults, not children.

1. Check to see if the person is responsive. Gently shake the person and shout, "Are you okay?"
2. If there is no response, call 911 immediately or send someone to call 911. Stay calm.
3. Kneel at the person's side near his or her head to start CPR.
4. Open the airway. Tilt the head back slightly. Lift the chin with one hand while pushing down on the forehead with the

other hand. (head tilt-chin lift method) (Fig. 7-1).

5. Hold the airway open and check for breathing:

- Look for the chest to rise and fall.
- Listen for sounds of breathing. Put your ear near the person's nose and mouth.
- Feel for the person's breath on your cheek.

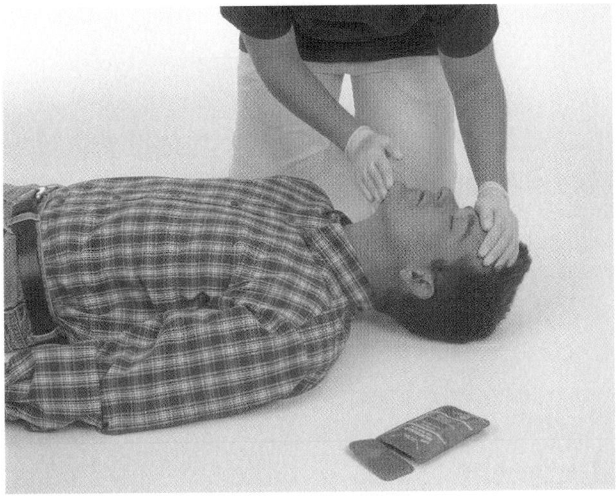

Fig. 7-1. **Opening the airway using the head tilt-chin lift method.**

6. If the person is not breathing, you will have to breathe for the person. Give two rescue breaths. To give rescue breaths:

- Pinch the nose to keep air from escaping. Cover the person's mouth completely with your mouth.
- If a barrier device, such as a special face mask, is available, use it to give rescue breathing (Fig. 7-2).

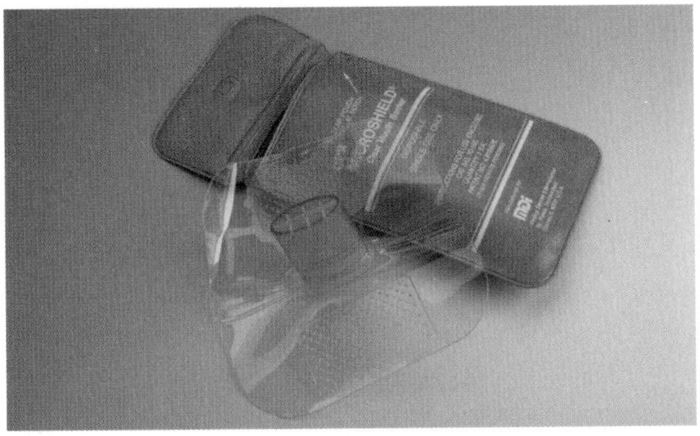

Fig. 7-2. **A barrier device protects you and the person you are helping from contact with body fluids.**

- Blow into the person's mouth slowly. Watch for the chest to rise (Fig. 7-3). Blow two full breaths, about two seconds each. Turn your head to the side to listen for air. If the chest does not rise when you give a rescue breath, reopen the airway. Use the head tilt-chin lift method. Try to give rescue breaths again.

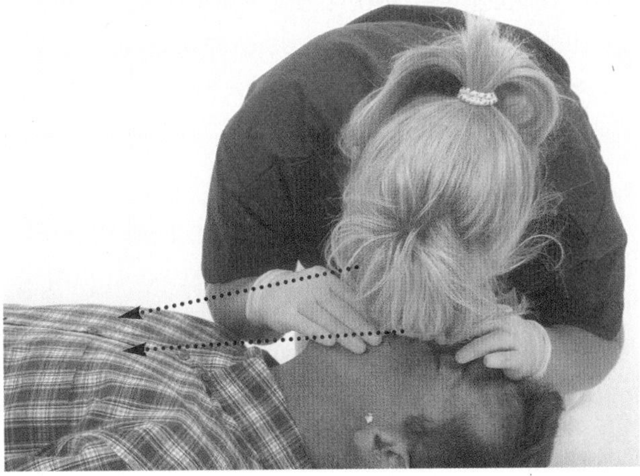

Fig. 7-3. **Blow into the person's mouth slowly, watching for the chest to rise.**

7. After giving rescue breaths, look for signs of response. The person may start moving, breathing normally, or coughing. If you do not see a response, give 15 chest compressions. Do this only if you have been trained to do so. Be sure the person is lying flat on a hard surface. To give chest compressions:

- Find the lower end of the person's sternum. Do this by following the rib cage up to the center of the chest.
- Place your index finger next to your middle finger where the ribs meet the sternum. Place the heel of your other hand next to the upper finger over the lower half of the sternum (Fig. 7-4).

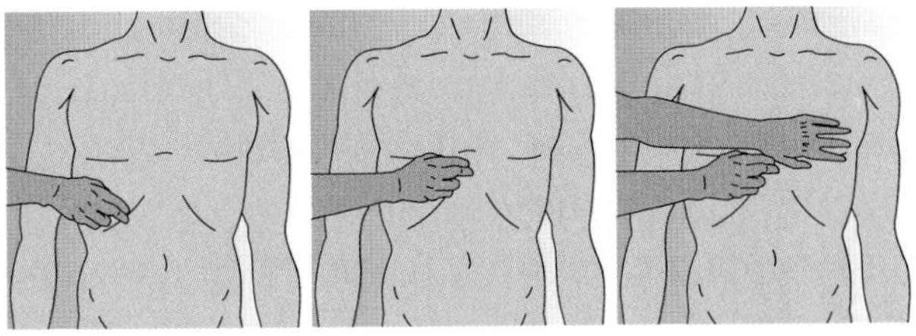

Fig. 7-4.

- Place the heel of your other hand on top of the positioned hand. Extend or interlace your fingers. Make sure your fingers are kept off the chest. Position your body directly over your hands. Keep your elbows straight. Look down at your hands.
- Use the heel of your hands to give 15 chest compressions. Push in 1 1/2 to 2 inches with each compression. Allow the chest to relax between compressions. Do not take your hands off the chest between compressions.

8. Give two more rescue breaths followed by 15 compressions. After about a minute of CPR, check for signs of response. If you see signs of response, stop compressions. Continue to provide rescue breathing as necessary (one breath every five seconds).

When medical help arrives follow their directions. Assist them as necessary. Report details of the incident.

Choking

When something is blocking the tube through which air enters the lungs, the person has an **obstructed airway**. When people are choking, they usually put their hands to their throat and cough (Fig. 7-5). As long as a person can speak, cough, or breathe, do nothing. Encourage him to cough as forcefully as possible to get the object out. Ask someone to get a nurse. Stay with the person until he stops choking or can no longer speak, cough, or breathe. Do not hit him on the back.

If a person can no longer speak, cough, or breathe, or turns blue, call for help immediately. Time is of extreme importance. The **Heimlich maneuver** is a procedure used for choking. It uses abdominal thrusts to move the blockage upward, out of the throat. Make sure the resident needs help before starting the Heimlich maneuver. If the resident cannot speak, cough, or breathe, or if his response is weak, start the Heimlich maneuver. Do this only if your facility allows you to perform this procedure.

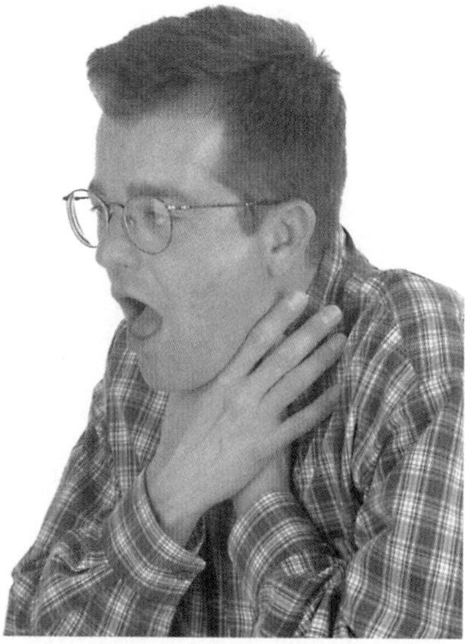

Fig. 7-5. **People who are choking usually put their hands to their throat and cough.**

Heimlich maneuver for the conscious person

1. Stand behind the person. Bring your arms under his arms. Wrap your arms around the person's waist.
2. Make a fist with one hand. Place the flat, thumb side of the fist against the person's abdomen, above the navel but below the breastbone.
3. Grasp the fist with your other hand. Pull both hands toward you and up, quickly and forcefully (Fig. 7-6).

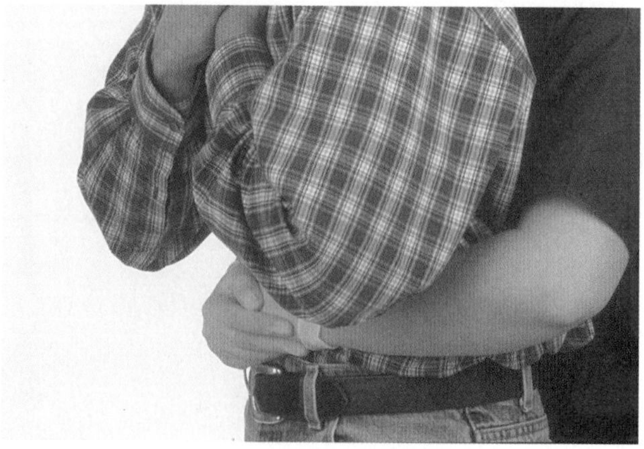

Fig. 7-6.

4. Repeat until the object is pushed out or the person loses consciousness.

Do not practice this procedure on a live person. This risks injury to the ribs or internal organs.

If the person becomes unconscious while choking, help him to the floor gently. Lie him on his back with his face up. Make sure help is on the way. He may have a completely blocked airway. He needs professional medical help immediately.

Heimlich maneuver for the unconscious person

1. Make sure the person is on his back.
2. Open the airway by tilting the head back and lifting the chin (head tilt-chin lift method).
3. Check for breathing.
4. If there is no breathing, open the mouth. Try to sweep the mouth with your finger to remove the blockage. Sweep along the inside of the mouth toward the base of the tongue (Fig. 7-7).

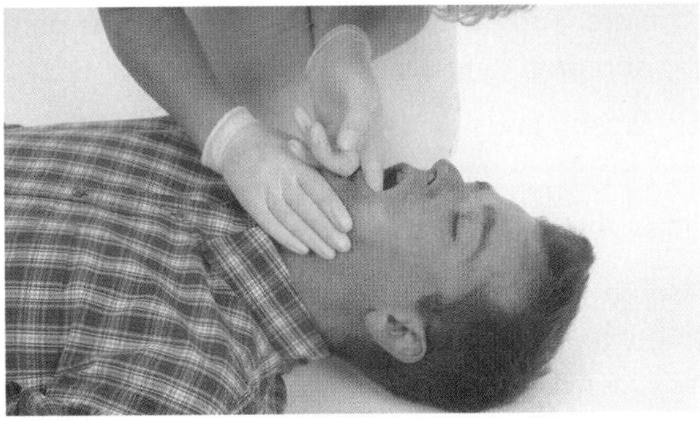

Fig. 7-7.

5. Pinch the nose closed. Give two full rescue breaths.
6. If air does not enter the airway, kneel and straddle the person's thighs, facing his face.
7. Place the heel of one hand on the person's abdomen, slightly above the navel. Your fingers should point toward the person's chest. Place your other hand over the first hand.
8. Give five abdominal thrusts by pushing your hands inward and upward (Fig. 7-8).

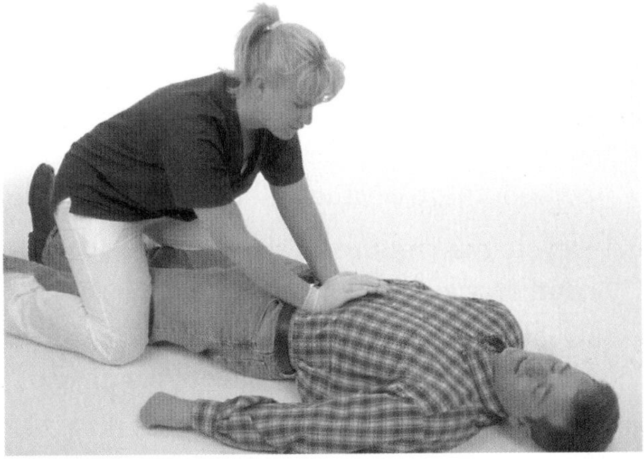

Fig. 7-8.

9. Check to see if the blockage is removed.
10. Try to sweep the object out with your fingers.
11. Repeat steps 5-9 if necessary.

Shock

Shock occurs when parts of the body do not receive an adequate blood supply. Bleeding, heart attack, severe infection, and falling blood pressure can lead to shock. Shock can become worse when the person is frightened or in severe pain.

Shock is a dangerous, life-threatening situation. Signs of shock include pale or bluish skin, staring, increased pulse and respiration rates, low blood pressure, and extreme thirst. Always call for help if you suspect a person is in shock. To prevent or treat shock, do the following:

Shock

1. Have the person lie down on her back. If the person is bleeding from the mouth or vomiting, place her on her side (unless you suspect that the neck, back, or spinal cord is injured).

2. Control bleeding. This procedure is described later in the chapter.
3. Check pulse and respirations if possible. (See chapter 17.)
4. Keep the person as calm and comfortable as possible.
5. Maintain normal body temperature. If the weather is cold, place a blanket around the person. If the weather is hot, provide shade.
6. Elevate the feet unless the person has a head or abdominal injury, breathing difficulties, or a fractured bone or back (Fig. 7-9). Elevate the head and shoulders if a head wound or breathing difficulties are present. Never elevate a body part if a broken bone exists.

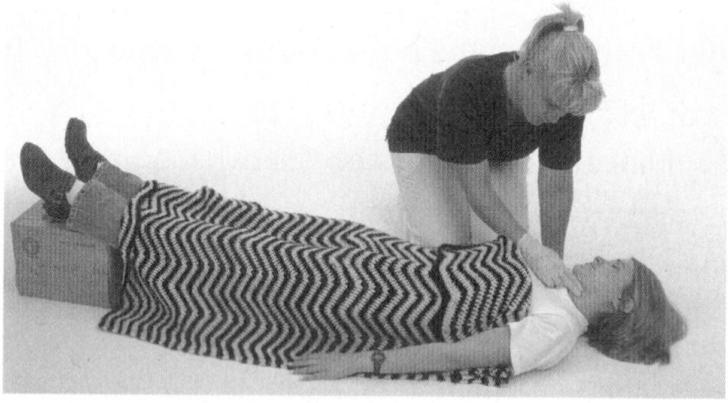

Fig. 7-9.

7. Do not give the person anything to eat or drink.
8. Call for help immediately. Victims of shock should always receive medical care as soon as possible.

Bleeding

Severe bleeding can cause death quickly. It must be controlled. Call the nurse immediately. Then follow these steps to control bleeding:

Bleeding

1. Put on gloves. Take time to do this. If the resident is able, he can hold his bare hand over the wound until you can put on gloves.
2. Hold a thick sterile pad, a clean pad, or a clean cloth, handkerchief, or towel against the wound.
3. Press down hard directly on the bleeding wound until help arrives. Do not decrease pressure (Fig. 7-10). Put additional pads over the first pad if blood seeps through. Do not remove the first pad.

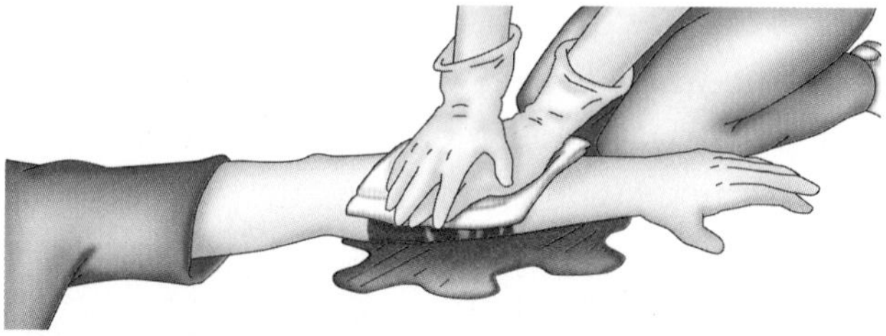

Fig. 7-10. **Hold pad over wound and press down hard. Do not decrease pressure.**

4. If you can, raise the wound above the level of the heart to slow down the bleeding. If the wound is on an arm, leg, hand, or foot, and there are no broken bones, prop up the limb. Use towels, blankets, coats, or other absorbent material.
5. When bleeding is under control, secure the dressing to keep it in place. Check for symptoms of shock (pale skin, increased pulse and respiration rates, low blood pressure, and extreme thirst). Stay with the person until help arrives.
6. Wash hands thoroughly when finished.

Poisoning

As you learned in chapter 6, facilities contain many harmful substances that should not be swallowed. Suspect poisoning when a resident suddenly collapses, vomits, and has heavy, difficult breathing. If you suspect poisoning, notify the nurse immediately. Look for a container that will help you find out what the resident has taken or eaten. Check the mouth for chemical burns. Use gloves to do this. Note the breath odor. The nurse may have you call the local or state poison control center. Follow instructions from poison control.

Burns

You first learned about preventing burns in chapter 6. Care of a burn depends on its depth, size, and location. There are three types of burns: first degree, second degree, and third degree burns (Fig. 7-11). First degree burns involve just the outer layer of skin. The skin becomes red, painful, and swollen, but no blisters occur. Second degree burns extend from the outer layer of skin to the next deeper layer of skin. The skin is red, painful, swollen, and blisters occur. Third degree burns involve all three layers of the skin. These burns may extend to the bone. If the nerves are destroyed, the person will not feel pain. The skin is shiny and appears hard. Skin may be white in color.

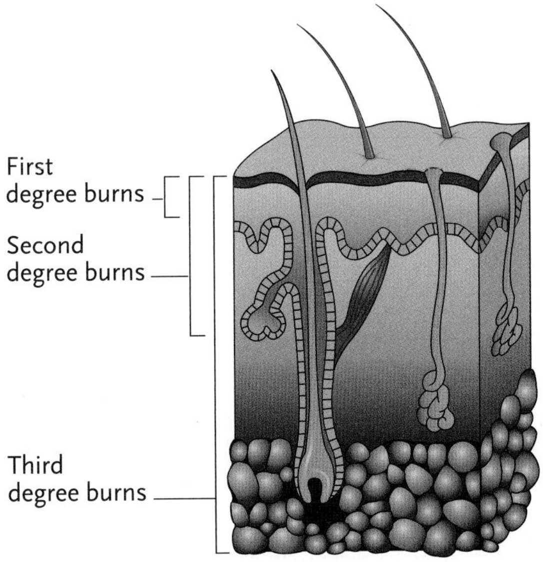

Fig. 7-11.

If a resident is burned, call or have someone else call for the nurse immediately.

Burns

To treat a minor burn:

1. Use cool, clean water (not ice) to decrease the skin temperature and prevent further injury (Fig. 7-12). Ice will cause further skin damage. Dampen a clean cloth and place it over the burn.
2. Once the pain has eased, you may cover the area with a dry, sterile gauze.

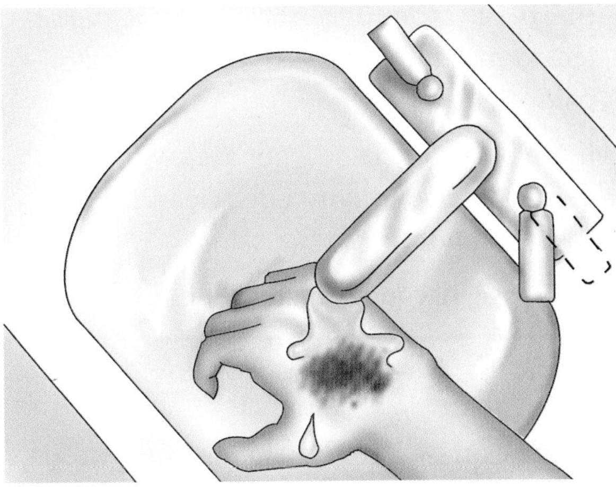

Fig. 7-12.

3. Never use any kind of ointment, salve, or grease on a burn.

For more serious burns:

1. Remove the person from the source of the burn. If clothing has caught fire, smother it with a blanket or towel to put out flames. Protect yourself from the source of the burn.
2. Call for emergency help.
3. Check for breathing, pulse, and severe bleeding.
4. Do not apply water. It may cause infection.
5. Remove as much of the person's clothing around the burned area as possible. Do not try to pull away clothing that sticks to the burn. Cover the burn with thick, dry, sterile gauze if available, or a clean cloth. A dry, insulated cool pack may be used over the dressing (Fig. 7-13). Again, never use any kind of ointment, salve, or grease on a burn.

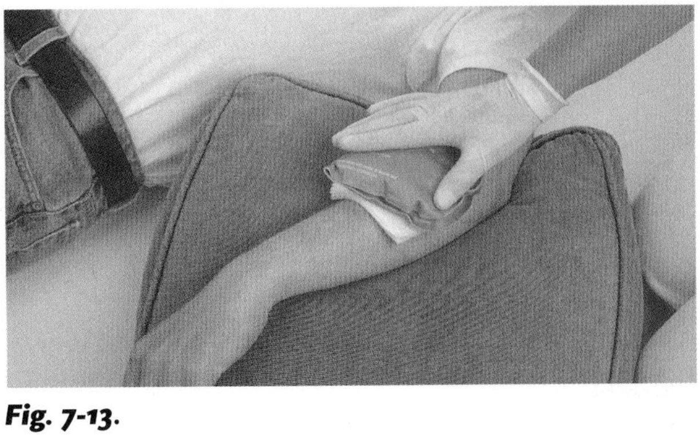

Fig. 7-13.

6. Ask the person to lie down. Elevate the affected part if this does not cause greater pain.
7. If the burn covers a larger area, wrap the person or the limb in a dry, clean sheet. Take care not to rub the skin.
8. Wait for emergency medical help.

Fainting

Fainting occurs when the blood supply drops, causing a loss of consciousness. Fainting may be the result of hunger, fear, pain, fatigue, standing for a long time, poor ventilation, or overheating. Signs and symptoms of fainting include dizziness, perspiration, pale skin, weak pulse, shallow respirations, and blackness in the visual field. If someone appears likely to faint, follow these steps:

Fainting

1. Have the person lie down or sit down before fainting occurs.
2. If the person is in a sitting position, have her bend forward and place her head between her knees (Fig. 7-14). If the person is lying flat on her back, elevate the legs.

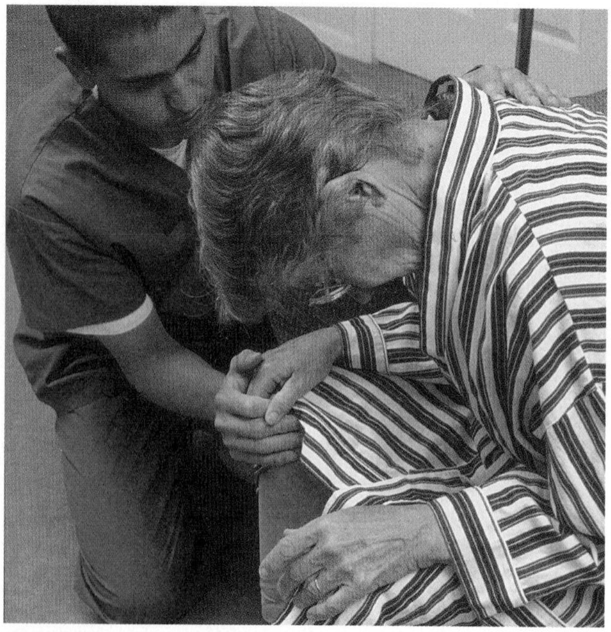

Fig. 7-14.

3. Loosen any tight clothing.
4. Have the person stay in position for at least five minutes after symptoms disappear.
5. Help the person get up slowly. Continue to observe her for symptoms of fainting. Stay with the person until she feels better. If you need help but cannot leave the person, use the call light.
6. Report the event to the nurse.

If a person does faint, lower him to the floor or other flat surface. Position him on his back. Elevate his legs eight to 12 inches. Loosen any tight clothing. Check to make sure the person is breathing. He should recover quickly, but keep him lying down for several minutes. Report the incident to the nurse immediately. Fainting may be a sign of a more serious medical condition.

Nosebleed

A nosebleed can occur suddenly when the air is dry or when injury has occurred. The medical term for a nosebleed is **epistaxis**. If a resident has a nosebleed, notify the nurse and take the following steps:

Nosebleed

1. Elevate the head of the bed. Tell the person to remain in a sitting position. Offer tissues or a clean cloth to catch the blood. Do not touch blood or bloody clothes, tissues or cloths without gloves.
2. Put on gloves. Apply firm pressure over the bridge of the nose. Squeeze the bridge of the nose with your thumb and forefinger (Fig. 7-15). You can have the resident do this until you are able to put on gloves.
3. Apply the pressure until the bleeding stops.
4. Use a cool cloth or ice wrapped in a cloth on the back of the neck, the forehead, or the upper lip to slow the flow of blood. Never apply ice directly to skin.

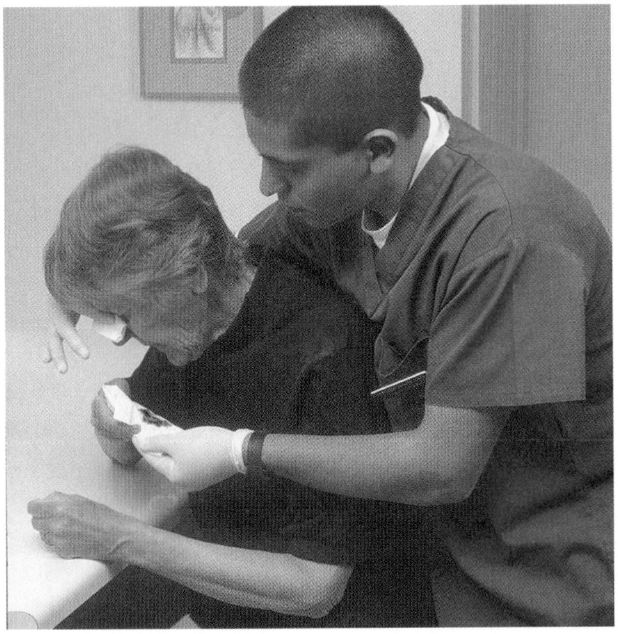

Fig. 7-15.

5. If the bleeding does not stop, tell the nurse immediately.

Myocardial Infarction or Heart Attack

When blood flow to the heart is completely blocked, oxygen and nutrients fail to reach its cells. Waste products are not removed. The muscle cells die. This is called a **myocardial infarction** (MI), or heart attack. You will learn more about MIs in chapter 18. A myocardial infarction is an emergency that can result in serious heart damage or death. The following are signs and symptoms of MI:

- sudden, severe pain in the chest, usually on the left side or in the center, behind the breastbone
- indigestion or heartburn
- nausea and vomiting
- dyspnea, or difficulty breathing
- dizziness
- pale, gray, or bluish (cyanotic) skin color, indicating lack of oxygen
- perspiration
- cold and clammy skin
- weak and irregular pulse rate
- low blood pressure
- anxiety and a sense of doom
- denial of a heart problem

The pain of a heart attack is commonly described as a crushing, pressing, squeezing, stabbing, piercing pain, or "like someone is sitting on my chest." The pain may go down the inside of the left arm. A person may also feel it in the neck and/or in the jaw. The pain usually does not go away.

You must take immediate action if a resident has any of these symptoms. Follow these steps:

Heart attack

1. Call or have someone call the nurse.
2. Place the person in a comfortable position. Encourage him to rest. Reassure him that you will not leave him alone.
3. Loosen clothing around neck (Fig. 7-16).

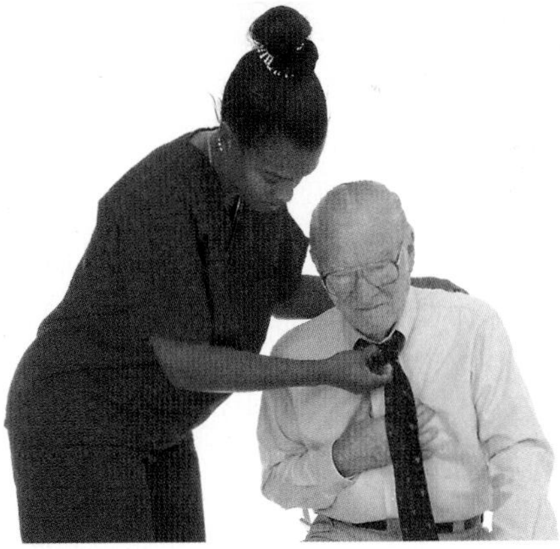

Fig. 7-16.

4. Do not give the person liquids or food.
5. Monitor the person's breathing and pulse. If the person stops breathing or has no pulse, perform rescue breathing or CPR only if you are trained and your facility permits you to do so.
6. Stay with the person until help arrives.

Some states allow NAs to offer heart medication to a person having a heart attack. Nitroglycerin is an example of heart medication. If you are allowed to do this, offer the medication only. Never place medication in someone's mouth.

Insulin Shock and Diabetic Coma

Insulin shock and diabetic coma are problems of diabetes that can be life-threatening. You will learn more about diabetes and related care in chapter 18.

Insulin shock, or hypoglycemia, can result from either too much insulin or too little food. It occurs when insulin is given and the person skips a meal or does not eat all the food required. Even when a regular amount of food is eaten, physical activity may rapidly absorb the food. This causes too much insulin to be in the body. Vomiting and diarrhea may also lead to insulin shock in people with diabetes.

The first signs of insulin shock include feeling weak or different, nervousness, dizziness, and perspiration. These signal that the resident needs food. The food should be in a form that can be rapidly absorbed. A lump of sugar, a hard candy, or a glass of orange juice should be consumed right away. A diabetic should always have a quick source of sugar handy. Call the nurse if the resident has shown signs of insulin shock. Signs and symptoms of insulin shock include:

- hunger
- weakness
- rapid pulse
- headache
- low blood pressure
- perspiration
- cold, clammy skin
- confusion
- trembling
- nervousness
- blurred vision
- numbness of the lips and tongue
- unconsciousness

Having too little insulin causes **diabetic coma**, also known as acidosis or hyperglycemia. It can result from undiagnosed diabetes, not enough insulin, eating too much, not getting enough exercise, and physical or emotional stress.

The signs of diabetic coma include increased thirst or urination, stomach pain, deep or difficult breathing, and breath that smells sweet or fruity. Other signs and symptoms of diabetic coma include:

- hunger
- weakness
- rapid, weak pulse
- headache
- low blood pressure
- dry skin
- flushed cheeks
- drowsiness
- slow, deep, and difficult breathing
- nausea and vomiting
- abdominal pain
- sweet, fruity breath odor
- air hunger, or resident gasping for air and being unable to catch his breath
- unconsciousness

Call the nurse immediately if you think your resident is experiencing diabetic coma.

Seizures

Seizures are involuntary, often violent, contractions of muscles. They can involve a small area or the entire body. Seizures are caused by a problem in the brain. They can occur in young children who have a high fever. Older children and adults who have a serious illness, fever, head injury, or a seizure disorder, such as epilepsy, may also have seizures.

The main goal of a caregiver during a seizure is to make sure the resident is safe. During a seizure, a person may shake severely and thrust arms and legs uncontrollably (Fig. 7-17). He may clench his jaw, drool, and be unable to swallow. The following emergency measures should be taken if a resident has a seizure:

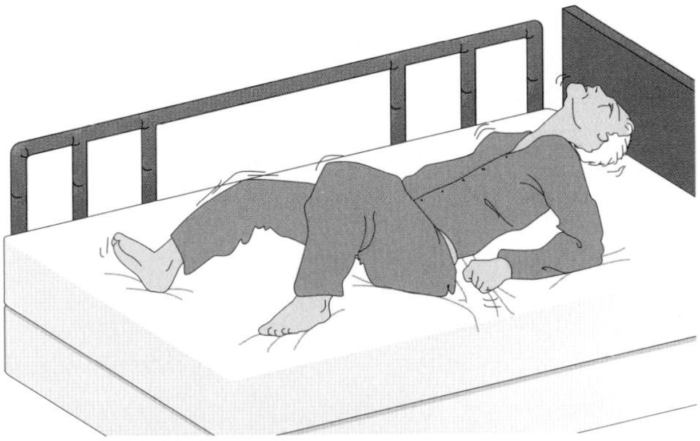

Fig. 7-17. **A person having a seizure may shake severely and thrust his arms and legs uncontrollably.**

Seizures

1. Lower the person to the floor.
2. Have someone call the nurse immediately. Do not leave the person unless you must do so to get medical help.
3. Move furniture away to prevent injury. If a pillow is nearby, place it under his or her head.
4. Do not try to restrain the person.
5. Do not force anything between the person's teeth. Do not place your hands in the person's mouth for any reason. You could be bitten.
6. Do not give liquids or food.
7. When the seizure is over, check breathing.
8. Report the length of the seizure and your observations to the nurse.

CVA or Stroke

You first learned about stroke, or cerebral vascular accident (CVA), in chapter 4. Symptoms of a stroke include dizziness, ringing in the ears, blurred vision, headache, nausea, vomiting, slurring of words, and loss of memory. These signs and symptoms should be reported immediately. A quick response is very important.

A **transient ischemic attack**, or TIA, is a warning sign of a stroke. TIA is also known as a "mini stroke." It is the result of a temporary lack of oxygen in the brain. Symptoms may last up to 24 hours. Symptoms include tingling, weakness, or some loss of movement in an arm or leg. These symptoms should not be ignored. Report them to the nurse immediately. Signs that a stroke is occurring include:

- loss of consciousness
- redness in the face
- noisy breathing
- dizziness
- blurred vision
- ringing in the ears
- headache
- nausea/vomiting
- seizures
- loss of bowel and bladder control
- paralysis on one side of the body
- weakness on one side of the body
- the inability to speak or to speak clearly
- use of strange words
- elevated blood pressure
- slow pulse rate

See chapter 18 for more information on stroke and related care.

Falls

You learned about the risk of falls and ways to prevent falls in chapter 6. Falls can be minor or severe. Report all falls to the nurse immediately. Complete an incident report. In the case of a severe fall, the nurse may ask you to call emergency medical services. Take the following steps to help a resident who has fallen:

- Widen your stance. Bring the resident's body close to you to break the fall. Bend your knees. Support the resident as you lower her to the floor.
- Do not try to reverse or stop a fall. You or the resident can suffer worse injuries if you do.
- Call for help. Do not attempt to get the resident up after the fall. Follow your facility's policies and procedures.

Vomiting

Vomiting, or emesis, is the act of ejecting stomach contents through the mouth. It can be a sign of a serious illness or injury. Because you may not know when a resident is going to vomit, you may not have time to explain what you will do and assemble supplies ahead of time. Talk to the resident soothingly as you help him clean up. Tell him what you are doing to help him. If a resident has vomited, notify the nurse and take the following steps:

Vomiting

1. Put on gloves.
2. Place an emesis basin under the chin. Remove it when vomiting has stopped.
3. Remove soiled linens or clothes. Replace with fresh linens or clothes.
4. If resident's intake and output (I&O) is being monitored (see chapter 16), measure and note amount of vomitus.
5. Flush vomit down the toilet and wash and store basin.
6. Remove gloves.
7. Wash your hands.
8. Put on fresh gloves.
9. Provide comfort to resident. Wipe face and mouth (Fig. 7-18). Position comfortably, and offer a drink of water. Provide oral care (see chapter 13). It helps get rid of the taste of vomit in the mouth.
10. Put soiled linen in proper containers.
11. Remove gloves.
12. Wash your hands again.
13. Document time, amount, color, odor and consistency of vomitus. Look for blood in vomitus or blood-tinged vomitus.

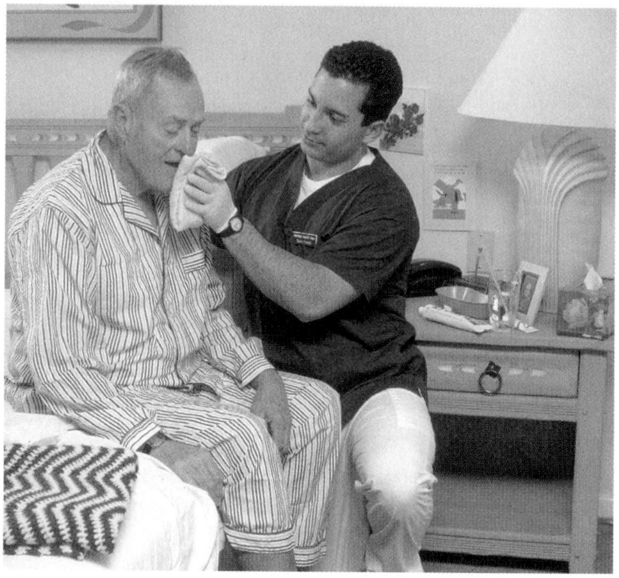

Fig. 7-18. **Be calm and comforting when helping a resident who has vomited.**

"Flying Ambulances"

Napoleon invaded Italy in 1796. During that invasion, Dominique Jean Larrey (1766-1842) developed "flying ambulances." These were horse-drawn vehicles that were able to quickly remove the wounded from the front lines for treatment. During the American Civil War, around 1863, "ambulance trains" similar to the legendary wagon trains appeared.

3. Describe disaster guidelines

Nursing assistants need to be skilled and responsible during a disaster. An emergency or disaster may occur during working hours. Disasters can include fire, flood, earthquake, hurricane, tornado, or severe weather. Today, many facilities also consider acts of terrorism as disasters.

Annual in-services and disaster drills are held at facilities. Take advantage of these sessions. Pay close attention to instructions.

During an emergency, a nurse or the administrator will give directions. Listen carefully to all directions. Follow instructions. Know the locations of all exits and stairways. Know where the fire alarms and extinguishers are located.

Know the appropriate action to take in any situation. This protects you and your residents. Each facility has a disaster plan available for employees to learn. Make sure you know your facility's plan. Your instructor will have specific guidelines for disasters that commonly occur in your area.

Chapter Review

1. List two steps to follow in an emergency situation.
2. What information should you be prepared to give when calling emergency services?
3. Why should you not perform CPR if you are not trained to do so?
4. How is the Heimlich maneuver used to help someone who is choking?
5. List the signs of shock.
6. Why should you not use ice on a burn?
7. List seven signs of a heart attack.
8. If a person feels like he is going to faint, in what position should he be placed?
9. Why should you put on gloves if a resident has a nosebleed?
10. Why should you not force anything into the mouth of a person who is having a seizure?
11. What causes insulin shock? What causes diabetic coma?
12. List the symptoms of a TIA.
13. What should you do if a resident starts to fall?
14. What are four things that should be documented about a resident's vomit?
15. What is an NA's role during a disaster?

Chapter 8
Human Needs and Human Development

1. Explain health and wellness

The World Health Organization has defined the word **health** as "a state of complete physical, mental, and social well-being, and not merely the absence of disease or infirmity." This view of health looks at the whole person. It also takes the focus off disease and changes it to healthy attitudes and lifestyle. In recent years, we have seen much information on health, wellness, and healthy living.

Wellness has to do with successfully balancing things that happen in our everyday lives. Five kinds of wellness have been defined: physical, social, emotional, intellectual, and spiritual. Physical wellness includes things like being able to complete everyday tasks. Social wellness has to do with relating to other people. Emotional wellness covers managing stress and expressing feelings. Intellectual wellness deals with growing and learning throughout life. Spiritual wellness includes religious beliefs, ethics, values, and morals.

2. Define "holistic care" and explain its importance in health care

The nursing profession takes a **holistic** view of resident care. The word "holistic" comes from Greek. It means "whole." Holistic means considering a whole system, such as a whole person. You do not divide the system up into parts. Holistic care is caring for the whole person. This includes his or her physical and **psychosocial needs** (Fig. 8-1). Psychosocial needs include social contact, emotions, thought, and spirituality. Meeting these needs can improve a resident's chances of living a better life.

A simple example of holistic care is taking time to talk with your residents while helping them bathe. You are taking care of the physical need with the bath. You are meeting the psychosocial need for contact with others at the same time.

The Roots of Psychology

The science of psychology started in the mid-1800s. Psychology is the science that deals with mental processes. An early philosopher named Wilhelm Wundt founded the first psychological laboratory in 1879. He was interested in studying the mind. Another early professor of psychology, Edward Titchener, said that psychology is "the science of consciousness." The work of Sigmund Freud did not become well-known until the 1920s. Freud developed "psychoanalysis." This is the idea that behavior is controlled by hidden motives and unconscious desires.

3. Explain why independence and self-care are important

Any big change in lifestyle, such as moving into a nursing home, requires a huge emotional adjustment. Think about some of the life-altering changes residents have had to make. The move into a facility may have been sudden due to health reasons. They may have had to sell their home, vehicles, and other personal belongings.

Residents experience fear, loss, and uncertainty with their decline in health and independence. These feelings may cause them to behave differently. Be aware that dramatic changes in a resident's life may cause anger, hostility, or depression. Be supportive and encouraging. Be patient, understanding, and empathic. **Empathy** is the ability to share an experience and feelings with another. This is done by putting yourself in his or her shoes.

To best understand feelings residents are having, you must understand how difficult it is to lose one's independence. Somebody else must now do what residents did for themselves all of their lives. It is also difficult for friends and family members. For example, a resident may have been the main provider for his or her family. A resident may have been the person who did all of the cooking for the family.

Residents may be experiencing some of the following losses:

- loss of spouse, family members, or friends due to death
- loss of workplace and its relationships due to retirement
- loss of ability to go to favorite places

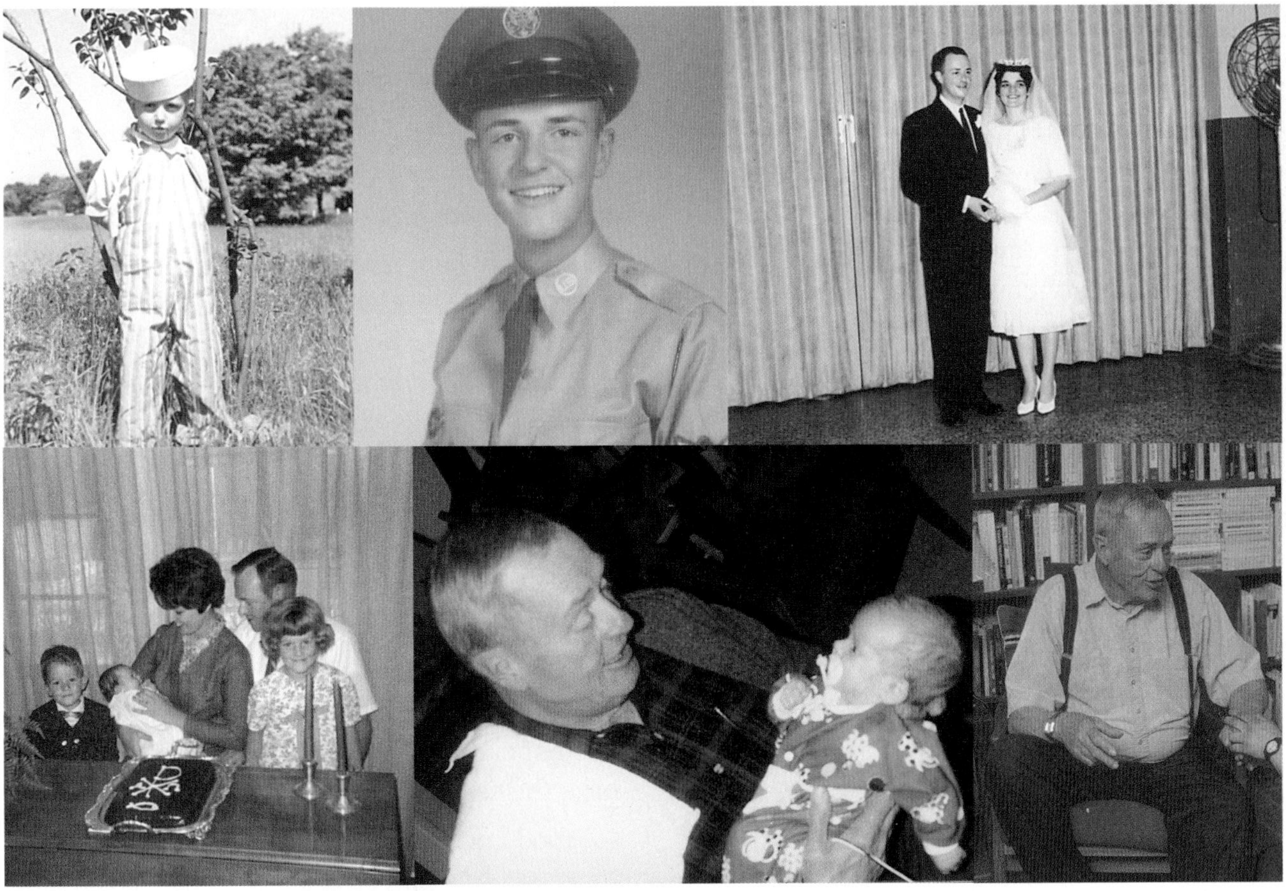

Fig. 8-1. **Remember that residents are people, not just lists of illnesses and disabilities. They have many needs, like you. Many have had rich and wonderful lives. Take time to know and care for your residents as whole people.**

- loss of home and personal possessions (Fig. 8-2)
- loss of ability to attend services and meetings at their faith communities
- loss of health and the ability to care for themselves
- loss of ability to move freely
- loss of pets

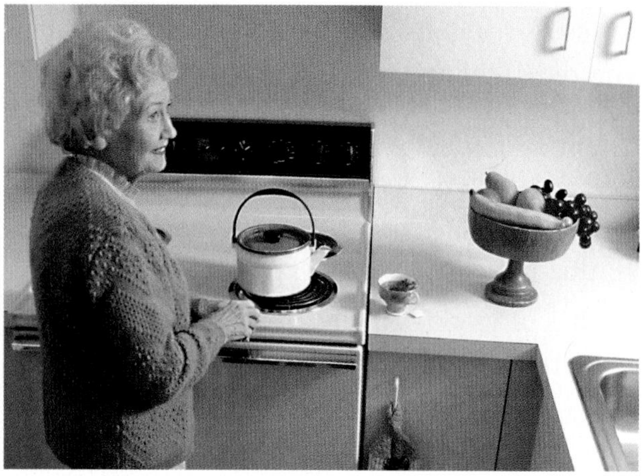

***Fig. 8-2.* Understand and be sympathetic that many residents had to leave familiar places.**

Independence often means not having to rely on others for money, daily routine care, or participation in social activities. **Activities of Daily Living** (ADLs) are the personal care tasks you do every day to care for yourself. People take these activities for granted until they can no longer do them for themselves. ADLs include bathing or showering, dressing, caring for teeth and hair, toileting, eating and drinking, and moving from place to place.

A loss of independence can cause:

- a poor self-image
- anger toward caregivers, others, and self
- feelings of helplessness, sadness, and hopelessness
- feelings of being useless
- increased dependence
- depression

To prevent these feelings, encourage residents to do as much as possible for themselves. Even if it seems easier for you to do things for residents, allow them to do tasks independently. Encourage self-care, regardless of how long it takes or how poorly they do it. Be patient (Fig. 8-3).

Allowing residents to make choices is another way to promote independence. For example, residents can choose where to sit while they eat. They can choose what they eat and in what order. Respect a resident's right to make choices.

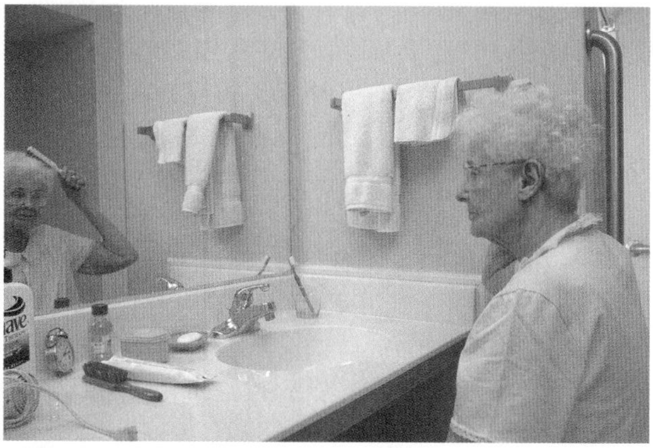

***Fig. 8-3.* Even if tasks take a long time, encourage residents to do what they can for themselves.**

STOP ***Promote independence and dignity.***

Never treat residents as children. They are adults. Encourage them to do self-care without rushing them. Remember that they have the right to refuse care and make their own choices. Maintaining your residents' dignity and independence is their legal right. It is also the proper and ethical way for you to work.

4. Identify basic human needs

People have different genes, physical appearances, cultural backgrounds, ages, and social or financial positions. But all human beings have the same basic physical needs:

- food and water
- protection and shelter
- activity

- sleep and rest
- safety
- comfort, especially freedom from pain

You will be helping residents meet these basic physical needs. By assisting with ADLs or helping residents learn to perform them independently, you help residents meet their basic needs.

People also have psychosocial needs. Psychosocial needs are not as easy to define as physical needs. However, all human beings have the following psychosocial needs:

- love and affection
- acceptance by others
- security
- self-reliance and independence in daily living
- contact with other people (Fig. 8-4)
- success and self-esteem

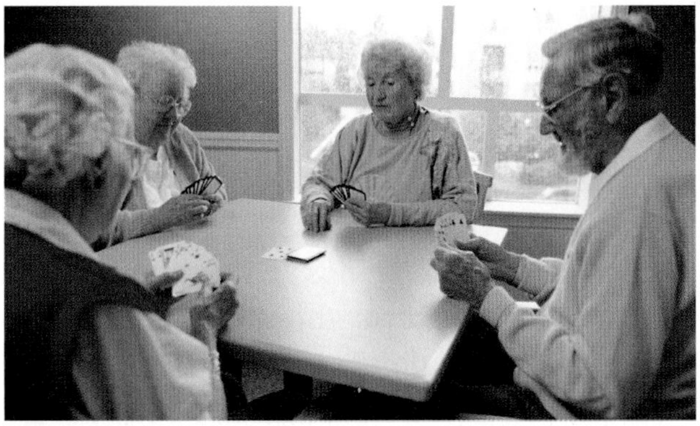

Fig. 8-4. **Social contact is an important psychosocial need.**

Health and well-being affect how well psychosocial needs are met. Stress and frustration occur when basic needs are not met. This can lead to fear, anxiety, anger, aggression, withdrawal, indifference, and depression. Stress can also cause physical problems that may eventually lead to illness.

Abraham Maslow was a researcher of human behavior. He wrote about physical and psychosocial needs. He arranged these needs into an order of importance. He thought that physical needs must be met before psychosocial needs can be met. His theory is called "Maslow's Hierarchy of Needs" (Fig. 8-5).

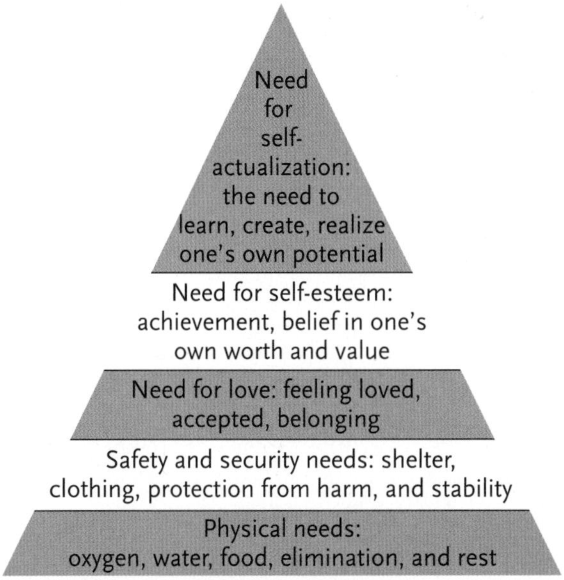
Need for self-actualization: the need to learn, create, realize one's own potential
Need for self-esteem: achievement, belief in one's own worth and value
Need for love: feeling loved, accepted, belonging
Safety and security needs: shelter, clothing, protection from harm, and stability
Physical needs: oxygen, water, food, elimination, and rest

Fig. 8-5. **Maslow's Hierarchy of Needs.**

STOP ***Ensure easy access to food and drink.***

Refusing to help residents meet their basic needs, such as eating and drinking, is abuse. When food is delivered to residents' rooms, trays must be set up in a timely manner. Residents must have their trays prepared so they can eat as easily as possible. Not bothering to open a milk carton or to cut meat on a plate can prevent a resident from eating all of the food needed. This can be considered abuse or neglect.

5. Identify ways to help residents meet their spiritual needs

Residents have spiritual needs. You can assist with these needs, too. Helping residents meet their spiritual needs can help them cope with illness or disability. Remember that spirituality is a sensitive area.

Residents may have strong beliefs in God or very little or no belief in a higher power. Residents may consider themselves spiritual, but may not believe in God or a higher power. The important thing for nursing assistants to remember is to respect all residents' beliefs, **whatever they are.** Do not make judgments about residents' spiritual beliefs or try to push your beliefs on residents.

Following are some ways you can help residents meet their spiritual needs:

- Learn about residents' religions or beliefs (Fig. 8-6). Listen carefully to what residents say.

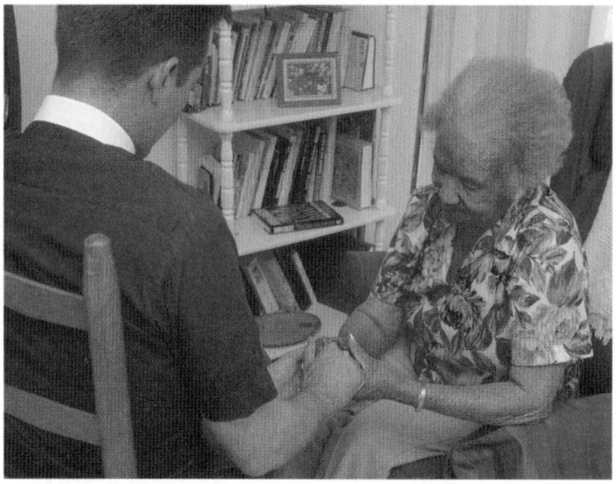

Fig. 8-6. **Be open to your residents' spiritual needs. Be welcoming when they receive visits from a spiritual leader.**

- Assist with practices such as dietary restrictions. Never judge them. Also, respect your resident's decision to refrain from food-related rituals.
- If they are religious, encourage participation in religious services.
- Respect all religious items.
- Report to the nurse (or social worker) if your resident expresses the desire to see clergy.
- Get to know the priest, rabbi, or minister who visits or calls your resident.
- Allow privacy for clergy visits.
- If asked, read religious materials aloud.
- If a resident asks you, help find spiritual resources available in the area. The yellow pages usually list churches, synagogues, and other houses of worship. You can also refer this request to the nurse or social worker.

You should never do any of the following:

- try to change someone's religion
- tell residents their belief or religion is wrong
- express judgments about a religious group
- insist residents join religious activities
- interfere with religious practices

Residents may simply want to talk to someone about their fears or concerns. Sometimes you are the single best person to meet this need. It is important to spend time listening to residents' concerns. You may want to speak only when it seems important, such as when the resident needs comfort.

Spiritual needs are different for each person. When you respect and support each resident's individual spiritual concerns, you are helping to meet their needs. You will learn more about religions and religious differences in learning objective 7.

6. Explain ways to accommodate sexual needs

Humans are sexual beings. They continue to have sexual needs throughout their lives (Fig. 8-7). Sexual urges do not end due to age or admission to a nursing home. The ability to engage in sexual activity, such as intercourse and masturbation, continues unless certain diseases or injuries occur. **Masturbation** means to touch or rub sexual organs in order to give oneself or another person sexual pleasure.

Residents have the right to choose how they express their sexuality. In all age groups, there is a variety of sexual behavior. This is true of your residents also. Do not judge any sexual behavior you see. An attitude that any expression of sexuality by the elderly is "disgusting" or "cute" is inappropriate. It deprives residents of their right to dignity and respect.

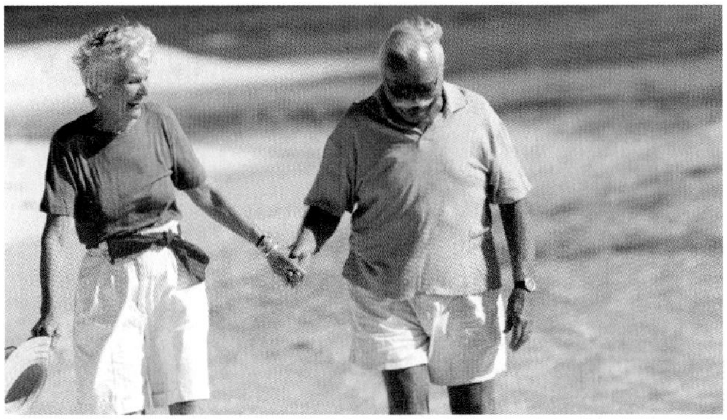

***Fig. 8-7.* Human beings continue to have sexual needs throughout their lives.**

Illness and disability can affect sexual desires, needs, and abilities. Residents may be sensitive about this. Sexual desire may not be lessened by a disability, although ability to meet sexual needs may be limited. Many people confined to wheelchairs can have sexual and intimate relationships. Do not assume you know what impact a physical disability has had on sexuality.

Sexual needs may also be affected by residents' living environments. A lack of privacy and no available partner are often reasons for a lack of sexual expression in nursing homes. Be sensitive to privacy needs.

To meet and respect residents' sexual needs, you can do the following:

- Always knock or announce yourself before entering residents' rooms. Listen and wait for a response before entering.
- If you encounter a sexual situation, provide privacy and leave the room.
- Be open and nonjudgmental about residents' sexual attitudes. Do not judge residents' sexual orientation. Do not judge any sexual behavior you see.
- Honor "Do Not Disturb" signs if your facility uses them.

If you encounter a sexual situation that is disturbing or inappropriate, ask a nurse for assistance. Tips on dealing with sexually-inappropriate behavior are in chapter 4.

Sexual Orientation

Sex and sexuality have been defined in separate ways. Sex is something a person does, while sexuality is something a person is. Sexual orientation is a person's desire for one gender or the other. Sexual orientation or identity plays a big part in human sexuality.

Terms defining sexual identity include:

Gay: 1. A person who has a desire for persons of the same sex. 2. A man whose sexual orientation is to men.

Heterosexual: A person who has a desire for persons of the opposite sex. This is also known as "straight."

Homosexual: A person who has a desire for persons of the same sex. The terms "gay" and "lesbian" are usually preferable.

Lesbian: A woman whose sexual orientation is to women.

Bisexual: A person who desires persons of both sexes.

Transsexual: 1. One who wishes to be accepted by society as a member of the opposite sex. 2. One who has undergone a sex change.

Sexual Abuse

Residents are to be protected from unwanted sexual advances of others. If you see sexual abuse happening, remove the resident from the situation. Take him or her to a safe place. Report to the nurse immediately after making sure the resident is safe and secure.

7. Identify ways to accommodate cultural and religious differences

You first learned about culture and cultural diversity in chapter 4. Cultural diversity has to do with the wide variety of people throughout the world. You will take care of residents with cultural backgrounds. They may have religious traditions different from your own. It is important to respect and value each person as an individual. Respond with acceptance, not prejudice. Sometimes it is easier to accept different practices or beliefs if you understand a little about them.

There are so many different cultures that they cannot all be listed here. One might talk about American culture being different from Japanese culture. But within American culture there are thousands of different groups with their own cultures. Japanese-Americans, African-Americans, and Native Americans are just a few. Even people from a particular region, state, or city can be said to have a different culture (Fig. 8-8). The culture of the South is not the same as the culture of New York City.

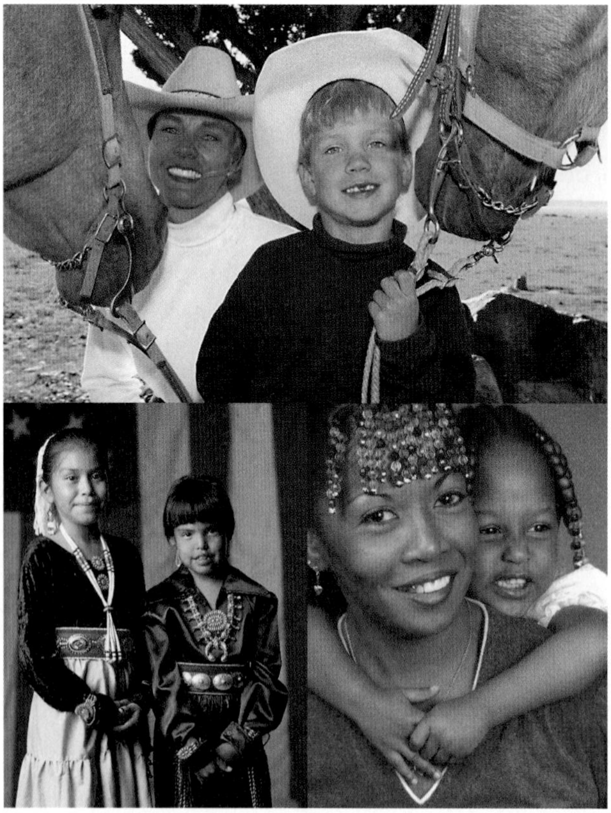

Fig. 8-8. **There are many different cultures in the United States.**

Cultural background affects how friendly people are to strangers. It can affect how close they want you to stand to them when talking. Be sensitive to your residents' backgrounds. You cannot expect to be treated the same way by all of your residents. You may have to adjust your behavior. You must treat all residents with respect and professionalism. Expect them to treat you respectfully as well.

A resident's first language may be different from yours. If he or she speaks a different language, an interpreter may be necessary. Take time to learn a few common phrases in a resident's native language. Picture cards and flash cards can assist with communication.

Religious differences also influence the way people behave. Religion can be very important in people's lives. You must respect the religious beliefs and practices of your residents, even if they are different from your own. Never question your residents' religious beliefs. Do not discuss your own beliefs with them. Understanding a little bit about common religious groups in America may be useful.

Christianity: Christians believe Jesus Christ was the son of God and that he died so their sins would be forgiven. Christians may be Catholic or Protestant. There are many subgroups or denominations (such as Baptists, Episcopalians, Evangelicals, Lutherans, Methodists, Mormons, or Presbyterians). Christians may go to church on Saturdays or Sundays. They may read the Bible, including the Old and New Testaments, take communion as a symbol of Christ's sacrifice, and be baptized. Religious leaders may be called priests, ministers, pastors, or deacons.

Judaism: Judaism is divided into Reform, Conservative and Orthodox movements. Jews believe that God gave them laws through Moses and in the Bible, and that these laws should order their lives. Jewish services are held on Friday evenings and sometimes on Saturdays, in synagogues or temples. Some Jewish men wear a yarmulke, or small skullcap, as a sign of their faith. Some Jews follow special dietary restrictions. Dietary restrictions are rules about what and when followers can eat. Jewish people may not do certain things, such as work or drive, on the Sabbath. This lasts from Friday sundown to Saturday sundown. Religious leaders are called rabbis.

Islam: Muslims, or followers of Mohammed, believe that Allah (God) wants people to follow the teachings of the prophet Mohammed in the Koran. Many Muslims pray five times a day facing Mecca, the holy city for their religion. Muslims worship at mosques and generally do not drink alcohol. There are other dietary restrictions, too.

Other major world religions include Hinduism, practiced in India and elsewhere. Confucianism is practiced in China and Japan. Buddhism started in Asia but has followers in other parts of the world. Native Americans follow many spiritual traditions throughout North America.

In addition to showing respect for different cultural and religious traditions, be aware of specific practices that affect your work. Many religious beliefs include dietary restrictions. Some examples are listed below:

- Many Jewish people eat kosher foods, do not eat pork, and do not eat meat products at the same meal with dairy products. Kosher food is food prepared in accordance with Jewish dietary laws. Respect and follow the resident's practices.
- Many Muslims do not eat pork or shellfish. They may not drink alcohol. Muslims may have regular periods of fasting. Fasting means not eating food or eating very little food.
- Some Catholics do not eat meat on Fridays during Lent.
- Some people are **vegetarians**. They do not eat any meat for religious, moral, or health reasons.
- Some people are vegans. **Vegans** do not eat any animals or animal products, such as eggs or dairy products.

8. Describe the need for activity

Activity is an essential part of a person's life. Activity improves and maintains physical and mental health. Inactivity and immobility can result in:

- loss of self-esteem
- depression
- boredom
- pneumonia
- urinary tract infection
- constipation
- blood clots
- dulling of the senses

Meaningful activities help promote independence, memory, self-esteem, and quality of life. In addition, physical activity can help manage illnesses, such as diabetes, high blood pressure, or high cholesterol. Regular physical activity can also help by:

- lessening the risk of heart disease, colon cancer, diabetes, and obesity
- relieving symptoms of depression
- improving mood and concentration
- improving body function
- lowering risk of falls
- improving sleep quality
- improving ability to cope with stress
- increasing energy
- increasing appetite and promoting better eating habits

Many facilities have an activity department. The activities are designed to help residents socialize and keep them physically and mentally active. Daily schedules are normally posted with activities for that particular day. Activities include exercise, arts and crafts, board games, newspapers, magazines, books, TV and radio, pet therapy, gardening, and group religious events.

One responsibility NAs have is to have residents ready to go when an activity is scheduled. They may need a reminder or encouragement, a trip to the bathroom, change of incontinent brief, or additional grooming. Make sure they feel comfortable before they leave their room.

Delta Society

Delta Society was founded in 1977 by a physician and a veterinarian. It is a national organization dedicated to the bond between animals and humans. It is a non-profit organization that unites people with disabilities and patients in healthcare facilities with professionally trained animals to help improve their health. The group welcomes donations and volunteers. You can contact the society by visiting their web site, www.deltasociety.org.

9. Discuss family roles and their significance in health care

Families are the most important unit within our social system (Fig. 8-9). Families play a huge role in many people's lives. Some examples of family types are listed below:

- Single-parent families include one parent with a child or children.
- Nuclear families include two parents with a child or children.
- Blended families include widowed or divorced parents who have remarried. There may be children from previous marriages as well as from this marriage.
- Multigenerational families include parents, children, and grandparents.
- Extended families may include aunts, uncles, cousins, or even friends.
- Families may also be made up of unmarried couples of the same sex or opposite sexes, with or without children.

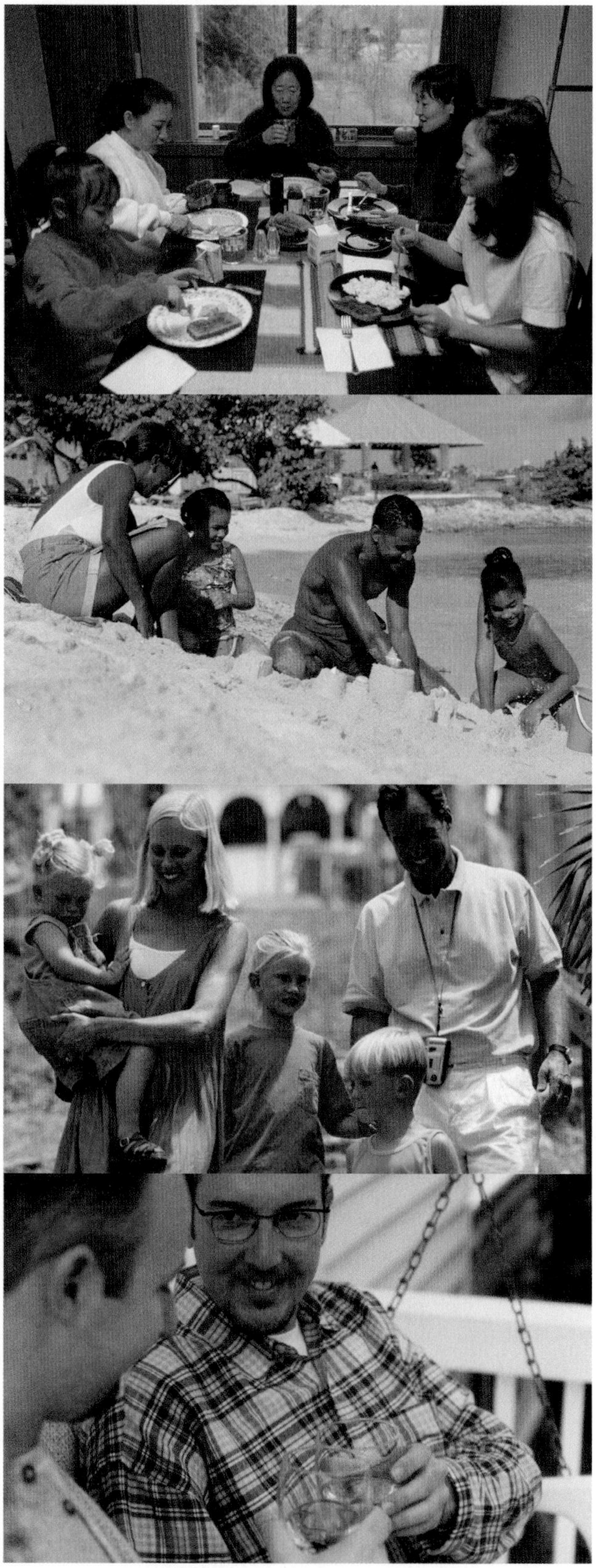

Fig. 8-9. **Families come in all shapes and sizes.**

Today a family is defined more by supporting each other than by the particular people involved. Your residents' families may not look like the kind of family you are used to. Residents with no living relatives may have friends or neighbors who act as a family. Whatever kinds of families your residents have, recognize the important part they can play. Family members help in many ways:

- helping residents make care decisions
- communicating with the care team
- giving support and encouragement
- connecting the resident to the outside world
- offering assurance to dying residents that family memories and traditions will be valued and carried on

Be respectful and nice to friends and family members. Allow privacy for visits. After any visitor leaves, observe the effect the visit had on the resident. Report any noticeable effects to the nurse. Some residents have good relationships with their families. Others do not. If you notice any abusive behavior from a visitor towards a resident, report it immediately to the nurse.

10. List ways to respond to emotional needs of residents and their families

Residents or family members may come to you with problems or needs. Changes in residents' health status can cause fear, uncertainty, stress, and anger. Your response will depend on many things. These include how comfortable you feel with emotions in general, how well you know the person, and what the need or problem is. Try to understand how the person feels.

The following are three good ways to respond in this situation:

Listen. Often just talking about a problem or concern can make it easier to handle. Sitting quietly and letting someone talk or cry may be the best help you can give (Fig. 8-10).

Families often seek out nursing assistants because they are closest to the residents. This is an important responsibility. Show families that you have time for them, too.

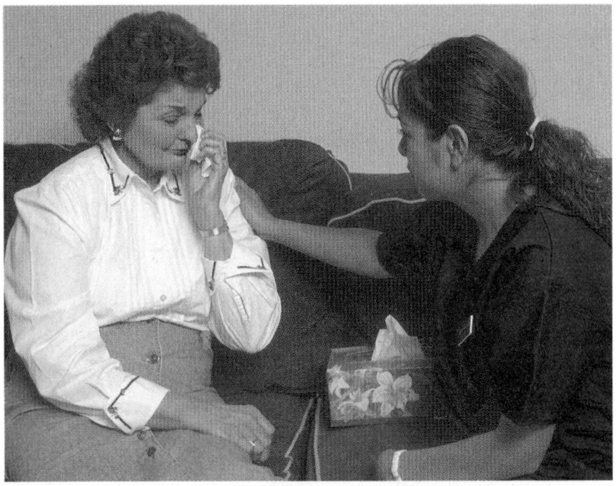

Fig. 8-10. **Sometimes listening to someone is the best way to provide emotional support.**

Offer support and encouragement. Saying things like, "You have really been under a lot of stress, haven't you?" or, "I can imagine that really is scary," can provide a lot of comfort. Avoid using clichés like, "It'll all work out." Things may not all work out. It is more comforting if you admit how hard the situation is. Do not simply dismiss feelings with a cliché.

Refer the problem to a nurse or social worker. When you feel that you cannot help someone, get someone else on the care team to handle the situation. Say something like, "Mrs. Pfeiffer, I think my supervisor would be better at getting you the help you need."

11. Describe the stages of human growth and development

Everyone will go through the same stages of development during his or her life. However, no two people will follow the exact same pattern or rate of development. Each resident must be treated as an individual and a whole person who is growing and developing. He or she should not be treated as someone who is merely ill or disabled.

Infancy, Birth to Twelve Months

Infants grow and develop very quickly in one year. A baby moves from total dependence to the relative independence of moving around, communicating basic needs, and feeding himself.

Physical development in infancy moves from the head down. For example, infants gain control over the muscles of the neck before the muscles in their shoulders. Control over muscles in the trunk area, such as the shoulders, develops before control of arms and legs (Fig. 8-11).

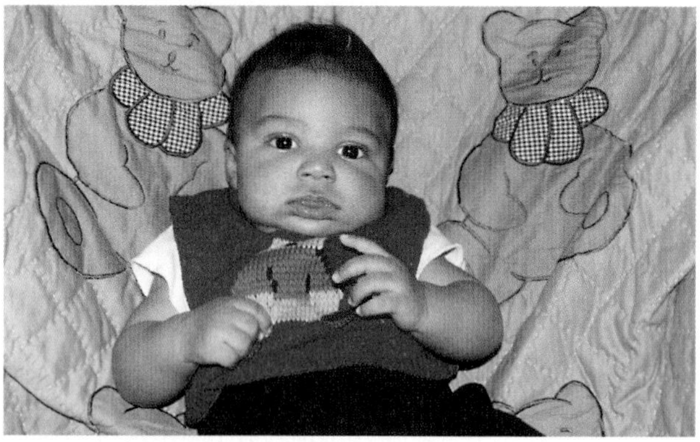

Fig. 8-11. **An infant's physical development moves from the head down.**

Childhood

The Toddler Period, Ages One to Three

During the toddler years, children gain independence. One part of this independence is new control over their bodies. Toddlers learn to speak, gain coordination of their limbs, and learn to control their bladders and bowels (Fig. 8-12).

Toddlers assert their new independence by exploring. Poisons and other hazards, such as sharp objects, must be locked away.

Psychologically, toddlers learn that they are individuals, separate from their parents. Children of this age may try to control their parents. They may try to get what they want by throwing tantrums, whining, or refusing to cooperate. This is a key time for parents to set rules and standards.

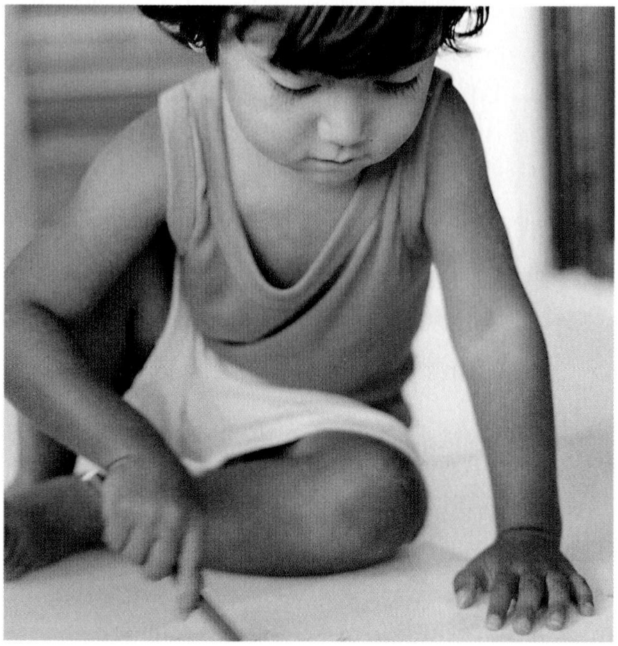

Fig. 8-12. **Toddlers gain coordination of their limbs.**

The Preschool Years, Ages Three to Six

Children in their preschool years develop new skills. These will help them become more independent and have social relationships (Fig. 8-13). They learn new words and language skills. They learn to play in groups. They become more physically coordinated. They learn to care for themselves. Preschoolers develop ways of relating to family members. They also begin to learn right from wrong.

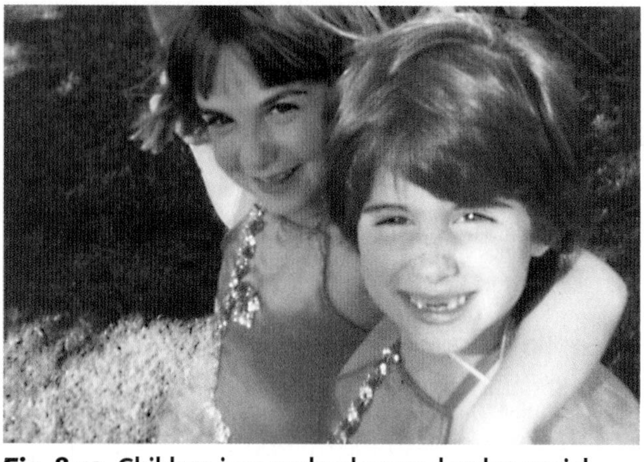

Fig. 8-13. **Children in preschool years develop social relationships.**

School-Age Children, Ages Six to Twelve

From ages six to about twelve years, children's development is centered on cognitive (related to thinking and learning) and social development. As children enter school, they also explore the world around them. They relate to other children through games, peer groups, and classroom activities. In these years, children learn to get along with each other. They also begin to behave in ways common to their sex. They begin to develop a conscience, morals, and self-esteem.

Adolescence

Puberty

During puberty, secondary sex characteristics, such as body hair, appear. Reproductive organs begin to function. The body begins to secrete reproductive hormones. The start of puberty occurs between the ages of ten and sixteen for girls and twelve and fourteen for boys.

Adolescence, Ages Twelve to Eighteen

Many teenagers have a hard time adapting to changes that occur in their bodies after puberty. Peer acceptance is important to them. Adolescents may be afraid that they are ugly or even abnormal.

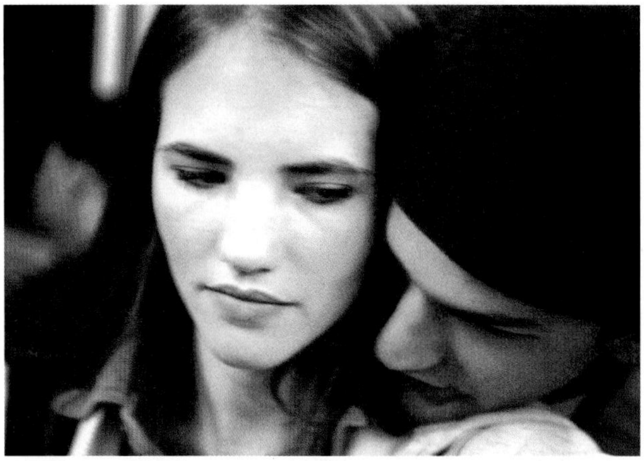

Fig. 8-14. **Adolescence is a time of adapting to change.**

This concern for body image and acceptance, combined with changing hormones that influence moods, can cause rapid mood swings. They remain dependent on their parents, but they need to express themselves socially and sexually. This causes conflict and stress. Social interaction between members of the opposite sex becomes very important.

Adulthood

Young Adulthood, Ages Eighteen to Forty

By the age of eighteen, most young adults have stopped growing. Adopting a healthy lifestyle in these years can make life better. This may also prevent health problems in later adulthood. Psychological and social development continues, however. The tasks of these years include:

- selecting an appropriate education
- selecting an occupation or career
- selecting a mate (Fig. 8-15)
- learning to live with a mate or others
- raising children
- developing a satisfying sex life

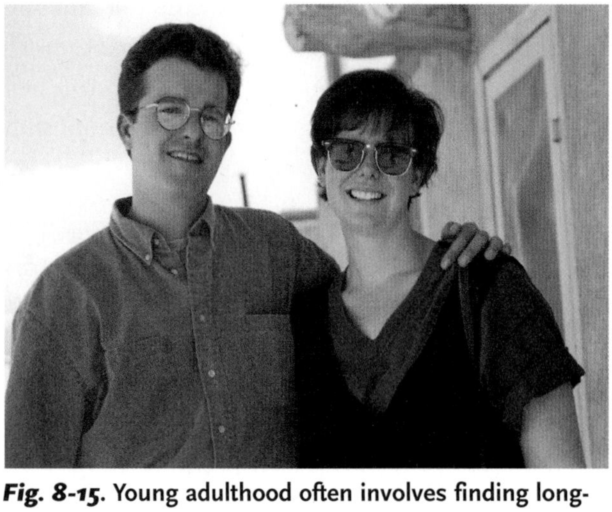

Fig. 8-15. **Young adulthood often involves finding long-term mates.**

Middle Adulthood: Forty to Sixty-five Years

In general, people in middle adulthood are more comfortable and stable than they were before. Many of their major life decisions have already been made. In the early years of middle adulthood people sometimes experience a "mid-life crisis." This is a period of unrest centered on an subconscious desire for change and fulfillment of unmet goals.

Late Adulthood: Sixty-five Years and Older

Persons in late adulthood must adjust to the effects of aging. These changes can include the loss of strength and health, the death of loved ones, retirement, and preparation for death. The developmental tasks of this age may seem to deal largely with loss. But solutions to these problems often involve new relationships, friendships, and interests.

Developmentally Disabled Residents

Some of the people you will care for will be developmentally disabled. This is a chronic condition that limits normal function. Causes vary from injury and disease to mental retardation. People who are developmentally disabled require the same respect, promotion of dignity, and good care as your other residents. Treat them as adults, regardless of their behavior. Praise and encourage them often. Repeat words to make sure they understand. Always be patient. You will learn more about developmental disabilities in chapter 18.

12. Distinguish between what is true and what is not true about the aging process

Geriatrics is the study of health, wellness, and disease later in life. It includes the health care of older people and the well-being of their caregivers. **Gerontology** is the study of the aging process in people from mid-life through old age. Gerontologists look at the impact of the aging population on society.

Later adulthood covers an age range of as many as 25 to 35 years. People in this age category can have very different abilities, depending on their health. Some 70- year-old people enjoy active sports, while others are not active. Many 85-year-old people can still live alone. Others may live with family members or in nursing homes.

Ideas about older people are often false. They create prejudices against the elderly. These are as unfair as prejudices against racial, ethnic, or religious groups. On television or in the movies older people are often shown as helpless, lonely, disabled, slow, forgetful, dependent, or inactive. However, research shows that most older people are active and engaged in work, volunteer activities, and learning and exercise programs. Aging is a normal process, not a disease. Most older people live independent lives and do not need assistance (Fig. 8-16). Prejudice toward, stereotyping of, and/or discrimination against older persons or the elderly is called **ageism.**

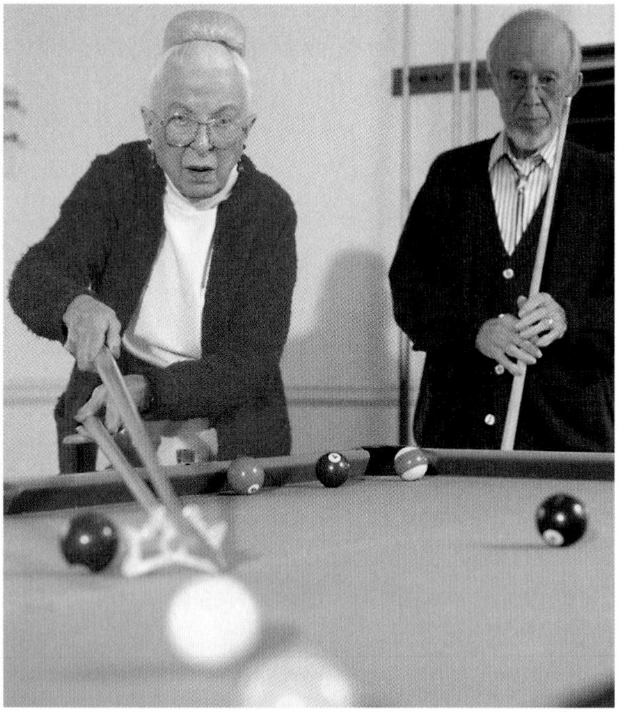

Fig. 8-16. **Older adults often remain active and engaged.**

As an NA you will spend much of your time working with elderly residents. You must know what is true about aging and what is not true. Aging causes many changes. Normal changes of aging do not mean an older person must become dependent, ill, or inactive.

Knowing normal changes of aging from signs of illness or disability will allow you to better help residents.

Normal changes of aging include:

- Skin is thinner, drier, more fragile, and less elastic.
- Muscles are not as strong.
- Senses of vision, hearing, taste, and smell change.
- Heart works less efficiently.
- Appetite decreases.
- Elimination is more frequent.
- Hormone production changes.
- Immunity weakens.
- Mild forgetfulness occurs.
- Lifestyle changes occur.

There are also changes that are NOT considered normal changes of aging and should be reported to the nurse. These include:

- signs of depression
- loss of ability to think logically
- poor nutrition
- shortness of breath
- incontinence

Keep in mind that this is not a complete list. Your job includes reporting any change, normal or not. You will learn more about normal changes of aging in chapter 9.

13. Identify community resources available to help the elderly

There are many community resources available to help your residents meet their different needs. Some of these resources are:

- local Area Agency on Aging
- Ombudsman program
- Alzheimer's Association
- local Hospice organization
- social workers
- resident advocacy organizations
- meal or transportation services

Chapter Review

1. What do the terms "health" and "wellness" mean?
2. What does holistic care involve?
3. What do psychosocial needs include?
4. List six examples of losses that residents may experience.
5. What can a lack of independence cause?
6. According to Maslow, which needs must be met first, physical or emotional?
7. List four ways you can help residents meet their spiritual needs.
8. List four ways to accommodate residents' sexual needs.
9. How can you show respect for different cultural and religious traditions?
10. What are some benefits of meaningful activity?
11. List four ways that families can help the resident.
12. Name three ways you can meet emotional needs of residents and their families.
13. Name one thing that happens at each stage of human development.
14. What stereotypes about older people do you think are most common? What can you do to avoid being prejudiced by these stereotypes?
15. List four community resources that can help residents meet their needs.

Chapter 9
The Healthy Human Body

1. Define key anatomical terms

Bodies are organized into body systems. Each system has conditions under which it works best. **Homeostasis** is the condition in which all of the body's systems are working their best. To be in homeostasis, our body's **metabolism**, or physical and chemical processes, must be working at a steady level. When disease or injury occur, the body's metabolism is disturbed. Homeostasis is lost.

Each system in the body has its own unique job. There are also normal, age-related changes for each body system. You need to understand what a normal change of aging is for each body system. This will help you better recognize any abnormal changes in your residents. This chapter also includes tips on how you can help residents with the normal changes of aging.

Body systems can be broken down in different ways. In this book we divide the human body into ten systems:

1. Integumentary, or skin
2. Musculoskeletal
3. Nervous
4. Circulatory or Cardiovascular
5. Respiratory
6. Urinary
7. Gastrointestinal
8. Endocrine
9. Reproductive
10. Immune and Lymphatic

Body systems are made up of organs. An **organ** has a specific function. Organs are made up of tissues. **Tissues** are made up of groups of cells that perform a similar task. For example, in the circulatory system, the heart is one of the organs. It is made up of tissues and cells. **Cells** are the building blocks of bodies. Living cells divide, grow, and die, renewing the tissues and organs of the body.

This section discusses the structure and function, as well as age-related changes, of each body system. Diseases and disorders of each system and their care will be discussed in chapter 18.

2. Describe the integumentary system

The largest organ and system in the body is the skin. The skin is a natural protective covering, or **integument**. Skin prevents injury to internal organs. It also protects the body against bacteria or germs. Skin also prevents the loss of too much water. Water is essential to life. Skin is made up of tissues and **glands**.

Glands secrete hormones. **Hormones** are chemical substances created by the body that control numerous body functions.

The skin is also a sense organ. It feels heat, cold, pain, touch, and pressure. It then tells the brain what it is feeling. Body temperature is controlled in the skin. Blood vessels in the skin **dilate**, or widen, when the outside temperature is too high. This brings more blood to the body surface to cool it off. The same blood vessels **constrict**, or narrow, when the outside temperature is too cold. By restricting the amount of blood reaching the skin, the blood vessels help the body retain heat (Fig. 9-1).

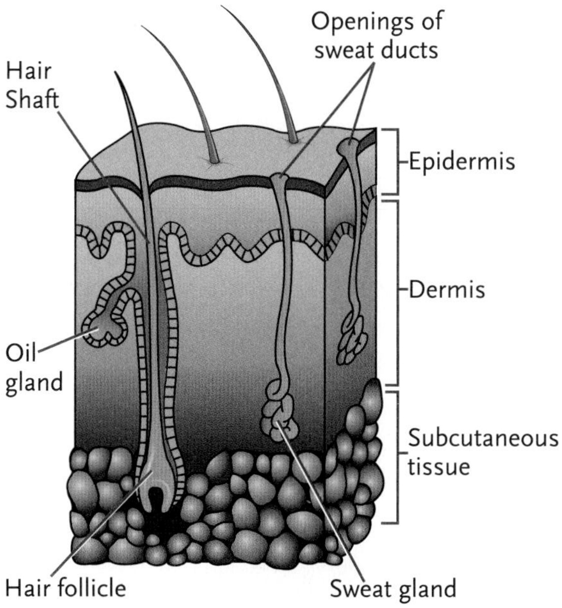

Fig. 9-1. **Cross-section showing the integumentary system.**

The blood vessels, called capillaries, are located in the dermis. The dermis is the inner layer of skin. The dermis also contains nerves, sweat glands, oil glands, and hair roots. Sweat glands help control body temperature by secreting sweat. Sweat contains mostly water, but also salt and a small amount of waste products. Sweat comes to the body surface through pores, or tiny openings in the skin. It cools the body as it evaporates. Oil glands in the dermis secrete oil. Oil comes to the skin surface through hair follicles, or roots. Oil keeps the skin and hair soft.

No blood vessels, and only a few nerve endings, are located in the epidermis. The epidermis is the outer layer of skin. Thinner than the dermis, the epidermis contains both dead and living cells. The dead cells begin deeper in the epidermis. They are pushed to the surface as other cells divide. They are eventually worn off. The epidermis also contains pigment cells that give the skin its color.

Hair grows from roots located in the dermis. It grows through hair follicles that extend through the epidermis to the outside of the body. Hair protects the body from heat and cold. Hair inside the nose and ears keeps out particles and germs trying to enter the body.

Normal changes of aging include:

- Skin gets thinner and more fragile. It is more easily damaged.
- Skin dries and is less elastic.
- Hair thins and turns gray.
- Wrinkles and brown spots appear.
- Protective fatty tissue gets thinner, so person feels colder.

How You Can Help: NA's Role

Keep residents' skin clean and dry. Use lotions as ordered for moisture. Layer clothing and bed covers for additional warmth. Keep sheets wrinkle-free. Provide careful nail care. If you are allowed to clip fingernails, do so with extreme care. Do not cut toenails. Encourage fluids.

OBSERVING AND REPORTING
Integumentary System

During daily care, a resident's skin should be observed for changes that may indicate disease. Observe and report these signs and symptoms:

- rashes or flakes of dry skin
- bruising
- cuts, boils, sores, wounds

- changes in color or moistness/dryness
- swelling
- scalp or hair changes
- skin that appears different from normal or that has changed

3. Describe the musculoskeletal system

Muscles, bones, ligaments, tendons, and cartilage give the body shape and structure. They work together to move the body.

Bones. The skeleton, or framework, of the human body has 206 bones (Fig. 9-2). Bones are hard and rigid, but are made up of living cells. Blood vessels supply oxygen and nutrients to the bones, as well as other tissues of the body. Another function of bones is to protect organs. For example, the skull protects the brain and the vertebrae protect the spinal cord.

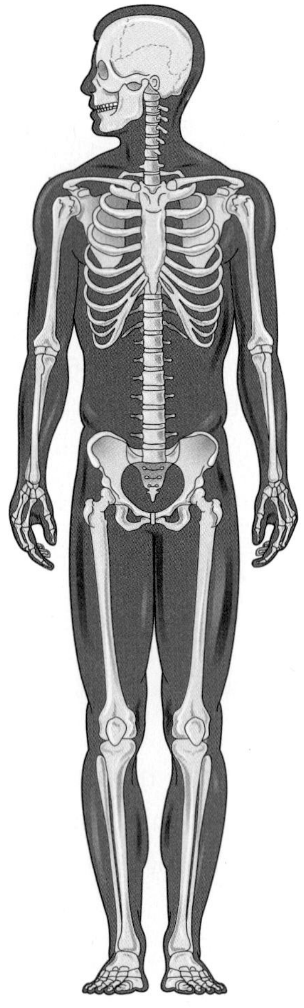

Fig. 9-2. **The skeleton is made of 206 bones that help movement and protect organs.**

Joints. Two bones meet at a joint. There are three major types of joints: fibrous, cartilaginous, and synovial. Different types of joints allow different types of movement (Fig. 9-3).

1. The ball and socket joint is a type of synovial joint. In this joint, the round end of one bone fits into the hollow end of the other bone. This makes movement possible in all directions. The hip and shoulder joints are examples.
2. The hinge joint is another example of a synovial joint. Like the hinge of a door, a hinge joint permits movement in one direction only. The elbow and knee are hinge joints. They only bend in one direction.

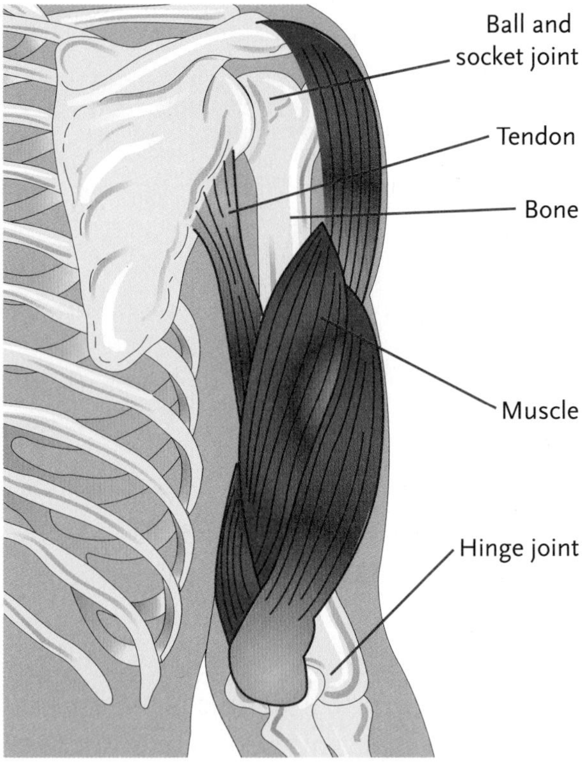

Fig. 9-3. **Muscles are connected to bone by tendons. Bones meet at different types of joints. The ball and socket joint and the hinge joint are shown here.**

Muscles. Muscles provide movement of body parts to maintain posture and to produce heat. Muscles can be voluntary or involuntary. Voluntary muscles are also called skeletal muscles. They are attached to bones. They can be moved when a person wants them to move. Examples of voluntary muscles are the arm and leg muscles, which are consciously controlled. Involuntary muscles cannot be consciously controlled. They automatically regulate the movement of organs and blood vessels. Examples of involuntary muscles are the heart and the diaphragm. The diaphragm is the muscle that makes humans breathe.

Exercise is important for improving and maintaining physical and mental health. For residents who are unable to exercise, range of motion (ROM) exercises can help. ROM exercises can prevent problems related to immobility (see chapter 21). These problems include a loss of self-esteem, depression, pneumonia, and urinary tract infections. A lack of activity can also lead to constipation, blood clots, dulling of the senses, and muscle atrophy or contractures. When **atrophy** occurs, the muscle wastes away, decreases in size, and becomes weak. When a **contracture** develops, the muscle shortens, becomes inflexible, and "freezes" in position. This causes permanent disability of the limb.

Normal changes of aging include:

- Muscles weaken and lose tone.
- Body movement slows.
- Joints become less flexible.
- Bones lose density. They become more brittle, making them more susceptible to breaks.
- Height is gradually lost.

How You Can Help: NA's Role

Falls can cause life-threatening complications, such as fractures. Prevent falls by keeping items out of residents' paths. Keep furniture in the same place. Keep walkers or canes where residents can easily get to them. Encourage regular movement and self-care. Help with range of motion (ROM) exercises as needed. Encourage residents to perform as many ADLs as possible.

OBSERVING AND REPORTING
Musculoskeletal System

Observe and report these signs and symptoms:

- changes in ability to perform routine movements and activities
- any changes in residents' ability to perform ROM exercises
- pain during movement
- any new or increased swelling of joints
- white, shiny, red, or warm areas over a joint
- bruising
- aches and pains reported to you

Be gentle when repositioning residents.
Pulling too hard on a resident's arm can easily dislocate the shoulder joints. Because of this, never jerk a resident's arm or attempt to lift or reposition a resident by pulling on his or her arm. Dislocations can cause extreme pain and even permanent damage.

4. Describe the nervous system

The nervous system is the control and message center of the body. It controls and coordinates all body functions. The nervous system also senses and interprets information from outside the human body (Fig. 9-4).

The neuron, or nerve cell, is the basic unit of the nervous system. Neurons send messages or sensations from the receptors in different parts of the body, through the spinal cord, to the brain.

The nervous system has two main parts: the central nervous system (CNS) and the peripheral nervous system (PNS). The CNS is the brain and spinal cord. The PNS deals with the outer part of the body via the nerves that extend throughout the body.

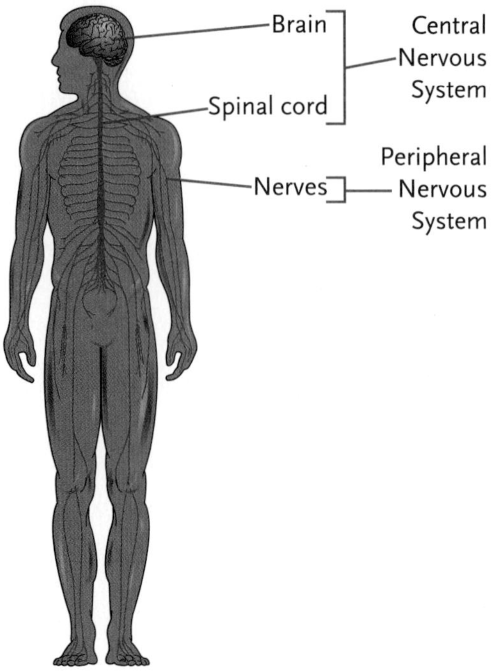

Fig. 9-4. **The nervous system includes the brain, spinal cord, and nerves throughout the body.**

The Central Nervous System

The brain is housed within the skull (Fig. 9-5). The spinal cord is housed within the spinal column. The spinal column extends from the brain into the trunk of the body. Both the brain and the spinal cord are covered by a protective membrane made up of three layers. Between two of these layers is the cerebrospinal fluid. This fluid circulates around the brain and spinal cord. It provides a cushion against injuries.

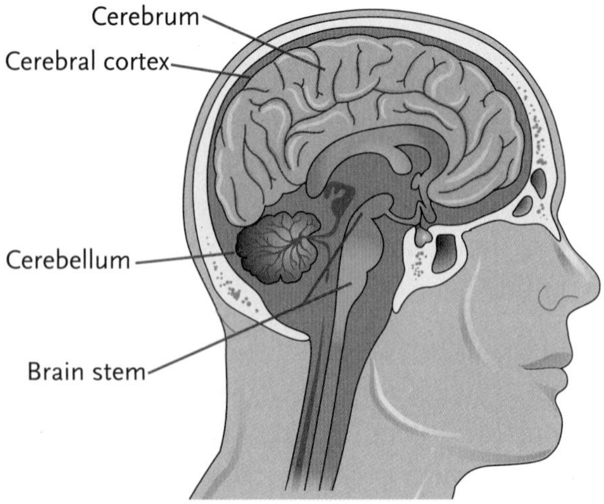

Fig. 9-5. **The three main sections of the brain are the cerebrum, brainstem, and the cerebellum.**

The brain has three main sections: the cerebrum, the cerebellum, and the brainstem. The largest section of the human brain is the cerebrum. The outside layer of the cerebrum is the cerebral cortex. The cerebral cortex is the part of the brain in which thinking, analysis, association of ideas, judgment, emotions, and memory occur. The cerebral cortex also:

- directs speech and emotions
- interprets messages from the eyes, ears, nose, tongue, and skin
- controls voluntary muscle movement

The cerebrum is divided into right and left hemispheres. The right hemisphere controls movement and function in the left side of the body. The left hemisphere controls movement and function in the right side of the body (Fig. 9-6). Any illness or injury to the right hemisphere affects functions on the left side of the body. Illness or injury to the left hemisphere disrupts function on the right side.

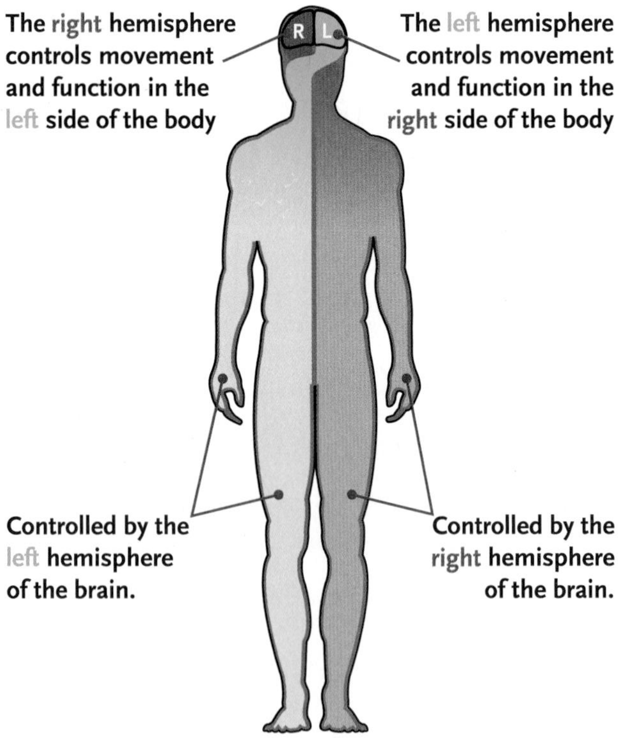

Fig. 9-6. **The right hemisphere controls movement and function in the left side of the body. The left hemisphere controls movement and function in the right side of the body.**

The cerebellum controls balance and regulates the body's voluntary muscles. It produces and coordinates smooth movements. Someone who has a problem in the cerebellum will be uncoordinated and have jerky movements and muscle weakness.

The cerebrum and cerebellum are connected to the spinal cord by the brainstem. The brainstem contains a kind of regulatory center. It controls heart rate, breathing, swallowing, coughing, vomiting, and closing or opening of blood vessels.

The spinal cord is connected to the brain. It is protected by the bones of the spinal column. Nerve pathways run through the spinal cord. They conduct messages between the brain and the body.

Normal changes of aging include:

- Responses and reflexes slow.
- Sensitivity of nerve endings in skin decreases.
- Person may show some memory loss, more often with short-term memory.

How You Can Help: NA's Role

Allow plenty of time for movement. Do not rush the person. Allow time for decision-making. Avoid sudden changes in schedule. Encourage reading and other mental activities.

OBSERVING AND REPORTING
Central Nervous System

Observe and report these signs and symptoms:

- fatigue or any pain with movement or exercise
- shaking or trembling
- inability to speak clearly
- inability to move one side of body
- disturbance or changes in vision or hearing
- changes in eating patterns and/or fluid intake
- difficulty swallowing
- bowel and bladder changes
- depression or mood changes
- memory loss or confusion
- violent behavior
- any unusual or unexplained change in behavior
- decreased ability to perform ADLs

The 3Rs vs. Art

The left hemisphere of the brain is usually involved in a person's ability to do the "3Rs," in this case, reading, writing and 'rithmetic, or mathematics. The right hemisphere of the brain is more involved in artistic and creative abilities.

The Nervous System: Sense Organs

The eyes, ears, nose, tongue, and skin are the body's major sense organs. They are part of the central nervous system because they receive impulses from the environment. They relay these impulses to the nerves.

The eye, which is about an inch in diameter, is located in a bony socket in the skull. The bony socket protects the eye, which is surrounded by muscles that control its movements (Fig. 9-7).

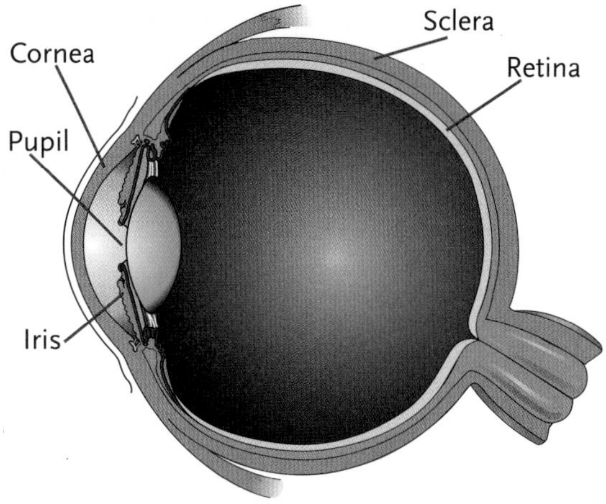

Fig. 9-7. **The parts of the eye.**

The outer part of the eye is called the sclera. The sclera appears white, except in front, where it is called the cornea. The cornea is actually clear, but it appears colored because it lies over the iris, or the colored part of the eye. The pupil, or black circle in the center of the iris, widens or narrows to adjust the amount of light that enters the eye. Inside the back of the eye is the retina. The retina contains cells that respond to light and send a message to the brain, where the picture is interpreted so you can "see."

The ear is a sense organ that provides balance and hearing. It is divided into three parts: the outer ear, the middle ear, and the inner ear (Fig. 9-8).

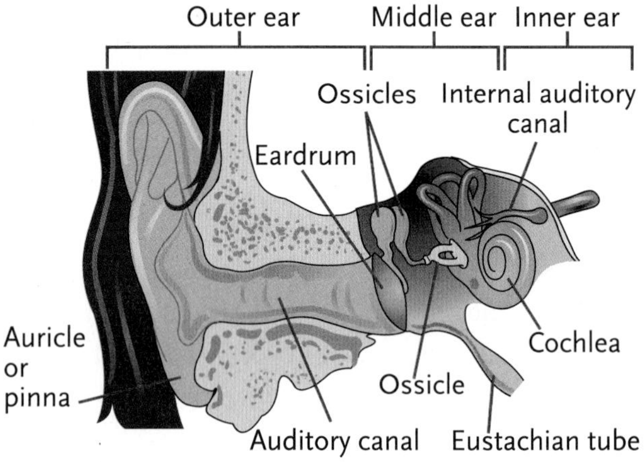

***Fig. 9-8.* The outer ear, middle ear, and inner ear are the three main divisions of the ear.**

The outer ear is the funnel-shaped outer part, sometimes called the auricle or pinna. It guides sound waves into the auditory canal. This canal is about one-inch long and contains many glands that secrete earwax. Earwax and hair in the ear protect the ear from foreign objects. The eardrum, or tympanic membrane, separates the outer ear from the middle ear.

The middle ear consists of the eustachian tube and three ossicles, small bones that amplify sound. The ossicles transmit sound to the inner ear. The eustachian tube connects the middle ear to the throat. It functions to allow air into the middle ear to equalize pressure on the tympanic membrane. The inner ear contains fluid that carries sound waves from the middle ear to the auditory nerve. The auditory nerve then transmits the impulse to the brain. The inner ear also contains structures that help in maintaining balance.

Normal changes of aging include:

- Vision and hearing decreases. Sense of balance may be affected.
- Sense of taste and smell decrease.
- Sensitivity to heat and cold decreases.

How You Can Help: NA's Role

Encourage the use of eyeglasses and hearing aids. Keep them clean. Speak slowly and clearly; do not shout. Loss of senses of taste and smell may lead to decreased appetite. Encourage good oral care. Foods with a variety of tastes and textures may be provided. Loss of smell may make resident unaware of increased body odor. Assist as needed with regular bathing.

OBSERVING AND REPORTING

Eyes and Ears

Observe and report these signs and symptoms:

- O&R changes in vision or hearing
- O&R signs of infection
- O&R dizziness
- O&R complaints of pain in eyes or ears

5. Describe the circulatory or cardiovascular system

The circulatory system is made up of the heart, blood vessels, and blood (Fig. 9-9). The heart pumps blood through the blood vessels to the cells. The blood carries food, oxygen, and other substances cells need to function properly.

The circulatory system performs these major functions:

- supplying food, oxygen, and hormones to cells
- producing and supplying infection-fighting blood cells
- removing waste products from cells
- controlling body temperature

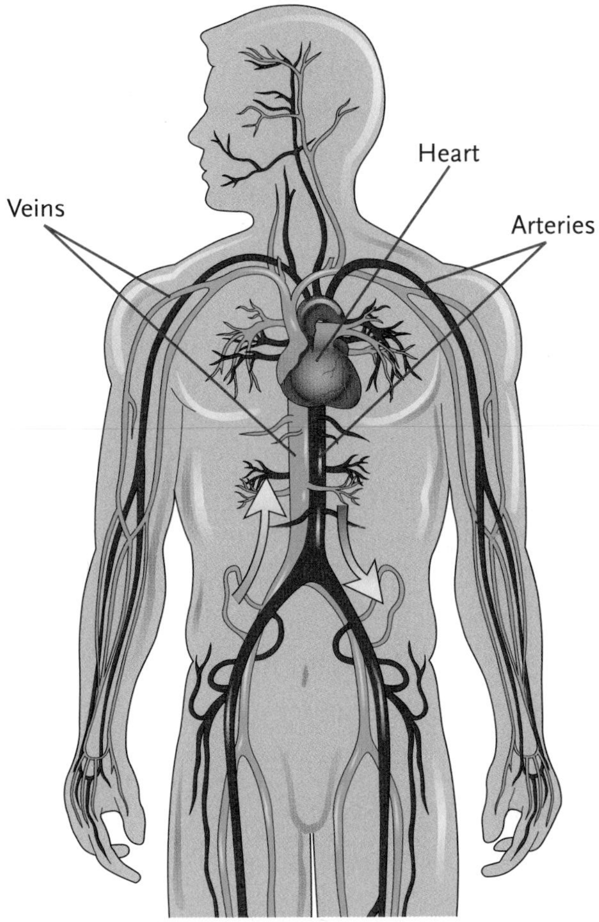

Fig. 9-9. **The heart, blood vessels, and blood are the main parts of the circulatory system.**

A healthy circulatory system is essential for life. Cells, tissues, and organs need good circulation to function well. If circulation is reduced, cells do not receive enough oxygen and nutrients. Waste products of cell metabolism are not removed. Organs become diseased.

Blood contains blood cells and plasma. Plasma is the liquid portion of the blood. It carries many substances, including blood cells, nutrients, and waste products. Analyzing these parts of blood samples can help identify illness and infection:

1. Red blood cells carry oxygen from the lungs to all parts of the body. Red blood cells are produced by bone marrow, a substance found inside hollow bones. Iron, found in bone marrow and red blood cells, is essential to blood. It gives it its red color. Red blood cells function for a short time, then die. They are filtered out of the blood by the liver and spleen. Iron in diets allows bodies to produce new red blood cells.
2. White blood cells defend the body against foreign substances, such as bacteria and viruses. When the body becomes aware of these invaders, white blood cells rush to the site of infection. They multiply rapidly. The bone marrow, spleen, and thymus gland produce white blood cells.
3. Platelets are also carried by the blood. They cause the blood to clot, preventing excess bleeding. Platelets are also produced by the bone marrow.

The heart is the pump of the circulatory system (Fig. 9-10). The heart is a muscle. It is located in the middle lower chest, on the left side. The heart muscle is made up of three layers: the pericardium, the myocardium and the endocardium.

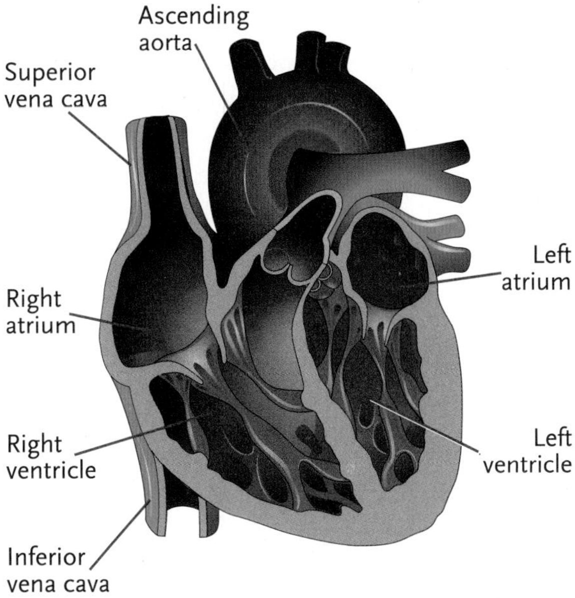

Fig. 9-10. **The four chambers of the heart connect to the body's largest blood vessels.**

The interior of the heart is divided into four chambers. The two upper chambers, called atria or the left atrium and right atrium, receive blood. The two lower chambers, or ventricles, pump blood. The right atrium receives blood from the veins. This blood, containing carbon dioxide, then flows into the right ventricle. It is pumped to the blood vessels in the lungs. Carbon dioxide is exchanged for oxygen. The heart's left atrium receives the oxygen-saturated blood. It then flows into the left ventricle. There it is pumped through the arteries to all parts of the body. Two valves, one located between the right atrium and right ventricle and the other between the left atrium and left ventricle, allow the blood to flow in only one direction (Fig. 9-11).

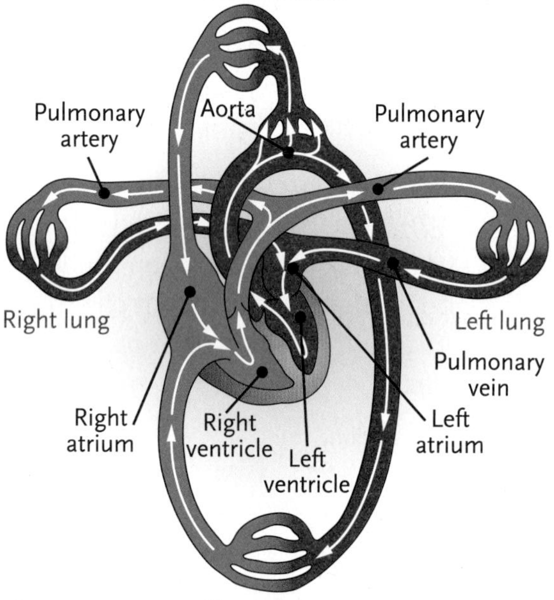

***Fig. 9-11.* The flow of blood through the heart.**

The heart functions in two phases:

1. The resting phase or diastole, when the chambers fill with blood; and
2. The contracting phase or systole, when the ventricles pump blood through the blood vessels. When a blood pressure is taken, the numbers measure these two phases. You will learn about taking blood pressure in chapter 17.

Three types of blood vessels are found in the body: arteries, capillaries, and veins.

Arteries carry oxygen-rich blood away from the heart. The blood is pumped from the left ventricle, through the aorta, the largest artery. Blood is then pumped through other arteries that branch off from it. The coronary arteries carry blood to the heart itself.

Capillaries are tiny blood vessels that receive blood from the arteries. Nutrients, oxygen, and other substances in the blood pass from the capillaries to the cells. Waste products, including carbon dioxide, pass from the cells into the capillaries.

Veins carry the blood containing waste products from the capillaries back to the heart. Near the heart, the veins come together to form the two largest veins, the inferior vena cava and the superior vena cava. These empty into the right atrium. The inferior vena cava carries blood from the legs and trunk. The superior vena cava carries blood from the arms, head, and neck.

Normal changes of aging include:

- Heart muscle loses strength.
- Blood vessels narrow.
- Blood flow decreases.

How You Can Help: NA's Role

Encourage movement and exercise. Allow enough time to complete activities. Prevent residents from tiring. Keep legs and feet warm.

OBSERVING AND REPORTING

Circulatory System

Observe and report these signs and symptoms:

- changes in pulse rate
- weakness, fatigue
- loss of ability to perform activities of daily living (ADLs)

- swelling of hands and feet
- pale or bluish hands, feet, or lips
- chest pain
- weight gain
- shortness of breath, changes in breathing patterns, inability to catch breath
- severe headache
- inactivity (which can lead to circulatory problems)

6. Describe the respiratory system

Respiration, the body taking in oxygen and removing carbon dioxide, involves breathing in (**inspiration**), and breathing out (**expiration**). The lungs accomplish this (Fig. 9-12).

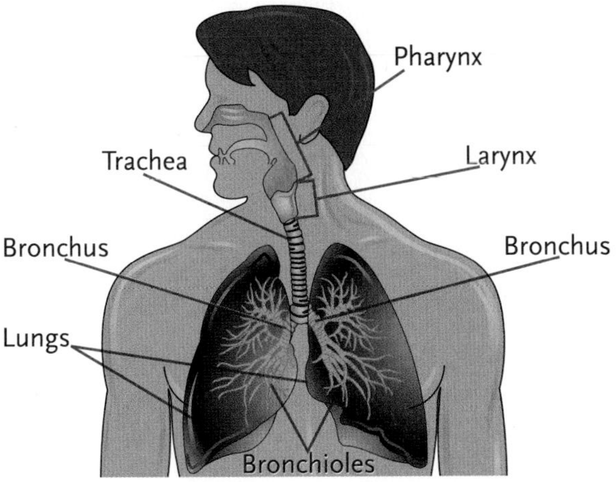

Fig. 9-12. **The respiratory process begins with inspiration through the nose or mouth. The air travels through the trachea and into the lungs via the bronchi, which then branch into bronchioles.**

The respiratory system has two functions:

1. It brings oxygen into the body.
2. It eliminates carbon dioxide produced as the body uses oxygen.

As the lungs inhale, the air is pulled in through the nose and into the pharynx, a tubular passageway for both food and air. From the pharynx, air passes into the larynx, or voice box. The larynx is located at the beginning of the trachea, or windpipe. The trachea divides into two branches at its lower portion, the right bronchus and the left bronchus, or bronchi. Each bronchus leads into each lung and then subdivides into bronchioles. These smaller airways subdivide further. They end in alveoli, tiny, one-cell sacs that appear in grape-like clusters. Blood is supplied to the alveoli by capillaries. Oxygen and carbon dioxide are exchanged between the alveoli and capillaries.

Oxygen-saturated blood then circulates through the capillaries and venules (small veins) of the lung, into the pulmonary vein and left side of the heart. The carbon dioxide is exhaled through the alveoli into the bronchioles and bronchi of the lungs, the trachea, through the larynx, the pharynx, and out the nose and mouth.

Each lung is covered by the pleura, a membrane with two layers. One is attached to the chest wall. One is attached to the surface of the lung. The space between the layers is filled with a thin fluid that lubricates the layers, preventing them from rubbing together during breathing.

Normal changes of aging include:

- Lung strength decreases.
- Lung capacity decreases.
- Oxygen in the blood decreases.
- Voice weakens.

How You Can Help: NA's Role

Encourage the person to get out of bed often. Encourage exercise and regular movement. Encourage and help with deep breathing exercises.

OBSERVING AND REPORTING

Respiratory System

Observe and report these signs and symptoms:

- change in respiratory rate
- shallow breathing or breathing through pursed lips
- coughing or wheezing

- nasal congestion or discharge
- sore throat, difficulty swallowing, or swollen tonsils
- the need to sit after mild exertion
- pale or bluish color of the lips and arms and legs
- pain in the chest area
- discolored **sputum**, or the fluid a person coughs up (green, yellow, blood-tinged, or gray)

7. Describe the urinary system

The urinary system has two vital functions:

1. It eliminates waste products created by the cells through urine.
2. It maintains water balance in the body.

The kidneys are located in the upper part of the abdominal cavity on each side of the spine. These two bean-shaped organs are protected by the muscles of the back and the lower part of the rib cage. When blood flows through the kidneys, waste products and excess water are filtered out. Necessary water and substances are reabsorbed into the bloodstream. Waste and the remaining fluid form urine. The body must maintain a proper balance between water absorbed in the body and waste fluids that are released from the body. You will learn more about fluid intake and output in chapter 16.

Each kidney has a ureter, which is attached to the bladder. Urine flows through the ureters to the bladder, a muscular sac in the lower part of the abdomen. Urine flows from the bladder through the urethra. It then passes out of the body through the meatus, the opening at the end of the urethra (Figs. 9-13 and 9-14).

In the female, the meatus is located in the genital area just in front of the opening of the vagina. In the male, the meatus is located at the end of the penis.

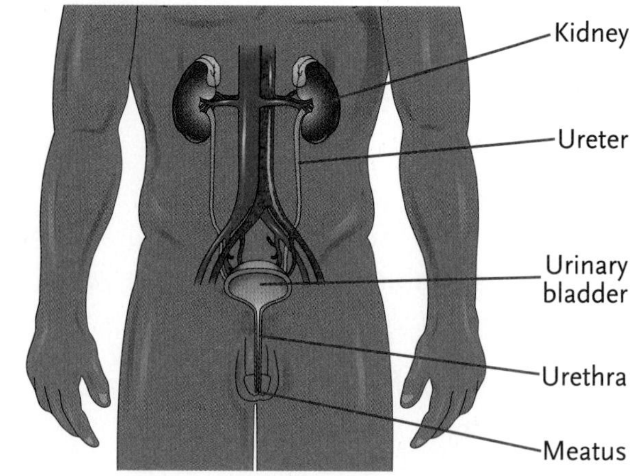

***Fig. 9-13*. The urinary system consists of two kidneys and their ureters, the bladder, the urethra, and the meatus.**

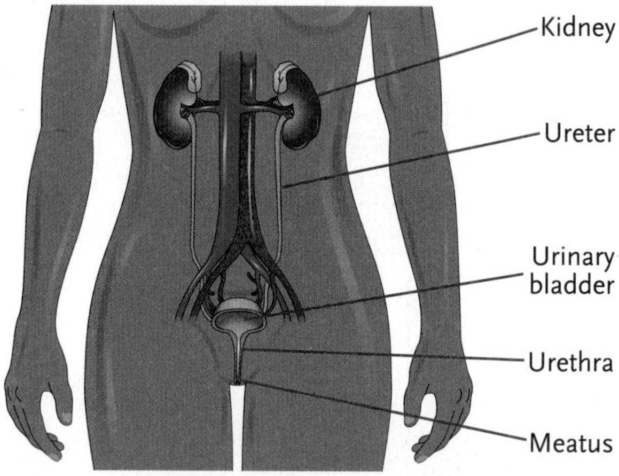

***Fig. 9-14*. The female urethra is shorter than the male urethra. Because of this, the female bladder is more likely to become infected by bacteria traveling up the urethra.**

Normal changes of aging include:

- The ability of kidneys to filter blood decreases.
- Bladder muscle tone weakens.
- Bladder holds less urine, which causes more frequent urination.
- Bladder may not empty completely, causing more chance of infection.

How You Can Help: NA's Role

Encourage residents to drink fluids. Offer frequent trips to the bathroom. If residents are incontinent, do not show frustration or anger. Keep residents clean and dry.

OBSERVING AND REPORTING
Urinary System

Observe and report these signs and symptoms:

- weight loss or gain
- swelling in the upper or lower extremities
- pain or burning during urination
- changes in urine, such as cloudiness, odor, or color
- changes in frequency and amount of urination
- swelling in the abdominal/bladder area
- complaints that bladder feels full or painful
- incontinence/dribbling
- pain in the kidney or back/flank region
- inadequate fluid intake

Tiny stones can be a big pain.

A kidney stone is a hard mass developed from crystals that separate from the urine and build up on the inner surfaces of the kidney. The stones themselves are also called renal calculi. They can block a ureter, which can cause extreme pain. Urine production may be decreased during a blockage because of a reflex that causes tiny vessels in the kidney to get smaller or constrict.

8. Describe the gastrointestinal system

The gastrointestinal (GI) system, also called the digestive system, has two functions:

1. **Digestion** is the process of breaking down food so that it can be absorbed into the cells.
2. **Elimination** is the process of expelling solid wastes that are not absorbed into the cells.

The GI system is made up of the alimentary canal and the other digestive organs (Fig. 9-15).

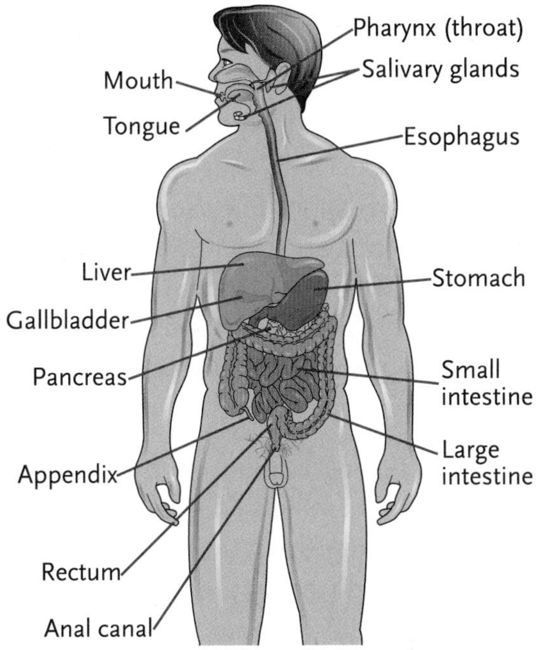

***Fig. 9-15.* The GI system consists of all the organs needed to digest food and process waste.**

The alimentary canal is a long passageway extending from the mouth to the anus, the opening of the rectum. Food passes from the mouth through the pharynx, esophagus, stomach, small intestine, large intestine, and out of the body as solid waste. The teeth, tongue, salivary glands, liver, gall bladder, and pancreas are the accessory organs to digestion. They help prepare the food so it can be absorbed.

Food is first placed in the mouth. The teeth chew it by cutting it, then chopping and grinding it into smaller pieces that can be swallowed. Saliva moistens the food and begins chemical digestion. The tongue helps with chewing and swallowing by pushing the food around between the teeth and then into the pharynx.

The pharynx is a muscular structure located at the back of the mouth. It extends into the throat. It contracts with swallowing and pushes food into the esophagus. The muscles of the esophagus then move food into the stomach through involuntary contractions called peristalsis.

The stomach is a muscular pouch located in the upper left part of the abdominal cavity. It provides physical digestion by stirring and churning the food to break it down into smaller particles. The glands in the stomach lining aid in digestion. They secrete gastric juices that chemically break down food. This process turns food into a semi-liquid substance called chyme. Peristalsis continues in the stomach, pushing the chyme into the small intestine.

The small intestine is about twenty feet long. Here enzymes secreted by the liver and the pancreas finish digesting the chyme. Bile, a green liquid produced by the liver, is stored in the gallbladder and released into the small intestine. Bile helps break down dietary fat. The liver converts fats and sugars into glucose, a sugar that can be carried to cells by the blood. The liver also stores glucose. The pancreas produces insulin, an enzyme that regulates the body's conversion of sugar into glucose.

The chyme is moved by peristalsis through the small intestine. There villi, tiny projections lining the small intestine, absorb the digested food into the capillaries.

Peristalsis moves the chyme that has not been digested through the large intestine. In the large intestine most of the water in the chyme is absorbed. What remains is feces, a semi-solid material of water, solid waste material, bacteria, and mucus. Feces passes by peristalsis through the rectum, the lower end of the colon. It moves out of the body through the anus, the rectal opening.

Normal changes of aging include:

- Saliva and digestive fluids decrease.
- Difficulty chewing and swallowing may occur.
- Absorption of vitamins and minerals decreases.
- Process of digestion is less efficient, causing more frequent constipation.

How You Can Help: NA's Role

Encourage fluids and nutritious, appealing meals. Allow time to eat. Make mealtime enjoyable. Provide good oral care. Make sure dentures fit properly and are cleaned regularly. Encourage daily bowel movements. Give residents the opportunity to have a bowel movement around the same time each day.

OBSERVING AND REPORTING

Gastrointestinal System

Observe and report these signs and symptoms:

- difficulty swallowing or chewing (including denture problems, tooth pain, or mouth sores)
- fecal incontinence (losing control of bowels)
- weight gain/weight loss
- anorexia (loss of appetite)
- abdominal pain and cramping
- diarrhea
- nausea and vomiting (especially vomitus that looks like coffee grounds)
- constipation
- gas
- hiccups, belching
- abnormally-colored stool (bloody, black, or hard)
- heartburn
- poor nutritional intake

9. Describe the endocrine system

The endocrine system is made up of glands that secrete hormones. Hormones are chemicals that control many of the organs and body systems (Fig. 9-16).

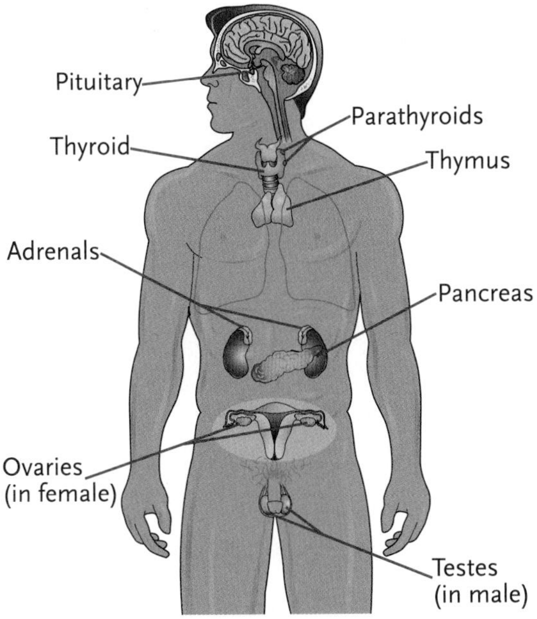

Fig. 9-16. **The endocrine system includes organs that produce hormones that regulate body processes.**

Hormones are carried in blood to the organs. Hormones regulate the body's processes, including:

- maintaining homeostasis
- influencing growth and development
- regulating levels of sugar in the blood
- regulating levels of calcium in the bones
- regulating the body's ability to reproduce
- determining how fast cells burn food for energy

The pituitary gland is located behind the eyes at the base of the brain. It is called the "master" gland. It secretes key hormones that cause other glands to produce other hormones. Some hormones secreted by the pituitary gland are:

- growth hormone, which regulates growth and development
- antidiuretic hormone (ADH), which controls the balance of fluids in the body
- oxytocin, which causes the uterus to contract during and after childbirth

It also produces hormones that regulate the thyroid gland and the adrenal glands.

The thyroid gland is located in the neck in front of the larynx. It produces thyroid hormone, which regulates metabolism, the burning of food for heat and energy.

The parathyroid glands secrete a hormone that regulates the body's use of calcium. Nerves and muscles require calcium to function smoothly. A deficiency of this hormone can cause severe muscle contractions and spasms. It can be fatal if untreated.

The pancreas, a gland located in the upper mid-section of the abdomen, secretes insulin. Insulin is a hormone that regulates the amount of sugar (glucose) available to the cells for metabolism. The cells cannot absorb sugar without insulin.

Two adrenal glands are located at the tops of the kidneys. They produce hormones that are essential to life. These hormones are important because they help the body

1. regulate carbohydrate metabolism
2. control the body's reaction to inflammation and stress
3. regulate salt and water absorption in the kidneys

Adrenal glands also produce the hormone adrenaline. It regulates muscle power, heart rate, blood pressure, and energy levels during stressful situations or emergencies.

Gonads, or sex glands, produce hormones that regulate the body's ability to reproduce. The testes in the male secrete testosterone. The ovaries in the female secrete estrogen and progesterone.

Normal changes of aging include:

- Levels of hormones, such as estrogen and progesterone, decrease.
- Insulin production lessens.
- Body is less able to handle stress.

How You Can Help: NA's Role

Encourage proper nutrition. Remove or reduce stressors. Stressors are anything that causes stress. Offer encouragement and listen to residents.

OBSERVING AND REPORTING
Endocrine System

Many endocrine illnesses can be treated with hormone supplements. These supplements must be given very precisely. For example, too much insulin administered to a diabetic can cause the sudden start of insulin shock.

Observe and report these symptoms:

- headache*
- weakness*
- blurred vision*
- dizziness*
- hunger*
- irritability*
- sweating/excessive perspiration*
- change in "normal" behavior*
- increased confusion*
- weight gain/weight loss
- loss of appetite/increased appetite
- increased thirst
- frequent urination
- dry skin
- sluggishness or fatigue
- hyperactivity

* indicates signs and symptoms that should be reported immediately

10. Describe the reproductive system

The reproductive system is made up of the reproductive organs. They are different in men and women. The reproductive system allows human beings to reproduce, or create new human life. Reproduction begins when a male's and female's sex cells (sperm and ovum) join. These sex cells are formed in the male and female sex glands. These sex glands are called the gonads.

The Male Reproductive System

In the male, the sex glands or gonads are the testes or testicles. The two oval glands are located outside the body in the scrotum. The scrotum is a sac made of skin and muscle. It is suspended between the thighs. The testes produce the male sex cells, called sperm, and testosterone (Fig. 9-17).

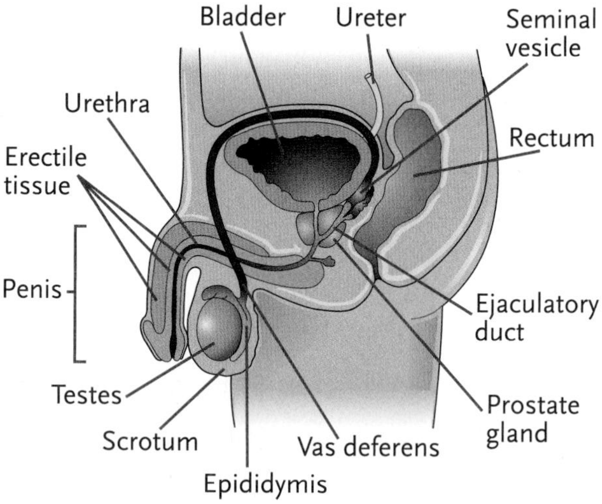

Fig. 9-17. **The male reproductive system.**

Testosterone is the male hormone needed for the reproductive organs to function properly. Testosterone also promotes development of male secondary sex characteristics. These include:

- facial hair
- pubic and underarm hair
- hair on the chest, legs, and arms
- deepening of the voice
- development of muscle mass

Sperm travel from the testes through a coiled tube, the epididymis, and another tube called the vas deferens. Sperm then pass into the seminal vesicle where semen is produced. Semen carries sperm out of the body.

The ducts coming from each seminal vesicle unite to form the ejaculatory ducts. They pass through the prostate gland, where more fluid is added to the semen. In the prostate, the ejaculatory ducts join the urethra, the tube through which both urine and semen pass. The urethra continues through the penis, the sex organ located outside the body, in front of the scrotum. The penis is composed of erectile tissue that becomes filled with blood during sexual excitement. As the penis fills with blood, it becomes enlarged and erect. It then can enter the vagina, the female reproductive tract, where semen containing sperm is released.

The Female Reproductive System

In the human female, the gonads are two oval glands called the ovaries. There are two ovaries, one on each side of the uterus. The ovaries make the female sex cells or eggs (ova). They release the female hormones, estrogen and progesterone. Each month from puberty to menopause, an egg is released from an ovary (Fig. 9-18). Menopause is when a female stops having menstrual periods.

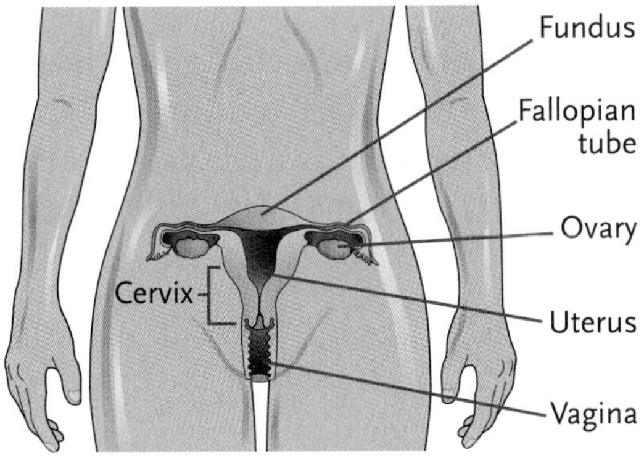

Fig. 9-18. **The female reproductive system.**

This cycle is maintained by estrogen and progesterone. These hormones control development of female secondary sex characteristics. These include:

- increased breast size
- wider and rounder hips
- axillary and pubic hair
- a slightly deeper voice

Once an egg is released from an ovary, it travels through the fallopian tube to the uterus. The uterus is a hollow, pear-shaped, muscular organ. It is located within the pelvis. It lies behind the bladder and in front of the rectum. If sexual intercourse takes place while the egg is in the fallopian tube, the egg may be fertilized by sperm in the fallopian tube. The fertilized egg then travels down into the uterus. It implants in the endometrium, the lining of the uterus. Stimulated by hormones, the endometrium builds up during the menstrual cycle. It has many blood vessels supplying it for the growth and feeding of an embryo. If the egg is not fertilized, the hormones decrease. The blood supply to the endometrium decreases. The endometrium then breaks up in a process called menstruation.

The main section of the uterus is the fundus. This is where a baby develops after the fertilized egg is implanted. The narrow neck of the uterus extending into the vagina is the cervix. The cervix has an opening through which menstrual fluid can pass and semen can enter the vagina. The vagina is the muscular canal that opens to the outside of the body. The external vaginal opening is partially closed by the hymen membrane. The vagina is kept moist by secretions from glands in the vaginal walls. The vagina receives the penis during sexual intercourse. It also serves as the birth canal. The baby passes through the cervix, which is made thin by pressure from the baby's head during contractions. Once the cervix opens, the baby can then move out through the vagina.

Normal changes of aging include:

Female

- Menstruation ends.
- Decrease in estrogen leads to loss of calcium. This causes brittle bones and, potentially, osteoporosis.
- Vaginal walls become drier and thinner.

Male

- Sperm production decreases.
- Prostate gland enlarges.

How You Can Help: NA's Role

Sexual needs continue as people age. Provide privacy whenever necessary for sexual activity. Respect your residents' sexual needs. Never make fun of or judge any sexual behavior.

OBSERVING AND REPORTING
Reproductive System

Observe and report these signs and symptoms:

- discomfort or difficulty with urination
- discharge from the penis or vagina
- swelling of the genitals
- changes in menstruation
- blood in urine or stool
- breast changes, including size, shape, lumps, or discharge from the nipple
- sores on the genitals
- resident reports of impotence, or inability of male to have sexual intercourse
- resident reports of painful intercourse

Sexual Expression and Privacy

Residents have the right to sexual freedom and expression. Residents have the right to privacy and to meet their sexual needs.

11. Describe the immune and lymphatic systems

The immune system protects the body from disease-causing bacteria, viruses, and organisms. The immune system protects the body in two ways:

1. Nonspecific immunity protects the body from disease in general.
2. Specific immunity protects against a particular disease that is invading the body at a given time.

Nonspecific Immunity

To protect itself against disease in general, the body has several defenses:

- Anatomic barriers include the skin and the mucous membranes. They provide a physical barrier to keep foreign materials—bacteria, viruses, or organisms—from invading the body. Saliva, tears, and mucus secretions also help protect the body by washing away substances.
- Physiologic barriers include body temperature and acidity of certain organs. Most organisms that cause disease cannot survive high temperatures or high acidity. When the body senses foreign organisms, it can raise its temperature (by running a fever) to kill off the invaders. The acidity of organs like the stomach keeps harmful bacteria from growing there.
- Inflammatory response refers to the body's ability to fight infection by inflammation or swelling of an infected area. When inflammation occurs, it indicates that the body has sent extra disease-fighting cells and extra blood to the infected area to fight the infection.

Bacteria beware.

The body protects itself against things that could cause harm if absorbed into the bloodstream. The lymphatic system kills many bacteria. Vomiting and diarrhea, symptoms of a GI system problem, are other responses that rid the body of irritating or harmful substances.

Specific Immunity

To protect itself against specific diseases, the body makes different types of cells that will fight a huge range of different invaders. Once it has successfully eliminated an invader, the immune system records the invasion in the form of antibodies. Antibodies are carried within cells. They prevent a disease from threatening the body a second time.

Acquired immunity is a kind of specific immunity. The body acquires it either by fighting an infection or by vaccination. For example, you can acquire immunity to a disease like the measles in two ways:

1. You get the measles. Your body forms antibodies to the disease to make sure you will not get it again; or
2. You get a vaccine for the measles. This causes your body to produce the same antibodies to protect you from the disease.

Hepatitis B vaccine

The three-step hepatitis B vaccine is normally given free of charge to NAs and other healthcare workers. When you begin your job, your employer must offer you the chance to take the vaccine. You must return for the second and third dose for maximum immunity.

The lymphatic system removes excess fluids and waste products from the body's tissues. It also helps the immune system fight infection. It is closely related to both the immune and the circulatory systems (Fig. 9-19).

The lymphatic system consists of lymph vessels and lymph capillaries in which a fluid called lymph circulates. Lymph is a clear yellowish fluid that carries disease-fighting cells called lymphocytes.

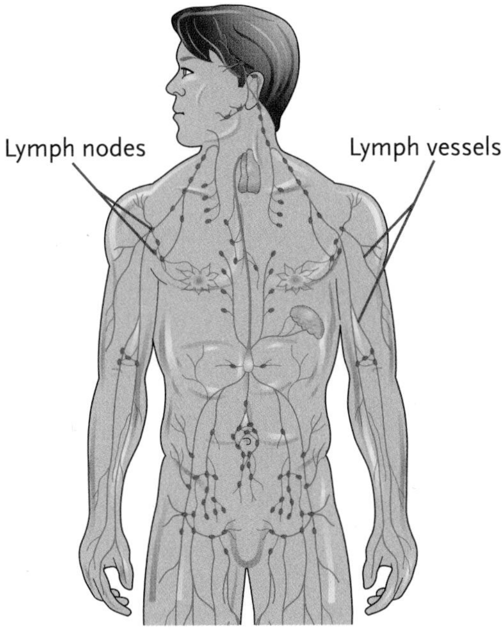

Fig. 9-19. **Lymph nodes are located throughout the body.**

When the body is fighting an infection, swelling may occur in the lymph nodes. These are oval-shaped bodies that can be as small as a pinhead or as large as an almond. Located in the neck, groin, and armpits, the lymph nodes filter out germs and waste products carried from the tissues by the lymph fluid. After lymph fluid has been purified in the lymph nodes, it flows into the bloodstream.

Unlike the circulatory system, in which the heart functions as a pump to move the blood, the lymph system has no pump. Lymph fluid is circulated by muscle activity, massage, and breathing. A sore muscle may feel better if you rub it. The rubbing action helps the lymph fluid circulate, carrying waste products away from the tired muscle.

Normal changes of aging include:

- Increased risk of all types of infections
- Decreased response to vaccines

How You Can Help: NA's Role

Follow rules for preventing infection. Wash hands often. Keep the resident's environment clean to prevent infection. Encourage and help with good personal hygiene. Encourage proper nutrition and fluid intake.

OBSERVING AND REPORTING
Immune and Lymphatic Systems

Observe and report these signs and symptoms:

- recurring infections (such as fevers and diarrhea)
- swelling of the lymph nodes
- increased fatigue

12. Define terms relating to position and location

It is important to be able to identify where an area or specific body part is located. Terms that deal with location and position may help you understand how body structures relate to each other. Some locations of the body are listed below:

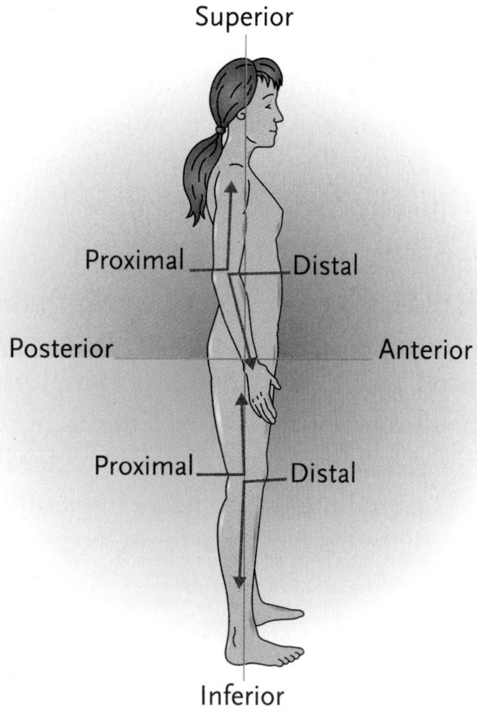

***Fig. 9-20.* Directions of the body.**

Superior: above, or higher
Example: The lungs are superior (above) to the knees.

Inferior: below, or lower
Example: The knees are inferior (below) to the lungs.

Anterior: toward the front
Example: The navel is on the anterior (front) surface of body.

Posterior: toward the back
Example: The buttocks are on the posterior (back) surface of body.

Ventral: toward the front
Example: The navel is on the ventral (toward the front) surface side of the body.

Dorsal: toward the back
Example: The buttocks are on the dorsal (toward the back) surface of the body.

Medial: toward the midline
Example: The lungs are medial to (at the midline of) the arms.

Lateral: away from the midline
Example: The arms are lateral to (away from midline of) the lungs.

Internal: within, or interior to
Example: The heart is internal (within, interior) to the rib cage.

External: outside, or exterior to
Example: The lips are external (outside, exterior) to the tonsils.

Superficial: toward the surface
Example: The skin is superficial (surface) to the ribs.

Deep: within, or interior to
Example: The ribs are deep (away from surface of) to the skin.

Central: the main part
Example: The brain is part of the central (main part of) nervous system.

Peripheral: extending from the main part
Example: Nerves in the arm are part of the peripheral (extending from main part of) nervous system.

Proximal: closer to the origin
Example: The shoulder is proximal (nearer to point of attachment) to the elbow.

Distal: further from the origin
Example: The elbow is distal (further to point of attachment) to the shoulder.

Parietal: pertaining to the wall
Example: The parietal pleura lines the chest cavity.

Visceral: pertaining to the organs
Example: The visceral pleura covers the lungs.

Chapter Review

1. What is homeostasis?
2. What does it mean to say that the skin is a "sense organ?"
3. List five signs and symptoms to observe and report about the integumentary system.
4. How many bones make up the skeleton of the human body?
5. What type of exercises can help prevent contractures and muscle atrophy?
6. List five signs and symptoms to observe and report about the musculoskeletal system.
7. What are two functions of the nervous system?
8. List nine signs and symptoms to observe and report about the nervous system.
9. List three signs and symptoms to observe and report about the eyes and ears.
10. What are four functions of the circulatory system?
11. List seven signs and symptoms to observe and report about the circulatory system.
12. What does "respiration" mean? What are the two parts involved in respiration?
13. List seven signs and symptoms to observe and report about the respiratory system.
14. What are two functions of the urinary system?
15. List seven signs and symptoms to observe and report about the urinary system.
16. What does "digestion" mean? What does "elimination" mean?
17. List nine signs and symptoms to observe and report about the gastrointestinal system.
18. List eight signs and symptoms to observe and report immediately about the endocrine system.
19. What is the function of the reproductive system?
20. List seven signs and symptoms to observe and report about the reproductive system.
21. What is the function of the lymphatic system?
22. List three signs and symptoms to observe and report about the immune system.
23. List and define ten terms relating to position and location.

Chapter 10
Moving, Lifting, and Positioning

1. Review the principles of body mechanics

You first learned about body mechanics in chapter 6. Always use good body mechanics when moving or positioning a resident. It helps protect both you and your residents. These ten rules will help you remember to use good body mechanics:

1. **Assess the load**. Before lifting, assess the weight of the load. Determine if you can safely move the object without help. Know the lift policies at your facility. Never attempt to lift someone you are not sure you can lift.
2. **Think ahead, plan, and communicate the move**. Check for any objects in your path. Look for any potential risks, such as a wet floor. Make sure the path is clear. Watch for hazards, like high-traffic areas, combative residents, or a loose toilet seat. Decide exactly what you are going to do together. Agree on the verbal cues you will use before attempting to transfer.
3. **Check your base of support. Be sure you have firm footing**. Use a wide but balanced stance to increase support. Keep this stance when walking. Have enough room to maintain a wide base of support. Make sure you and your resident wearing non-skid shoes.
4. **Face what you are lifting**. Your feet should always face the direction you are moving. Twisting at the waist increases the likelihood of injury.
5. **Keep your back straight**. Keep your head up and shoulders back. This will keep the back in the proper position. Take a deep breath to help you regain correct posture.
6. **Begin in a squatting position. Lift with your legs**. Bend at the hips and knees. Use the strength of your leg muscles to stand and lift the object. You will need to push your buttocks out to do this. Before you stand with the object you are lifting, remember that your legs, not your back, will enable you to lift. You should be able to feel your leg muscles work. Lift with the large leg muscles to decrease stress on the back.
7. **Tighten your stomach muscles when beginning the lift**. This will help to take weight off the spine and maintain alignment.
8. **Keep the object close to your body**. This decreases stress to your back. Lift objects to your waist. Carrying them any higher can affect your balance.

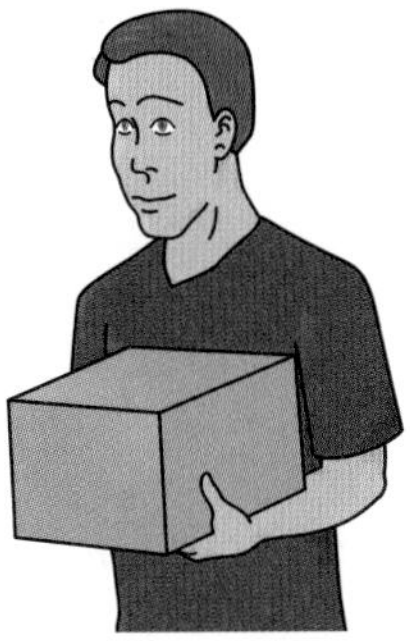

Fig. 10-1. Keeping objects close while carrying them decreases stress on the back.

9. **Do not twist.** Turn and face the area you are moving the object to. Then set the object down. Twisting increases the stress on your back. It should always be avoided.
10. **Push or pull when possible rather than lifting.** When you lift an object, you must overcome gravity to balance the load. Try to push or pull the object instead. Then you only need to overcome the friction between the surface and the object. Use your body weight to move the object, not your lifting muscles. Push rather than pull whenever possible. Stay close to the object.

2. Explain beginning and ending steps in care procedures

Within most care procedures, there are beginning and ending steps that are repeated. Understand why each step is important. It will help you remember to perform them every time care is provided.

Beginning Steps

Wash your hands. Handwashing provides for infection control. Nothing fights infection like consistent, proper handwashing.

Identify yourself by name. Identify the resident by name. Residents have the right to know the identity of their caregivers. Addressing residents by name shows respect (Fig. 10-2). It also establishes correct identification. This prevents care from being performed on the wrong person.

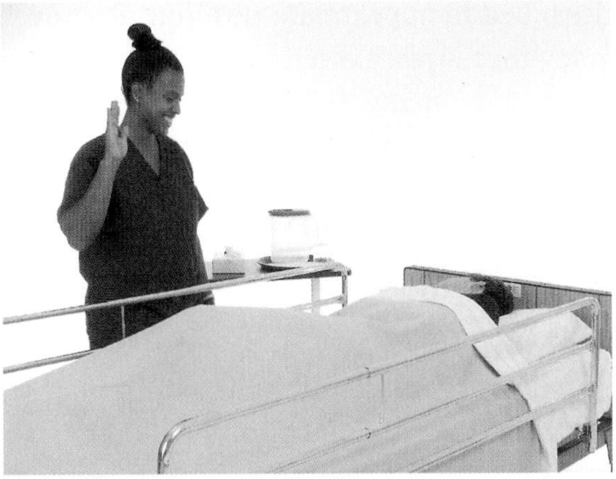

Fig. 10-2. Identify yourself to each resident. Identify each resident before performing care.

Explain procedure to the resident. Speak clearly, slowly, and directly. Maintain face-to-face contact whenever possible. Residents have a right to know exactly what care you will provide. This also promotes understanding, cooperation, and independence. Encouraging residents' independence is important. Residents are more able to do things for themselves if they know what needs to happen.

Provide for the resident's privacy with curtain, screen, or door. Doing this maintains residents' rights to privacy and dignity. Providing for privacy is not simply a courtesy; it is a legal right.

If the bed is adjustable, adjust bed to a safe level, usually waist high. If the bed is movable, lock bed wheels. This prevents injury to you and to residents. Locking bed wheels is an important safety measure. It ensures that the bed will not move as you are performing care.

Ending Steps

Make resident comfortable. Make sure sheets are free from wrinkles and the bed free from crumbs. Sheets that are damp, wrinkled, or bunched up are uncomfortable to be on. They may prevent the resident from resting or sleeping well. Sheets that do not lie flat under the resident's body increase the risk of pressure sores because they cut off circulation. Other comfort measures include replacing bedding and pillows.

Return bed to appropriate position. Remove privacy measures. Lowering the bed provides for residents' safety. In some facilities, the bed will be returned to the lowest position. Remove any extra privacy measures added during the procedure. This includes anything you may have draped over and around residents, as well as privacy screens.

Before leaving, place call light within resident's reach. A call light allows residents to communicate with staff as necessary. Remember that the decision not to respond to a call light is considered neglect. Unless residents are on fluid restrictions, provide fresh water before leaving the room. Keeping beverages close by encourages residents to drink more often. Make sure that the pitcher and cup are light enough for residents to lift.

Wash your hands. Again, handwashing is the most important thing you can to do to prevent the spread of infection.

Report any changes in resident to the nurse. Reporting promptly and accurately provides the nurse with information to assess resident. Care plans are made based on your reports.

Document procedure using facility guidelines. What you write is a legal record of what you did. If you do not document it, legally it did not happen.

3. Explain why position changes are important for bedbound residents and describe five basic positions

Residents who spend a lot of time in bed often need help getting into comfortable positions. They also need to change positions periodically. Too much pressure on one area for too long can cause a decrease in circulation. This increases the risk of pressure sores and other problems like muscle contractures. Constant pressure causes the greatest risk of pressure sores, a major problem in nursing homes. You will learn much more about pressure sores and prevention in chapter 13.

Positioning means helping residents into positions that will be comfortable and healthy for them. Bedbound residents should be repositioned every two hours. Document the position and time every time there is a change. The care plan will give specific instructions. Always keep principles of body mechanics and alignment in mind when positioning residents. Also, check skin for whiteness or redness, especially around bony areas, each time you reposition a resident.

These are tips for positioning residents in the five basic body positions:

1. **Supine**: In this position, the resident lies flat on his back. To maintain correct body position, support the head and shoulders with a pillow (Fig. 10-3). You may also use pillows, rolled towels, or washcloths to support his arms (especially a weak or immobilized arm) or hands. The heels should be "floating." This means you must place a firm pillow under the calves. The heels do not touch the bed. Pillows or a footboard can be used to keep the feet flexed.

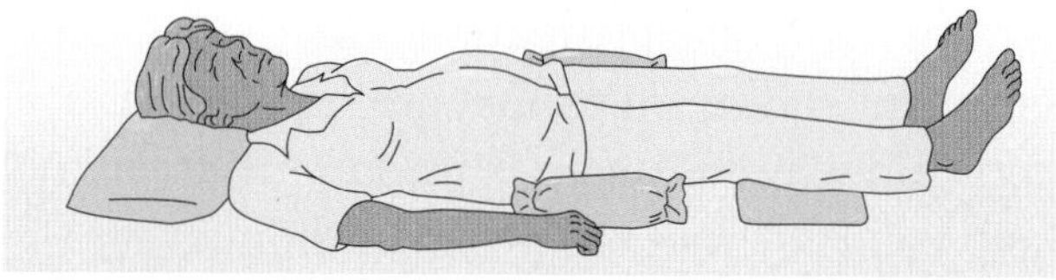

Fig. 10-3. **A person in the supine position is lying flat on his or her back.**

2. **Lateral/Side**: A resident in the lateral position is lying on either side. There are many ways to do this. Pillows can support the arm and leg on the upper side, the back, and the head (Fig. 10-4). Ideally, the knee on the upper side of the body should be flexed. The leg is brought in front of the body and supported on a pillow. There should be a pillow under the bottom foot. The toes should not touch the bed. If the top leg cannot be brought forward, it rests on the bottom leg. Pillows should be

used between the two legs. This relieves pressure and avoids skin breakdown.

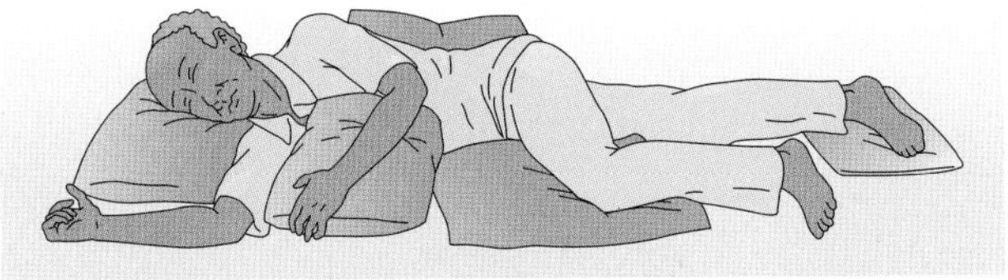

Fig. 10-4. **A person in the lateral position is lying on his or her side.**

3. **Prone**: A resident in the prone position is lying on the abdomen, or front side of the body (Fig. 10-5). This is not comfortable for many people, especially elderly people. Never leave a resident in a prone position for very long. In this position, the arms are either at the sides or raised above the head. The head is turned to one side. A small pillow may be used under the head and under the legs. This keeps the feet from touching the bed.

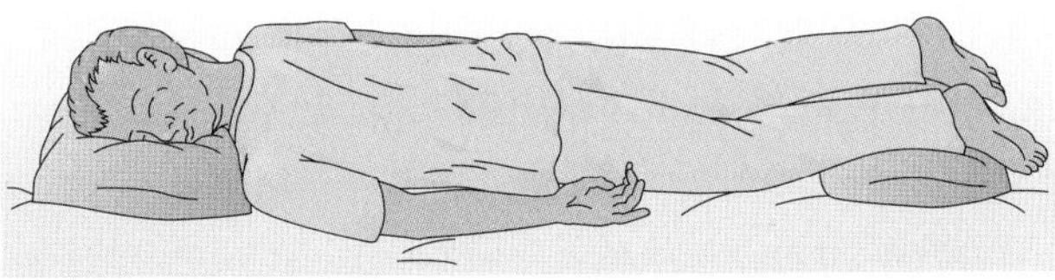

Fig. 10-5. **A person lying in the prone position is lying on his or her abdomen.**

4. **Fowler's**: A resident in the Fowler's position is in a semi-sitting position. The head and shoulders are elevated. The resident's knees may be flexed and elevated. Use a pillow or rolled blanket as a support (Fig. 10-6). The feet may be flexed and supported using a footboard or other support. The spine should be straight. In a true Fowler's position, the upper body is raised halfway between sitting straight up and lying flat. In a semi-Fowler's position, the upper body is not raised as high.

5. **Sims'**: The Sims' position is a left side-lying position. The lower arm is behind the back. The upper knee is flexed and raised toward the chest, using a pillow as support. There should be a pillow under the bottom foot so that the toes do not touch the bed (Fig. 10-7).

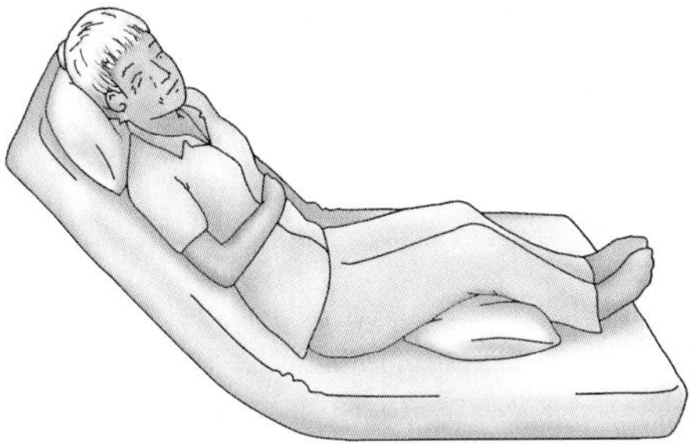

Fig. 10-6. **A person lying in the Fowler's position is partially reclined.**

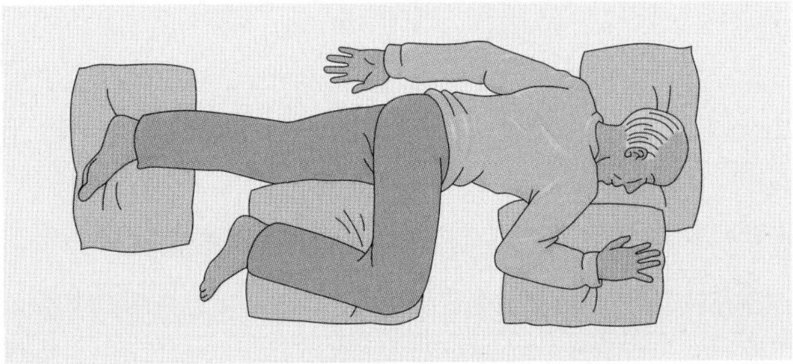

Fig. 10-7. **A person in the Sims' position is lying on his or her left side with one leg drawn up.**

The Trendelenburg and Reverse Trendelenburg are used with residents with special needs. For example, Trendelenburg may be used for a resident who has gone into shock and has poor blood flow (Fig. 10-8). Reverse Trendelenburg may be used for a resident who needs a faster emptying of the stomach due to a digestive problem (Fig. 10-9). These positions always require a doctor's order. Some electric beds have buttons or levers that place the bed in these two positions. You will learn more about beds in chapter 12.

Always check the skin for signs of irritation whenever you reposition a resident.

STOP

Safety, not speed!

Repositioning residents can be challenging. The simple act of turning a resident may break a bone, tear fragile skin, or pull on tubing. Be very careful when moving and positioning residents. Moving too quickly can cause serious injury and potential complications. Moving residents in a hasty or rough manner is abusive behavior.

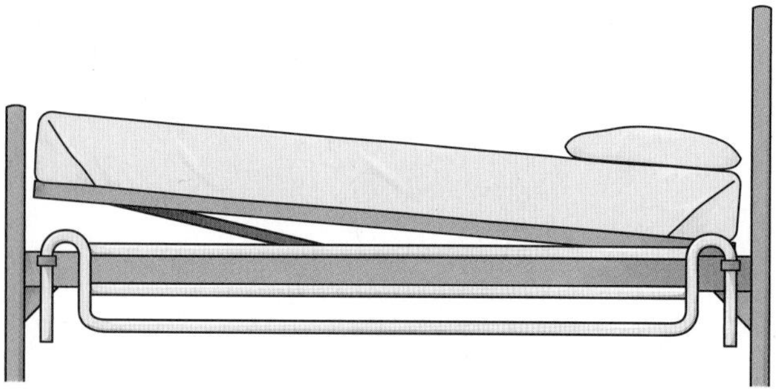

Fig. 10-8. **The Trendelenburg position. This position is only used with a doctor's order.**

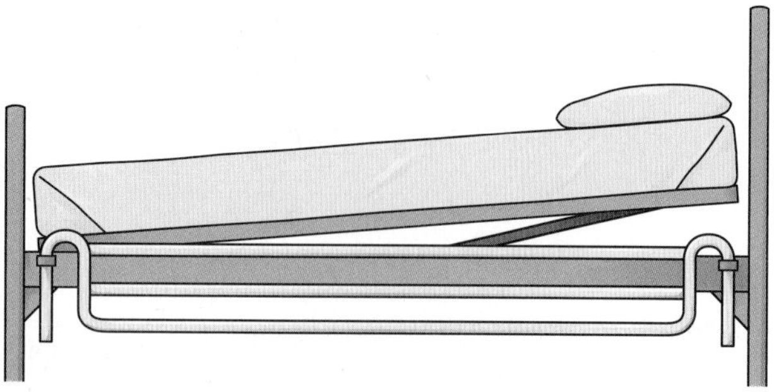

Fig. 10-9. **The Reverse Trendelenburg position. This position is only used with a doctor's order.**

Locking arms with a resident and raising head and shoulders

1. Wash your hands.
2. Identify yourself by name. Identify the resident by name.
3. Explain procedure to the resident. Speak clearly, slowly, and directly. Maintain face-to-face contact whenever possible.
4. Provide for the resident's privacy with curtain, screen, or door.
5. If the bed is adjustable, adjust bed to a safe level, usually waist high. Lock bed wheels.
6. Place pillow at the head of bed against the headboard.
7. Stand at the side of the bed. Face the head of bed.
8. Gently slide one hand under the resident's closest shoulder.
9. Gently slide the other hand under the resident's upper back.
10. At the count of three, slowly raise the resident's head and shoulders. Give necessary care (Fig. 10-10).

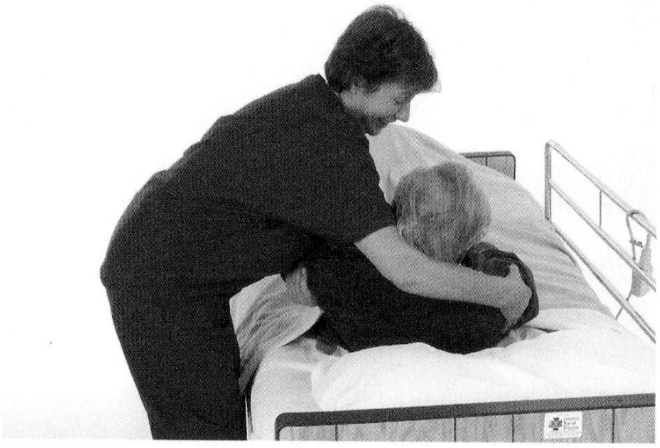

Fig. 10-10.

11. Replace pillow under the resident's head.
12. Make resident comfortable. Make sure sheets are free from wrinkles and the bed free from crumbs.
13. Return bed to appropriate position. Remove privacy measures.
14. Before leaving, place call light within resident's reach.
15. Wash your hands.
16. Report any changes in resident to the nurse.
17. Document procedure using facility guidelines.

Helping a resident move up in bed helps prevent skin irritation that can lead to pressure sores. You can use a helper if one is available. Get help if you think it is not safe to move the resident by yourself. If a resident cannot help you, use a draw sheet or turning sheet (Fig. 10-11). A **draw sheet** is an extra sheet placed on top of the bottom sheet. It allows you to reposition the resident without causing shearing. **Shearing** is friction and pressure on the skin from rubbing or dragging it across surfaces (the bottom sheet).

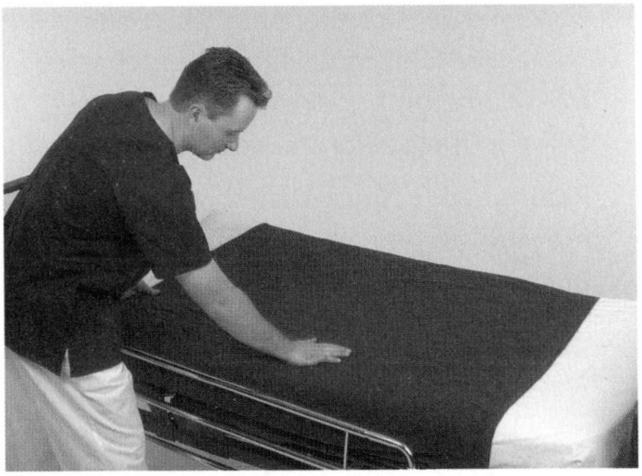

Fig. 10-11. **A draw sheet is a special sheet (or a regular bed sheet folded in half) is used to move residents in bed without causing shearing.**

Assisting a resident to move up in bed

1. Wash your hands.
2. Identify yourself by name. Identify the resident by name.
3. Explain procedure to the resident. Speak clearly, slowly, and directly. Maintain face-to-face contact whenever possible.
4. Provide for the resident's privacy with curtain, screen, or door.
5. If the bed is adjustable, adjust bed to a safe level, usually waist high. Lock bed wheels.
6. Lower the head of bed. Move pillow to head of the bed.
7. Lower the side rail (if not already lowered) on side nearest you.
8. Stand by bed with feet apart. Face the resident.
9. Place one arm under resident's shoulder blades. Place the other arm under resident's thighs.
10. Ask resident to bend knees, brace feet on mattress, and push feet on the count of three.
11. On three, shift body weight. Move resident while resident pushes with her feet (Fig. 10-12).

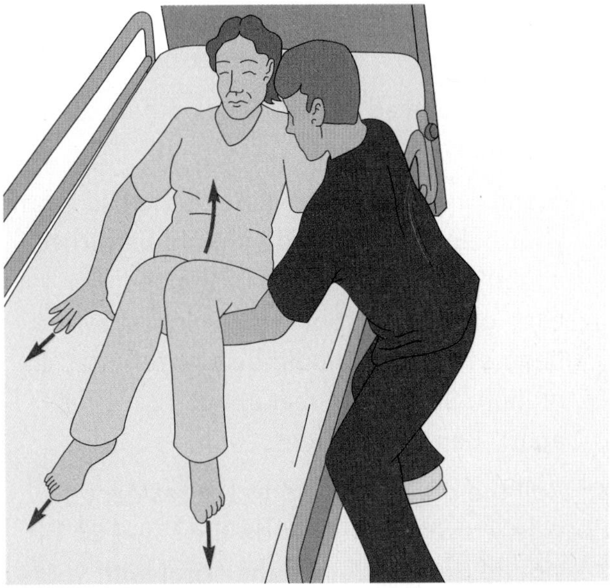

Fig. 10-12. **Keep your back straight and your knees bent.**

12. Place pillow under resident's head.
13. Make resident comfortable. Make sure sheets are free from wrinkles and the bed free from crumbs.
14. Return bed to appropriate position. Remove privacy measures.
15. Before leaving, place call light within resident's reach.
16. Wash your hands.
17. Report any changes in resident to the nurse.
18. Document procedure using facility guidelines.

Assisting a resident to move up in bed with one assistant (using draw sheet)

Equipment: draw sheet

1. Wash your hands.
2. Identify yourself by name. Identify the resident by name.
3. Explain procedure to the resident. Speak clearly, slowly, and directly. Maintain face-to-face contact whenever possible.
4. Provide for the resident's privacy with curtain, screen, or door.

5. If the bed is adjustable, adjust bed to a safe level, usually waist high. Lock bed wheels.
6. Lower the head of bed. Move pillow to head of the bed.
7. Stand on the opposite side of the bed from your helper. Each of you should be turned slightly toward the head of the bed. For each of you, the foot that is closest to the head of the bed should be pointed that direction. Stand with feet about 12 inches apart. Bend your knees.
8. Roll the draw sheet up to the resident's side. Have your helper do the same on his side of the bed. Grasp the sheet with your palms up. Have your helper do the same.
9. Shift your weight to your back foot (the foot closer to the foot of the bed). Have your helper do the same (Fig. 10-13). On the count of three, both shift your weight to your forward feet. Slide the resident toward the head of the bed (Fig. 10-14).

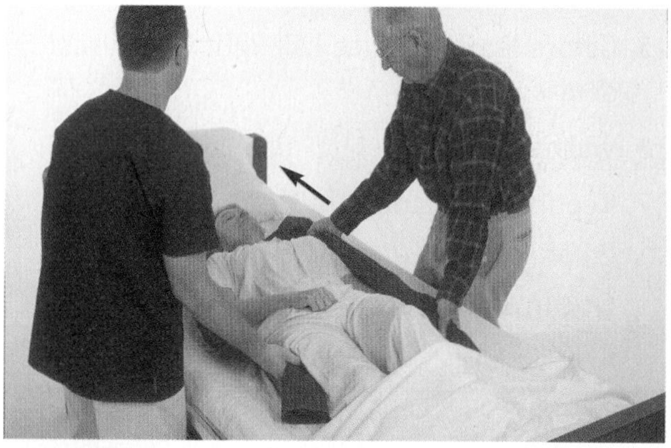

Fig. 10-13.

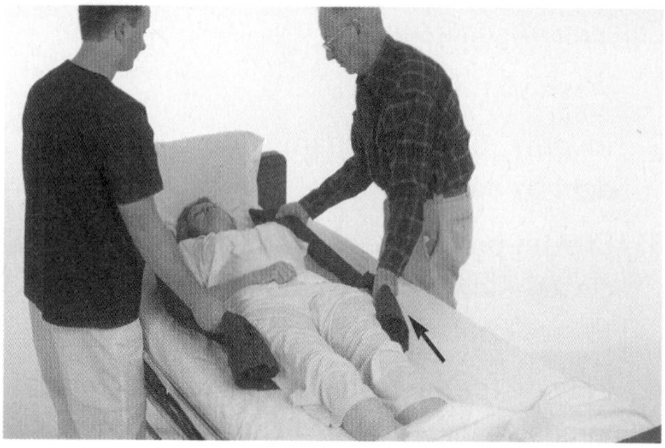

Fig. 10-14.

10. Make resident comfortable. Make sure sheets are free from wrinkles and the bed free from crumbs. Unroll the draw sheet. Leave it in place for the next repositioning.
11. Return bed to appropriate position. Remove privacy measures.
12. Before leaving, place call light within resident's reach.
13. Wash your hands.
14. Report any changes in resident to the nurse.
15. Document procedure using facility guidelines.

Moving a resident to the side of the bed

1. Wash your hands.
2. Identify yourself by name. Identify the resident by name.
3. Explain procedure to the resident. Speak clearly, slowly, and directly. Maintain face-to-face contact whenever possible.
4. Provide for the resident's privacy with curtain, screen, or door.
5. If the bed is adjustable, adjust bed to a safe level, usually waist high. Lock bed wheels.
6. Lower the head of bed.
7. Gently slide your hands under the head and shoulders and move toward you (Fig. 10-15). Gently slide your hands under midsection and move toward you. Gently slide your hands under hips and legs and move toward you (Fig. 10-16).
8. Make resident comfortable. Make sure sheets are free from wrinkles and the bed free from crumbs.
9. Return bed to appropriate position. Remove privacy measures.
10. Before leaving, place call light within resident's reach.
11. Wash your hands.

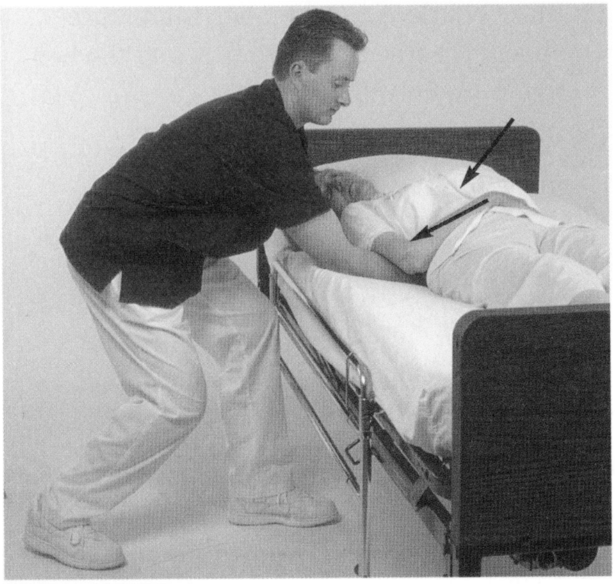

Fig. 10-15.

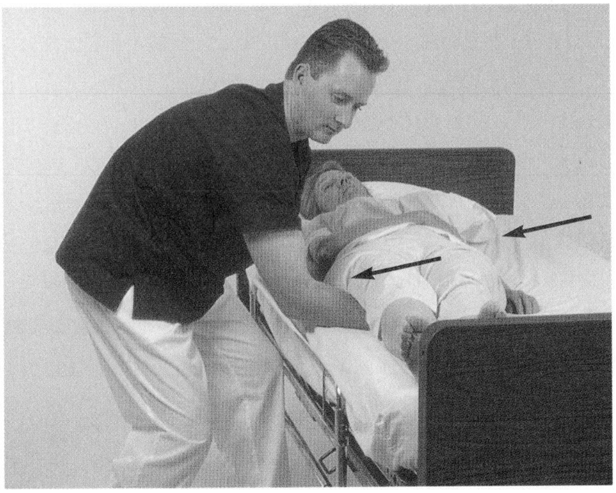

Fig. 10-16.

12. Report any changes in resident to the nurse.
13. Document procedure using facility guidelines.

Turning a resident

1. Wash your hands.
2. Identify yourself by name. Identify the resident by name.
3. Explain procedure to the resident. Speak clearly, slowly, and directly. Maintain face-to-face contact whenever possible.
4. Provide for the resident's privacy with curtain, screen, or door.
5. If the bed is adjustable, adjust bed to a safe level, usually waist high. Lock bed wheels.
6. Lower the head of bed.
7. Stand on side of bed opposite to where person will be turned. The far side rail should be raised.
8. Lower side rail nearest you.
9. Move resident to side of bed nearest you using previous procedure.

Turning resident away from you:

10. Cross resident's arm over his or her chest. Cross the leg nearest you over the far leg.

    a. Stand with feet about 12 inches apart. Bend your knees.

    b. Place one hand on the resident's shoulder. Place the other hand on the resident's nearest hip.

    c. Gently push the resident toward the other side of the bed. Shift your weight from your back leg to your front leg (Fig. 10-17).

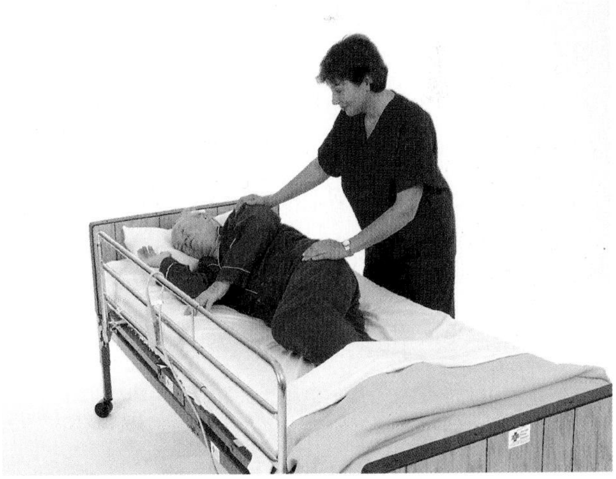

Fig. 10-17.

Turning resident toward you:

10. Cross resident's arm over his or her chest. Cross the leg furthest from you over the near leg.

    a. Raise both side rails.

    b. Stand with feet about 12 inches apart. Bend your knees.

c. Place one hand on the resident's far shoulder. Place the other hand on the resident's far hip.

d. Gently roll the resident toward you (Fig. 10-18).

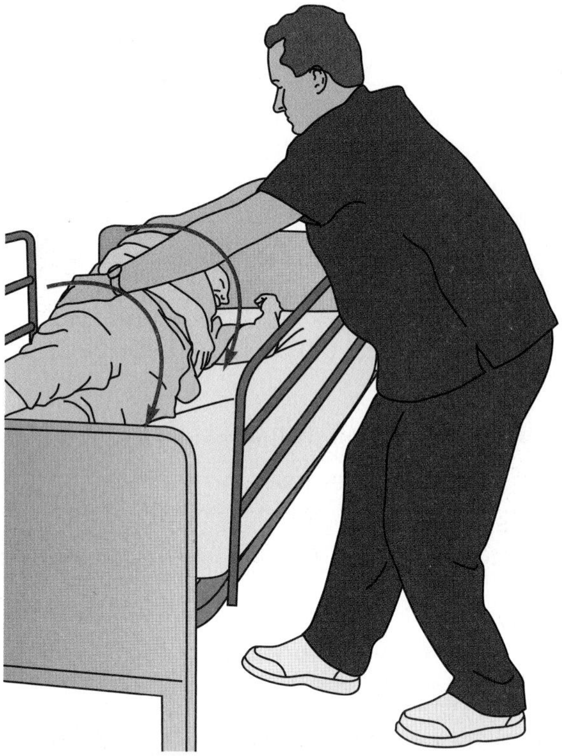

Fig. 10-18.

12. Position resident properly. Use proper body alignment:

- head supported by pillow
- shoulder adjusted so resident is not lying on arm
- top arm supported by pillow
- back supported by supportive device
- top knee flexed
- top leg supported by supportive device with hip in proper alignment (Fig. 10-19)

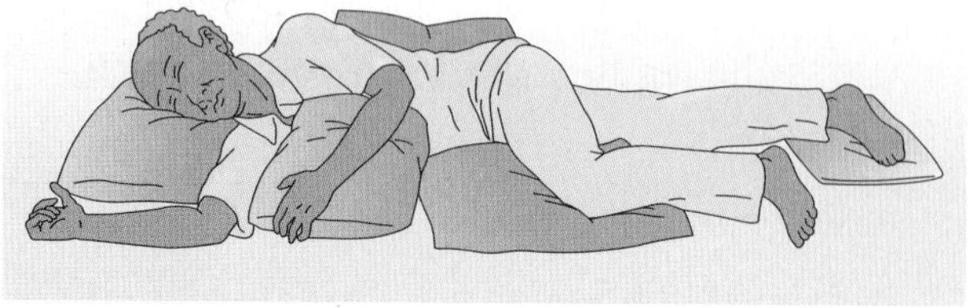

Fig. 10-19.

12. Make resident comfortable. Make sure sheets are free from wrinkles and the bed free from crumbs.
13. Return bed to appropriate position. Remove privacy measures.
14. Before leaving, place call light within resident's reach.
15. Wash your hands.
16. Report any changes in resident to the nurse.
17. Document procedure using facility guidelines.

Logrolling means moving a resident as a unit, without disturbing the alignment of the body. The head, back and legs must be kept in a straight line. This is necessary in case of neck or back problems, spinal cord injuries, or back or hip surgeries. A draw sheet helps with moving. Be very careful when logrolling residents. Stand next to the bed to prevent the resident from rolling out of bed.

Logrolling a resident with one assistant

Equipment: draw sheet

1. Wash your hands.
2. Identify yourself by name. Identify the resident by name.
3. Explain procedure to the resident. Speak clearly, slowly, and directly. Maintain face-to-face contact whenever possible.
4. Provide for the resident's privacy with curtain, screen, or door.
5. If the bed is adjustable, adjust bed to a safe level, usually waist high. Lock bed wheels.
6. Lower the head of bed.
7. Lower the side rail on side nearest you.
8. Both co-workers stand on the same side of the bed. One person stands at the resident's head and shoulders. The other stands near the resident's midsection.

9. Place the resident's arms across his or her chest. Place a pillow between the knees.
10. Stand with feet about 12 inches apart. Bend your knees.
11. Grasp the draw sheet on the far side (Fig. 10-20).

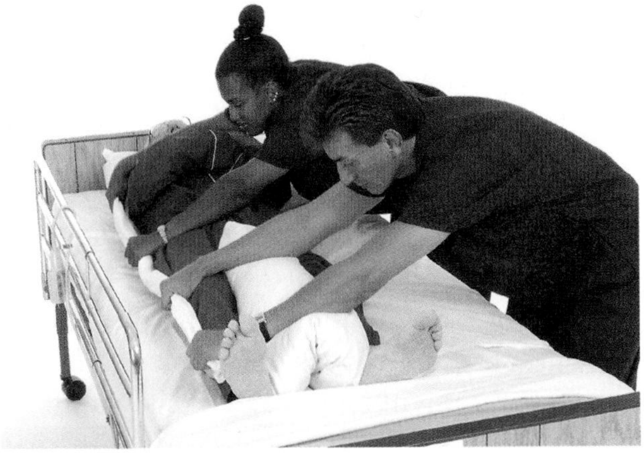

Fig. 10-20.

12. On the count of three, gently roll the resident toward you. Turn the resident as a unit (Fig. 10-21).

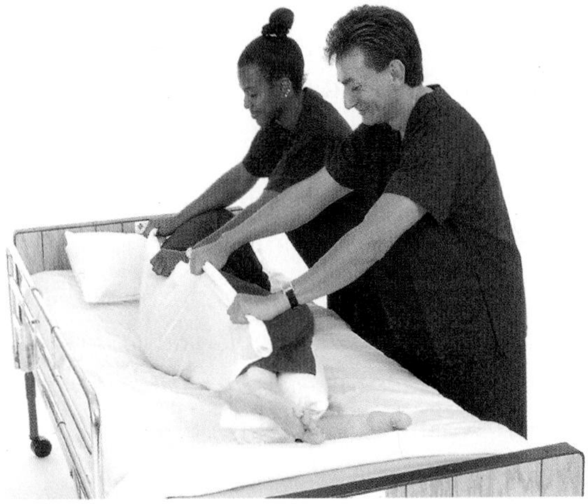

Fig. 10-21.

13. Make resident comfortable. Make sure sheets are free from wrinkles and the bed free from crumbs.
14. Return bed to appropriate position. Remove privacy measures.
15. Before leaving, place call light within resident's reach.
16. Wash your hands.
17. Report any changes in resident to the nurse.
18. Document procedure using facility guidelines.

Before a resident who has been lying down stands up, she should dangle. To **dangle** means to sit up with the feet over the side of the bed to regain balance. For residents unable to walk, dangling the legs for a few minutes may be ordered.

Assisting a resident to sit up on side of bed: dangling

1. Wash your hands.
2. Identify yourself by name. Identify the resident by name.
3. Explain procedure to the resident. Speak clearly, slowly, and directly. Maintain face-to-face contact whenever possible.
4. Provide for the resident's privacy with curtain, screen, or door.
5. Adjust bed height to lowest position. Lock bed wheels.
6. Raise the head of bed to sitting position.
7. Place one arm under resident's shoulder blades. Place the other arm under resident's thighs (Fig. 10-22).

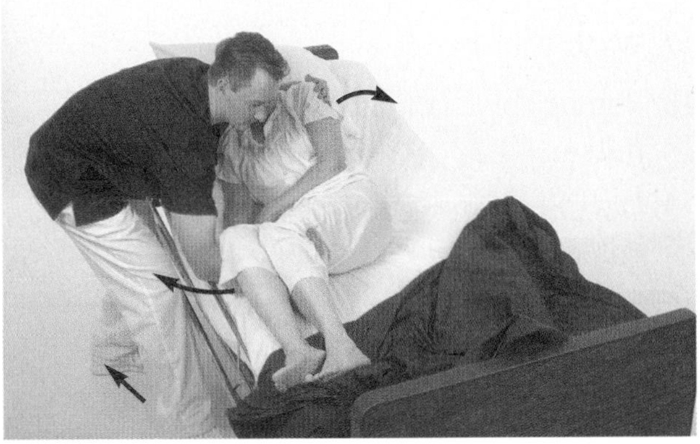

Fig. 10-22.

8. On the count of three, slowly turn resident into sitting position with legs dangling over side of bed (Fig. 10-23).

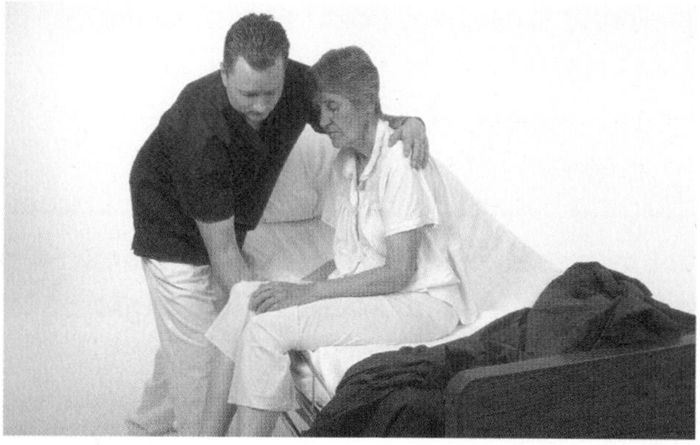

Fig. 10-23.

9. Ask resident to hold onto edge of mattress with both hands. Assist resident to put on nonskid shoes or slippers.
10. Have resident dangle as long as ordered. Stay with the resident at all times. Check for dizziness. If resident feels dizzy or faint, help her lie down again. Tell the nurse at once.
11. Take vital signs as ordered.
12. Remove slippers or shoes.
13. Gently assist resident back into bed. Place one arm around resident's shoulders. Place the other under resident's knees. Slowly swing resident's legs onto bed.
14. Make sure resident is comfortable.
15. Remove privacy measures.
16. Before leaving, place call light within resident's reach.
17. Wash your hands.
18. Report any changes in resident to the nurse.
19. Document procedure using facility guidelines.

4. Describe how to safely transfer residents

Transfers allow a resident to move from one place to another. Examples of transfers are from bed to chair or toilet, bed to stretcher, or wheelchair to toilet or vehicle.

It is important to know that some residents have a strong side and a weak side. The weak side is called the "involved" or "affected" side. Plan the move so that the strong side moves first. The weak side follows. It is hard for a resident to move a weak arm and leg first and bear enough weight for the move.

The strong arm transfers.

When transferring a resident with one weak side, the strong arm transfers.

One of the most important things during resident transfers is safety. In 2002, OSHA announced new ergonomic guidelines for transfers. **Ergonomics** is the science of designing equipment and work tasks to suit the worker's abilities. OSHA now says that manual lifting of residents should be reduced in all cases and eliminated when possible. Manual lifting, transferring, and repositioning of residents may increase risks of pain and injury. For facilities, this means buying equipment to help aides perform these tasks. For NAs, this means using equipment properly. Always get help when you need it.

Communicate.

Any time you help a resident, talk to them about what you would like to do. Promote their independence by letting them do what they can. The two of you must work together, especially during transfers.

Some transfers require the use of devices. A **transfer belt** is a safety device used to transfer residents who are weak, unsteady, or uncoordinated. It is called a **gait belt** when used to help residents walk. The belt is made of canvas or other heavy material. It sometimes has handles. It fits around the resident's waist outside his or her clothing. When putting a belt on, leave enough room to insert two fingers into the belt. The transfer belt gives you something firm to hold on to. Transfer belts cannot be used if a resident has fragile bones or recent fractures.

Applying a transfer belt

1. Wash your hands.
2. Identify yourself by name. Identify the resident by name.
3. Explain procedure to the resident. Speak clearly, slowly, and directly. Maintain face-to-face contact whenever possible.
4. Provide for the resident's privacy with curtain, screen, or door.
5. Assist the resident to a sitting position.
6. Place the belt over the resident's clothing and around the waist. Do not put it over bare skin.
7. Tighten the buckle until it is snug. Leave enough room to insert two fingers into the belt. The fingers should fit comfortably under the belt.
8. Check to make sure that a female's breasts are not caught under the belt.
9. For comfort, place the buckle off-center in the front or back (Fig. 10-24).

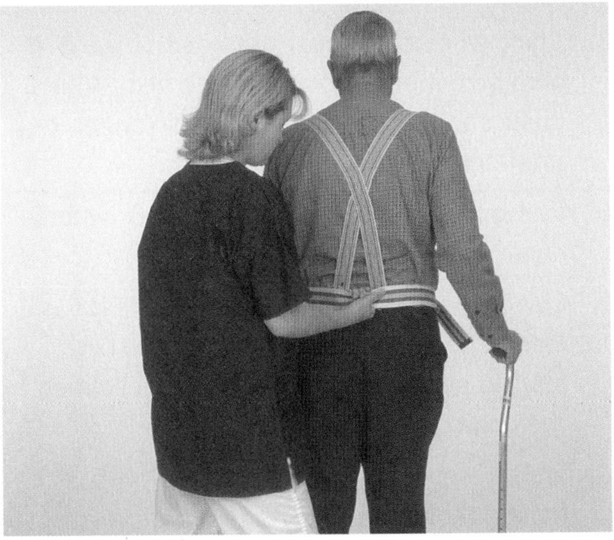

Fig. 10-24. **An NA helping a resident walk using a transfer belt. You will learn more about helping residents walk in chapter 21.**

A sliding or transfer board may be used to help transfer residents who cannot bear weight on their legs. Slide boards can be used for almost any transfer that involves moving from one sitting position to another. For example, transfers from a bed to a chair (Fig. 10-25).

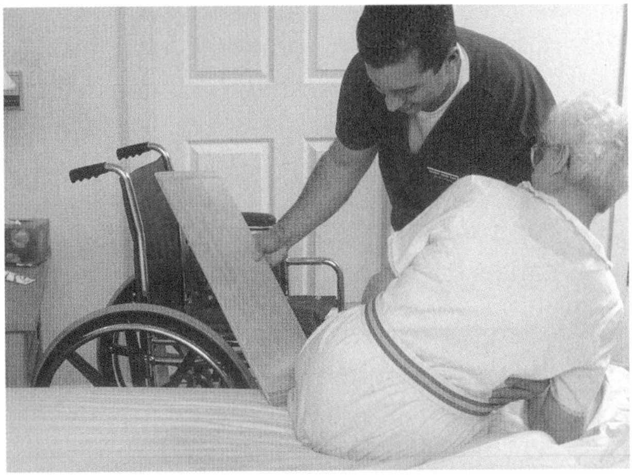

Fig. 10-25. **A sliding board can help with bed-to-chair transfers.**

Wheelchairs/Geriatric Chairs

Learn how a wheelchair works (Fig. 10-26). You should know how to apply and release the brake and how to work the footrests. The wheelchair should be locked before helping a resident into or out of it. After a transfer, a wheelchair should be unlocked.

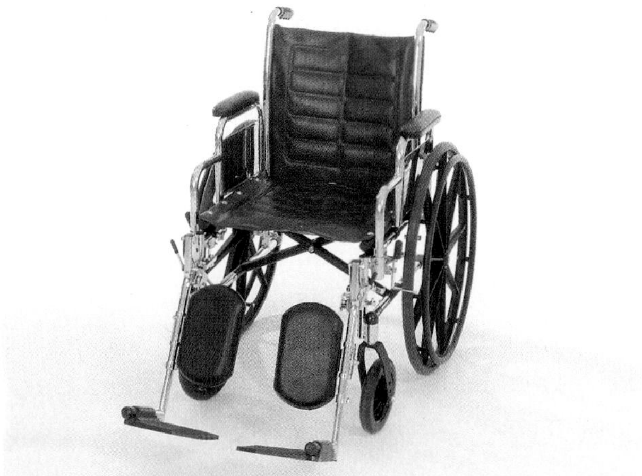

Fig. 10-26. **A standard wheelchair.**

To open a standard wheelchair, pull on both sides. Make the armrests separate and the seat flatten. To close the wheelchair, lift the center of the seat. Pull upward until the chair collapses.

To remove an armrest, press a button, usually by the armrest, and lift it. To attach an armrest, line up the button. Slip into place until the buttons click.

To remove the footrest, locate the lever. Pull back, and pull the footrest off the knobs. To reattach the footrest, line up the knobs. Slide footrest into place until it clicks.

To lift or lower footrest, support the leg or foot. Squeeze lever and pull up or push down.

Make sure the resident is safe and comfortable during transfers. When moving down a ramp, go backwards. The resident should face the top of the ramp, also going backwards. When using an elevator, turn the chair around before entering it, so the resident faces forward in the elevator.

If the resident needs to be moved back in the wheelchair or geriatric chair (geri-chair), go to the back of the chair. Reach forward and down under the resident's arms. Ask the resident to place his feet on the ground and push up. Pull the resident up in the chair while the resident pushes.

Ask the resident how you can help with wheelchairs. Some residents may only want you to bring the chair to the bedside. Others may want you to be more involved.

The tray table on geri-chairs can be heavy. Use caution when raising and lowering this table. Do not catch your fingers or the resident's fingers in the tray when attaching or releasing the tray table. Remember that geri-chairs can be considered restraints (chapter 6).

Before any transfer, make sure the resident is wearing non-skid footwear and it is securely fastened. This promotes residents' safety and reduces the risk of falls.

Falls

Remember these tips if a resident starts to fall during a transfer:

- *Widen your stance. Bring the resident's body close to you to break the fall. Bend your knees. Support the resident as you lower her to the floor.*
- *Do not try to stop a fall. You or the resident can be injured if you try to stop it rather than break the fall.*
- *Call for help. Do not try to get the resident up after the fall.*

Transferring a resident from bed to wheelchair

Equipment: wheelchair, transfer belt, non-skid footwear

1. Wash your hands.
2. Identify yourself by name. Identify the resident by name.
3. Explain procedure to the resident. Speak clearly, slowly, and directly. Maintain face-to-face contact whenever possible.
4. Provide for the resident's privacy with curtain, screen, or door.
5. Place wheelchair near the head of the bed with arm almost touching the bed. Wheelchair should be on resident's stronger, or unaffected, side.
6. Remove wheelchair footrests. Lock wheelchair wheels.
7. Lower the head of the bed to make it flat. Adjust bed level. The height of the bed should be equal to or slightly higher than the chair. Lock bed wheels.
8. Help resident to sitting position with feet flat on the floor.
9. Put non-skid footwear on resident and securely fasten.
10. **With transfer (gait) belt:**

a. Stand in front of resident.

b. Stand with feet about 12 inches apart. Bend your knees.

c. Place belt around resident's waist. Grasp belt securely on both sides.

Without transfer belt:

a. Stand in front of resident.

b. Stand with feet about 12 inches apart. Bend your knees.

c. Place your arms around resident's torso under the arms. Ask resident to place his hands on your shoulders if possible.

11. Provide instructions to allow resident to help with transfer. Instructions may include:

    "When you start to stand, push with your hands against the bed."

    "Once standing, if you're able, you can take small steps in the direction of the chair."

    "Once standing, reach for the chair with your stronger hand."

12. With your legs, brace resident's lower legs to prevent slipping (Fig. 10-27).

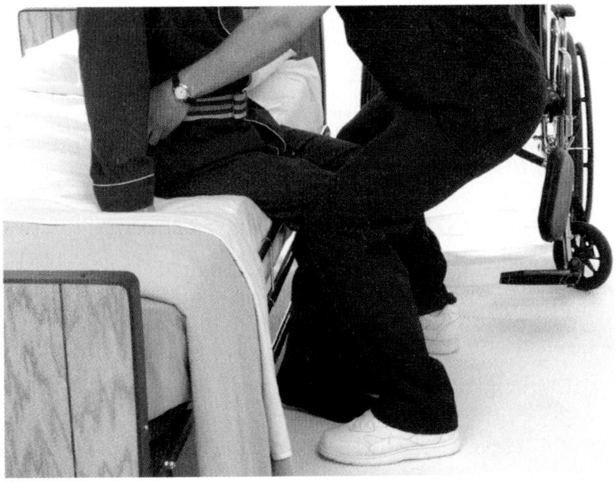

Fig. 10-27.

13. Count to three to alert resident.
14. On three, slowly help resident to stand.
15. Help resident to pivot to front of wheelchair with back of resident's legs against wheelchair.
16. Lower resident into wheelchair.
17. Reposition resident with hips touching back of wheelchair. Remove transfer belt, if used.
18. Place resident's feet on footrests.
19. Make resident comfortable. Remove privacy measures.
20. Before leaving, place call light within resident's reach.
21. Wash your hands.
22. Report any changes in resident to the nurse.
23. Document procedure using facility guidelines.

When a resident is in a wheelchair, he or she should be repositioned every two hours or as needed. The reasons for doing this are:

- It promotes comfort.
- It reduces pressure.
- It increases circulation.
- It exercises the joints.
- It promotes muscle tone.

The resident's body should be kept in good alignment while in the wheelchair. Special cushions, pillows, and soft blankets can be used for support. The hips should be positioned well back in the chair.

Stretchers

Stretchers move residents within facilities or to other facilities. Stretchers are used when residents must lie down and/or are very ill. Stretchers have safety straps that are used when the resident is on the stretcher. Residents should never be left alone on a stretcher.

A draw sheet is used to transfer a resident to a stretcher. The procedure below shows a transfer to a stretcher from a bed using four workers. At least three workers are necessary to safely transfer a resident to a stretcher.

Transferring a resident from bed to stretcher

1. Wash your hands.
2. Identify yourself by name. Identify the resident by name.
3. Explain procedure to the resident. Speak clearly, slowly, and directly. Maintain face-to-face contact whenever possible.
4. Provide for the resident's privacy with curtain, screen, or door.
5. Lower the head of bed so that it is flat. Lock bed wheels.
6. Lower the side rail on side to which you will move resident.
7. Move the resident to the side of the bed. Have your co-workers help you do this. Refer back to the procedure "Moving a resident to the side of the bed" in this chapter.
9. Lower the side rail on the other side of the bed. Keep a hand on the resident at all times.
10. Place stretcher solidly against the bed. Lock stretcher wheels. Bed height should be equal to the height of the stretcher. Remove stretcher safety belts.
11. Two workers should be on one side of resident. Two workers should be standing behind the stretcher.
12. Each worker should roll up the sides of the draw sheet and prepare to move the resident (Fig. 10-28). Protect the resident's arms and legs during the transfer.

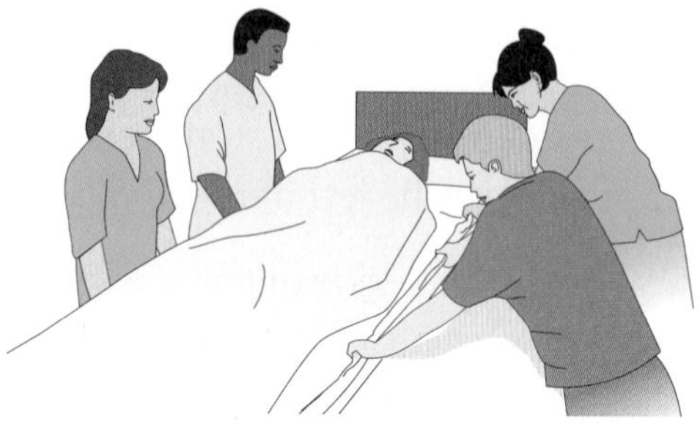

Fig. 10-28.

13. On the count of three, the workers should lift and move the resident to the stretcher. All should move at once. Make sure the resident is centered on the stretcher (Fig. 10-29).

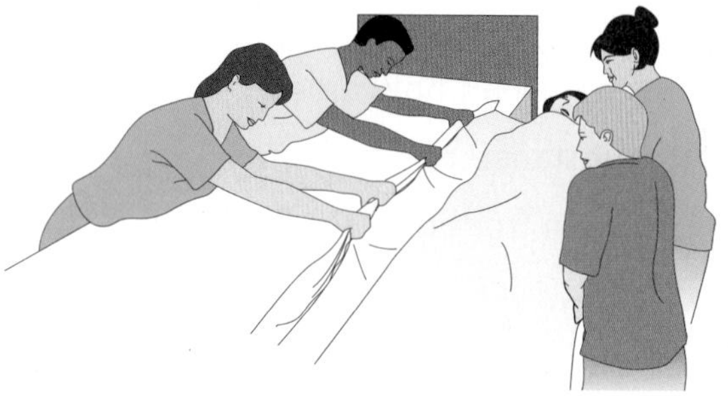

Fig. 10-29.

14. Place a pillow under the resident's head if allowed. Cover resident.
15. Place safety straps across the resident. Raise side rails on stretcher.
16. Unlock stretcher's wheels. Take resident to appropriate site. Stay with the resident until another team member takes over.
17. Wash your hands.
18. Report any changes in resident to the nurse.
19. Document procedure using facility guidelines.

   To return the resident to bed, reverse the above procedure.

Mechanical Lifts

You may help the resident with many types of transfers with the mechanical or hydraulic lift if you are trained to do so. This lift avoids wear and tear on your body. Lifts help prevent injury to you and the resident.

Never use equipment you have not been trained to use. You or your resident could get hurt if you use lifting equipment improperly.

There are many different types of mechanical lifts. You must be trained on the specific lift you will be using. Using these devices helps prevent common workplace injuries. Please understand and use provided equipment (Fig. 10-30).

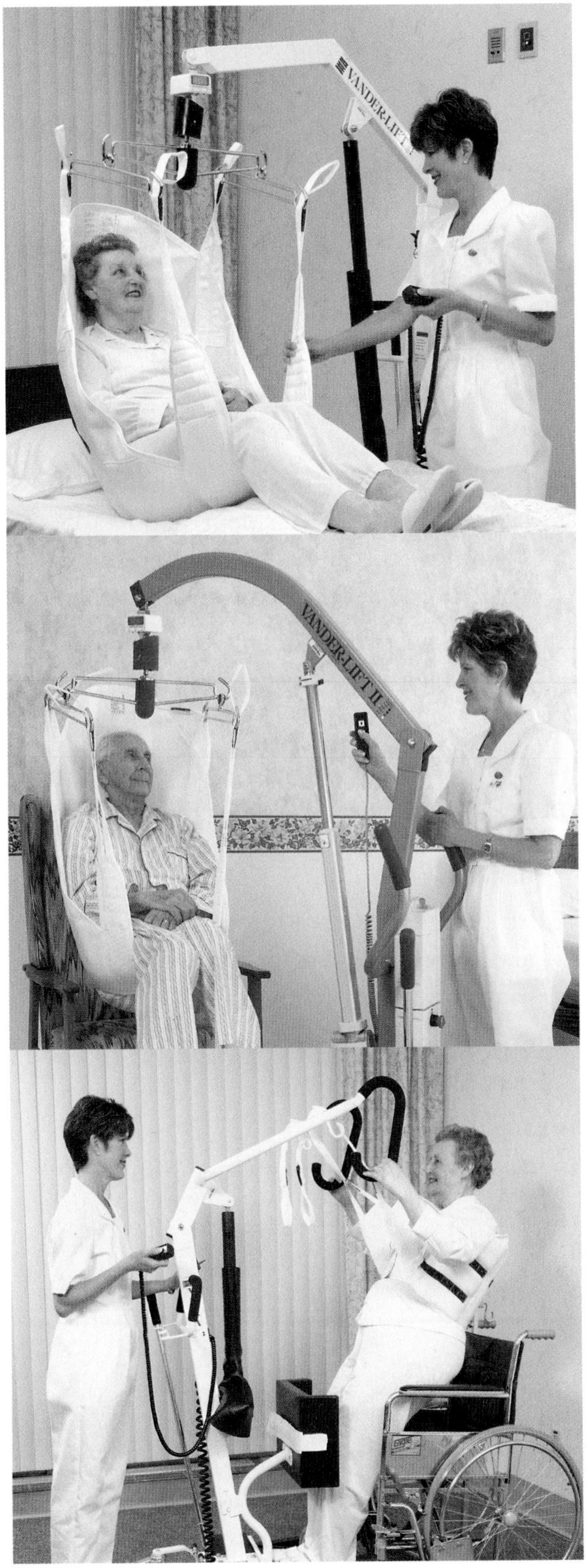

Fig. 10-30. **Today, there are lifts for transferring both completely dependent residents and residents who can bear some weight. (Photo courtesy of VANCARE Inc., 800-694-4525)**

Transferring a resident using a mechanical lift

This is a basic procedure for transferring using a mechanical lift.

Equipment: wheelchair or chair, co-worker, mechanical or hydraulic lift

1. Wash your hands.
2. Identify yourself by name. Identify the resident by name.
3. Explain procedure to the resident. Speak clearly, slowly, and directly. Maintain face-to-face contact whenever possible.
4. Provide for the resident's privacy with curtain, screen, or door.
5. Lock bed wheels.
6. Position wheelchair next to bed. Lock brakes.
7. Help the resident turn to one side of the bed. Position the sling under the resident, with the edge next to the resident's back. Fanfold if necessary. Fanfolding means folding several times into pleats. Make the bottom of the sling even with the resident's knees. Help the resident roll back to the middle of the bed. Spread out the fanfolded edge of the sling.
8. Roll the mechanical lift to bedside. Make sure the base is opened to its widest point. Push the base of the lift under the bed.
9. Place the overhead bar directly over the resident (Fig. 10-31).
10. With the resident lying on his back, attach one set of straps to each side of the sling. Attach one set of straps to the overhead bar (Fig. 10-32). If available, have a co-worker support the resident at the head, shoulders, and knees while being lifted. The resident's arms should be folded across his chest (Fig. 10-33). If the device has "S" hooks, they should face away from resident (Fig. 10-34). Make sure all straps are connected properly.

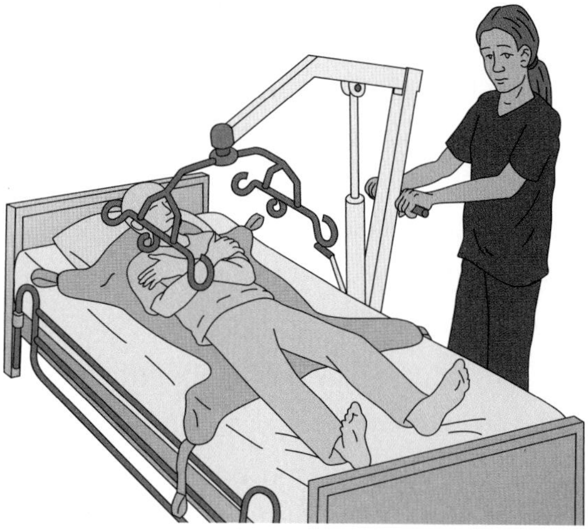

Fig. 10-31.

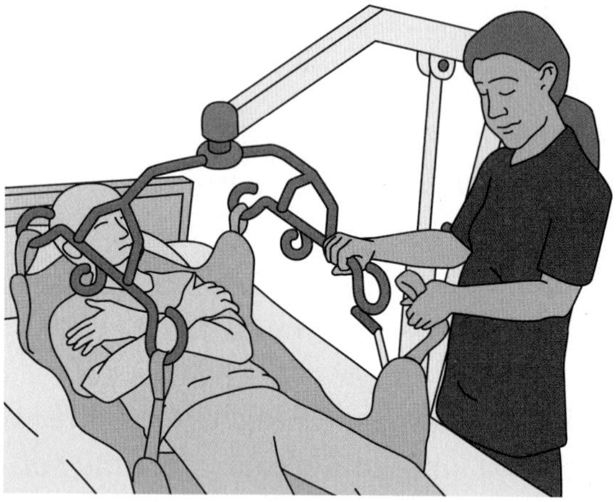

Fig. 10-32.

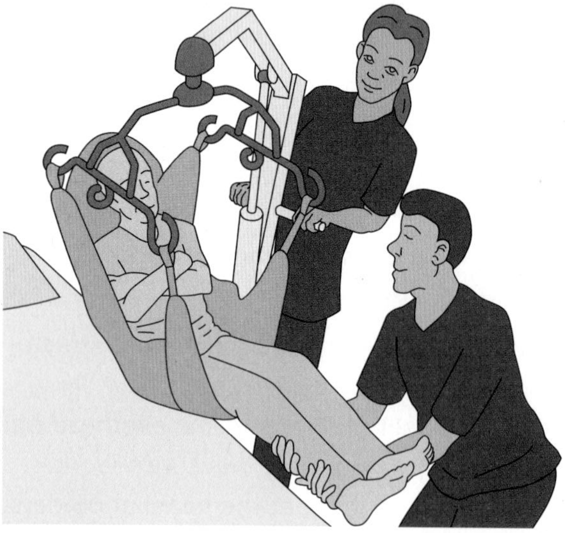

Fig. 10-33.

11. Following manufacturer's instructions, raise the resident two inches above the bed. Pause a moment for the resident to gain balance.

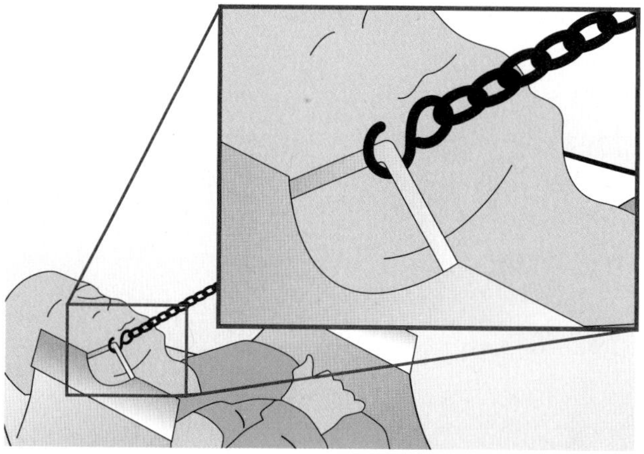

Fig. 10-34.

12. If available, a lifting partner can help support and guide the resident's body. You can then move the lift so that the resident is positioned over the chair or wheelchair.
13. Slowly lower the resident into the chair or wheelchair. Push down gently on the resident's knees to help the resident into a sitting position.
14. Undo the straps from the overhead bar. Leave the sling in place for transfer back to bed.
15. Be sure the resident is seated comfortably and correctly in the chair or wheelchair. Remove privacy measures.
16. Before leaving, place call light within resident's reach.
17. Wash your hands.
18. Report any changes in resident to the nurse.
19. Document procedure using facility guidelines.

Toilet Transfers

If residents are able to use the toilet, the bladder empties more efficiently. You will learn more about bedpans and urinals in chapter 14. Offer trips to the toilet often. Respond to call lights quickly.

In order to use the toilet, residents must be able to bear some weight on their legs. Falls may occur in and on the way to the bathroom. Use a transfer belt to assist. Do not leave a resident alone if you feel it is unsafe.

Transferring a resident onto and off of a toilet

Equipment: disposable gloves, toilet tissue, wheelchair, transfer belt, non-skid shoes

1. Wash your hands.
2. Identify yourself by name. Identify the resident by name.
3. Explain procedure to the resident. Speak clearly, slowly, and directly. Maintain face-to-face contact whenever possible.
4. Provide for the resident's privacy with curtain, screen, or door.
5. Position wheelchair at a right angle to the toilet to face the hand bar/wall rail.
6. Remove wheelchair footrests. Lock wheels.
7. Apply a transfer belt around the resident's waist. Grasp the belt. Put one of your hands toward the resident's back and one toward the resident's front.
8. Ask resident to push against the armrests of the wheelchair and stand, reaching for and grasping the hand bar (Fig. 10-35).

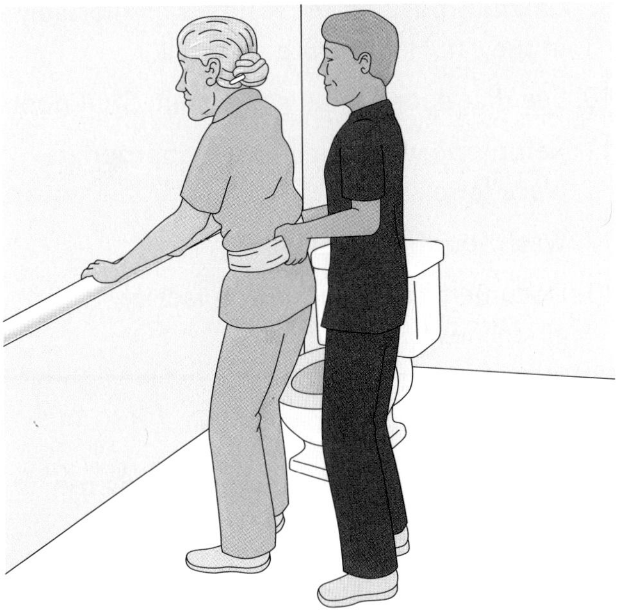

Fig. 10-35.

9. Ask resident to pivot her foot and back up so that she can feel the front of the toilet with the back of her legs (Fig. 10-36).

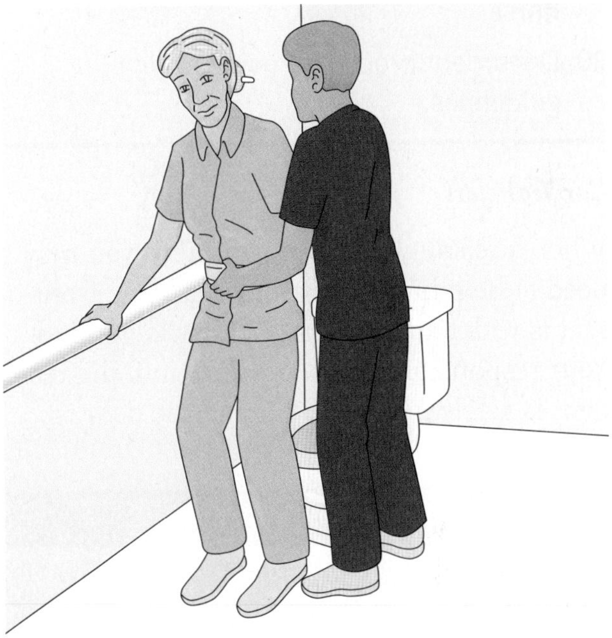

Fig. 10-36.

10. Help resident to pull down underwear and pants. You may need to keep one hand on the transfer belt while helping to remove clothing.
11. Help resident to slowly sit down onto the toilet. Allow privacy unless resident cannot be left alone.
12. When the resident is finished, apply gloves. Assist with perineal care as necessary (see chapter 13). Ask her to stand and reach for the hand bar.
13. Use toilet tissue or damp cloth to clean the resident. Make sure he or she is clean and dry before pulling up clothing. Remove and dispose of gloves.
14. Pull up resident's clothing. Help resident to the sink to wash hands.
15. Help resident back into wheelchair.
16. Wash your hands.
17. Help resident to leave the bathroom. Make sure resident is comfortable. Remove privacy measures.

18. Before leaving, place call light within resident's reach.
19. Report any changes in resident to the nurse.
20. Document procedure using facility guidelines.

Car Transfers

When a resident is leaving a facility, you may need to help him or her into a car. The front seat is wider and is usually easier to get into. Your responsibilities do not end until the resident is safely inside the car and the door is closed.

Transferring a resident into a car

Equipment: car, wheelchair

1. Wash your hands.
2. Identify yourself by name. Identify the resident by name.
3. Explain procedure to the resident. Speak clearly, slowly, and directly. Maintain face-to-face contact whenever possible.
4. Place wheelchair close to the car at a 45 degree angle. Open the door on the resident's stronger side.
5. Lock wheelchair.
6. Ask the resident to push against the arm rests of the wheelchair and stand (Fig. 10-37).

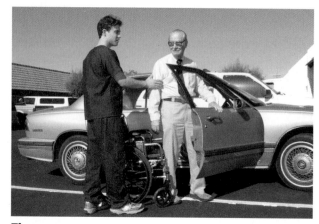

Fig. 10-37.

7. Ask the resident to stand, grasp the car, and pivot his foot so the side of the car seat touches the back of the legs.
8. The resident should then sit in the seat and lift one leg, and then the other, into the vehicle (Fig. 10-38).

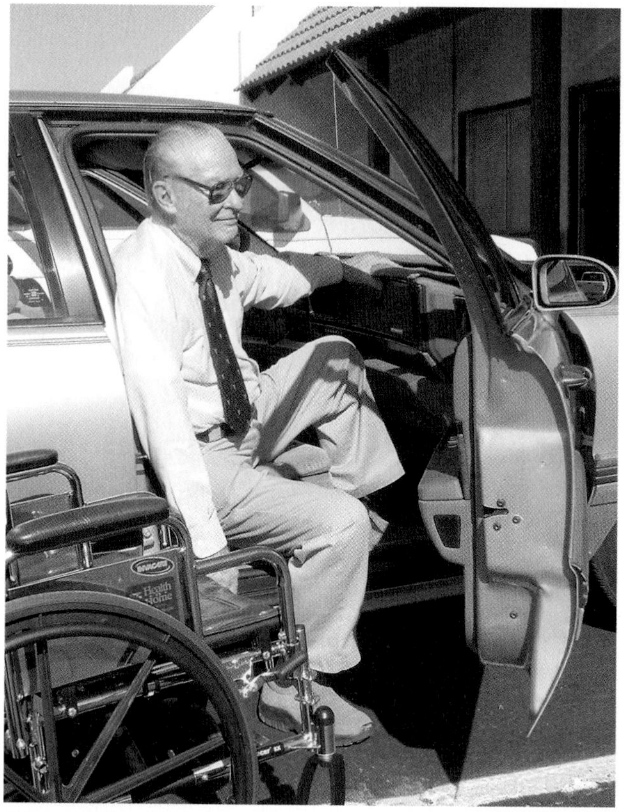

Fig. 10-38.

9. Carefully position the resident comfortably in the car. Help secure seat belt.
10. See that door can be safely shut. Shut door.
11. Return the wheelchair to the appropriate place for cleaning.
12. Wash your hands.
13. Document procedure using facility guidelines.

Chapter Review

1. List ten rules for using proper body mechanics.
2. Why do residents who spend a lot of time in bed need to change positions often?

3. In which position is a resident lying on his/her side?
4. In which position is a resident lying on his/her stomach?
5. In which position is a resident lying flat on his/her back?
6. In which position is a resident lying on his/her side with the lower arm behind the back and the upper knee bent and raised toward the chest?
7. In which position is a resident in a semi-sitting position with the head and shoulders up?
8. What is a draw sheet?
9. What is shearing?
10. When is logrolling necessary?
11. What is a transfer belt?
12. Before helping a resident into or out of a wheelchair, what should you do?
13. Describe what you should you do if a resident starts to fall.
14. When are stretchers used for residents?
15. What can the proper use of mechanical lifts help prevent?
16. What is better about a resident being able to use the toilet rather than a bedpan or urinal?

Chapter 11
Admitting, Transferring, and Discharging

1. Describe how residents may feel when entering a facility

As you learned in chapter 8, moving into a facility requires a big adjustment. New residents may have been independent for a long time. They may be moving from a family member's home. Either way, there is a huge emotional adjustment to be made (Fig. 11-1). Residents may experience fear, uncertainty, anger, and loss. They may have lost their health, mobility, independence, family, friends, pets, plants, and other things.

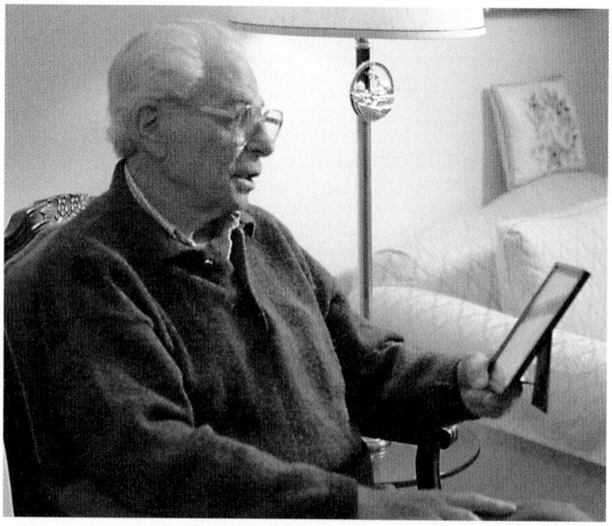

Fig. 11-1. **New residents must leave familiar places and things.**

Empathize with new residents. Think about how you would feel if you had to give up many of your things to move into an unfamiliar place full of strangers.

NAs have an important role when new residents move into a facility. This includes supporting residents emotionally. NAs will be the team members most involved with the resident.

2. Explain the nursing assistant's role in the admission process

Admission is often the first time you meet a new resident. This is a time of first impressions. Make sure a resident has a good impression of you and your facility. Explain what to expect. Answer all questions a resident has. Ask questions. Find out the resident's personal preferences and routines.

Your facility will have a procedure for admitting residents to their new home. These guidelines will help make the experience pleasant and successful.

GUIDELINES
Admission

- Prepare the room before the resident arrives. He or she will feel expected and welcome. Know the condition of the resident. Know if he or she is bed-bound or is able to walk.

- Introduce yourself. State your position. Always call the person by his formal name until he tells you what he wants to be called.
- Never rush the process or the new resident. He should not feel like he is an inconvenience.
- Make sure that the new resident feels welcome and wanted.
- Explain day-to-day life in the facility. Offer to take the resident on a tour (Fig. 11-2).

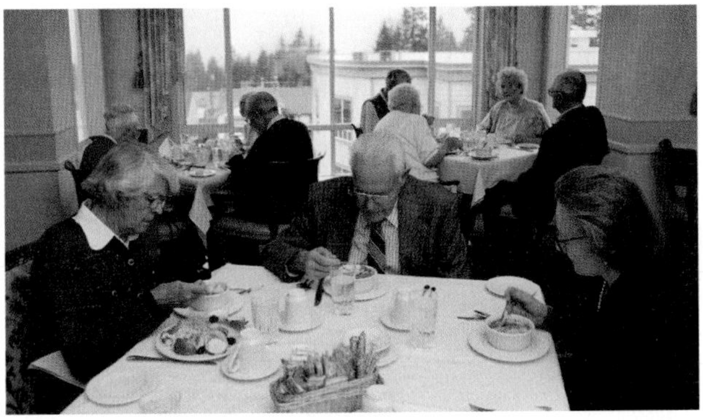

Fig. 11-2. Make sure you include the dining room when taking a new resident on a tour.

- Introduce the resident to everyone you see (Fig. 11-3).

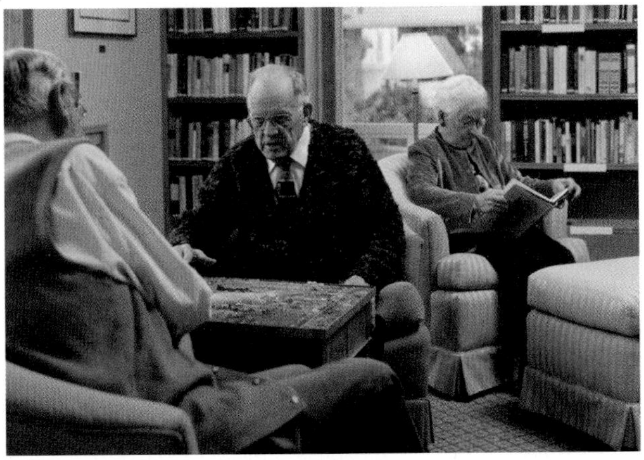

Fig. 11-3. Introduce new residents to all other residents you see.

- Handle personal items with care and respect. A resident has a legal right to have his personal items treated carefully. These items are special things he has chosen to bring with him. When setting up the room, ask him what he likes. Place personal items where the resident wants them (Fig. 11-4).

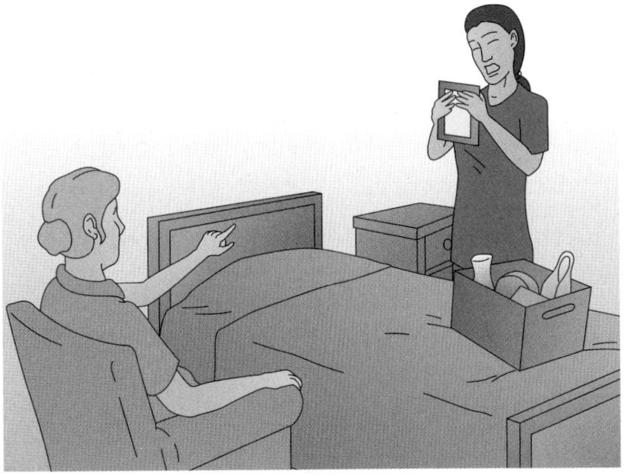

Fig. 11-4. Handle personal items carefully. Set up the room as she prefers.

- Follow your facility's rules regarding your tasks.

STOP *Upon admission, residents must be told of their rights. They must be provided with a written copy of these rights. This includes rights about funds and the right to file a complaint with the state survey agency.*

Admitting a resident

Equipment: may include admission paperwork (checklist and inventory form), gloves and vital signs equipment

Often an admission kit will contain a urine specimen cup and transport bag, and personal care items, such as bath basin, water pitcher, drinking glass, toothpaste and soap.

1. Wash your hands.
2. Identify yourself by name. Identify the resident by name.
3. Explain procedure to the resident. Speak clearly, slowly, and directly. Maintain face-to-face contact whenever possible.
4. Provide for the resident's privacy with curtain, screen, or door. If the family is present, ask them to step outside until the admission process is over.

5. If part of facility procedure, do these things:

   Take the resident's height and weight (see procedure below).

   Take the resident's baseline vital signs (see chapter 17). **Baseline** signs are initial values that can then be compared to future measurements.

   Obtain a urine specimen if required (see chapter 14).

   Complete the paperwork. Take an inventory of all the personal items.

   Help the resident put personal items away.

   Provide fresh water.
6. Show the resident the room and bathroom. Explain how to work the bed (and television if there is one). Show the resident how to work the call light and explain its use.
7. Introduce the resident to his roommate, if there is one. Introduce other residents and staff.
8. Make sure resident is comfortable. Remove privacy measures.
9. Before leaving, place call light within resident's reach.
10. Wash your hands.
11. Document procedure using facility guidelines.

In addition to measuring weight and height at admission, you will check them as part of your care. Height is checked less often than weight. Weight changes can be signs of illness. You must report any weight loss or gain, no matter how small.

Measuring and recording weight of an ambulatory resident

Equipment: standing scale, pen and paper to record your findings

1. Wash your hands.
2. Identify yourself by name. Identify the resident by name.
3. Explain procedure to the resident. Speak clearly, slowly, and directly. Maintain face-to-face contact whenever possible.
4. Provide for resident's privacy with curtain, screen, or door.
5. Start with scale balanced at zero.
6. Help resident to step onto the center of the scale.
7. Weigh resident. This is done by balancing the scale by making the balance bar level. Move the small and large weight indicators until the bar balances (Fig. 11-5).

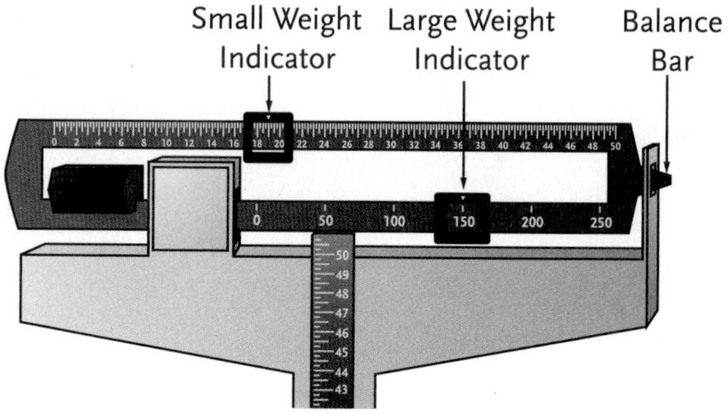

Fig. 11-5.

8. Help resident off scale before recording weight.
9. Record weight.
10. Remove privacy measures.
11. Before leaving, place call light within resident's reach.
12. Wash your hands.
13. Document procedure using facility guidelines.

Some residents will not be able to get out of a wheelchair easily. These residents may be weighed on a wheelchair scale. With this scale, wheelchairs are rolled onto the scale (Fig. 11-6). On some wheelchair scales, you will need to subtract the weight of the wheelchair from a resident's weight. In this case, weigh the empty wheelchair first. Then subtract the wheelchair's weight from the total. Some wheelchairs are marked with their weight.

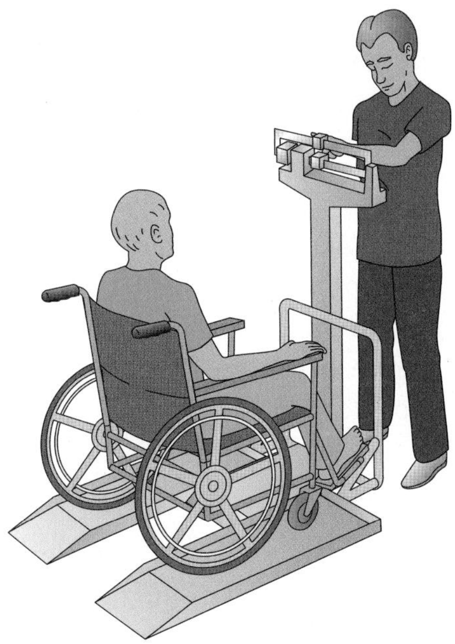

Fig. 11-6. A type of wheelchair scale.

Some residents will not be able to get out of bed. Weighing these residents requires a special scale (Fig. 11-7). Before using a bed scale, know how to use it properly and safely. Follow your facility's procedure and any manufacturer's instructions.

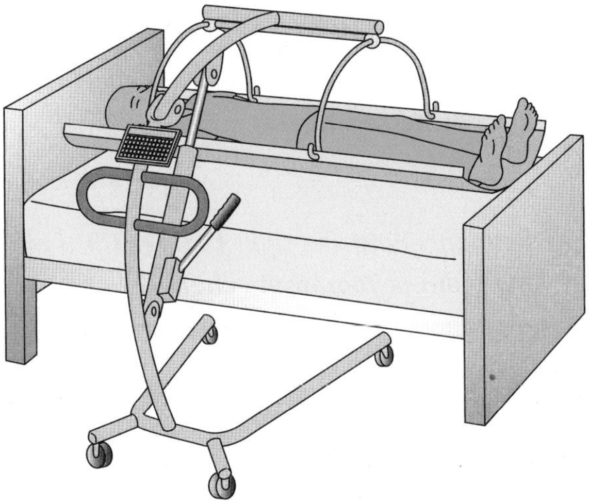

Fig. 11-7. A type of bed scale.

Measuring and recording height of an ambulatory resident

Equipment: standing scale, pen and paper to record your findings

1. Wash your hands.
2. Identify yourself by name. Identify the resident by name.
3. Explain procedure to the resident. Speak clearly, slowly, and directly. Maintain face-to-face contact whenever possible.
4. Provide for resident's privacy with curtain, screen, or door.
5. Help resident to step onto scale, facing away from the scale.
6. Ask resident to stand straight. Help as needed.
7. Pull up measuring rod from back of scale. Gently lower measuring rod until it rests flat on resident's head (Fig. 11-8).

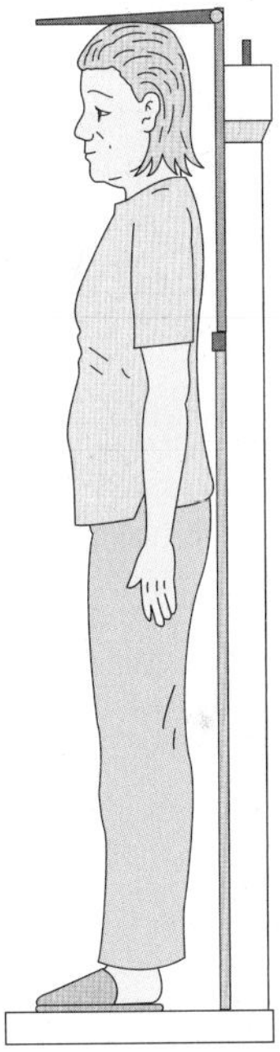

Fig. 11-8.

8. Check resident's height.
9. Help resident off scale before recording height. Make sure measuring rod does not hit the resident's head while helping resident off the scale.
10. Record height.
11. Remove privacy measures.
12. Before leaving, place call light within resident's reach.
13. Wash your hands.
14. Document procedure using facility guidelines.

The rod measures height in inches and fractions of inches. Record the total number of inches. If you have to change inches into feet, remember that there are 12 inches in a foot.

If residents cannot get out of bed, measure height by with a tape measure (Fig. 11-9). Position the resident lying straight in bed. Mark the sheet with a pencil at the top of the head and at the bottom of the feet (Fig. 11-10). Measure the distance between the marks. Record the height.

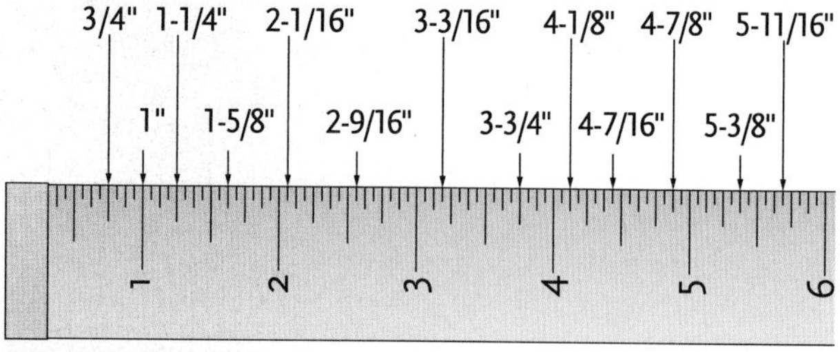

Fig. 11-9. A tape measure.

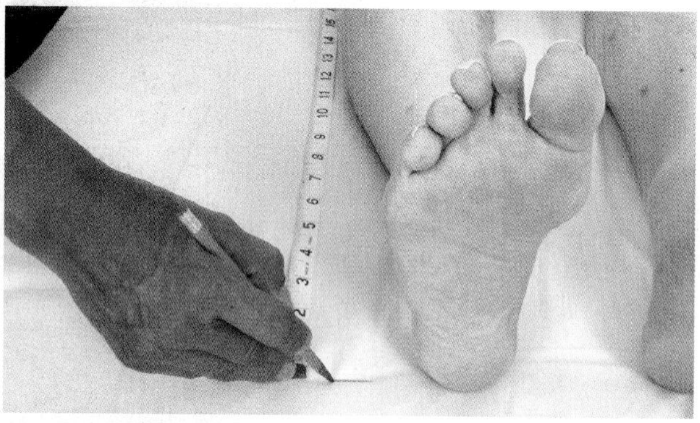

Fig. 11-10. To record the height of a resident in bed, mark the sheet at the resident's head and feet.

New residents may have good days followed by not-so-good days. Let residents adapt to their new homes at their own pace. Everyone is different. Getting used to a new home may take quite some time.

3. Explain the nursing assistant's role during an in-house transfer of a resident

Residents may be transferred to a different area of the facility. In cases of acute illness, they may be transferred to a hospital. Change is difficult. This is especially true when a person has an illness or his or her condition gets worse. Make the transfer as smooth as possible for the resident. Try to lessen the stress. Inform the resident of the transfer as soon as possible. He can then begin to adjust to the idea. Explain how, where, when and why the transfer will occur.

For example, "Mrs. Jones, you will be moving to a private room. You will be transferred to your new room in a wheelchair. This will happen on Wednesday around 10 a.m. The staff will take good care of you and your things. We will make sure you are comfortable. Do you have any questions?"

NAs will usually pack all of the resident's belongings. Packing up all of the items may take some time. Pack personal items carefully.

The resident may be transferred in a bed, in a stretcher, or in a wheelchair. Find out the method from the nurse so that you can plan the move.

When you arrive at a new unit, introduce the resident to everyone. It is a good idea to check on the resident later in the day to make sure he is settled. After that, it is nice to stop in sometimes to say hello. This helps the resident stay connected to you.

STOP *Residents have the right to be notified of any room or roommate change.*

Transferring a resident

Equipment: may include a wheelchair, cart for belongings, the medical record, all of the resident's personal care items

1. Wash your hands.
2. Identify yourself by name. Identify the resident by name.
3. Explain procedure to the resident. Speak clearly, slowly, and directly. Maintain face-to-face contact whenever possible.
4. Provide for resident's privacy with curtain, screen, or door.

5. Collect the items to be moved onto the cart. Take them to the new location. If the resident is going into the hospital, the facility may want them placed in temporary storage.
6. Help the resident into the wheelchair (stretcher may be used for some residents). Take him or her to proper area.
7. Introduce new residents and staff.
8. Help the resident to put personal items away.
9. Make sure that the resident is comfortable. Remove privacy measures.
10. Before leaving, place call light within resident's reach.
11. Wash your hands.
12. Report any changes in resident to the nurse.
13. Document procedure using facility guidelines.

4. Explain the nursing assistant's role in the discharge of a resident

The day of discharge is usually a happy day for a resident who is going home. You will collect the resident's belongings and pack them. Know the condition of the resident. Find out if he will be using a wheelchair or stretcher for discharge. Ask the resident which personal care items to bring. Be positive. Assure the resident he is ready for this important change. He may have doubts about not being cared for at the facility anymore. Remind him that his doctor believes he is ready.

The nurse may cover important information with the resident and family. Some of these areas may be discussed:

- future doctor or physical therapy appointments (Fig. 11-11)
- medications
- the ambulation instructions from the doctor
- any restrictions on activities
- special exercises to keep the resident functioning at the highest level
- any special nutrition or dietary requirements
- community resources

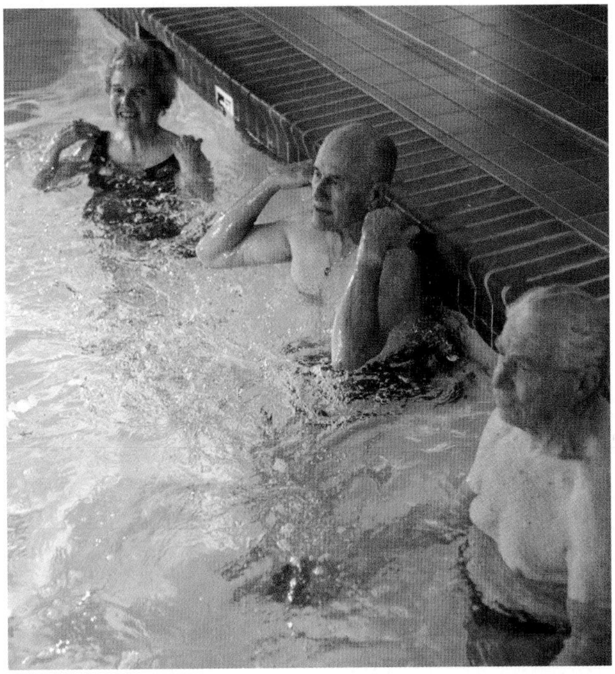

Fig. 11-11. **After a resident is discharged, she may continue to receive physical therapy.**

AMA

Sometimes a resident decides to leave a facility without the approval of the doctor. This is called leaving AMA or "against medical advice." A process must then be followed to protect the facility and staff. The resident usually signs a form that says he or she knows the risks of leaving. If you see signs that a resident might be leaving the facility, notify the charge nurse.

Discharging a resident

Equipment: may include a wheelchair, cart for belongings, the discharge paperwork, including the inventory list done on admission, all of the resident's personal care items

1. Wash your hands.

2. Identify yourself by name. Identify the resident by name.
3. Explain procedure to the resident. Speak clearly, slowly, and directly. Maintain face-to-face contact whenever possible.
4. Provide for resident's privacy with curtain, screen, or door.
5. Compare the checklist to the items there. If all items are there, ask the resident to sign.
6. Put the items to be taken onto the cart and take them to pick-up area.
7. Help the resident dress and then into the wheelchair (stretcher may be used for some residents).
8. Help the resident to say his goodbyes to the staff and residents.
9. Help the resident into the wheelchair. Take him to the pick-up area. Help him into vehicle. You are responsible for the resident until he or she is safely in the car and the door is closed.
10. Wash your hands.
11. Document procedure using facility guidelines.

5. Describe the nursing assistant's role in physical exams

Some residents need a physical exam when arriving at a facility. Others need a physical exam after they have been there for a while. Know your role during a physical exam so the process runs smoothly. Doctors or nurses will do part or all of the exam. NAs may be asked to help.

You can help residents with their emotional needs by being there for them. Exams can make people anxious. They may fear what the examiner will do or what he or she will find. Exams can cause discomfort and embarrassment. Help residents by listening to them, talking to them, or even holding their hand.

You will get equipment for the nurse or doctor. Examples of equipment are:

- sphygmomanometer (used to measure blood pressure; you will learn about this in chapter 17)
- stethoscope
- alcohol wipes
- flashlight
- thermometer
- tongue depressor
- eye chart
- tuning fork (tests hearing with vibrations)
- reflex hammer (taps body parts to test reflexes)
- otoscope (lighted instrument that examines the outer ear and eardrum)
- ophthalmoscope (lighted instrument that examines the eye)
- specimen containers
- lubricant
- Hemoccult card (tests for blood in stool)
- vaginal speculum for females (opens the vagina so that it and the cervix can be examined)
- gloves
- drape

Place the resident in the correct position. Stay with the resident as needed. Some positions are embarrassing and uncomfortable. You can help by explaining why the position is needed. Explain how long the resident can expect to stay in the position.

The **dorsal recumbent** position is used to examine the breasts, chest, and abdomen. It is also used to examine the perineal area (Fig. 11-12). A resident in the dorsal recumbent position is flat on his or her back. The knees are flexed and feet flat on the bed. The drape is put over the resident, covering her body. Her head remains uncovered.

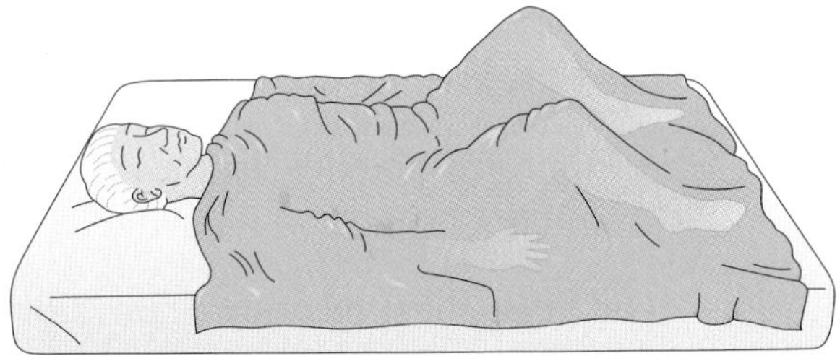

Fig. 11-12. **The dorsal recumbent position.**

A **lithotomy** position is used to examine the vagina (Fig. 11-13). The resident lies on her back. Her hips are brought to the edge of the exam table. Her legs are flexed. Feet are in padded stirrups. The drape is put over the resident, covering her body. Her head remains uncovered. The drape is also brought down to cover the perineal area.

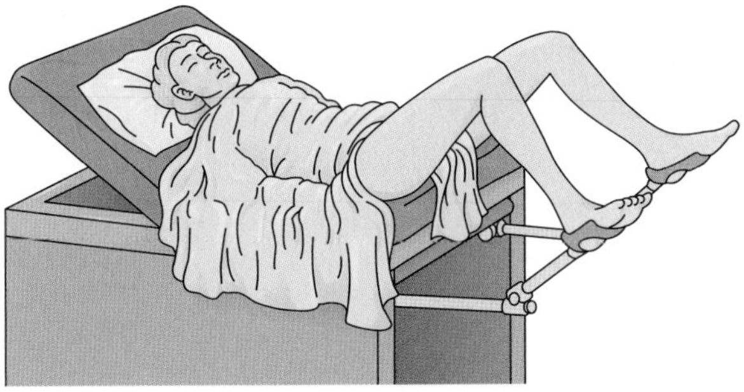

Fig. 11-13. **The lithotomy position.**

The **knee-chest** position is used to examine the rectum, or sometimes, the vagina (Fig. 11-14). A resident in the knee-chest position is lying on his or her abdomen. The knees are pulled towards the abdomen and legs are separated. Arms are pulled up and flexed. The head is turned to one side. In the knee-chest position, the resident will be wearing a gown and possibly socks. The drape should be applied in a diamond shape to cover the back, buttocks and thighs.

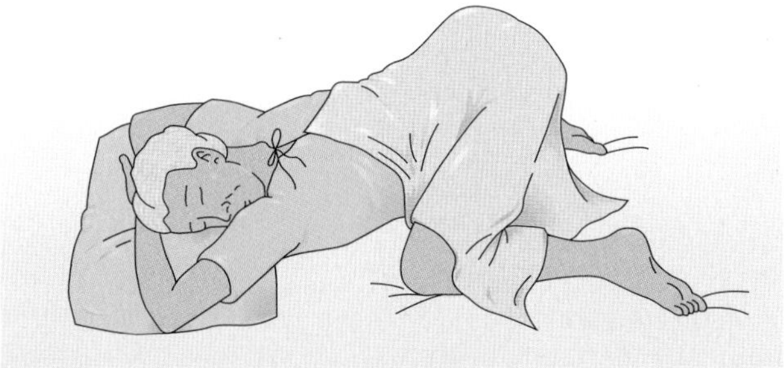

Fig. 11-14. **The knee-chest position.**

Provide a drape for the resident. Offer other privacy measures, such as closing the privacy screen or curtain and closing the door to the room. Promote the resident's right to privacy. Tell the resident that he or she will not be exposed more than necessary during the exam.

GUIDELINES
Physical Exams

- Wash your hands before and after the exam.
- Ask the resident to urinate before the exam. Collect any urine needed for a specimen at this time.
- Provide privacy throughout the exam. Use drapes and privacy screens for privacy. Expose only the body part being examined.
- Listen to and calm the resident throughout the exam.
- Follow the directions of the examiner.
- Help the resident into the proper positions as needed.
- Protect the resident from falling.
- Provide enough light for examiner.
- Put instruments in the proper place for the examiner. Hand instruments to the examiner as needed.
- Take and label specimens as needed.
- Follow Standard Precautions.
- After the exam, the NA's responsibilities include:
  - Help the resident clean up and get dressed. Help the resident safely back to his or her room.
  - Dispose of any trash and disposable equipment in the exam area.
  - Bring all reusable equipment to the appropriate cleaning room. Clean and store reusable equipment according to facility policy.
  - Label and bring any specimens to the desk to take to the lab.

Residents have the right to know why exams are being done and who is doing them. Residents have the right to choose examiners and to have family members present during the exam.

Chapter Review

True or False. Mark each statement with either a "T" for true or "F" for false.

1. _____ Moving into a nursing home is a big change.
2. _____ It is important to never rush the admission process for a new resident.
3. _____ It is not necessary to introduce a new resident to staff members and other residents.
4. _____ You should handle a new resident's personal items carefully.
5. _____ If a resident loses one pound, you do not need to report the weight loss.
6. _____ Residents who are unable to get out of bed cannot have their height measured.
7. _____ On some wheelchair scales, you will need to subtract the weight of the wheelchair before recording a resident's weight.
8. _____ To lessen the stress of a transfer, inform the resident as soon as possible so he can begin to adjust to the idea.
9. _____ You may leave a discharged resident before you have helped him into a vehicle.
10. _____ Exams can cause discomfort and embarrassment.
11. _____ The dorsal recumbent position is used to examine the vagina.
12. _____ A lithotomy position is used to examine the breasts.
13. _____ The knee-chest position is used to examine the rectum.
14. _____ Draping a resident promotes privacy and dignity.
15. _____ You must follow Standard Precautions while helping with physical exams.

Chapter 12
The Resident's Unit

1. Describe a standard resident unit

A resident's unit is the room or area where the resident lives. It contains furniture and personal items. The unit is the resident's home. It must be treated with respect. Always knock. Wait for permission before entering.

Once personal items are in place within a room or unit, do not move them without permission. If a safety hazard exists, inform the nurse. He or she will handle the situation.

Each unit may have slightly different equipment. Personal items that bring the resident happiness should be encouraged. Resident rooms should be personal and home-like.

Standard unit equipment includes:

- Bed
- Bedside stand
- Overbed table
- Chair
- Emesis basin
- Bedpan
- Urinal
- Bath basin
- Call light
- Privacy curtain

Residents can store small items in bedside stands. The water pitcher and cup are often placed on top of the bedside stand. A telephone and/or a radio, and other items, such as photos, may also be placed there. These items may be stored inside the bedside stand:

- Urinal/bedpan and covers
- Wash basin
- Emesis basin
- Soap dish and soap
- Bath blanket
- Toilet paper
- Personal hygiene items

The overbed table may be used for meals or personal care. It is a clean area. It must be kept clean and free of clutter (Fig. 12-1). Bedpans and urinals and soiled linen should not be placed on overbed tables.

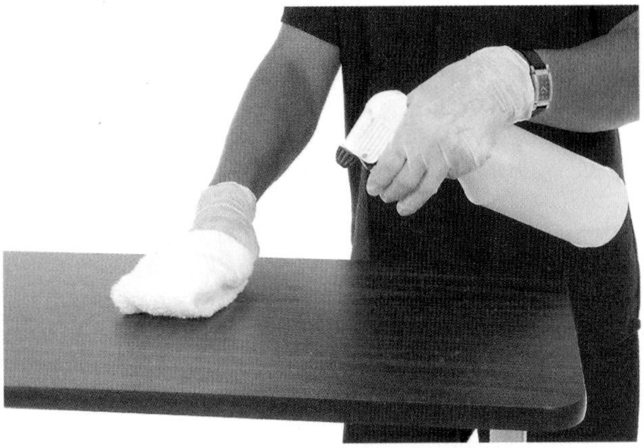

Fig. 12-1. **Overbed tables must be kept clean and free of clutter.**

The intercom system is the most common call system. When the resident presses the button, a light will be seen and/or a bell will be heard at the nurses' station. The call light allows the resident to contact staff anytime. It is important to always place the call light within the resident's reach. Answer all call lights immediately.

STOP ***Making fun is not funny.***

Making fun of any resident's personal items is wrong and cruel. If an NA or any staff member makes fun of residents or their belongings, it is verbal abuse.

2. Discuss how to care for and clean unit equipment

You will be taught the right way to use many pieces of equipment. Know how to use and care for all equipment. This prevents infection and injury. If you do not know how to use a piece of equipment, ask for help. Do not try to operate equipment that you do not know how to use.

Some equipment you will use will be **disposable**. This means it is thrown out after use. Disposable razors and latex gloves are two examples. Disposable equipment prevents the spread of microorganisms. Discard disposable equipment in proper containers.

Some equipment will need to be cleaned after each use. Bedpans and wash basins are examples. Rinse them with water before cleaning them. Wear gloves while rinsing and cleaning this equipment so that you do not touch infectious wastes.

After cleaning and drying equipment, you may need to disinfect it. Disinfection is the use of chemicals to destroy pathogens. It does not kill all microorganisms. Sterilization means all microorganisms are destroyed, not just pathogens. Some equipment will need to be sterilized. An autoclave is usually used to sterilize equipment. This machine creates steam or a type of gas that kills microorganisms.

You will need to keep a resident's unit neat and clean.

GUIDELINES

Resident's Unit

- Clean the overbed table after use. Place it within the resident's reach before leaving.
- Keep the call light within the resident's reach at all times. Check to see that the resident can reach the call light every time you leave the room.
- Remove crumbs from the bed right after meals. Straighten bed linens as needed.
- Before leaving a resident's room, re-stock supplies. This includes facial tissues, bathroom tissue, paper towels, soap, or any other needed item.
- Check equipment daily. Make sure it is working properly and not damaged. If you find any damaged equipment, such as frayed or cracked cords, report it to the nurse or appropriate department.
- Refill water pitchers regularly unless resident has a fluid restriction. Promptly report to a nurse if a resident is not drinking his fluids.
- Remove anything that might cause odors or safety hazards, like trash, clutter or spills. Clean up spills promptly. Throw out disposable supplies. Empty trash at least daily. Replace any equipment that is stained or has an odor.
- Report signs of insects or pests immediately.
- Do not move resident's belongings. Do not discard resident's items. Respect the resident's things.

After providing care, tidy the area. Clean and put away equipment. Providing a clean, safe, and orderly environment is part of your job.

Watch those fingers and toes.

Being careless or moving quickly with equipment can cause injury. Toes and fingers may be jammed when moving the overbed table. Move equipment carefully. Tell residents exactly what you will be doing.

3. Identify factors affecting a resident's comfort

Many things affect residents' comfort within their rooms. The more you pay attention and try to improve things, the more comfortable residents may feel.

Noise Level

Common nursing home noises can upset and/or irritate residents. You can help by keeping noise level low:

- Do not bang equipment or meal trays.
- Keep your voice low.
- Promptly answer ringing telephones and call lights.
- If allowed, close doors when asked by residents.

Odors

Odors in a facility may be caused by many things. Urine, feces, vomit, certain diseases, and wound drainage all cause bad odors. Body and breath odors may be offensive, too. You can help control odors.

- Promptly clean up after incontinence (inability to control urine or bowels).
- Change incontinent briefs as soon as they are soiled. Dispose of them properly.
- Empty and clean bedpans, urinals, commodes, and emesis basins (kidney-shaped basins) promptly.
- Change soiled bed linens and clothing as soon as possible.
- Give personal care regularly to help avoid body and breath odors.

Temperature

Older and ill persons may feel cold often. Temperature in nursing homes should range between 71° and 81° F. You can help residents stay comfortable.

- Layer clothing and bed covers for warmth.
- Remove residents from any drafts.
- Offer blankets to persons in wheelchairs.
- Keep residents covered while giving personal care.

Lighting

Good lighting is important to safety and fall prevention. Good lighting also helps make a room pleasant. Residents may prefer darker rooms when they are ill, have a headache, or are sleeping. Blinds or shades help darken a room. Other residents prefer to sleep with a light on. Keep lighting controls within the resident's reach.

4. Explain the importance of sleep and factors affecting sleep

Sleep is a natural period of rest for the mind and body. Energy may be restored. Sleep and rest are two basic needs, as described in chapter 8. Bodies cannot live long without sleep. Sleep is needed to replace old cells with new ones. Sleep provides new energy to organs. Sleep performs these functions:

- It repairs the body and mind.
- Dreams help the brain sort out all the things that it has been dealing with during the day.
- Deep sleep helps the body to renew.

The elderly may require longer to go to sleep. They can have more irregular sleep patterns. Some will need short naps during the day.

Many elderly persons, especially those who are living away from their homes, have sleep problems. Many things can affect sleep. Fear, stress, noise, diet, medications, and illness all affect sleep. Sharing a room with another person can disturb sleeping. When a resident complains of lack of sleep, staff should observe for:

- sleeping too much in daytime
- too much caffeine late in the day
- wearing night clothes during day instead of day wear
- eating too late at night
- not taking medication ordered for sleep
- taking new medications
- TV or light on late at night
- pain

Lack of sleep causes many problems. These include decreased mental function, reduced reaction time, and irritability. Sleep deprivation also decreases immune system function. The elderly may be less able to tolerate sleep deprivation.

5. Discuss two types of beds

Residents' rooms should have comfortable beds. There are different types of facility beds. Two common types are electric and manual beds (Fig. 12-2).

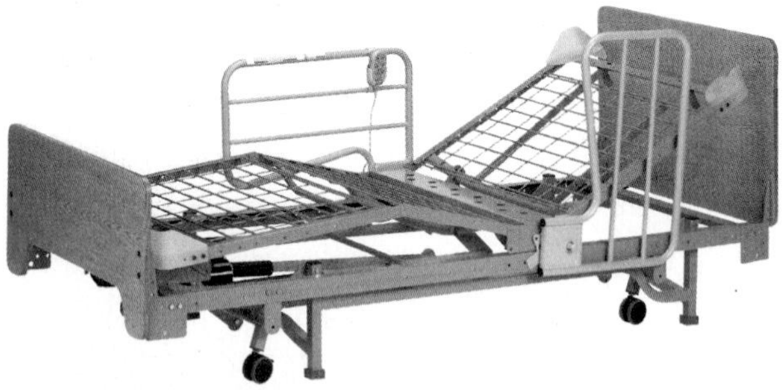

Fig. 12-2. **One type of electric bed. (Photo courtesy of Invacare Continuing Care Group, 1-800-347-5440, www.invacare-ccg.com.)**

Both are adjustable. Raising a bed horizontally while giving care reduces bending and stretching. Normally, beds are kept in their lowest horizontal position. This is so residents can get in and out of beds more easily.

Operation of electric beds tends to be simple (Fig 12-3). Controls are attached to the bed. Electric beds usually have half-side rails and openings for equipment such as IVs.

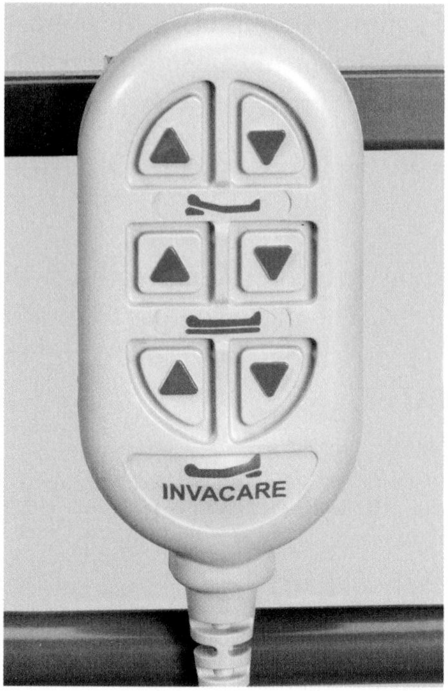

Fig. 12-3. **Controls for an electric bed. (Photo courtesy of Invacare Continuing Care Group, 1-800-347-5440, www.invacare-ccg.com.)**

Manual beds may be more difficult to use. They have cranks at the foot of the bed that move different parts of the bed. The left crank moves the head of the bed up and down. The center crank moves the entire bed up and down. The right crank moves the foot of the bed up and down. Keep cranks down at all times unless they are being used. This prevents injury. Manual beds may have full or partial side rails. These beds may not have some features that an electric bed has, such as attached controls and special openings.

6. Describe bedmaking guidelines and perform proper bedmaking

Some residents spend much or all of their time in bed. Careful bedmaking is essential to comfort, cleanliness, and health. Sheets should always be changed after personal care, such as bed baths. Change them when bedding or sheets are damp, soiled, or in need of straightening. Residents' bed linens must be changed often for three reasons:

1. Sheets that are damp, wrinkled, or bunched up are uncomfortable. They may keep the resident from sleeping well.
2. Microorganisms live in moist, warm places. Bedding that is damp or unclean may cause infection and disease.
3. Residents who spend long hours in bed are at risk for pressure sores. Sheets that do not lie flat increase this risk by cutting off circulation.

GUIDELINES
Bedmaking

- Before getting clean linen, wash your hands.
- When collecting bed linen, carry it away from you. If linen touches your uniform, it is contaminated (Fig. 12-4).

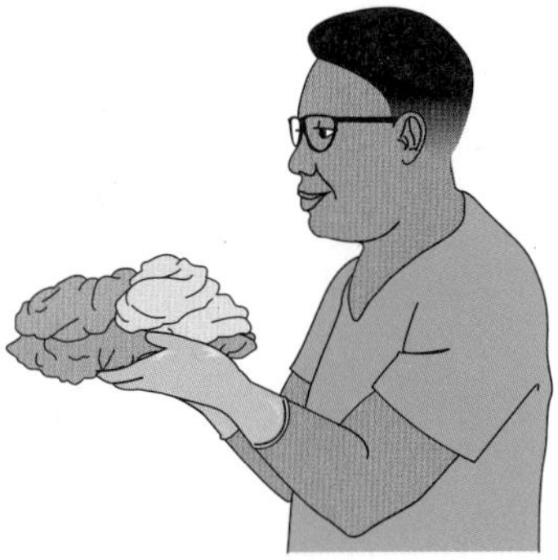

Fig. 12-4. **Carry dirty linen away from your uniform.**

- Do not shake linen. It may spread airborne contaminants.
- Do not take linen from one resident's room to another resident's room. This can spread pathogens.
- When removing dirty linen, roll it away from you. Rolling puts the dirtiest surface of the linen inward. This lessens contamination.
- Wear gloves when removing linens.
- Look for personal items, such as dentures, hearing aids, jewelry, and glasses, before removing linens.
- Change linens when wet, soiled, or too wrinkled for comfort. Residents can develop pressure sores if left in wet, soiled, or wrinkled linen.
- Keep beds smooth and wrinkle- and crumb-free. Lumps, crumbs, and wrinkles irritate skin and cause pressure sores.
- Change disposable pads whenever they become soiled or wet (Fig. 12-5). Dispose of them properly.

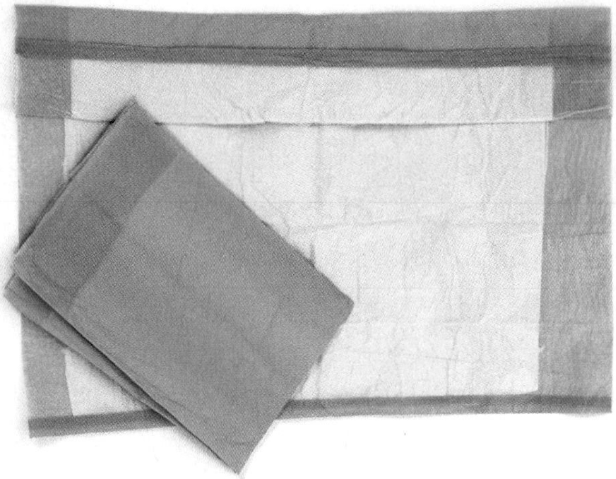

Fig. 12-5. **Absorbent pads.**

If a resident cannot get out of bed, you must change the linens with the resident in bed. An **occupied bed** is a bed made while the resident is in the bed. When making the bed, use a wide stance. Bend your knees. Avoid bending from the waist, especially when tucking sheets or blankets under the mattress. Raise the height of the bed. Mattresses can be heavy. Bend your knees to avoid injury. It is easier to make an empty bed than one with a resident in it. An **unoccupied bed** is a bed made while no resident is in the bed. If the resident can be moved, your job will be easier.

Making an occupied bed

Equipment: clean linen: mattress pad, fitted or flat bottom sheet, waterproof bed protector if needed, cotton draw sheet, flat top sheet, blan-

ket(s), bath blanket, pillowcase(s), gloves (if you are going to be touching linens soiled with body fluids)

1. Wash your hands.
2. Identify yourself by name. Identify the resident by name.
3. Explain procedure to the resident. Speak clearly, slowly, and directly. Maintain face-to-face contact whenever possible.
4. Provide for the resident's privacy with curtain, screen, or door.
5. Place clean linen on clean surface within reach (e.g., bedside stand, overbed table, or chair).
6. Adjust bed to a safe working level, usually waist high. Lock bed wheels. Lower head of bed.
7. Put on gloves if linens are soiled with body fluids.
8. Loosen top linen from the end of the bed or working side. Cover the resident with a cotton bath blanket or the loosened top sheet on the bed.
9. You will make the bed one side at a time. Raise side rail on far side of bed. After raising side rail, help resident to turn onto side, moving away from you toward raised side rail (Fig. 12-6).

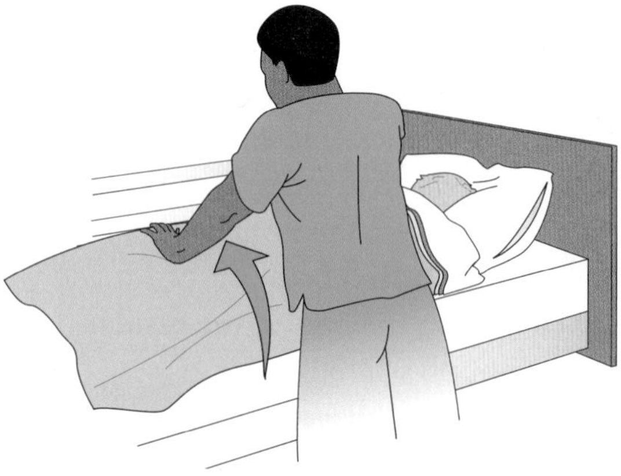

Fig. 12-6.

10. Loosen bottom soiled linen on working side.
11. Roll bottom soiled linen toward resident. Tuck it snugly against resident's back.
12. Place and tuck in clean bottom linen. Finish with bottom sheet free of wrinkles. If you are using a flat bottom sheet, leave enough overlap on each end to tuck under the mattress. If the sheet is only long enough to tuck in at one end, tuck it in securely at the top of the bed. Make hospital corners to keep bottom sheet wrinkle-free (Fig. 12-7).

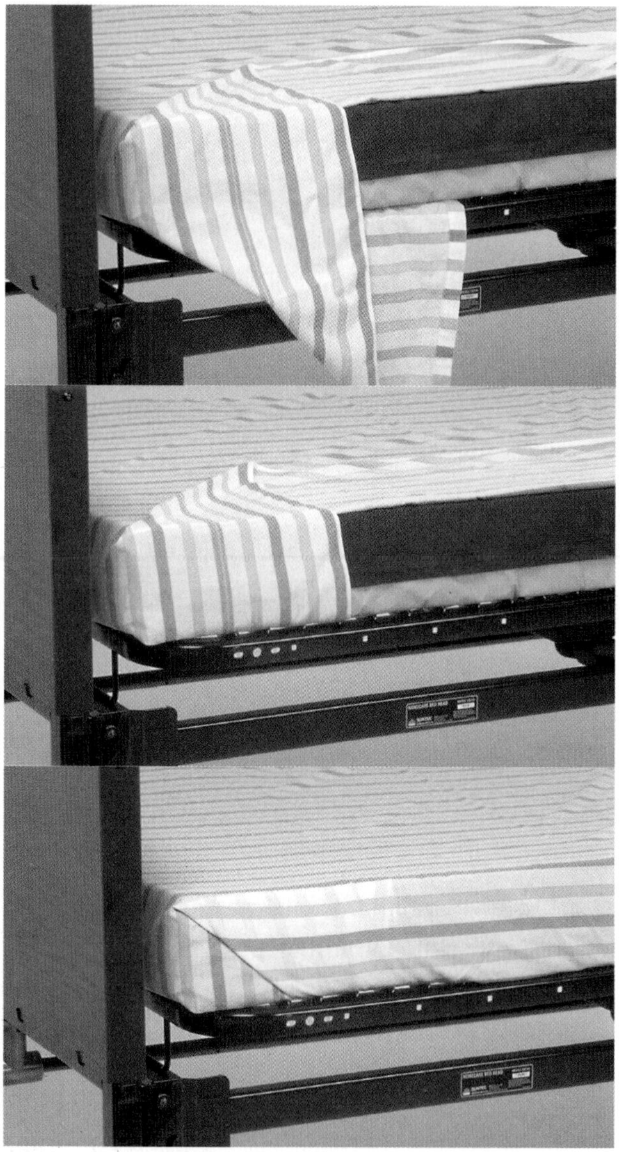

***Fig. 12-7.* Hospital corners help keep the flat sheet smooth.**

13. Smooth the bottom sheet out toward the resident. Be sure there are no wrinkles in the mattress pad. Roll the extra material to-

ward the resident. Tuck it under the resident's body.

14. If using a waterproof pad, unfold it and center it on the bed. Tuck the side near you under the mattress. Smooth it out toward the resident. Tuck as you did with the sheet.
15. If using a draw sheet, place it on the bed. Tuck in on your side, smooth, and tuck as you did with the other bedding.
16. Help resident to turn onto clean bottom sheet (Fig. 12-8). Raise side rail nearest you.

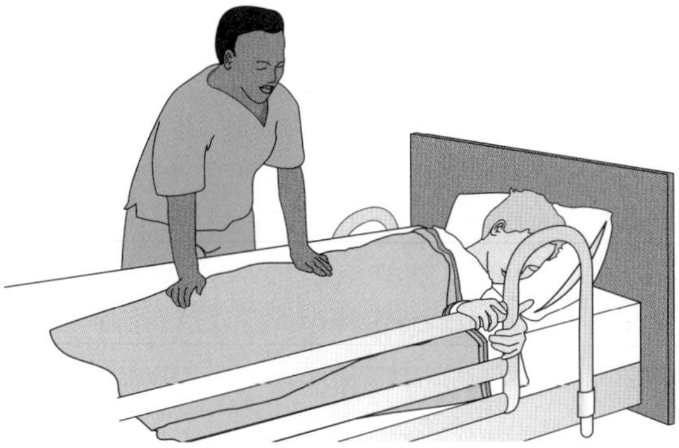

Fig. 12-8.

17. Move to other side of bed and lower side rail.
18. Turn resident away from you toward side rail.
19. Loosen soiled linen. Look for personal items. Roll linen from head to foot of bed. Avoid contact with your skin or clothes. Place it in a hamper/bag, at foot of the bed, or in a chair.
20. Pull and tuck in clean bottom linen just like the other side. Finish with bottom sheet free of wrinkles (Fig. 12-9).
21. Place resident on his back. Keep resident covered and comfortable, with a pillow under the head. Raise side rail.
22. Unfold the top sheet. Place it over the resident. Ask the resident to hold the top sheet. Slip the blanket or old sheet out from underneath (Fig. 12-10). Put it in the hamper/bag.

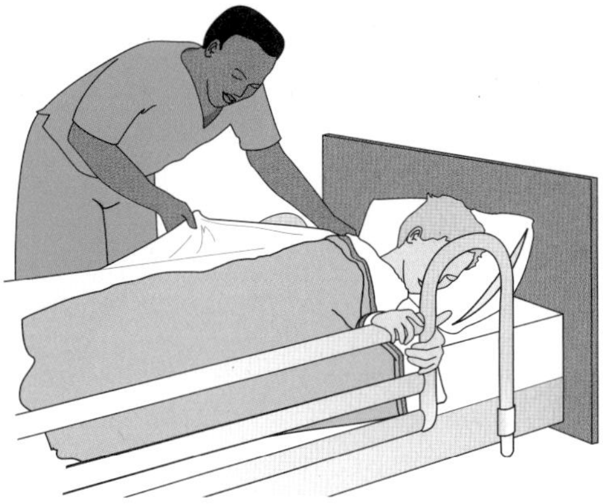

Fig. 12-9.

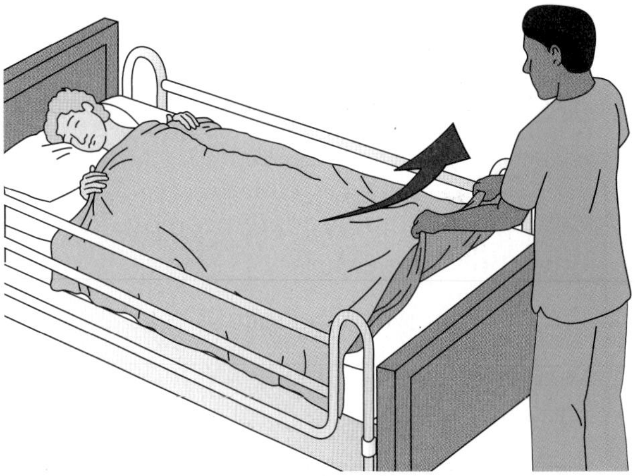

Fig. 12-10.

23. Place a blanket over the top sheet. Tuck the bottom edges of top sheet and blanket under the bottom of the mattress. Make hospital corners on each side. Loosen the top linens over the resident's feet. This prevents pressure on the feet. At the top of the bed, fold the top sheet over the blanket about six inches.
24. Remove the pillow. Do not hold it near your face. Remove the soiled pillowcase by turning it inside out. Place it in the hamper/bag.
25. With one hand, grasp the clean pillowcase at the closed end. Turn it inside out over your arm. Next, using the same hand that has the pillowcase over it, grasp one narrow edge of the pillow. Pull the pillowcase over it with your free hand (Fig. 12-11). Do the same for any other pillows. Place them under resident's head with open end away from door.

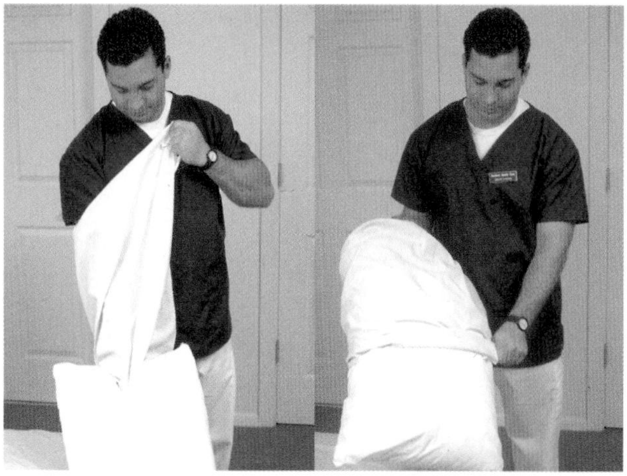

Fig. 12-11.

26. Make resident comfortable. Make sure sheets are free from wrinkles and the bed free from crumbs.
27. Return bed to appropriate position. Remove privacy measures.
28. Put call light within resident's reach.
29. Dispose of soiled linen in the proper container.
30. Remove gloves if worn.
31. Wash your hands.
32. Report any changes in resident to the nurse.
33. Document procedure using facility guidelines.

Making an unoccupied bed

Equipment: clean linen: mattress pad, fitted or flat bottom sheet, waterproof bed protector if needed, blanket(s), cotton draw sheet, flat top sheet, pillowcase(s), gloves (if you are going to be touching linens soiled with body fluids)

1. Wash your hands.
2. Place clean linen on clean surface within reach (e.g., bedside stand, overbed table, or chair).
3. Adjust bed to a safe working level, usually waist high. Lock bed wheels. Put bed in flattest position.
4. Put on gloves if linens are soiled with body fluids.
5. Loosen soiled linen. Roll soiled linen (soiled side inside) from head to foot of bed. Avoid contact with your skin or clothes. Place it in a hamper/bag, at foot of the bed, or in chair.
6. Remove gloves. Wash your hands.
7. Remake the bed. Spread mattress pad and bottom sheet, tucking under. Make hospital corners to keep bottom sheet wrinkle-free. Put on mattress protector and draw sheet. Smooth, and tuck under sides of bed.
8. Place top sheet and blanket over bed. Center these, tuck under end of bed and make hospital corners. Fold down the top sheet over the blanket about six inches. Fold both top sheet and blanket down so resident can easily get into bed (Fig. 12-12). If resident will not be returning to bed immediately, leave bedding up.

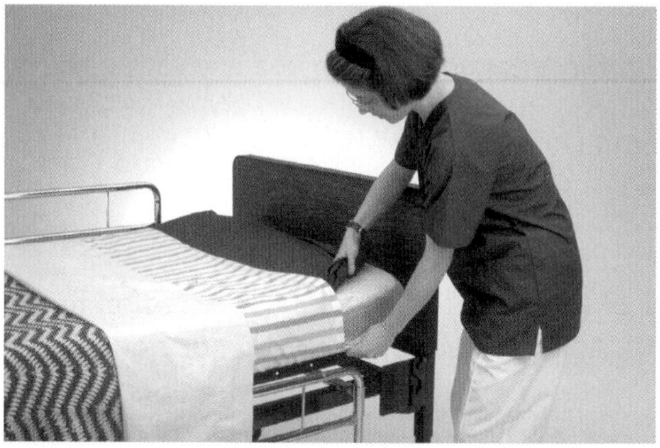

Fig. 12-12. **The top sheet and blanket are folded down so that residents can more easily get into bed.**

9. Remove pillows and pillowcases. Put on clean pillowcases (as described above). Replace pillows.
10. Return bed to appropriate position.
11. Dispose of soiled linen in the proper container.
12. Remove gloves if worn.
13. Wash your hands.

14. Document procedure using facility guidelines.

A **closed bed** is a bed completely made with the bedspread and blankets in place. A closed bed is turned into an **open bed** by folding the linen down to the foot of the bed. Most residents are out of bed much of the day. A closed bed is made until it is time for the resident to go to sleep. Then an open bed is made.

Give prompt, compassionate care.

Some residents will unintentionally soil or wet the bed. Change the sheets, along with all clothing and pads, immediately when this happens. Do so with compassion and respect. Be professional. Do not draw attention to the resident or tell other residents. Clean the resident. Make him feel comfortable. When residents are left in soiled beds, it may be considered physical and emotional abuse, as well as neglect.

A **surgical bed** is made to easily accept residents who must return to bed on stretchers. Residents on stretchers are usually returning from treatment or hospital visits. Use caution when transferring residents from stretchers to beds. Lock bed and stretcher wheels. The bed and stretcher must be close together during the transfer (see chapter 10).

Making a surgical bed

Equipment: clean linen (see procedure: making an unoccupied bed), gloves

Discuss the preparation for the arrival of a resident on a stretcher with the nurse. When preparing the room, you may need to set up equipment in the room. Check with the nurse for instructions on gathering any extra equipment/supplies.

1. Wash your hands.
2. Place clean linen on clean surface within reach (e.g., bedside stand, overbed table, or chair).
3. Adjust bed to a safe working level, usually waist high. Lock bed wheels.
4. Put on gloves.
5. Remove all soiled linen, rolling it (soiled side inside) from head to foot of bed. Avoid contact with your skin or clothes. Place it in a hamper/bag, at foot of the bed, or in chair.
6. Remove gloves. Wash your hands.
7. Make an unoccupied bed with bedding left up (a closed bed). Do not tuck top linens under the mattress.
8. Fold top linens down from the head of the bed and up from foot of the bed. (Fig. 12-13)

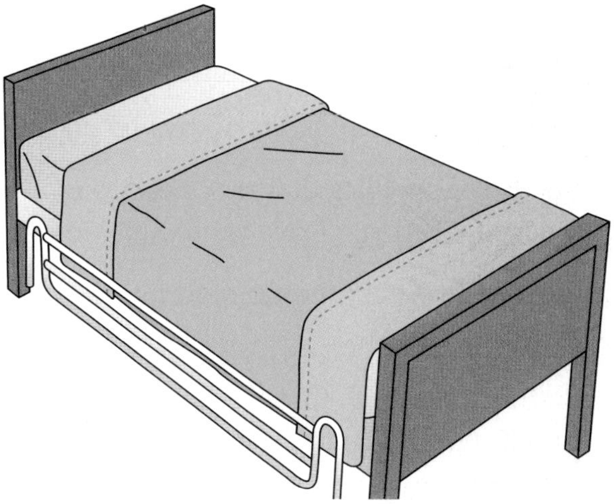

Fig. 12-13.

9. Fanfold linens lengthwise to the side away from door. Fanfolded means folded several times into pleats (Fig 12-14).

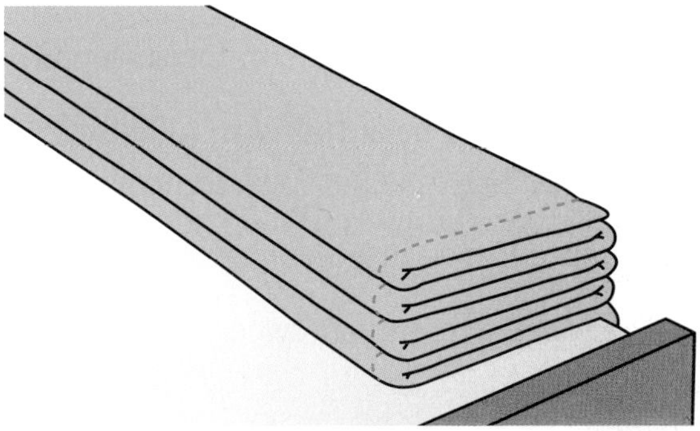

Fig. 12-14.

10. Put on clean pillowcases. Place the pillows on a clean surface off the bed (e.g., bedside stand, overbed table, or chair).
11. Leave bed in its highest position. Leave both side rails down.
12. Move all furniture to make room for the stretcher.
13. Do not place call light on bed. That is placed after the resident returns to bed.
14. Dispose of soiled linen in the proper container.
15. Wash your hands.
16. Document procedure using facility guidelines.

Chapter Review

1. What is the overbed table used for? Can you place bedpans and soiled linen on it?
2. Where should call lights always be placed?
3. List three supplies that may need to be restocked when you leave residents' rooms.
4. Why is disposable equipment used?
5. List four things that may affect residents' comfort. For each thing you list, describe one thing you can do to help promote comfort.
6. List two functions that sleep performs for the body.
7. When a resident is not sleeping well, what may be affecting his sleep?
8. What can happen if a person loses sleep?
9. List two types of beds found in a facility. Which type has attached bed controls?
10. When should bed linens be changed?
11. Explain the difference between an open and a closed bed.
12. What problem can wet, soiled, or wrinkled sheets cause?
13. Which way should pillows face while under residents' heads?

Chapter 13
Personal Care Skills

1. Explain personal care of residents

Hygiene is the term used to describe ways to keep bodies clean and healthy. Bathing and brushing teeth are two examples. **Grooming** means practices like caring for fingernails and hair. Hygiene and grooming, as well as dressing and eating, are called activities of daily living (ADLs). You will help residents every day with these tasks.

These activities are often called "A.M. care" or "P.M. care." This refers to the time of day when they are done.

A.M. care includes:

- offering a bedpan or urinal or helping the resident to the bathroom
- helping the resident to wash face and hands
- helping with mouth care before or after breakfast, as the resident prefers

P.M. care includes:

- offering a bedpan or urinal or helping the resident to the bathroom
- helping the resident to wash face and hands
- giving a snack (if allowed)
- performing mouth care
- giving a back rub (if allowed)

The way you help residents with personal care plays a large part in promoting their independence and dignity. The tasks you help with and how much help you give will be different for each resident. It will depend on each resident's ability to do self-care and/or his or her physical or mental limitations. For example, a resident who has recently had a stroke will need more help than one who has a broken foot that is almost healed. Promoting independence is an important part of the care you give.

Personal care is a very private experience. It may be embarrassing for some residents. You must be professional when helping with these tasks. Before you start, explain to the resident exactly what you will be doing. Ask if he or she would like to use the bathroom or bedpan first. Give the resident privacy. Let him or her make as many decisions as possible about when, where, and how a task is done (Fig. 13-1). This promotes dignity and independence. Encourage a resident to do as much as he or she is able to do while giving care.

Here are other ways to provide respect, dignity, and privacy when helping with care:

- Do not interrupt them while a resident is in the bathroom.
- Leave the room when a resident receives or makes phone calls.

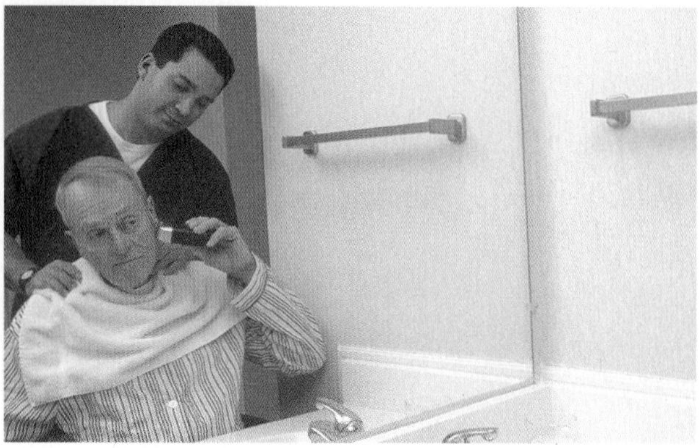

***Fig. 13-1.* Let the resident make as many decisions as possible about the personal care you will perform.**

- Respect residents' private time and personal things.
- Do not interrupt a resident while dressing.
- Encourage residents to do things for themselves. Be patient.
- Be patient while residents choose their clothing. Keep them covered whenever possible when you help with dressing.

During personal care, look for any problems or changes that have occurred. Personal care gives you a chance to talk with residents. Some residents will share feelings and concerns with you. You can also observe a resident's environment. Look for physical and mental changes. Look for unsafe or unhealthy surroundings. Report these to the nurse.

If the resident seems tired, stop and take a short rest. Never rush him or her. After care, always ask if the resident would like anything else. Leave the resident's area clean and tidy. Make sure the call light is within reach. Leave the bed in its lowest position unless instructed otherwise.

OBSERVING AND REPORTING
Personal Care

- skin color, temperature, redness (more information listed in next learning objective)
- mobility
- flexibility
- comfort level, or pain or discomfort
- strength and the ability to perform ADLs
- mental and emotional state
- resident complaints

2. Identify guidelines for providing good skin care and preventing pressure sores

Immobility reduces the amount of blood that circulates to the skin. Residents who have less mobility have more risk of skin deterioration at pressure points. **Pressure points** are areas of the body that bear much of its weight. Pressure points are mainly located at bony prominences. **Bony prominences** are areas of the body where the bone lies close to the skin. These areas include elbows, shoulder blades, tailbone, hip bones, ankles, heels, and the back of the neck and head. The skin here is at a much higher risk for skin breakdown.

Other areas at risk are the ears, the area under the breasts, and the scrotum (Fig. 13-2). The pressure on these areas reduces circulation, decreasing the amount of oxygen the cells receive. Warmth and moisture also add to skin breakdown. Once the surface of the skin is weakened, pathogens can invade and cause infection. When infection occurs, the healing process slows down. (Refer to chapter 5 for information on pathogens and infection.)

When skin begins to break down, it becomes pale, white, or a reddened color. Darker skin may look purple. The resident may also feel tingling or burning in the area. This discoloration does not go away, even when the resident's position is changed. If pressure is allowed to continue, the area will further break down. The resulting wound is called a **pressure sore**, **bed sore**, or **decubitus ulcer**.

Once a pressure sore forms, it can get bigger, deeper, and infected. Most pressure sores occur within a few weeks of admission to a

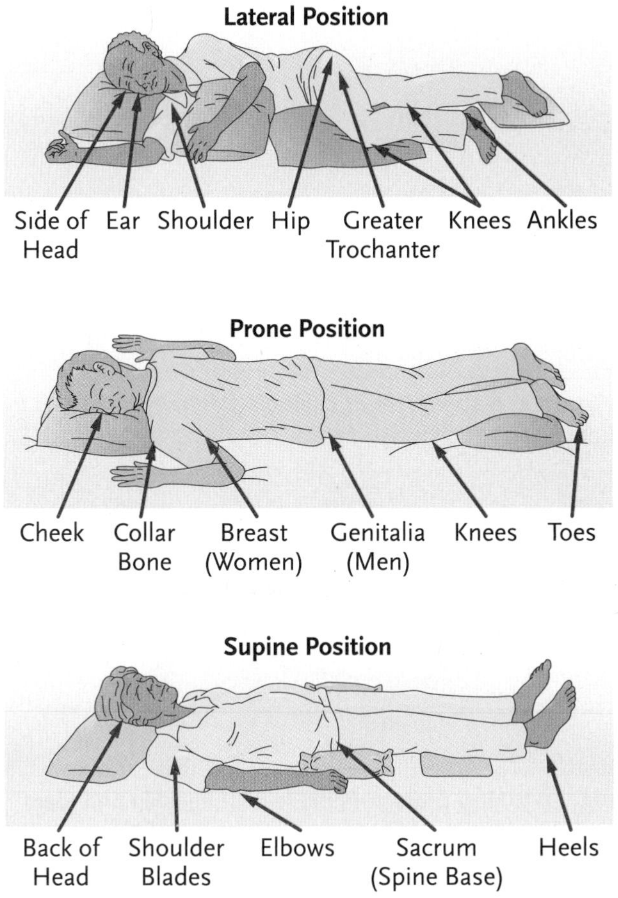

***Fig. 13-2.* Pressure sore danger zones.**

nursing home. Pressure sores are painful and difficult to heal. They can lead to life-threatening infection. Prevention is very important.

There are four accepted stages of pressure sores (Fig. 13-3):

Stage 1: Area where skin is intact but there is redness that is not relieved within 15 to 30 minutes after removing pressure.

Stage 2: Partial skin loss involving the outer and/or inner layer of skin. The ulcer is superficial. It looks like a blister or a shallow crater.

Stage 3: Full skin loss involving damage or death of tissue that may extend down to but not through the tissue that covers muscle. The ulcer looks like a deep crater.

Stage 4: Full skin loss with major destruction, tissue death, damage to muscle, bone, or supporting structures.

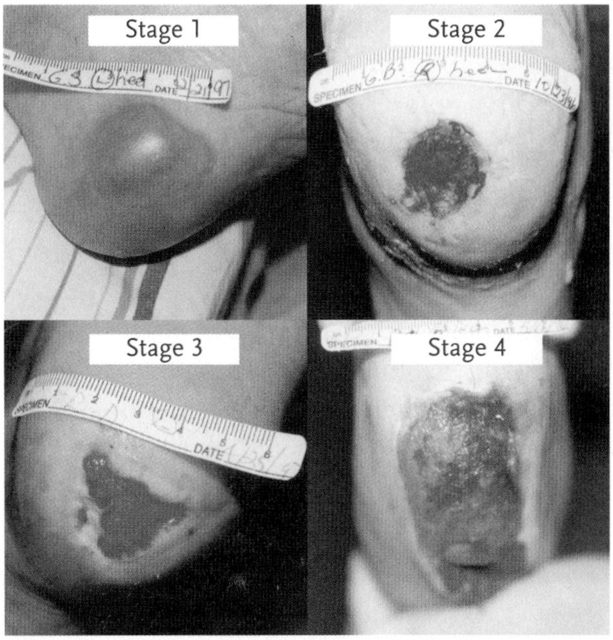

***Fig. 13-3.* Pressure sores are categorized by four stages. (Photos courtesy of Dr. Tamara D. Fishman and The Wound Care Institute, Inc.)**

OBSERVING AND REPORTING

Resident's Skin

Report any of these to the nurse:

- pale, white, reddened, or purple areas, blisters or bruises on the skin
- tingling, warmth, or burning of the skin
- dry or flaking skin
- itching or scratching
- rash or any skin discoloration
- swelling
- blisters
- fluid or blood draining from skin
- broken skin
- wounds or ulcers on the skin
- changes in wound or ulcer (size, depth, drainage, color, odor)
- broken skin between toes or around toenails

GUIDELINES

Basic Skin Care

- Report changes in a resident's skin.

- Provide regular care for skin to keep it clean and dry. When complete baths are not taken every day, check the resident's skin. Give skin care daily.
- Reposition immobile residents at least every two hours.
- Give frequent and thorough skin care as often as needed for incontinent residents. Change clothing and linens often as well. Check on them every two hours or as needed.
- Do not scratch or irritate the skin in any way. Report to the nurse if a resident wears shoes or slippers that cause blisters or sores.
- Massage the skin often. Use light, circular strokes to increase circulation. Use little or no pressure on bony areas. Do not massage a white, red, or purple area or put any pressure on it. Massage the healthy skin and tissue around the area.
- Be careful during transfers. Avoid pulling or tearing fragile skin.

For residents who are not mobile or cannot change positions easily, remember:

- Keep the bottom sheet tight and free from wrinkles. Keep the bed free from crumbs.
- Do not pull the resident across sheets during transfers or repositioning. This causes shearing, or pressure, when the surfaces rub against each other.
- Place a sheepskin, chamois skin, or bed pad under the back and buttocks to absorb moisture or perspiration that may build up and to protect the skin from irritating bed linens (Fig. 13-4).
- Relieve pressure under bony prominences. Place foam rubber or sheepskin pads under them. Heel and elbow protectors made of foam and sheepskin are available (Fig. 13-5).

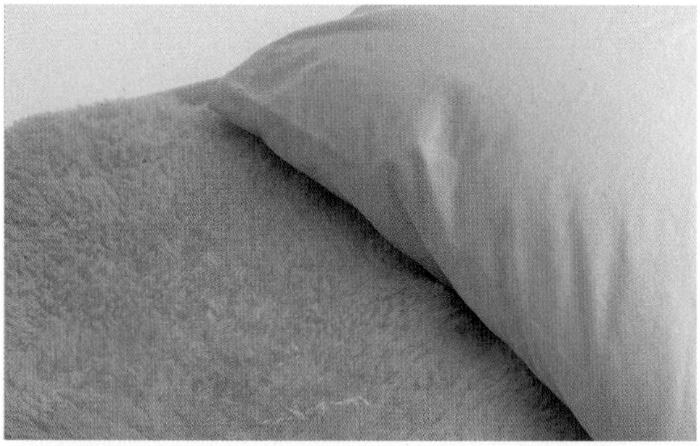

Fig. 13-4. **A sheepskin or chamois skin may be placed to help absorb moisture.**

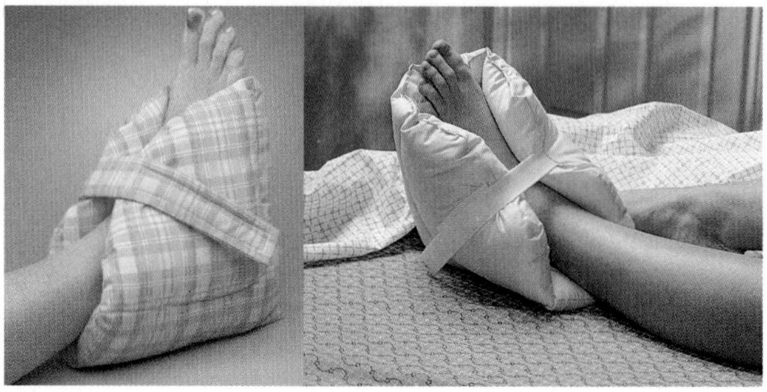

Fig. 13-5. **Heel protectors made of sheepskin and foam are available. (Reprinted with permission of Briggs Corporation, 800-247-2343)**

- A bed or chair can be made softer with flotation pads or an egg-crate mattress (Fig. 13-6).

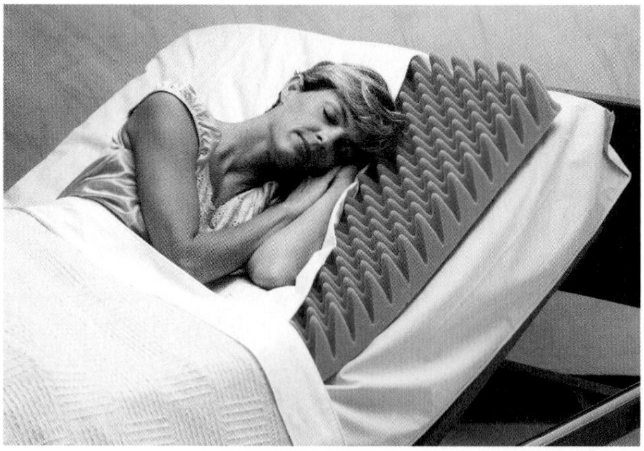

Fig. 13-6. **An egg-crate mattress can make a bed softer. (Reprinted with permission of Briggs Corporation, 800-247-2343)**

- Residents in chairs or wheelchairs need to be repositioned often, too.

Many positioning devices are available to help make residents more comfortable and safe.

GUIDELINES
Using Positioning Devices

- Backrests can be regular pillows or special wedge-shaped foam pillows.
- Bed cradles are used to keep the bed covers from pushing down on a resident's feet.
- Use draw sheets, or turning sheets, under residents who cannot help with turning, lifting, or moving up in bed. Draw sheets help prevent skin damage from shearing.
- Footboards are padded boards placed against the resident's feet to keep them flexed (Fig. 13-7).

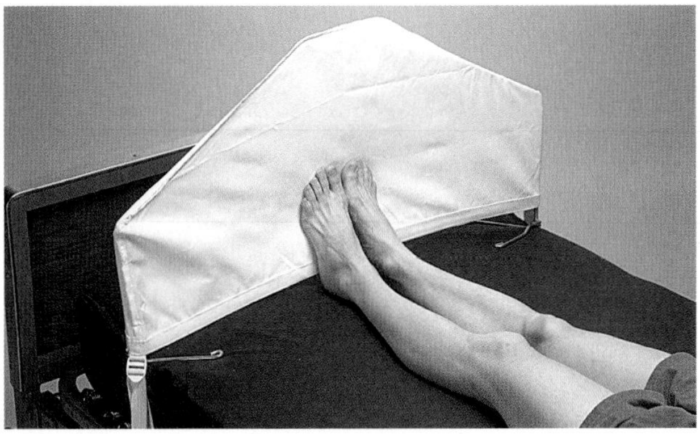

Fig. 13-7. **Footboards help prevent pressure sores. (Reprinted with permission of Briggs Corporation, 800-247-2343)**

- Hand rolls keep the fingers from curling tightly. A rolled washcloth, gauze bandage, or a rubber ball placed inside the palm may be used to keep the hand in a natural position (Fig. 13-8).

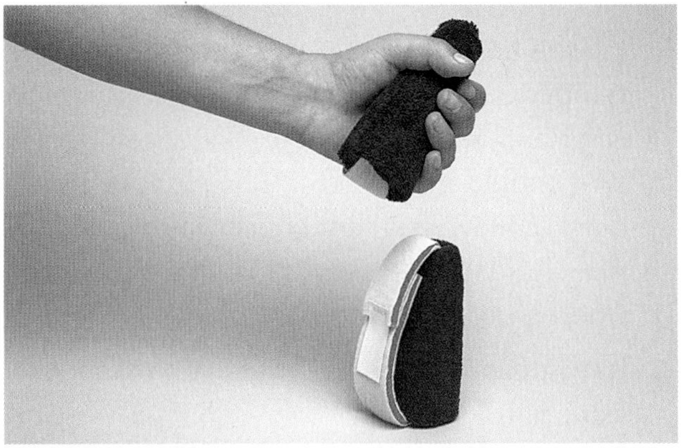

Fig. 13-8. **A handroll. (Reprinted with permission of Briggs Corporation, 800-247-2343)**

- Splints may be prescribed by a doctor to keep a resident's joints in the correct position (Fig. 13-9). Splints and the skin area around them should be cleaned at least once daily and as needed.

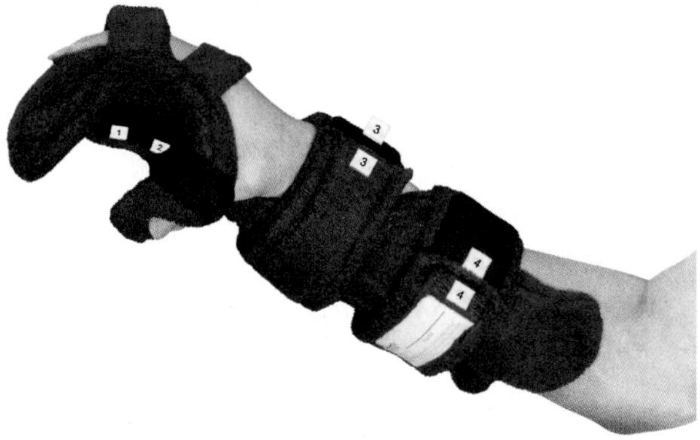

Fig. 13-9. **One type of splint. (Photo courtesy of Lenjoy Medical Engineering "Comfy Splints™" 800-582-5332, www.comfysplints.com.)**

- Trochanter rolls keep a resident's hips from turning outward. A rolled towel works well, too (Fig. 13-10).

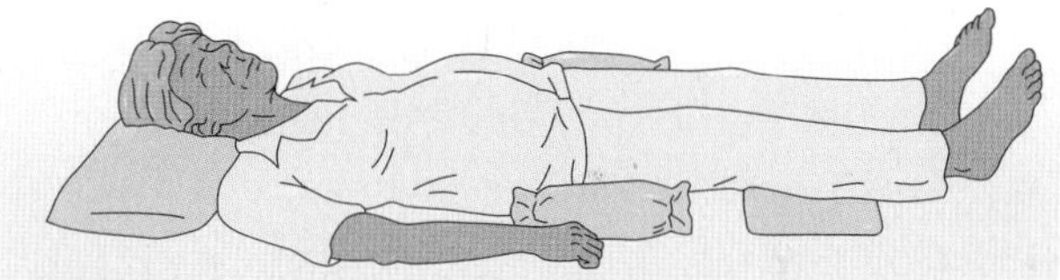

Fig. 13-10. **Trochanter rolls help keep the hips from turning outward.**

3. Explain guidelines for assisting with bathing

Bathing promotes good health and well-being. It removes perspiration, dirt, oil, and dead skin cells from the skin. Bathing gives you the chance to observe a resident's skin.

There are four basic types of baths. These are a partial bath, a shower, a tub bath, or a complete bed bath. A **partial bath** is performed on days when a complete bed bath, tub bath, or shower is not done. It includes washing the face, underarms, and hands, and performing perineal care.

The decision on which bath to give a resident rests first with the doctor, then with the resident. A doctor may write an order for "no shower" until a wound has healed. Some residents are confined to bed. This makes a bed bath necessary. For bed-bound residents, bed baths will also move arms and legs. This increases body movement and circulation.

A doctor may order a special bath using an additive. An **additive** is a substance added to another substance changing its effect. Examples of bath additives include bran, oatmeal, sodium bicarbonate, and epsom salts.

GUIDELINES
Bathing

- The face, hands, underarms, and perineum should be washed every day. The **perineum** includes the genitals and anus and the area between them. A complete bath or shower can be taken every other day or even less often.
- Older skin produces less perspiration and oil. Elderly people with dry and fragile skin should bathe only once or twice a week. This prevents further dryness.
- Use only products approved by the facility or that the resident prefers.
- Before bathing a resident, make sure the room is warm enough.
- Before bathing, make sure the water temperature is safe and comfortable. Test the water temperature to make sure it is not too hot. Then have the resident test the water temperature. His or her sense of touch may be different than yours. The resident is best able to choose a comfortable water temperature.
- Gather supplies before giving a bath so a resident is not left alone.
- Make sure all soap is removed from the skin before completing the bath.
- Keep a record of the bathing schedule for each resident. Follow the care plan.

Giving a complete bed bath

Equipment: bath blanket, bath basin, soap, bath thermometer, 2-4 washcloths, 2-4 bath towels, orangewood stick or emery board, lotion, deodorant, clean gown or clothes, gloves

1. Wash your hands.
2. Identify yourself by name. Identify the resident by name.
3. Explain procedure to the resident. Speak clearly, slowly, and directly. Maintain face-to-face contact whenever possible.
4. Provide for the resident's privacy with curtain, screen, or door. Be sure the room is a comfortable temperature and there are no drafts.
5. Adjust bed to a safe level, usually waist high. Lock bed wheels.
6. Adjust position of side rails to ensure resident safety at all times.
7. Place a bath blanket or towel over resident (Fig. 13-11). Ask him to hold onto it as you remove or fold back top bedding. Keep resident covered with bath blanket (or top sheet).

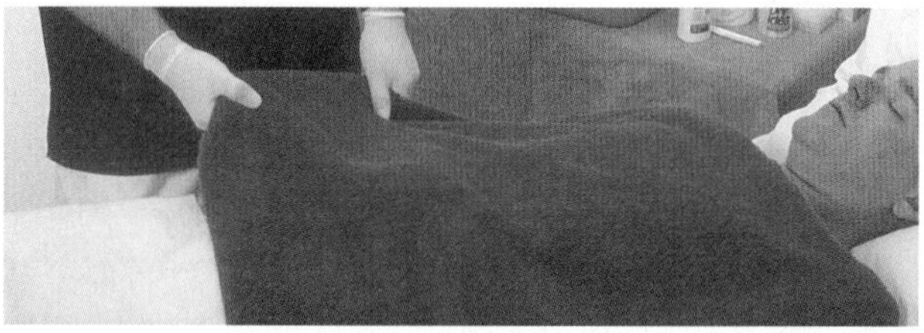

Fig. 13-11.

8. Fill the basin with warm water. Test water temperature with thermometer or your wrist and ensure it is safe. Water temperature should be 105° to 110° F. It cools quickly. Have resident check water temperature. Adjust if necessary. Change the water when it becomes too cool, soapy, or dirty.
9. If resident has open wounds or broken skin, put on gloves.
10. Ask and help resident to participate in washing.

11. Uncover only one part of the body at a time. Place a towel under the body part being washed.
12. Wash, rinse, and dry one part of the body at a time. Start at the head. Work down, and complete the front first. Fold the washcloth over your hand like a mitt and hold it in place with the thumb (Fig. 13-12).

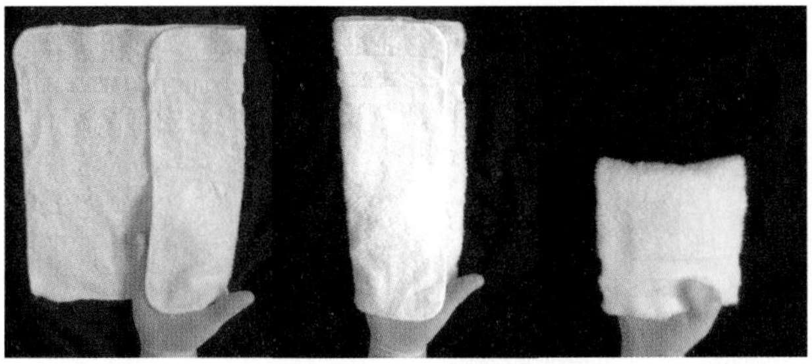

Fig. 13-12.

Eyes and Face: Wash face with wet washcloth (no soap). Begin with the eye farther away from you. Wash inner aspect to outer aspect (Fig. 13-13). Use a different area of the washcloth for each eye. Wash the face from the middle outward. Use firm but gentle strokes. Wash the neck and ears and behind the ears. Rinse and pat dry.

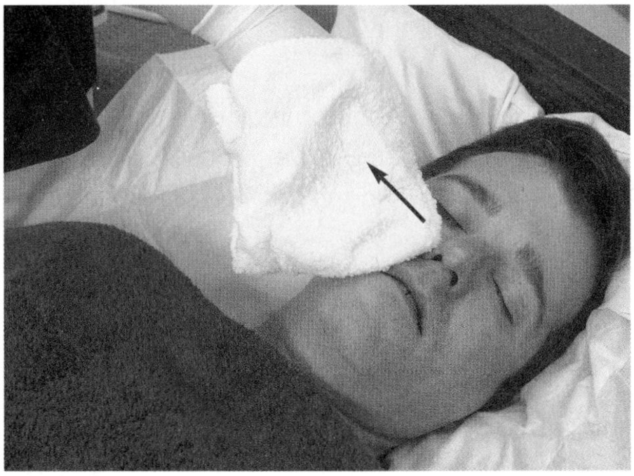

Fig. 13-13.

Arms: Remove the resident's top clothing. Cover him with the bath blanket or towel. With a soapy washcloth, wash the upper arm and underarm. Use long strokes from the shoulder to the elbow. Rinse and pat dry. Wash the elbow. Wash, rinse, and dry from the elbow down to the wrist (Fig. 13-14).

Wash the hand in a basin: Clean under the nails with an orangewood stick or nail brush if available (Fig. 13-15). Rinse and pat dry. Give nail care (see procedure later in this chapter) only if it has been assigned.

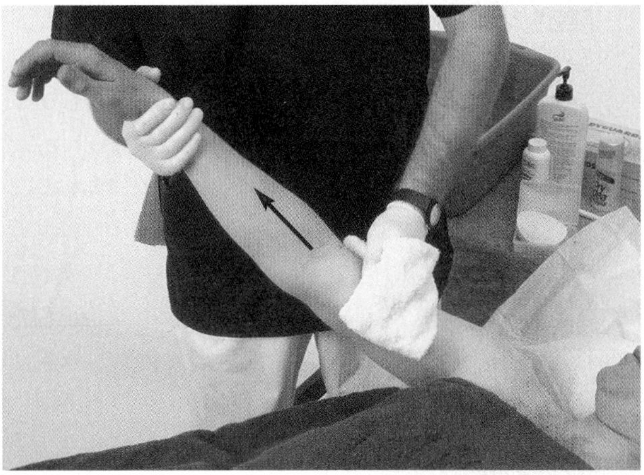

Fig. 13-14.

Do not give nail care for a diabetic resident. Repeat for the other arm. Put lotion on the resident's elbows and hands if ordered.

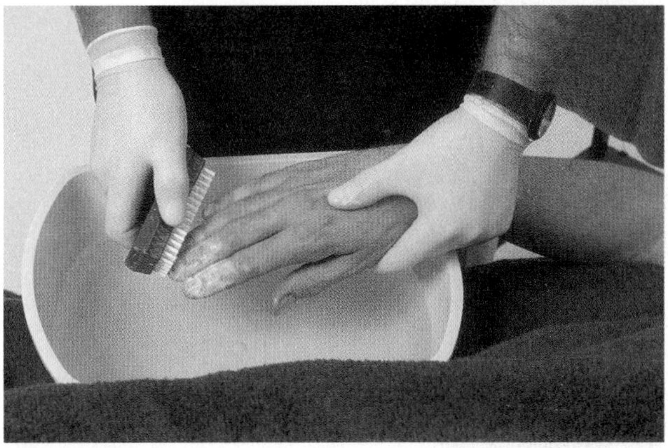

Fig. 13-15.

Chest: Place the towel again across the resident's chest. Pull the blanket down to the waist. Lift the towel only enough to wash the chest. Rinse it, and pat dry. For a female resident, wash, rinse, and dry breasts and under breasts. Check the skin in this area for signs of irritation and chafing.

Abdomen: Fold the blanket down so that it still covers the pubic area. Wash the abdomen, rinse, and pat dry. If the resident has an ostomy, or opening in the abdomen for getting rid of body wastes, give skin care around the opening (chapter 15 includes more information about ostomies). Cover with the towel. Pull the cotton blanket up to the resident's chin. Remove the towel.

Legs and Feet: Expose one leg. Place a towel under it. Wash the thigh. Use long downward strokes. Rinse and pat dry. Do the same from the knee to the ankle (Fig. 13-16). Place another towel under the foot. Move the basin to the towel. Place the foot into the basin. Wash the foot and between the toes (Fig. 13-17). Rinse foot and pat dry. Make sure area between toes is dry. Give nail care (see procedure later in this chapter) only if it has been assigned. Do not give nail care for a diabetic resident. Never clip a resident's toenails. Apply lotion to the foot if ordered, especially at the heels. Repeat steps for the other leg and foot.

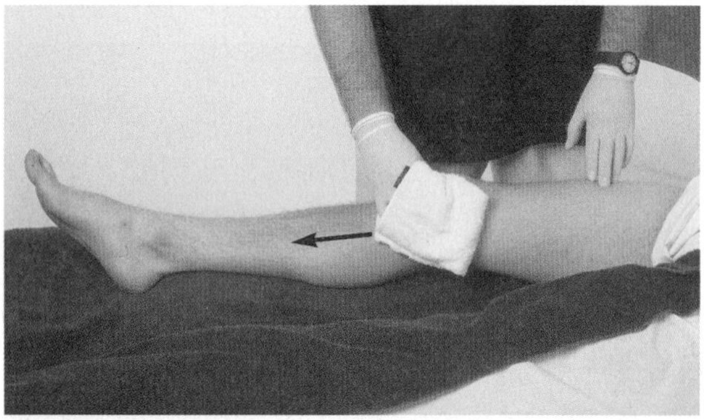

Fig. 13-16.

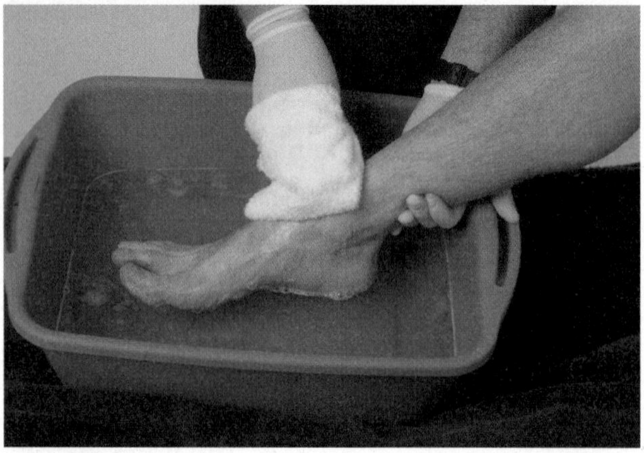

Fig. 13-17.

Back: Help resident move to the center of the bed. Ask resident to turn onto his side so his back is facing you. If the bed has rails, raise the rail on the far side for safety. Fold the blanket away from the back. Place a towel lengthwise next to the back. Wash the back, neck, and buttocks with long, downward strokes. Rinse and pat dry (Fig. 13-18). Apply lotion if ordered.

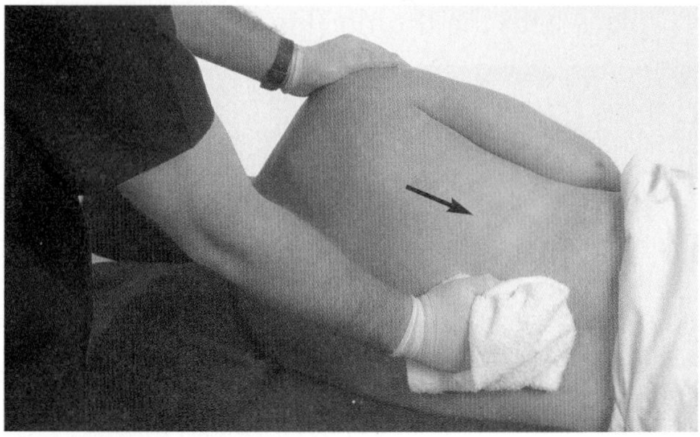

Fig. 13-18.

13. Place the towel under the buttocks and upper thighs. Help the resident turn onto his back. Ask if he is able to wash the perineal area. If the resident is able to do this, place a basin of clean, warm water and a washcloth and towel within reach. Leave the room if the resident desires. If the resident has a urinary catheter in place, remind him not to pull it.
14. If the resident cannot provide perineal care, you must do so. Put on gloves (if you haven't already done so) first. Provide privacy at all times.
15. Change bath water. Wash, rinse, and dry perineal area. Work from front to back.

    For a female resident: Wash the perineum with soap and water. Work from front to back, using single strokes (Fig. 13-19). Do not wash from the back to the front. This may cause infection. Use a clean area of washcloth or a clean washcloth for each stroke. First wipe the center of the perineum, then each side. Then spread the labia majora, the outside folds of perineal skin that protect the urinary meatus and the vaginal opening. Wipe from front to back on each side. Rinse the area in the same way. Dry entire perineal area. Move from front to back. Use a blotting motion with towel. Ask resident to turn on her side. Wash, rinse, and dry buttocks and anal area. Clean the anal area without contaminating the perineal area.

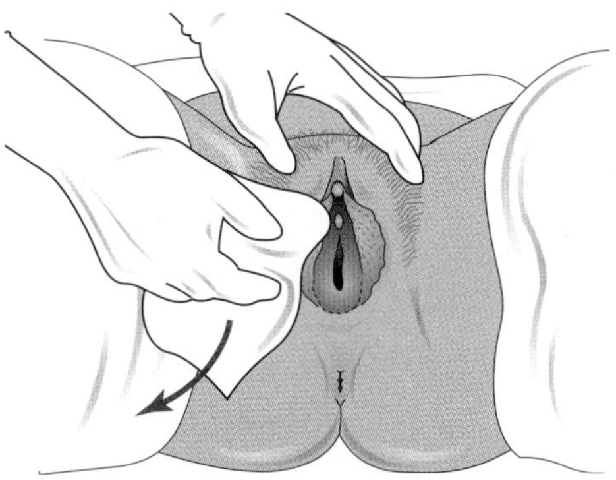

Fig. 13-19.

For a male resident: If the resident is uncircumcised, pull back the foreskin first. Gently push skin towards the base of penis. Hold the penis by the shaft. Wash in a circular motion from the tip down to the base. Use a clean area of washcloth or clean washcloth for each stroke (Fig. 13-20). Rinse the penis. If resident is uncircumcised, gently return foreskin to normal position. Then wash the scrotum and groin. The **groin** is the area from the pubis (area around the penis and scrotum) to the upper thighs. Rinse and pat dry. Ask the resident to turn on his side. Wash, rinse, and dry buttocks and anal area. Clean the anal area without contaminating the perineal area.

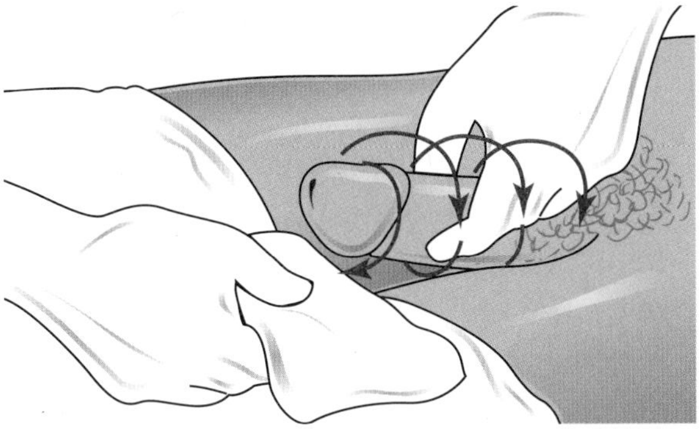

Fig. 13-20.

16. Provide deodorant.
17. Remove and dispose of gloves properly.
18. Put clean gown on resident. Brush or comb the resident's hair (see procedure later in this chapter).
19. Make resident comfortable. Make sure sheets are dry and free from wrinkles and the bed free from crumbs.
20. Return bed to appropriate position. Remove privacy measures.
21. Put call light within resident's reach.
22. Place soiled clothing and linens in proper containers.
23. Empty, rinse, and wipe bath basin. Return to proper storage.
24. Wash your hands.
25. Report any changes in resident to the nurse.
26. Document procedure using facility guidelines.

A back rub can help relax your resident. It can make him more comfortable and increase circulation. Back rubs are often given after baths.

Giving a back rub

Equipment: cotton blanket or towel, lotion

1. Wash your hands.
2. Identify yourself by name. Identify the resident by name.
3. Explain procedure to the resident. Speak clearly, slowly, and directly. Maintain face-to-face contact whenever possible.
4. Provide for resident's privacy with curtain, screen, or door.
5. Adjust bed to a safe working level, usually waist high. Lock bed wheels.
6. Position resident lying on his stomach (Fig. 13-21). If this is uncomfortable, have him lie on his side. Cover with a cotton blanket.

Expose back to the top of the buttocks. Back rubs can also be given with the resident sitting up.

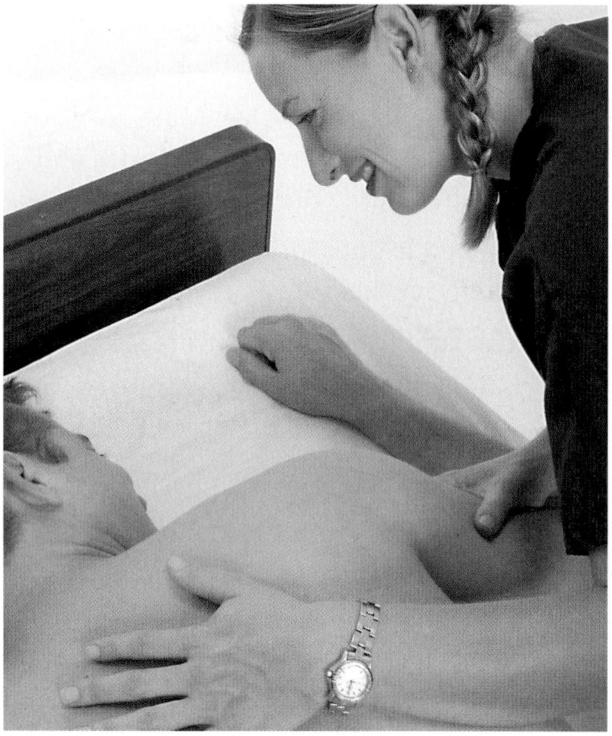

Fig. 13-21.

7. Warm lotion by putting bottle in warm water for five minutes. Run your hands under warm water. Pour lotion on your hands. Rub them together. Always put lotion on your hands rather than on resident's skin.
8. Place hands on each side of upper part of the buttocks. Make long, smooth upward strokes with both hands. Move along each side of the spine, up to the shoulders (Fig. 13-22). Circle hands outward. Move back along outer edges of the back. At buttocks, make another circle. Move hands back up to the shoulders. Without taking hands from resident's skin, repeat for three to five minutes.
9. Knead with the first two fingers and thumb of each hand. Place them at base of the spine. Move upward together along each side of the spine. Apply gentle downward pressure with fingers and thumbs. Follow same direction as with the long smooth strokes, circling at shoulders and buttocks (Fig. 13-23).

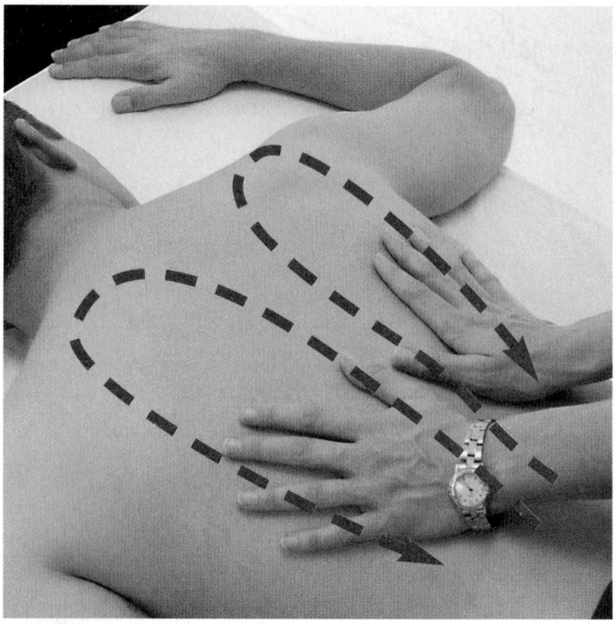

Fig. 13-22.

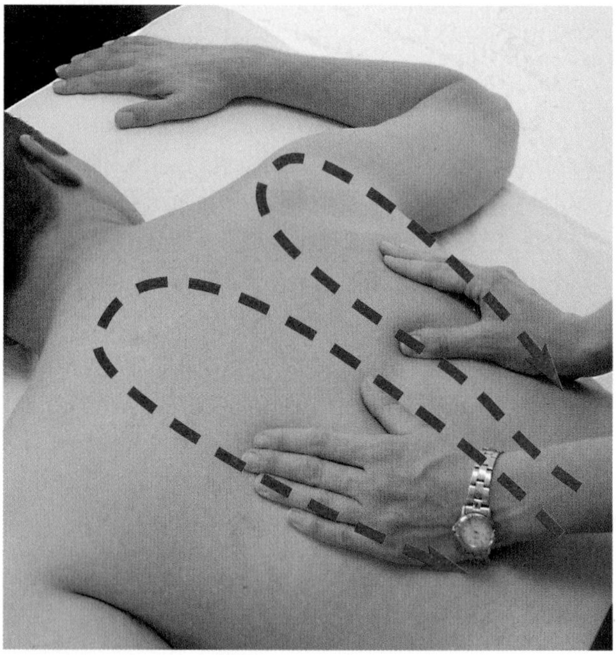

Fig. 13-23.

10. Gently massage bony areas (spine, shoulder blades, hip bones). Use circular motions of fingertips. If any of these areas are red, massage around them.
11. Finish with some long, smooth strokes.
12. Dry the back if extra lotion remains on it.

13. Remove blanket and towel.
14. Help the resident get dressed. Make resident comfortable. Make sure sheets are free from wrinkles and the bed free from crumbs.
15. Store supplies. Place soiled clothing and linens in proper containers.
16. Return bed to proper position. Remove privacy measures.
17. Before leaving, place call light within resident's reach.
18. Wash your hands.
19. Report any changes in resident to the nurse.
20. Document procedure using facility guidelines.

Shampooing resident's hair in bed

Equipment: shampoo, hair conditioner if requested, 2 bath towels, washcloth, bath thermometer, pitcher or handheld shower or sink attachment, waterproof pad, bath blanket, trough, basin, comb and brush, hair dryer

1. Wash your hands.
2. Identify yourself by name. Identify the resident by name.
3. Explain procedure to the resident. Speak clearly, slowly, and directly. Maintain face-to-face contact whenever possible.
4. Provide for the resident's privacy with curtain, screen, or door. Be sure the room is a comfortable temperature and there are no drafts.
5. Adjust bed to a safe level, usually waist high. Lock bed wheels. Remove pillows. Place resident in a flat position.
6. Test water temperature with thermometer or your wrist. Ensure it is safe. Water temperature should be 105° F. Have resident check water temperature. Adjust if necessary.
7. Raise the side rail farthest from you.
8. Place the waterproof pad under the resident's head and shoulders. Cover the resident with the bath blanket. Fold back the top sheet and regular blankets.
9. Place collection container under resident's head (e.g., trough, basin). Place one towel across the resident's shoulders.
10. Protect resident's eyes with dry washcloth.
11. Using the pitcher or attachment, wet hair thoroughly. Apply small amount of shampoo to your hands. Rub them together. Using both hands, massage shampoo to a lather in resident's hair.
12. With your fingertips, lather and massage scalp. Use a circular motion, from front to back (Fig. 13-24). Do not scratch the scalp.

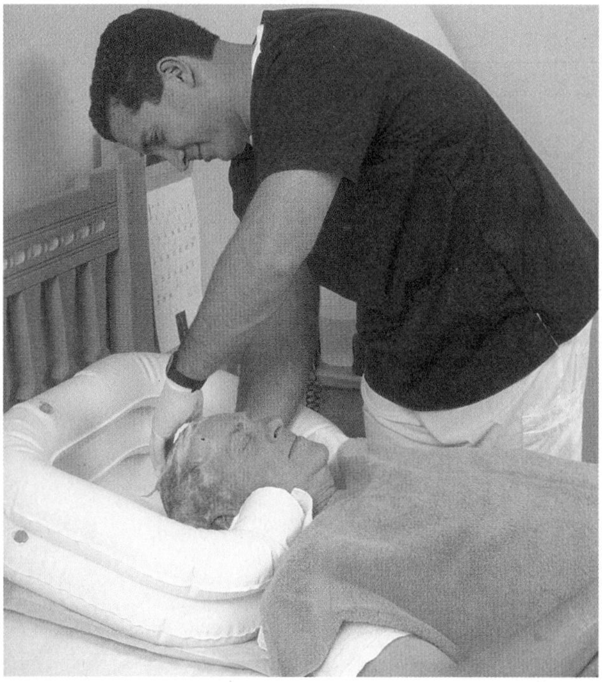

Fig. 13-24.

13. Rinse hair until water runs clear. Apply conditioner. Rinse as directed on container.
14. Cover resident's hair with clean towel. Dry his face with washcloth used to protect eyes.
15. Remove trough and waterproof covering.
16. Raise head of bed.

17. Gently rub the scalp and hair with the towel.
18. Dry and comb resident's hair as he or she prefers (see procedure later in the chapter).
19. Make resident comfortable. Make sure sheets are free from wrinkles and the bed free from crumbs.
20. Return bed to proper position. Remove privacy measures.
21. Before leaving, place call light within resident's reach.
22. Empty, rinse, and wipe bath basin/ pitcher. Return to proper storage.
23. Clean comb/brush. Return hairdryer and comb/brush to proper storage.
24. Place soiled linen in proper container.
25. Wash your hands.
26. Report any changes in resident to nurse.
27. Document procedure using facility guidelines.

Many people prefer showers or tub baths to bed baths (Fig. 13-25 and Fig. 13-26). Check with the nurse first to make sure a shower or tub bath is allowed.

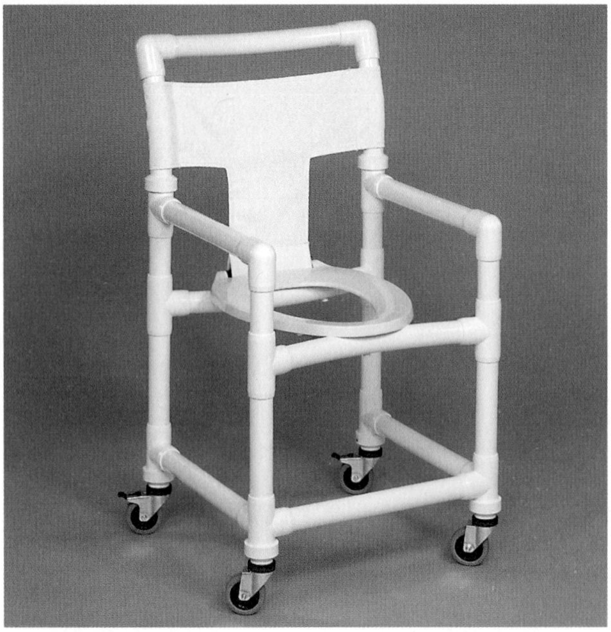

Fig. 13-25. **A shower chair helps residents who take showers (Photo courtesy of Nova Ortho Med, Inc.).**

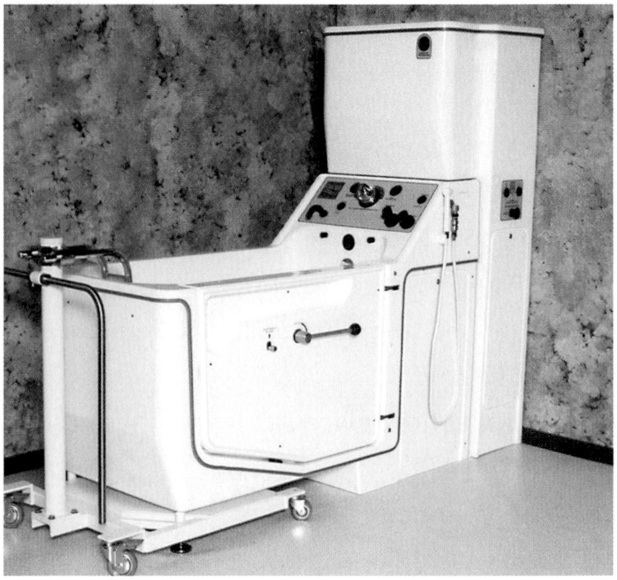

Fig. 13-26. **A common style of tub in nursing homes. (Photo courtesy of Lee Penner of Penner Tubs)**

GUIDELINES
Safety for Showers and Tub Baths

- Clean tub or shower before and after use.
- Make sure bathroom or shower room floor is dry.
- Be familiar with available safety and assistive devices. Check that hand rails, grab bars, and lifts are in working order.
- Have resident use safety bars to get into or out of the tub or shower.
- Some facilities have a policy that requires you to undress residents in their rooms before moving them to the shower room. If so, cover resident while going to and from shower or tub room. It provides warmth and privacy. In other facilities, policy requires you to move residents to the shower room and undress them there.
- Place all needed items within reach.
- Do not leave the resident alone.
- Avoid using bath oils. They make surfaces slippery.
- Test water temperature with thermometer or your wrist before resident gets into shower. Water temperature should be no

more than 105° F. Make sure temperature is comfortable for resident.

Do not overexpose.

Privacy is very important when moving residents to the shower or tub room and during the shower or tub bath. Make sure the resident's body is not unnecessarily exposed.

Giving a shower or a tub bath

Equipment: bath blanket, soap, shampoo, bath thermometer, 2-4 washcloths, 2-4 bath towels, clean gown and robe or clothes, nonskid footwear, gloves, lotion, deodorant

1. Wash your hands.
2. Place equipment in shower or tub room. Clean shower or tub area and shower chair.
3. Wash your hands.
4. Go to resident's room. Identify yourself by name. Identify the resident by name.
5. Explain procedure to the resident. Speak clearly, slowly, and directly. Maintain face-to-face contact whenever possible.
6. Provide for resident's privacy with curtain, screen, or door.
7. Help resident to put on nonskid footwear. Transport resident to shower or tub room.

For a shower:

8. If using a shower chair, place it into position. Lock wheels. Safely transfer resident into shower chair.
9. Turn on water. Test water temperature with thermometer. Water temperature should be no more than 105° F. Have resident check water temperature.

For a tub bath:

8. Safely transfer resident onto chair.
9. Fill the tub halfway with warm water. Test water temperature with thermometer. Water temperature should be no more than 105°F. Have resident check water temperature.
10. Put on gloves.
11. Help resident remove clothing and shoes.
12. Help the resident into shower or tub. Put shower chair into shower and lock wheels.
13. Stay with resident during procedure.
14. Let resident wash as much as possible. Help to wash his or her face.
15. Help resident shampoo and rinse hair.
16. Help to wash and rinse the entire body. Move from head to toe.
17. Turn off water or drain the tub. Cover resident with bath blanket while tub drains.
18. Unlock shower chair wheels if used. Roll resident out of shower, or help resident out of tub and onto a chair.
19. Give resident towel(s) and help to pat dry. Pat dry under the breasts, between skin folds, in the perineal area, and between toes.
20. Apply lotion and deodorant as needed.
21. Place soiled clothing and linens in proper containers.
22. Remove gloves and dispose of them.
23. Wash your hands.
24. Help resident dress and comb hair before leaving shower room. Put on nonskid footwear. Return resident to his or her room.
25. Make sure resident is comfortable and safe.
26. Before leaving, place call light within resident's reach.
27. Report any changes in resident to nurse.
28. Document procedure using facility guidelines.

Some residents will have whirlpool baths. In a whirlpool bath, the action of the water cleanses. It also helps stimulate circulation and wound healing. To take a whirlpool bath, a resident is covered, placed in a chairlift, and lowered into the whirlpool. If you assist with this type of bath, do not leave the resident alone. The resident may feel faint or dizzy after the bath. Help the resident as needed. Do not rush him or her. The tub and chair must be cleaned after use.

4. Explain guidelines for assisting with grooming

Good grooming affects the way residents feel about themselves, and how they look to others. A well-groomed person is likely to feel better physically and emotionally. When helping with grooming, always let residents do all they can for themselves. Let them make as many choices as possible. Follow the care plan's instructions for what care to give. Some residents may have particular ways of grooming themselves. They may have routines. These routines are important even when people are elderly, sick, or disabled (Fig. 13-27). Remember, some residents may be embarrassed or depressed because they need help with grooming tasks they have done for themselves most their lives. Be sensitive to this.

Nail care should only be given if assigned. Never cut a resident's toenails. Poor circulation can lead to infection if skin is accidentally

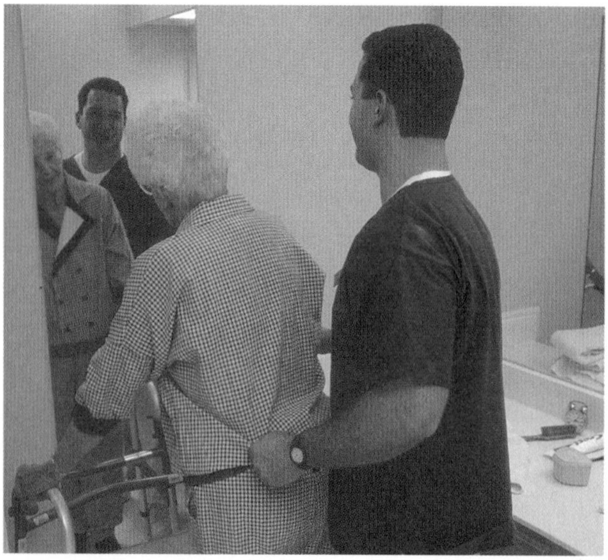

Fig. 13-27. **A well-groomed appearance helps people feel good about themselves.**

cut while caring for nails. In a diabetic resident, such an infection can lead to a severe wound or even amputation. See chapter 18 for more information on diabetes. If you are told to give nail care, know exactly what care you are to provide. Never use the same nail equipment on more than one resident.

Providing fingernail care

Equipment: orangewood stick, emery board, lotion, basin, soap, washcloth, 2 towels, bath thermometer

1. Wash your hands.
2. Identify yourself by name. Identify the resident by name.
3. Explain procedure to the resident. Speak clearly, slowly, and directly. Maintain face-to-face contact whenever possible.
4. Provide for resident's privacy with curtain, screen, or door.
5. If resident is in bed, adjust bed to a safe level, usually waist high. Lock bed wheels.
6. Fill the basin halfway with warm water. Test water temperature with thermometer or your wrist. Ensure it is safe. Water temperature should be 105° F. Have resident check water temperature. Adjust if necessary.
7. Place basin at a comfortable level for the resident. Soak the resident's nails in basin of water. Soak all ten fingertips for two to four minutes.
8. Remove hands. Wash hands with soapy washcloth. Rinse. Pat hands dry with towel, including between fingers.
9. Place the resident's hands on the towel. Use the pointed end of the orangewood stick or a nail brush to remove dirt from under the nails (Fig. 13-28).
10. Wipe orangewood stick on towel after cleaning each nail. Wash resident's hands again. Dry them thoroughly.

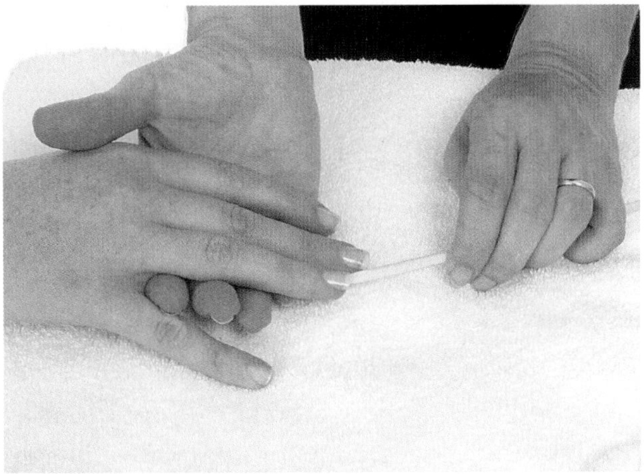

Fig. 13-28.

11. Groom nails with file or emery board. File in a curve.
12. Finish with nails smooth and free of rough edges.
13. Apply lotion from fingertips to wrist.
14. Make sure resident is comfortable and safe.
15. Make sure sheets are free from wrinkles and the bed free from crumbs.
16. Before leaving, place call light within resident's reach.
17. Empty, rinse, and wipe basin. Return to proper storage.
18. Dispose of soiled linen in the proper container.
19. Wash your hands.
20. Report any changes in resident to the nurse.
21. Document procedure using facility guidelines.

Quality foot care is extremely important. It should be a part of daily care of residents. Keeping the feet clean and dry helps prevent complications.

OBSERVING AND REPORTING
Foot Care

Report any of these to the nurse:

- excessive dryness of the skin of the feet
- breaks or tears in the skin
- ingrown nails
- reddened areas on the feet
- drainage or bleeding
- change in color of the skin or nails, especially blackening
- soft, fragile heels
- corns and blisters

Providing foot care

Equipment: basin, bath mat, soap, lotion, washcloth, 2 towels, bath thermometer, clean socks

Support the foot and ankle throughout procedure.

1. Wash your hands.
2. Identify yourself by name. Identify the resident by name.
3. Explain procedure to the resident. Speak clearly, slowly, and directly. Maintain face-to-face contact whenever possible.
4. Provide for resident's privacy with curtain, screen, or door.
5. If resident is in bed, adjust bed to a safe level, usually waist high. Lock bed wheels.
6. Fill the basin halfway with warm water. Test water temperature with thermometer or your wrist. Ensure it is safe. Water temperature should be 105° F. Have resident check water temperature. Adjust if necessary.
7. Place basin on the bath mat.
8. Remove resident's socks. Completely submerge resident's feet in water. Soak the feet for five to ten minutes.
9. Remove one foot from water. Wash entire foot, including between the toes and around nail beds, with soapy washcloth (Fig. 13-29).
10. Rinse entire foot, including between the toes.

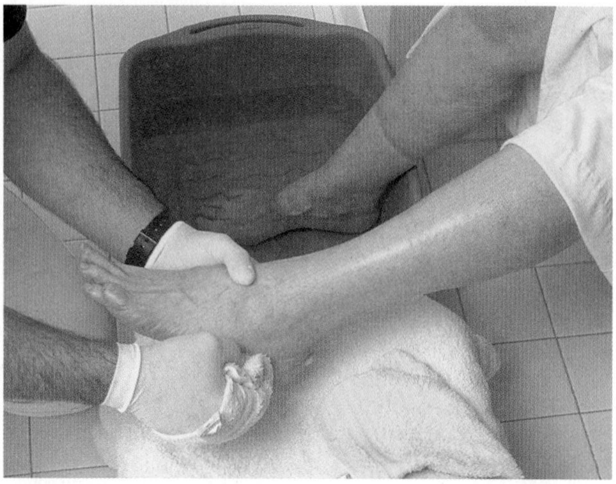

Fig. 13-29.

11. Dry entire foot, including between the toes.
12. Repeat steps 9 through 11 for the other foot.
13. Put lotion in hand. Warm lotion by rubbing hands together.
14. Massage lotion into entire foot (top and bottom), except between the toes. Remove excess (if any) with a towel.
15. Help resident to replace socks. Make resident comfortable. Make sure sheets are free from wrinkles and the bed free from crumbs.
16. Return bed to appropriate position. Remove privacy measures.
17. Before leaving, place call light within resident's reach.
18. Empty, rinse, and wipe basin. Return to proper storage.
19. Dispose of soiled linen in the proper container.
20. Wash your hands.
21. Report any changes in resident to the nurse.
22. Document procedure using facility guidelines.

Shaving is an important part of daily grooming. However, keep in mind that some residents will not want to be shaved. Respect personal preferences for shaving. If a resident has a beard or mustache, it will need daily care. Washing and combing a beard or mustache every day is usually enough. Ask the person how he would like it done. Do not trim or shave a beard or mustache without the resident's permission.

When shaving residents, be careful. Avoid nicks and cuts. Follow Standard Precautions. Always wear gloves. Shaving may cause bleeding. Wearing gloves promotes infection control.

Types of Razors

A safety razor has a sharp blade, but with a special safety casing to help prevent cuts. This type of razor requires shaving cream or soap.

An electric razor is the safest and easiest type of razor to use. It does not require soap or shaving cream.

A disposable razor requires shaving cream or soap. It is discarded after use.

GUIDELINES
Shaving

- Always wear gloves when shaving residents.
- When using a safety or disposable razor, soften hair on face first with a warm, wet cloth.
- Shave in the direction of the hair growth. This maximizes hair removal.
- Use after-shave if a resident wants it.
- Discard disposable shaving products in the biohazard container.
- Do not use an electric razor near any water, when oxygen is in use, or if resident has a pacemaker. Electricity near water may cause electrocution. Electricity near oxygen may cause an explosion. Electricity

near some pacemakers may cause an irregular heartbeat.

Shaving a resident

Be sure the resident wants you to shave him or help him shave before you begin.

Equipment: basin, 2 towels, washcloth, bath thermometer, mirror, shaving cream or soap, after-shave (for male residents), gloves, razor

1. Wash your hands.
2. Identify yourself by name. Identify the resident by name.
3. Explain procedure to the resident. Speak clearly, slowly, and directly. Maintain face-to-face contact whenever possible.
4. Provide for resident's privacy with curtain, screen, or door.
5. If the bed is adjustable, adjust bed to a safe level, usually waist high. Lock bed wheels.
6. Raise head of bed so resident is sitting up.

Shaving using a safety or disposable razor:

7. Fill bath basin halfway with warm water.
8. Drape towel under resident's chin.
9. Apply gloves.
10. Wet beard with warm washcloth. Put shaving cream or soap over area.
11. Hold skin taut. Shave beard in downward strokes on face and upward strokes on neck. Rinse razor often in warm water to keep it clean and wet (Fig. 13-30).

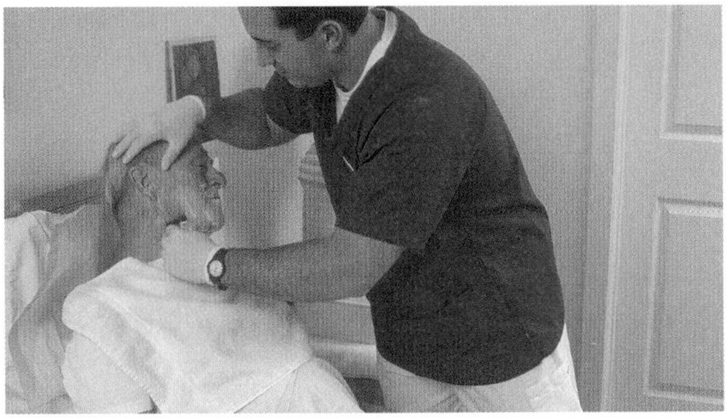

Fig. 13-30.

12. Offer mirror to resident.
13. Wash, rinse, and dry face after the shave. Apply after-shave lotion as requested.
14. Remove towel.
15. Remove gloves.

Shaving using an electric razor:

7. Do not use an electric razor near any water, when oxygen is in use, or if resident has a pacemaker.
8. Drape towel under resident's chin.
9. Apply gloves.
10. Apply pre-shave lotion as resident wishes.
11. Hold skin taut. Shave with smooth, even strokes. Shave beard in circular motion.
12. Offer mirror to resident.
13. Apply after-shave lotion as resident wishes.
14. Remove towel.
15. Remove gloves.

Final steps:

16. Make sure that resident and area are free of loose hairs. Make resident comfortable. Make sure sheets are free from wrinkles and the bed free from crumbs.
17. Return bed to appropriate position. Remove privacy measures.
18. Before leaving, place call light within resident's reach.
19. *For safety razor*: Rinse safety razor. *For disposable razor*: Dispose of a disposable razor in biohazard container. *For electric razor*: Clean head of electric razor. Remove whiskers from razor. Re-cap shaving head. Return razor to case.
20. Return supplies and equipment to proper storage.
21. Wash your hands.
22. Report any changes in resident to the nurse.
23. Document procedure using facility guidelines.

NAs help keep residents' hair clean and styled (Fig. 13-31). You must let residents choose their own hairstyles. Use hair ornaments only as requested. Do not comb or brush residents' hair into a childish style.

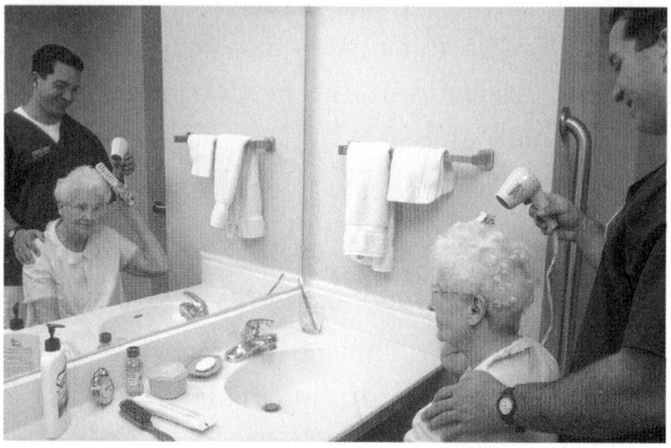

Fig. 13-31. **Allowing residents to choose their own hairstyles helps maintain independence and dignity.**

Handle residents' hair gently. Hair usually thins as people age. Pieces of hair can be pulled out of the head while combing or brushing it. Also, the skin on residents' heads is fragile. Handle hair carefully.

Never cut residents' hair. Many facilities have a barber, beautician, and/or hairstylist available to residents.

Dandruff is an excessive shedding of dead skin cells from the scalp. It is the result of the normal growing process of the skin cells of the scalp. The most common symptom is flaking of small, round, white patches from the head. Itching can also occur.

Dandruff is a natural process. It cannot be stopped. It can only be controlled. Regular shampooing with a medicated dandruff shampoo can help control it.

Combing or brushing hair

Use hair care products that the resident prefers for his or her type of hair.

Equipment: comb, brush, towel, mirror, hair care items requested by resident

1. Wash your hands.
2. Identify yourself by name. Identify the resident by name.
3. Explain procedure to the resident. Speak clearly, slowly, and directly. Maintain face-to-face contact whenever possible.
4. Provide for resident's privacy with curtain, screen, or door.
5. If the bed is adjustable, adjust bed to a safe level, usually waist high. Lock bed wheels.
6. Raise head of bed so resident is sitting up. Place a towel under the head or around the shoulders.
7. Remove any hair pins, hair ties, and clips.
8. Remove tangles first by dividing hair into small sections. Put a small amount of detangler or leave-in conditioner on the tangle. Hold lock of hair just above the tangle so you do not pull at the scalp. Gently comb or brush through the tangle.
9. After tangles are removed, brush two-inch sections of hair at a time. Brush from roots to ends (Fig. 13-32).

   Residents who have dry, brittle hair may require a special treatment with oil or hair lotion. Residents whose hair is tightly curled may use a comb with large teeth, or a pick.
10. Style hair as resident prefers. Avoid childish hairstyles. Each resident may like different styles and different hair products. Offer mirror to resident.

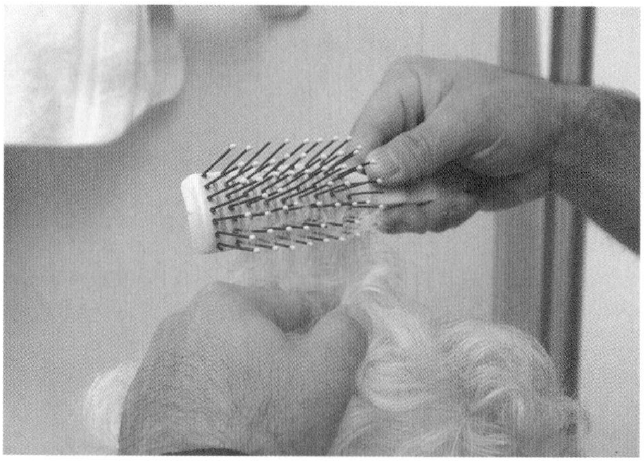

Fig. 13-32.

11. Make resident comfortable. Make sure sheets are free from wrinkles and the bed free from crumbs.
12. Return bed to appropriate position. Remove privacy measures.
13. Before leaving, place call light within resident's reach.
14. Return supplies to proper storage. Clean hair from brush/comb.
15. Dispose of soiled linen in the proper container.
16. Wash your hands.
17. Report any changes in resident to nurse.
18. Document procedure using facility guidelines.

Pediculosis is an infestation of lice. Lice are tiny bugs that bite into the skin and suck blood to live and grow. Three types of lice are head lice, body lice, and crab or pubic lice. Head lice are usually found on the scalp.

Lice are hard to see. Symptoms include itching, bite marks on the scalp, skin sores, and matted, bad-smelling scalp and hair. If you notice any of these symptoms, tell the nurse immediately. They can spread very quickly. Special lice cream, shampoo, or lotion may be used to treat the lice. People who have lice spread it to others. They can spread very quickly. To help prevent the spread of lice, do not share residents' combs, brushes, clothes, wigs, and hats.

Cosmetics

Cosmetics are things used to enhance beauty or cleanse and improve the skin. Women usually use them more, although some men use them.

Help to apply cosmetics as residents request. The application of makeup, including type and amount, should be based on residents' wishes.

5. List guidelines for assisting with dressing

When helping a resident with dressing, know what limitations he or she has. If he or she has a weakened side from a stroke or injury, that side is called the **affected side**. It will be weaker. Never refer to the weaker side as the "bad side," or talk about the "bad" leg or arm. Use the terms **weaker** or **involved** to refer to the affected side. The weaker arm is usually placed through a sleeve first (Fig. 13-33). When a leg is weak, it is easier if the resident sits down to pull the pants over both legs.

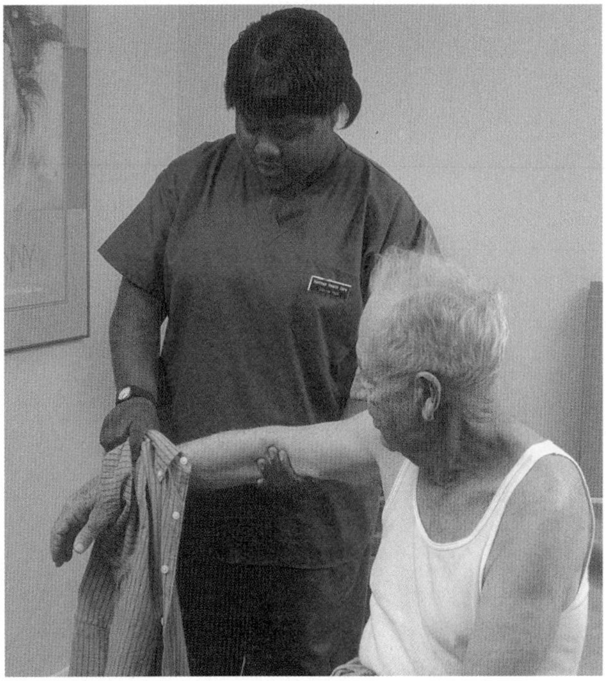

Fig. 13-33. **When dressing, start with the affected (weaker) side first.**

GUIDELINES

Dressing and Undressing

- As with all care, the resident's wishes should be asked and followed. Remember: resident-directed care is the resident's right and your responsibility.
- Let the resident to choose clothing for the day. Check to see if it is clean, appropriate for the weather, and in good condition. Encourage the resident to dress in regular clothes rather than nightclothes. Wearing

regular daytime clothing encourages more activity and out-of-bed time. Elastic-waist pants or skirts are easy to pull on over legs and hips. Be sure the waistband of underpants, slip, pantyhose, pants, or skirt fits comfortably at the waist. Clothing that is a size larger than the resident would normally wear is easier to put on.

- The resident should do as much to dress or undress himself as possible. It may take longer, but it helps maintain independence and regain self-care skills. Ask where your help is needed.
- Provide privacy. If the resident has just had a bath, cover him with the bath blanket. Put on undergarments first. Never expose more than needed.
- When putting on socks or stockings, roll or fold them down. They can then be slipped over the toes and foot, then unrolled up into place. Make sure toes, heels, and seams of socks or stockings are in the right place.
- For a female resident, make sure bra cups fit over the breasts. Front-fastening bras are easier for residents to work by themselves.
- Bras that fasten in back can be put around the waist and fastened first. Then rotate around and move up bra. Put arms through the straps last. This can be reversed for undressing.
- For residents who have weakness or paralysis on one side, place the weaker, or affected, arm or leg through the garment first. Then help with the strong arm or leg. When undressing, do the opposite—start with the stronger, or unaffected side.

Several types of adaptive aids for dressing are available. These help residents maintain independence in dressing themselves (Fig. 13-34). An occupational therapist may teach residents to perform ADLs using adaptive equipment.

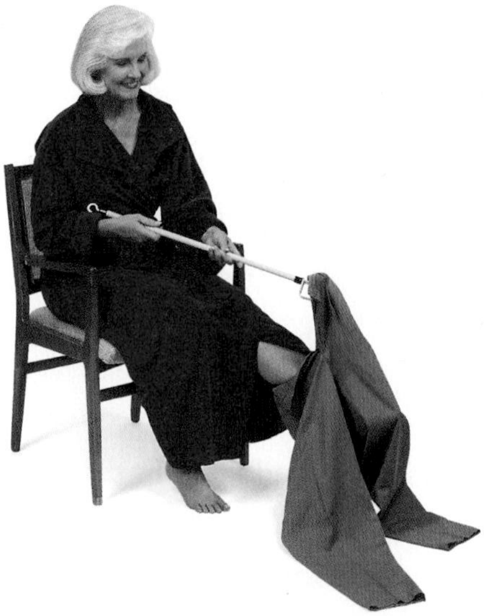

***Fig. 13-34.* Special dressing aids can help residents dress themselves. (Photo courtesy of North Coast Medical, Inc., www.ncmedical.com, 800-821-9319)**

Dressing a resident with an affected right arm

When putting on all items, move resident's body gently and naturally. Avoid force and overextension of limbs and joints.

Equipment: clean clothes of resident's choice, non-skid footwear

1. Wash your hands.
2. Identify yourself by name. Identify the resident by name.
3. Explain procedure to the resident. Speak clearly, slowly, and directly. Maintain face-to-face contact whenever possible.
4. Provide for resident's privacy with curtain, screen, or door.
5. Ask resident what she would like to wear. Dress her in outfit of choice (Fig 13-35).
6. Remove resident's gown. Do not completely expose resident. Take off stronger side first when undressing.
7. Help resident to put the right (affected) arm through the right sleeve of the shirt, sweater, or slip before placing garment on left (unaffected) arm.
8. Help resident put on skirt, pants, or dress.

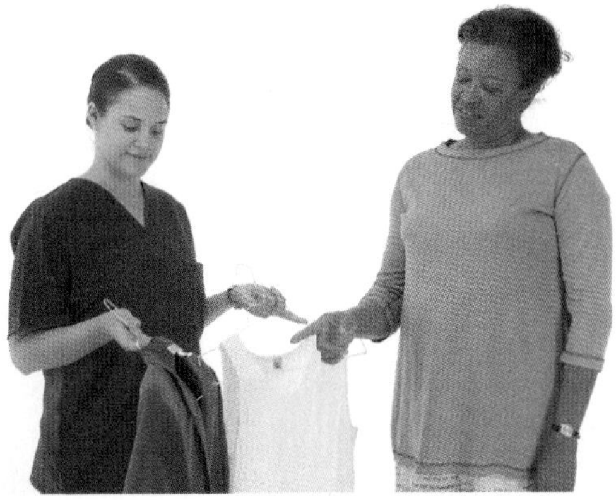

Fig. 13-35.

9. Place bed at the lowest position.
10. Help to apply non-skid footwear. Tie laces.
11. Finish with resident dressed appropriately. Make sure clothing is right-side-out and zippers/buttons are fastened.
12. Remove privacy measures. Place gown in soiled linen container.
13. Before leaving, place call light within resident's reach.
14. Wash your hands.
15. Report any changes in resident to the nurse.
16. Document procedure using facility guidelines.

6. Identify guidelines for good oral care

Oral care, or care of the mouth, teeth, and gums, is done at least twice each day. Oral care should be done after breakfast and after the last meal or snack of the day. It may also be done before a resident eats. Oral care includes brushing teeth and tongue, flossing, and caring for dentures (Fig. 13-36). When giving oral care, wear gloves. Follow Standard Precautions.

Serious problems, like gum disease, can occur when proper oral care is not done. An unhealthy mouth can also lead to a poor appetite and weight loss.

Plaque is a substance that forms in a brief period of time if oral care is not done regularly. Plaque can turn into hard deposits, called tartar, if left on the teeth too long. **Tartar** is filled with bacteria. It may cause gum disease and loose teeth if it is not removed by a dentist. **Gingivitis** is an inflammation of the gums. This can lead to periodontal disease when the areas around the teeth, such as the gums, become diseased. Oral care also helps prevent bad breath (**halitosis**). When you give oral care, observe the resident's mouth to help prevent these problems.

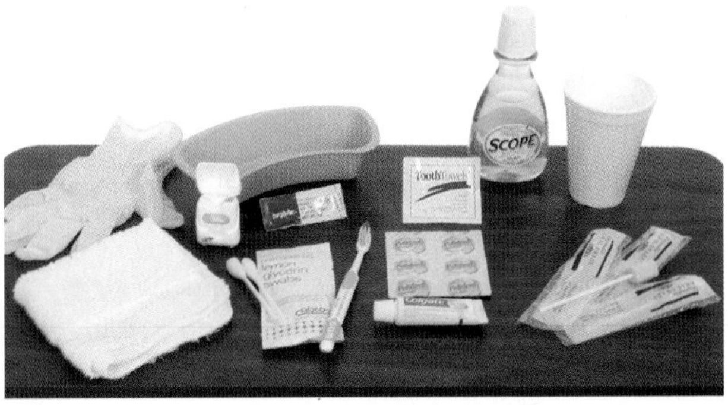

***Fig. 13-36.* Some supplies needed for oral care.**

OBSERVING AND REPORTING
Oral Care

- irritation
- infection
- raised areas
- coated or swollen tongue
- ulcers, such as canker sores or small, painful, white sores
- flaky, white spots
- dry, cracked, bleeding, or chapped lips
- loose, chipped, broken, or decayed teeth
- swollen, irritated, bleeding, or whitish gums
- breath that smells bad or fruity
- resident reports of mouth pain

Providing oral care

Equipment: toothbrush, toothpaste, emesis basin, gloves, towel, glass of water

1. Wash your hands.
2. Identify yourself by name. Identify the resident by name.
3. Explain procedure to the resident. Speak clearly, slowly, and directly. Maintain face-to-face contact whenever possible.
4. Provide for resident's privacy with curtain, screen, or door.
5. Adjust bed to a safe level, usually waist high. Lock bed wheels. Make sure resident is in an upright sitting position.
6. Put on gloves.
7. Place towel across resident's chest.
8. Wet brush. Put on small amount of toothpaste.
9. Clean entire mouth (including tongue and all surfaces of teeth). Use gentle strokes. First brush upper teeth, then lower teeth. Use short strokes. Brush back and forth.
10. Hold emesis basin to the resident's chin.
11. Have resident rinse mouth with water and spit into emesis basin (Fig. 13-37).

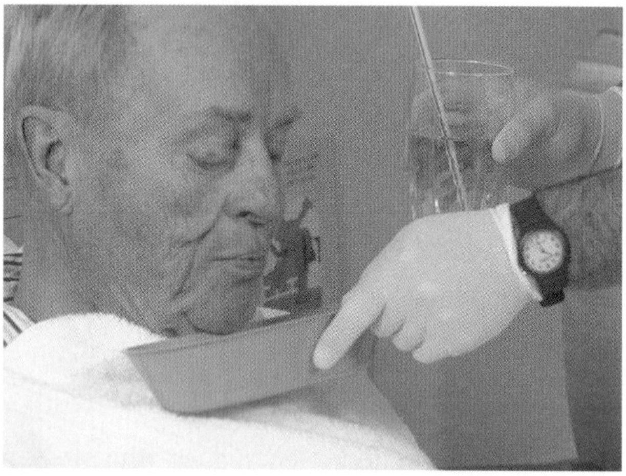

Fig. 13-37.

12. Wipe resident's mouth and remove towel.
13. Dispose of soiled linen in the proper container.
14. Clean and return supplies to proper storage.
15. Remove gloves. Dispose of gloves properly.
16. Make resident comfortable. Make sure sheets are free from wrinkles and the bed free from crumbs.
17. Return bed to appropriate position. Remove privacy measures.
18. Before leaving, place call light within resident's reach.
19. Wash your hands.
20. Report any problems with teeth, mouth, tongue, and lips to nurse. This includes odor, cracking, sores, bleeding, and any discoloration.
21. Document procedure using facility guidelines.

Dental floss is a special kind of string used to clean between teeth. Flossing the teeth removes plaque and tartar buildup around the gum line and between the teeth. Teeth may be flossed right after or before they are brushed, as the resident prefers. Flossing should not be done for certain residents. Follow the care plan's instructions.

Flossing teeth

Equipment: floss, cup with water, emesis basin, gloves, towel

1. Wash your hands.
2. Identify yourself by name. Identify the resident by name.
3. Explain procedure to the resident. Speak clearly, slowly, and directly. Maintain face-to-face contact whenever possible.
4. Provide for resident's privacy with curtain, screen, or door.
5. Adjust the bed to a safe level, usually waist high. Lock bed wheels. Make sure the resident is in an upright sitting position.
6. Put on gloves.
7. Wrap the ends of floss securely around each index finger (Fig. 13-38).

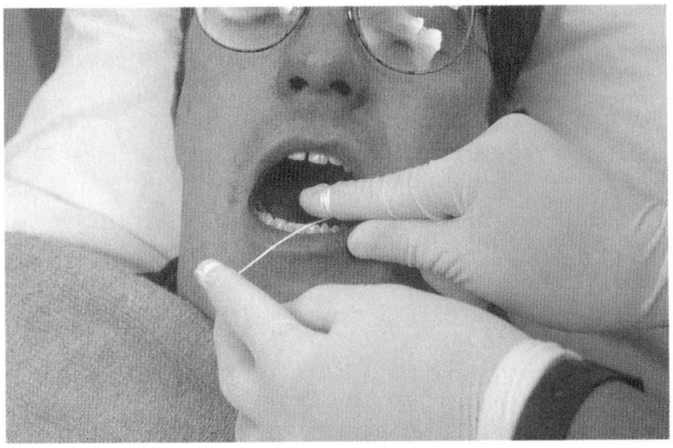

Fig. 13-38.

8. Starting with the back teeth, place floss between teeth. Move it down the surface of the tooth. Use a gentle sawing motion (Fig. 13-39).

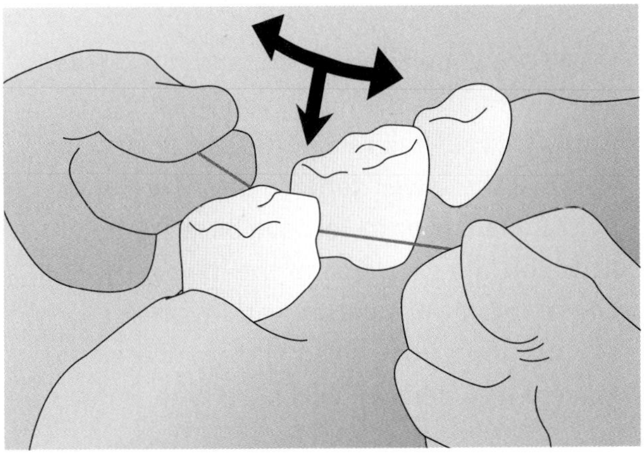

Fig. 13-39.

Continue to the gum line. At the gum line, curve the floss into a letter C. Slip it gently into the space between the gum and tooth. Then go back up, scraping that side of the tooth (Fig. 13-40).

Repeat this on the side of the other tooth.

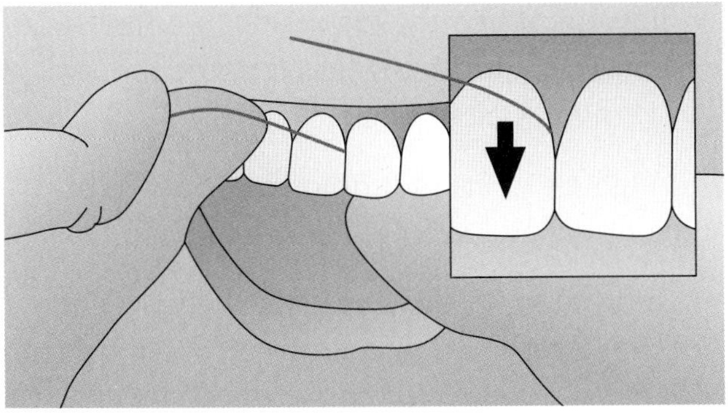

Fig. 13-40.

9. After every two teeth, unwind floss from your fingers. Move it so you are using a clean area. Floss all teeth.
10. Offer water to rinse the mouth. Ask the resident to spit it into the basin.
11. Offer resident a face towel when done flossing all teeth.
12. Dispose of soiled linen in the proper container.
13. Clean and return supplies to proper storage.
14. Remove and dispose of gloves properly.
15. Make resident comfortable. Make sure sheets are free from wrinkles and the bed free from crumbs.
16. Return bed to appropriate position. Remove privacy measures.
17. Before leaving, place call light within resident's reach.
18. Wash your hands.
19. Report any problems with teeth, mouth, tongue, and lips to nurse. This includes odor, cracking, sores, bleeding, and any discoloration.
20. Document procedure using facility guidelines.

7. Define "dentures" and explain guidelines for good denture care

Dentures are artificial teeth. They are expensive. Take good care of them. Handle dentures carefully to avoid breaking or chipping them. Remember, if a resident's dentures break, he or she cannot eat. When cleaning dentures, wear gloves. Notify the nurse if a resident's dentures do not fit properly, are chipped, or are missing.

When storing dentures, place them in a denture cup with the resident's name on it. Make sure you match the dentures to the correct resident.

Cleaning and storing dentures

Equipment: denture brush or toothbrush, denture cleanser or tablet, labeled denture cup, 2 towels, gloves

1. Wash your hands.
2. Put on gloves.
3. Line sink/basin with a towel(s).
4. Rinse dentures in cool running water before brushing them. Do not use hot water. Hot water may damage dentures.
5. Apply toothpaste or cleanser to toothbrush.
6. Brush dentures on all surfaces (Fig. 13-41).

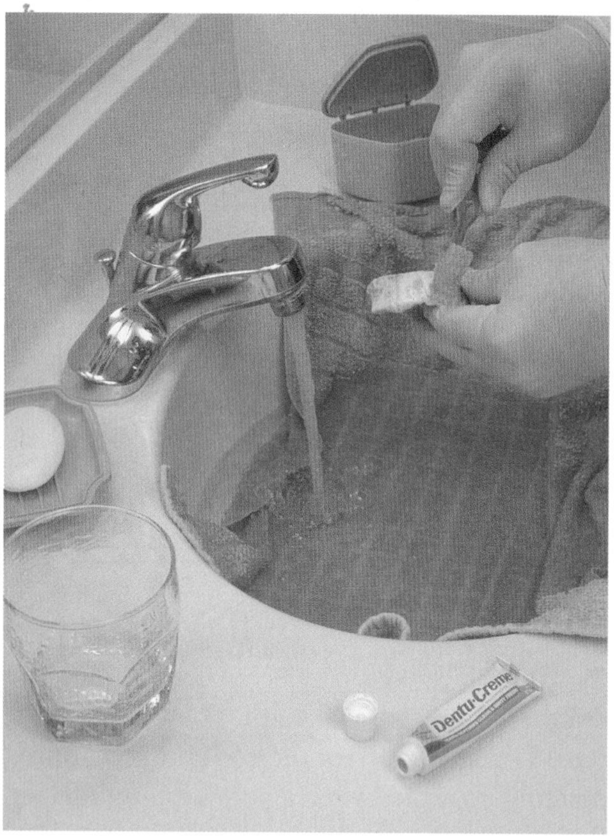

Fig. 13-41.

7. Rinse all surfaces of dentures under cool running water. Do not use hot water.
8. Rinse denture cup before placing clean dentures in it.
9. Place dentures in clean denture cup. Cover dentures completely with solution or cool water. Make sure cup is labeled with resident's name.
10. Clean and return the equipment to proper storage.
11. Dispose of towels in proper container.
12. Remove your gloves. Dispose of gloves properly.
13. Wash your hands.
14. Report any changes in appearance of dentures to the nurse.
15. Document procedure using facility guidelines.

Removing and Reinserting Dentures

If you are allowed to do so, and if a resident cannot remove dentures, you must do it. Apply gloves. Ask resident to sit upright. Remove the lower denture first. The lower denture is easier to remove because it floats on the gum line of the lower jaw. Grasp the lower denture with a gauze square (for a good grip) and remove it. Place it in a denture cup filled with water.

The upper denture is sealed by suction. Firmly grasp the upper denture with a gauze square. Give a slight downward pull to break the suction. Turn it at an angle to take it out of the mouth.

When inserting dentures, ask resident to sit as upright as possible. Apply gloves. Apply denture cream or adhesive to the dentures if needed. When the resident's mouth is open, place upper denture into the mouth by turning it at an angle.

Straighten it. Press it onto the upper gum line firmly and evenly (Fig. 13-42).

Insert the lower denture onto the gum line of the lower jaw. Press firmly.

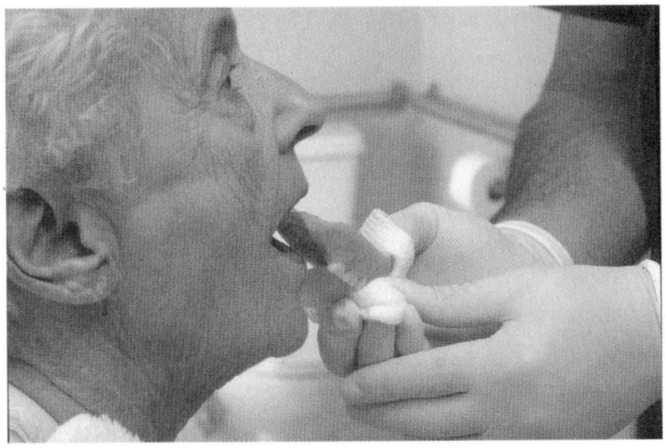

Fig. 13-42.

8. Describe guidelines for performing oral care for an unconscious resident

Although residents who are unconscious cannot eat, breathing through the mouth causes saliva to dry in the mouth. Good mouth care needs to be performed more frequently to keep the mouth clean and moist. Swabs with a mixture of lemon juice and glycerine are sometimes used to soothe the gums. But these may further dry the gums if used too often. Follow the care plan regarding the use of swabs.

With unconscious residents, use as little liquid as possible when giving mouth care. Because the person's swallowing reflex is weak, he or she is at risk for aspiration. **Aspiration** is the inhalation of food or drink into the lungs. Aspiration can cause pneumonia or death. Turning unconscious residents on their sides before giving oral care can also help prevent aspiration. Chapter 16 has more information on aspiration.

Providing oral care for the unconscious resident

Equipment: sponge swabs, padded tongue blade, towel, emesis basin, gloves, lip moisturizer, cleaning solution (check the care plan)

1. Wash your hands.
2. Identify yourself by name. Identify the resident by name. Even residents who are unconscious may be able to hear you. Always speak to them as you would to any resident.
3. Explain procedure to the resident. Speak clearly, slowly, and directly. Maintain face-to-face contact whenever possible.
4. Provide for resident's privacy with curtain, screen, or door.
5. Adjust bed to a safe level, usually waist high. Lock bed wheels.
6. Put on gloves.
7. Turn resident's head to the side. Place a towel under his cheek and chin. Place an emesis basin next to the cheek and chin for excess fluid.
8. Hold mouth open with padded tongue blade (Fig. 13-43).

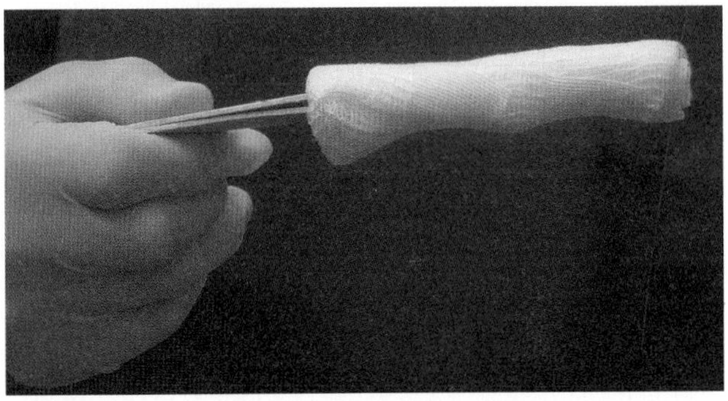

Fig. 13-43. **To make a padded tongue blade, place two wooden tongue blades together and wrap the upper half with gauze. Tape the gauze in place.**

9. Dip swab in cleaning solution. Wipe teeth, gums, tongue, and inside surfaces of mouth. Change swab often. Repeat until the mouth is clean (Fig. 13-44).
10. Rinse with clean swab dipped in water.
11. Remove the towel and basin. Pat lips or face dry if needed. Apply lip moisturizer.
12. Dispose of soiled linen in the proper container.
13. Clean and return supplies to proper storage.
14. Remove your gloves. Dispose of gloves properly.

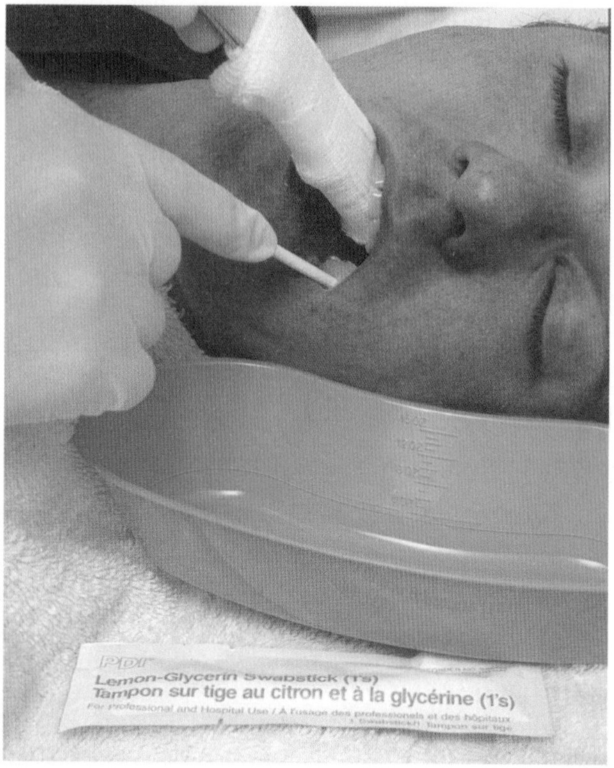

Fig. 13-44.

15. Make sure sheets are free from wrinkles and the bed free from crumbs.
16. Return bed to appropriate position. Remove privacy measures.
17. Before leaving, place call light within resident's reach.
18. Wash your hands.
19. Report any changes in resident to the nurse.
20. Document procedure using facility guidelines.

STOP

Unconscious Residents

Even when people are unconscious, they still may be able to hear what is going on around them. Unconscious people have been known to "wake up" and relate many of the things they heard while they were unconscious. Limit your discussions to appropriate subjects. Speak respectfully. Explain what you are doing. Do not talk about anything personal while giving care. Speak to unconscious residents as you would to any resident.

Chapter Review

1. List four examples of activities of daily living (ADLs).
2. Give two examples of how to promote dignity and independence while giving personal care.
3. Why is prevention of pressure sores so important?
4. List ten signs to report about a resident's skin.
5. At a minimum, how often should residents be repositioned?
6. List four examples of positioning devices and explain how they can help.
7. Why is it unnecessary for many residents to have a complete bath or shower every day?
8. How often should the perineum be washed?
9. Why should residents, as well as NAs, test the water temperature before bathing?
10. List two benefits of back rubs.
11. Why should residents be covered while being transported to and from shower or tub rooms?
12. In what ways can good grooming affect a resident?
13. Explain why NAs must be especially careful while giving nail care to diabetic residents.
14. Why should gloves be worn while shaving residents?

15. List the reasons why electric razors should not be used near water, when oxygen is in use, or if a resident has a pacemaker.
16. What is dandruff?
17. If a resident has an affected side due to a stroke or an injury, how should an NA refer to that side?
18. Why should daytime clothing, rather than nightwear, be encouraged when dressing a resident?
19. What is the minimum number of times per day that oral care is done?
20. Explain why hot water should not be used when handling or cleaning dentures.
21. How can NAs help prevent aspiration during oral care of unconscious residents?

Chapter 14
Urinary Elimination

1. List qualities of urine and identify signs and symptoms about urine to report

Urination is the process of **voiding**, or emptying the bladder of urine. Urine is made of water and waste products from the blood. Humans must urinate several times a day. Regular urination is vital to keep the urinary system, including the kidneys, ureters, bladder, and urethra, healthy.

Urine will normally be light, pale yellow or amber in color. Medication and some foods can cause urine to change color. Urine should be clear or transparent. It can become cloudy as it stands. If it is cloudy when freshly voided, it can be a sign of infection. Report this to the nurse. Urine should have a faint smell. If it smells fruity or bad, report it right away. It could be a sign of an infection or illness.

Normal urine output varies with age and the amount and type of liquids consumed. Adults should produce about 1200 to 1500 cc of urine per day. Elderly adults may produce less.

OBSERVING AND REPORTING
Urine

Report any of these to the nurse:

- cloudy urine
- dark or rust-colored urine
- strong-, offensive-, or fruity-smelling urine
- pain, burning, or pressure when urinating
- blood, pus, mucus, or discharge in urine
- protein or glucose in urine (you will learn more about these things later in the chapter)
- **incontinence** (the inability to control the bladder muscles)

The Bladder: Exposed

In 1879, Nitze and Leiter developed the first cystoscope. This instrument is used to examine the inside of the bladder and the ureters. The electric light bulb had not been invented. They used an exposed platinum wire lit by an electric current for light. By the 1920s, an IV for looking at the urological tract was made. This became known as angiography. It uses a special dye injected into the bloodstream to view and examine blood vessels.

2. List factors affecting urination and demonstrate how to assist with elimination

There are many things that affect normal urination:

Growth and Development: The bladder is not able to hold the same amount of urine as it did when people were younger. Elderly people may need to urinate more frequently. Many awaken several times during the night to urinate. The bladder may not empty completely, causing susceptibility to infection. Adults void approximately 1200 to 1500 cc per day.

Psychological factors: A lack of privacy can affect urination. Stress affects urination. It can cause frequent, small amounts of urine output. It may also tense the sphincter muscle. A **sphincter** is a ring-like muscle that opens and closes an opening in the body. The flow of urine from the bladder is controlled by a group of muscles collectively called the urethral sphincter. The muscles are called this because they are close to the urethra.

Fluid intake: The amount of fluid a person drinks affects urinary output. Alcohol and caffeine increase urine output.

Muscle tone: A lack of activity lessens sphincter control, which can increase urinary incontinence. Muscle tone can be affected by whether or not a woman has had children. Trauma and indwelling catheters can affect muscle tone.

Medications: Certain medications cause urine production to increase or decrease. A resident who has high blood pressure may be taking diuretics. Diuretics are drugs that reduce fluid in the body by increasing urine output. This can cause frequent urination.

Disorders that affect urination:

- Bladder disease
- Infection
- Arthritis *
- Cognitive defects
- Fever and heavy sweating
- Congestive heart failure (CHF) *
- Diabetes *

* You will learn more about these disorders in chapter 18.

Residents who cannot get out of bed to go to the bathroom may be given a bedpan, a urinal, or a fracture pan. A **fracture pan** is flatter than the regular bedpan. It is used for residents who cannot assist to raise their hips onto a regular bedpan (Fig. 14-1).

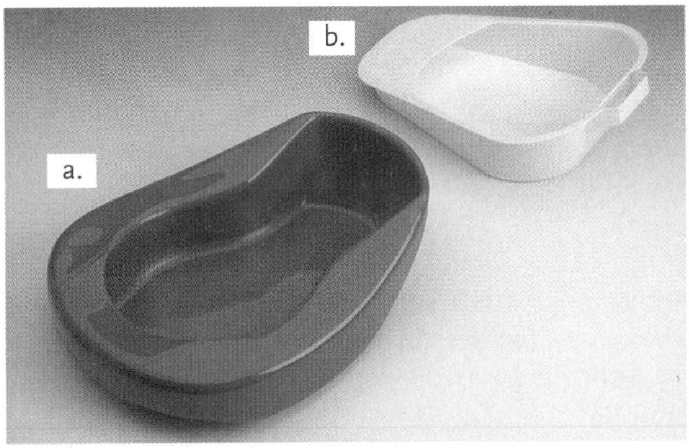

Fig. 14-1. **a) Standard pan and b) fracture pan.**

Women will use a bedpan for urination and bowel movements. Men will generally use a urinal for urination and a bedpan for a bowel movement (Fig. 14-2). This equipment should be rinsed with a facility-approved disinfectant after each use. It is kept in the bathroom or another location between uses. Residents who share bathrooms may need to have urinals and bedpans labeled. Follow your facility's policy for storage. Never place this equipment on an overbed table or on top of a side table.

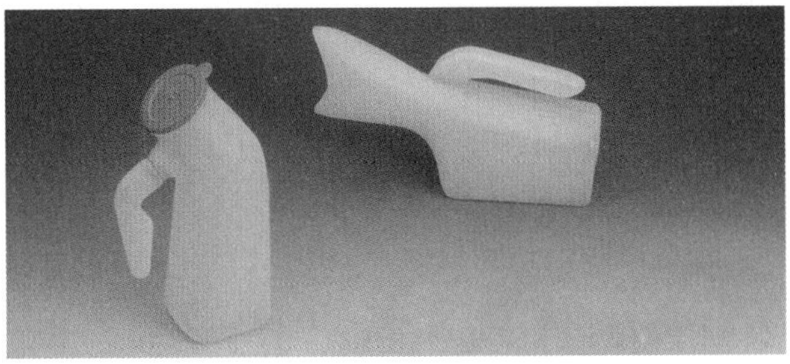

Fig. 14-2. **Urinals.**

Residents who can get out of bed but cannot walk to the bathroom may use a portable commode. A **portable commode** is a chair with a toilet seat and a removable container under it (Fig. 14-3).

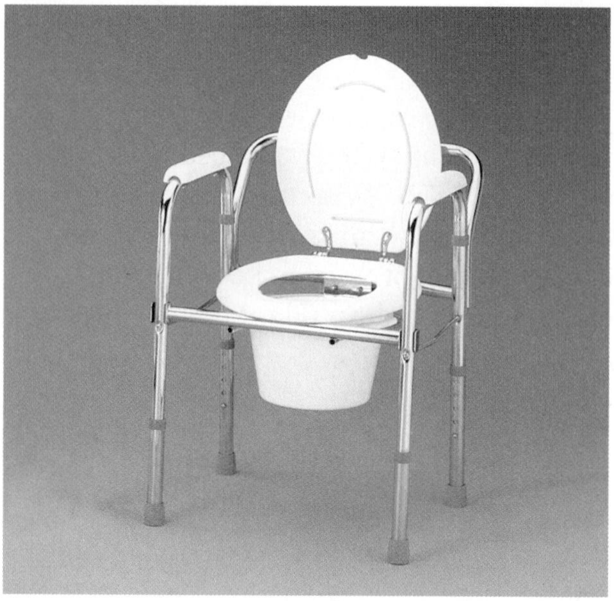

Fig. 14-3. **A portable commode can be used for residents who can get out of bed but may not be able to move to the bathroom easily. (Photo courtesy of Nova Ortho Med, Inc.)**

Wastes such as urine and feces can carry infection. Always dispose of wastes in the toilet. Be careful not to spill or splash. Wear gloves when handling bedpans, urinals, or basins that contain wastes. This includes dirty bath water. Wash these containers thoroughly with an approved disinfectant. Rinse and dry. Return to storage.

Assisting a resident with use of a bedpan

Equipment: bedpan, bedpan cover, protective pad or sheet, bath blanket, toilet paper, washcloths or wipes, gloves

1. Wash your hands.
2. Identify yourself by name. Identify the resident by name.
3. Explain procedure to the resident. Speak clearly, slowly, and directly. Maintain face-to-face contact whenever possible.
4. Provide for resident's privacy with curtain, screen, or door.
5. Before placing bedpan, lower head of bed. Lock bed wheels.
6. Apply gloves.
7. Cover the resident with a bath blanket and ask him to hold it while you pull down the top covers underneath it.
8. Place a protective pad under the resident's buttocks and hips. To do this, have the resident roll toward you. If the resident cannot do this, you must turn him toward you (see chapter 10). Be sure resident cannot roll off the bed. Move to empty side of bed. Place protective sheet on the area where the resident will lie on his back. The side of protective sheet nearest the resident should be fanfolded (folded several times into pleats) (Fig. 14-4). Ask resident to roll onto his back, or roll him as you did before. Unfold rest of protective sheet so it completely covers the area under and around the resident's hips. (Fig. 14-5)

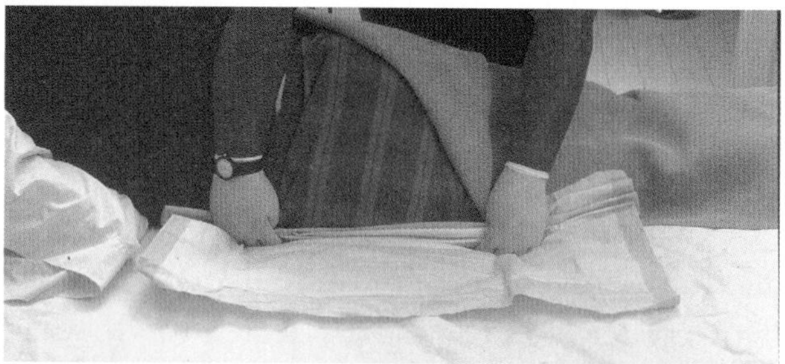

Fig. 14-4.

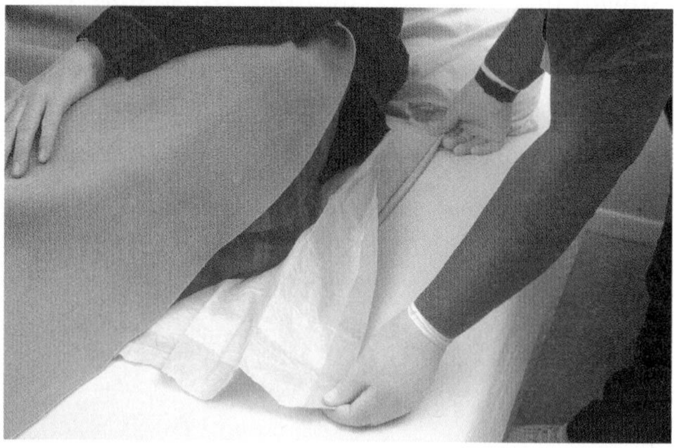

Fig. 14-5.

9. Ask resident to remove undergarments or help him do so.
10. If resident is able, ask him to raise hips by pushing with feet and hands. Place bedpan correctly under resident's buttocks [Standard bedpan: Position bedpan so wider end

of pan is aligned with resident's buttocks (Fig. 14-6); Fracture pan: Position bedpan with handle toward foot of bed (Fig. 14-7)].

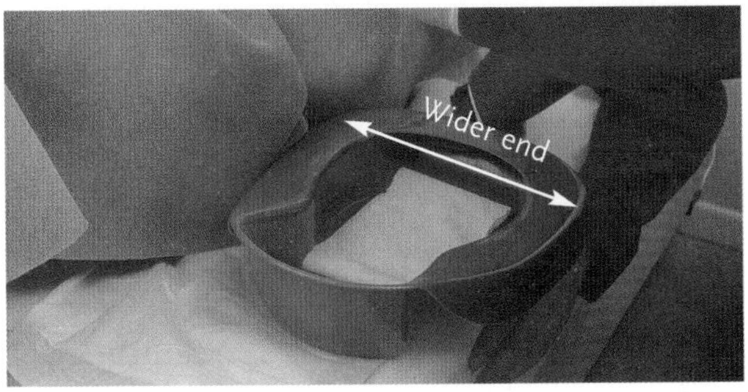

Fig. 14-6.

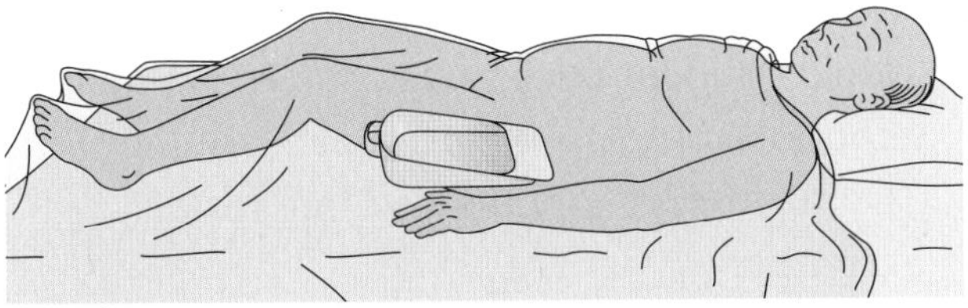

Fig. 14-7.

11. If resident cannot help in getting on the bedpan, take these steps:

    Turn the resident away from you, onto his or her side. Slip the bedpan under the hips and gently roll the resident back onto the bedpan. Keep bedpan centered underneath.
12. Raise the head of bed.
13. Put toilet tissue within reach.
14. Leave call light within reach while resident is using bedpan. Ask resident to signal when done.
15. Return. Lower head of bed.
16. Remove bedpan carefully. Cover bedpan.
17. Provide perineal care if help is needed. Wipe female residents from front to back.
18. Empty bedpan into toilet. Note color, odor, and consistency of contents.
19. Rinse bedpan. Pour rinse water into toilet. Use approved disinfectant. Return to proper storage.
20. Remove and dispose of gloves properly.
21. Help resident to wash hands after using bedpan. Dispose of soiled washcloth or wipes properly. Help resident put on undergarment.
22. Make resident comfortable. Make sure sheets are free from wrinkles and the bed free from crumbs.
23. Return bed to appropriate position. Remove privacy measures.
24. Before leaving, place call light within resident's reach.
25. Wash your hands.
26. Report any changes in resident to the nurse.
27. Document procedure using facility guidelines.

Assisting a male resident with a urinal

Equipment: urinal, protective pad or sheet, washcloths or wipes, gloves

1. Wash your hands.
2. Identify yourself by name. Identify the resident by name.
3. Explain procedure to the resident. Speak clearly, slowly, and directly. Maintain face-to-face contact whenever possible.
4. Provide for resident's privacy with curtain, screen, or door.
5. Lock bed wheels. Apply gloves.
6. Place a protective pad under the resident's buttocks and hips.
7. Hand the urinal to the resident. If the resident cannot do so himself, place urinal between his legs and position penis inside the urinal (Fig. 14-8). Replace bed covers.

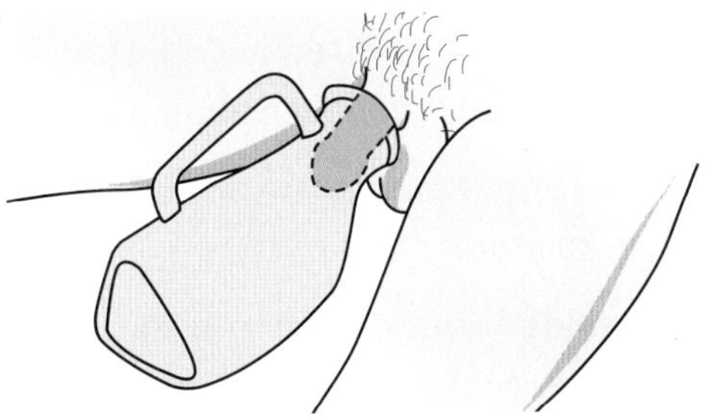

Fig. 14-8.

8. Leave call light within reach while resident is using urinal. Ask resident to signal when done.
9. Remove urinal. Empty contents into toilet. Note color, odor, and qualities (e.g., cloudy) of contents.
10. Rinse urinal. Pour rinse water into toilet. Use approved disinfectant. Return to proper storage.
11. Remove and dispose of gloves.
12. Help resident to wash hands after using urinal. Dispose of soiled washcloth or wipes properly.
13. Make resident comfortable. Make sure sheets are free from wrinkles and the bed free from crumbs.
14. Return bed to appropriate position if adjusted. Remove privacy measures.
15. Before leaving, place call light within resident's reach.
16. Wash your hands.
17. Report any changes in resident to the nurse.
18. Document procedure using facility guidelines.

Helping a resident use a portable commode

Equipment: portable commode with basin, toilet paper, washcloths or wipes, gloves

1. Wash your hands.
2. Identify yourself by name. Identify the resident by name.
3. Explain procedure to the resident. Speak clearly, slowly, and directly. Maintain face-to-face contact whenever possible.
4. Provide for resident's privacy with curtain, screen, or door.
5. Help resident out of bed and to portable commode. Make sure resident is wearing non-skid shoes.
6. If needed, help resident remove clothing and sit comfortably on toilet seat. Put toilet tissue within reach.
7. Leave call light within reach while resident is using commode. Ask resident to signal when done.
8. Return. Apply gloves.
9. Give perineal care if help is needed. Wipe female residents from front to back.
10. Help resident to wash hands after using commode. Dispose of soiled washcloth or wipes properly.
11. Help resident back to bed. Make resident comfortable. Make sure sheets are free from wrinkles and the bed free from crumbs.
12. Remove waste container. Empty into toilet. Note color, odor, and consistency of contents.
13. Rinse container. Pour rinse water into toilet. Use approved disinfectant. Return to proper storage.
14. Remove and dispose of gloves properly.
15. Return bed to appropriate position. Remove privacy measures.
16. Before leaving, place call light within resident's reach.
17. Wash your hands.
18. Report any changes in resident to the nurse.
19. Document procedure using facility guidelines.

3. Identify reasons for incontinence

When people cannot control the muscles of the bowels or bladder, they are said to be incontinent. This is not a normal part of aging. Incontinence can occur in residents who are bedbound, ill, elderly, paralyzed, or have circulatory or nervous system diseases or injuries. Different types of incontinence are:

- **Stress incontinence**: loss of urine due to an increase in intra-abdominal pressure; for example when sneezing, laughing, or coughing
- **Urge incontinence**: involuntary voiding from an abrupt urge to void
- **Mixed incontinence**: symptoms of both urge and stress incontinence are present
- **Functional incontinence**: urine loss caused by things outside urinary tract
- **Overflow incontinence**: due to overflow or over-distention of the bladder

Residents who are incontinent need reassurance and understanding.

GUIDELINES
Preventing Incontinence

- Offer a bedpan or take residents to the bathroom often.
- Follow toileting schedules.
- Know residents' routines and urinary habits. Know signs, such as holding the lower abdomen, which might indicate the need to urinate.
- Answer call lights promptly. This may prevent avoidable accidents.
- Walking can stimulate the need to go to the bathroom. Take daily walks close to a bathroom.

Keep residents clean, dry, and free from odor. Give good skin care as well. Urine irritates the skin. It should be washed off completely by bathing and good perineal care.

Residents who are bedbound should have a plastic, latex, or disposable sheet placed under them to protect the bed. Place a draw sheet over it to absorb moisture and protect skin.

Disposable incontinence pads or briefs for adults are available. They keep body wastes away from the skin (Fig. 14-9). Change wet briefs immediately. Never refer to an incontinence brief or pad as a "diaper." Residents are not children. This is disrespectful.

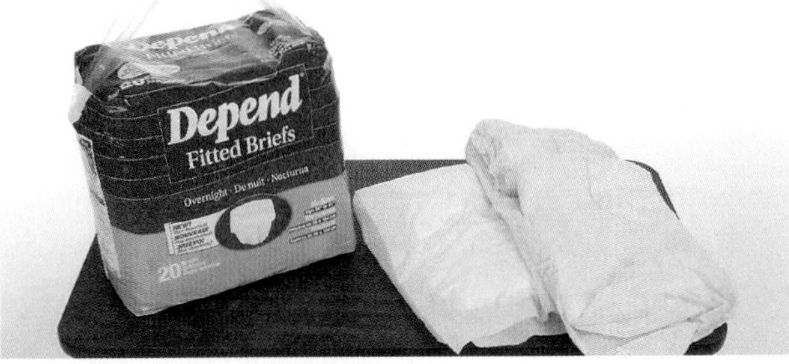

Fig. 14-9. **A type of incontinent pad.**

Providing perineal care for an incontinent resident

Equipment: 2 clean protective pads, 4 washcloths or wipes, 1 towel, gloves, basin with warm water, soap, bath blanket, bath thermometer

1. Wash your hands.
2. Identify yourself by name. Identify the resident by name.
3. Explain procedure to the resident. Speak clearly, slowly, and directly. Maintain face-to-face contact whenever possible.
4. Provide for resident's privacy with curtain, screen, or door.
5. Adjust bed to a safe level, usually waist high. Lock bed wheels.
6. Lower head of bed. Position resident lying flat on his or her back. Raise the side rail farthest from you.
7. Test water temperature with thermometer or your wrist to ensure safety. Water temperature should be 105° to 109° F. Have resident check water temperature. Adjust if necessary.
8. Put on gloves.
9. Remove soiled protective pad from under resident by turning resident on his side, away from you. (See procedure "Turning a resident" in chapter 10.) Roll soiled pad into itself with wet side in/dry side out.
10. Place clean protective pad under his or her buttocks.

11. Return resident to lying on his back.
12. Cover resident with bath blanket.
13. Expose perineal area only. Clean perineal area.

   For a female resident: Wash the perineum with soap and water. Move from front to back. Use single strokes (Fig. 14-10). Do not wash from the back to the front. This may cause infection. Use a clean area of washcloth or clean washcloth for each stroke. First wipe the center of the perineum, then each side. Spread the labia majora, the outside folds of perineal skin that protect the urinary meatus and the vaginal opening. Wipe from front to back on each side. Rinse the area in the same way. Dry entire perineal area. Move from front to back, using a blotting motion with towel. Ask resident to turn on her side. Wash, rinse, and dry buttocks and anal area. Cleanse the anal area without contaminating the perineal area.

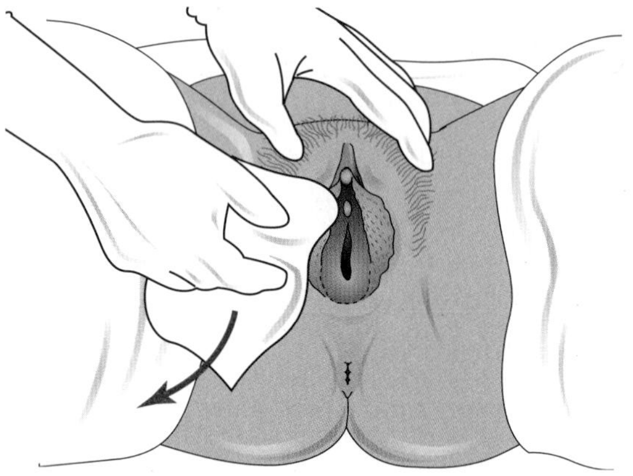

Fig. 14-10.

   For a male resident: If the resident is uncircumcised, retract the foreskin. Gently push skin towards the base of penis.

   Hold the penis by the shaft. Wash in a circular motion from the tip down to the base (Fig. 14-11). Use a clean area of washcloth or clean washcloth for each stroke. Rinse the penis. If resident is uncircumcised, gently return foreskin to normal position. Then wash the scrotum and groin. Rinse and pat dry. Ask the resident to turn on his side. Wash, rinse, and dry buttocks and anal area. Cleanse the anal area without contaminating the perineal area.

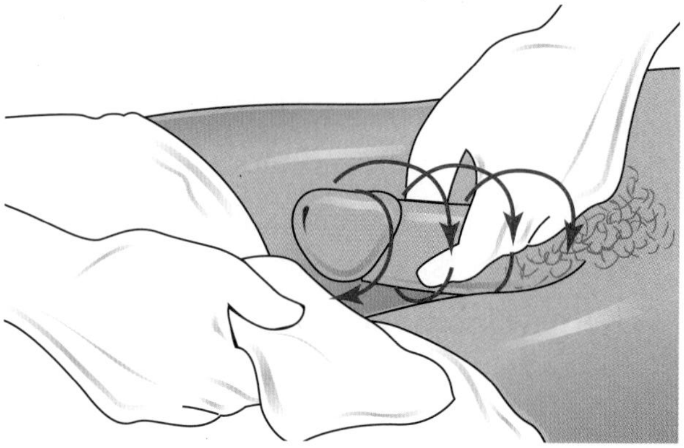

Fig. 14-11.

14. Turn resident on his side away from you. Remove the wet protective pad after drying buttocks.
15. Place a dry protective pad under the resident.
16. Reposition the resident.
17. Empty, rinse, and wipe basin. Return to proper storage.
18. Place soiled clothing and linens in proper containers.
19. Dispose of soiled protective pads in proper containers.
20. Remove and dispose of gloves properly.
21. Make resident comfortable. Make sure sheets are free from wrinkles and the bed free from crumbs.
22. Return bed to appropriate position. Remove privacy measures.
23. Before leaving, place call light within resident's reach.
24. Wash your hands.
25. Report any changes in resident to the nurse.
26. Document procedure using facility guidelines.

No shortcuts with resident care!

Residents are sometimes incontinent in bed. Do not take shortcuts when changing bed linen after incontinence. If you replace a disposable pad without changing the wet linen, it may be considered neglect. Remove all wet linen and disposable pads. Replace them with clean ones.

4. Describe how to promote normal urination

You play an important role in helping residents with urination.

GUIDELINES
Promoting Normal Urination

- Offer trips to the bathroom often. Try to have residents empty bladders regularly.
- Follow a toileting schedule if there is one.
- Offer privacy whenever possible.
- The best position for women to have normal urination is sitting. For men, it is standing. Avoid the lying position if possible. A person in the lying position cannot put pressure on the bladder. This works against gravity.
- Promote proper hygiene. If a resident cannot do it alone, help with perineal care. Wipe from front to back for women. Have resident wash hands.
- Report any changes in appearance or frequency of urination.
- Encourage residents to drink enough water daily. Generally, a healthy person needs to take in from 64 to 96 ounces (oz.) of fluid each day. Provide fresh water and juices often (Fig. 14-12).
- Be aware of excessive caffeine, sodium, and sugar in a resident's diet.
- Follow any fluid restrictions.

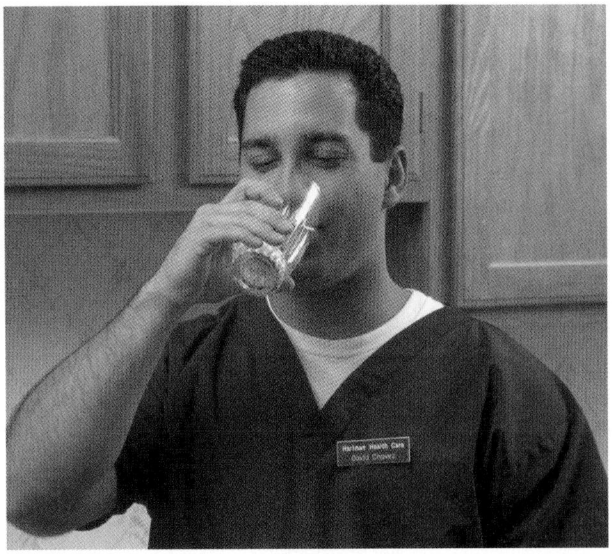

Fig. 14-12. **Drinking plenty of fluids is important to promoting a healthy urinary system.**

- To strengthen muscle tone, encourage Kegel exercises. Kegel exercises use the pelvic floor muscles. When urinating, stop the flow once or twice. This will help you recognize your Kegel muscles. To do Kegel exercises, squeeze the muscles for ten seconds. Relax ten seconds. These can be done 20-80 times a day. They can be done anywhere. They need to be a part of a woman's daily routine.

Help residents promptly.

Do your residents wait to go to the bathroom? This is unhealthy for their urinary systems. Residents should be taken to the bathroom as soon as they need to urinate. They should never have to wait. Accidents are not the only problem with waiting. Holding urine in the bladder for too long can cause bacteria to grow. This leads to infection.

5. Describe guidelines for catheter care

A **catheter** is a tube used to drain urine from the bladder. A **straight catheter** does not stay inside the person. It is removed immediately after urine is drained. An **indwelling**

catheter stays inside the bladder for a period of time (Fig. 14-13). The urine drains into a bag. NAs do not usually insert, remove, or irrigate catheters. You may be asked to provide daily care for the catheter, cleaning the area around the urethral opening and emptying the drainage bag.

a.

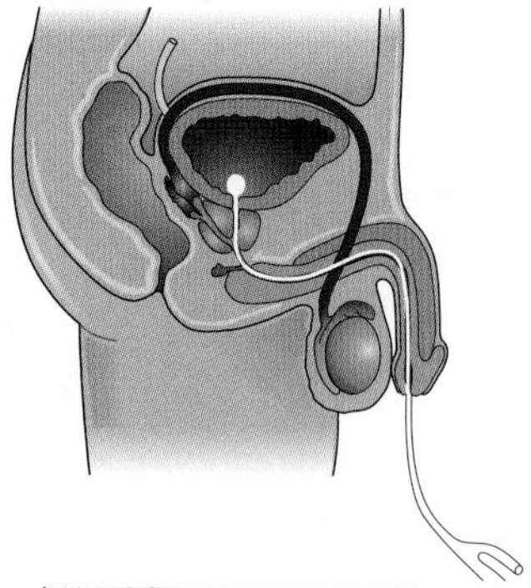

b.

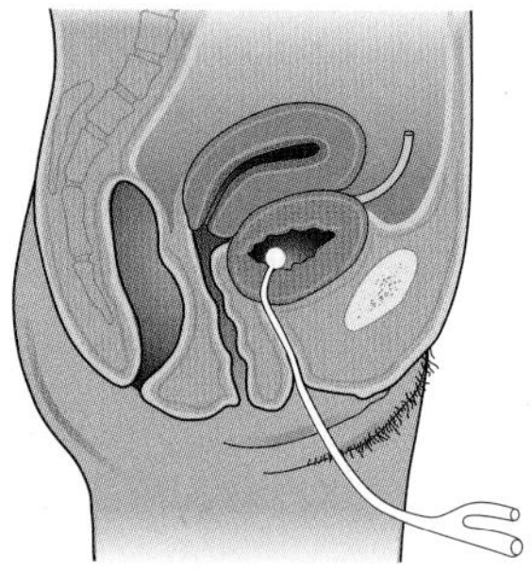

Fig. 14-13. **a) An indwelling catheter (male). b) An indwelling catheter (female).**

An external, or **condom catheter** (also called a Texas catheter), has an attachment on the end that fits onto the penis (Fig. 14-14). The attachment is fastened with tape. The external catheter is changed daily or as needed.

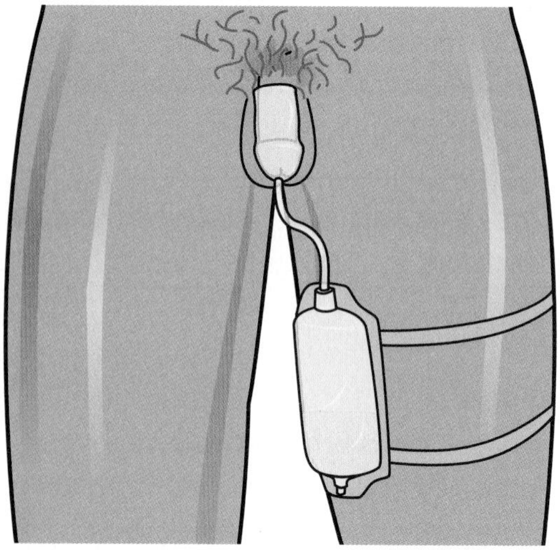

Fig. 14-14. **An external or condom catheter.**

GUIDELINES

Catheters

- Always make sure that the drainage bag is lower than the hips or bladder. Urine must never flow from the bag or tubing back into the bladder. This can cause infection.
- Keep the drainage bag off the floor.
- Tubing should be kept as straight as possible. It should not be kinked. Kinks, twists, or pressure on the tubing (such as from the resident sitting or lying on the tubing) can keep urine from draining.
- The genital area must be kept clean to prevent infection. Because the catheter goes all the way into the bladder, germs can enter more easily. Daily care of the genital area is very important.

OBSERVING AND REPORTING

Catheter Care

Report any of these to the nurse:

- blood in the urine or any other unusual appearance
- catheter bag does not fill after several hours
- catheter bag fills suddenly
- catheter is not in place
- urine leaks from the catheter
- resident reports pain or pressure
- odor

Providing catheter care

Equipment: bath blanket, protective pad, bath basin, soap, bath thermometer, 2-4 washcloths or wipes, 1 towel, gloves

1. Wash your hands.
2. Identify yourself by name. Identify the resident by name.
3. Explain procedure to the resident. Speak clearly, slowly, and directly. Maintain face-to-face contact whenever possible.

4. Provide for resident's privacy with curtain, screen, or door.
5. Adjust bed to a safe working level, usually waist high. Lock bed wheels.
6. Lower head of bed. Position resident lying flat on his back. Raise the side rail farthest from you.
7. Remove or fold back top bedding. Keep resident covered with bath blanket.
8. Test water temperature with thermometer or your wrist and ensure it is safe. Water temperature should be 105° to 109° F. Have resident check water temperature. Adjust if necessary.
9. Put on gloves.
10. Ask the resident to flex his knees and raise the buttocks off the bed by pushing against the mattress with his feet. Place clean protective pad under his buttocks.
11. Expose only the area necessary to clean the catheter.
12. Place towel or pad under catheter tubing before washing.
13. Apply soap to wet washcloth.
14. Hold catheter near meatus. Avoid tugging the catheter.
15. Clean at least four inches of catheter nearest meatus. Move in only one direction, away from meatus. Use a clean area of the cloth for each stroke.
16. Rinse at least four inches of catheter nearest meatus. Move in only one direction, away from meatus (Fig. 14-15). Use a clean area of the cloth for each stroke.
17. Dispose of linen properly.
18. Empty, rinse, and wipe basin. Return to proper storage.
19. Remove and dispose of gloves.
20. Help resident dress. Make resident comfortable. Make sure sheets are free from wrinkles and the bed free from crumbs. Check that the catheter tubing is free from kinks and twists.

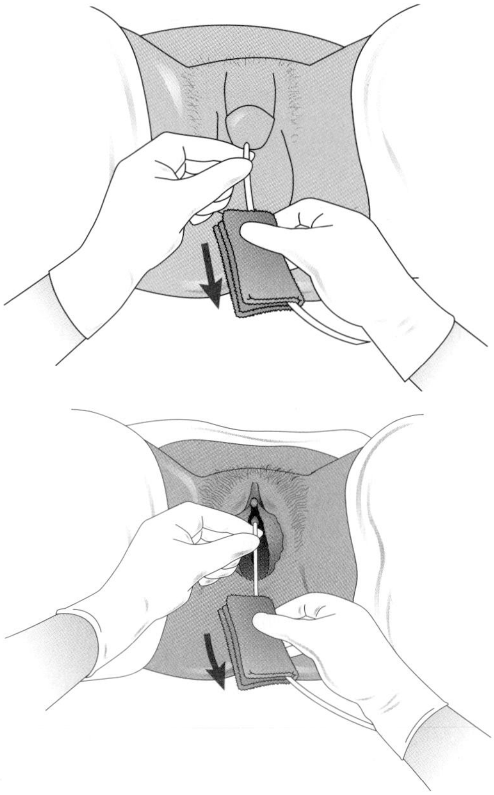

Fig. 14-15.

21. Return bed to appropriate position. Remove privacy measures.
22. Before leaving, place call light within resident's reach.
23. Place soiled clothing and linens in proper containers.
24. Wash your hands.
25. Report any changes in resident to the nurse.
26. Document procedure using facility guidelines.

Emptying the catheter drainage bag

Equipment: **graduate** *(measuring container), alcohol wipes, paper towels, gloves*

1. Wash your hands.
2. Identify yourself by name. Identify the resident by name.

3. Explain procedure to the resident. Speak clearly, slowly, and directly. Maintain face-to-face contact whenever possible.
4. Provide for resident's privacy with curtain, screen, or door.
5. Put on gloves.
6. Place paper towel on the floor under the drainage bag. Place measuring container on the paper towel.
7. Open the drain or spout on the bag. Allow urine to flow out of the bag into the measuring container (Fig. 14-16). Do not let spout touch the measuring container.

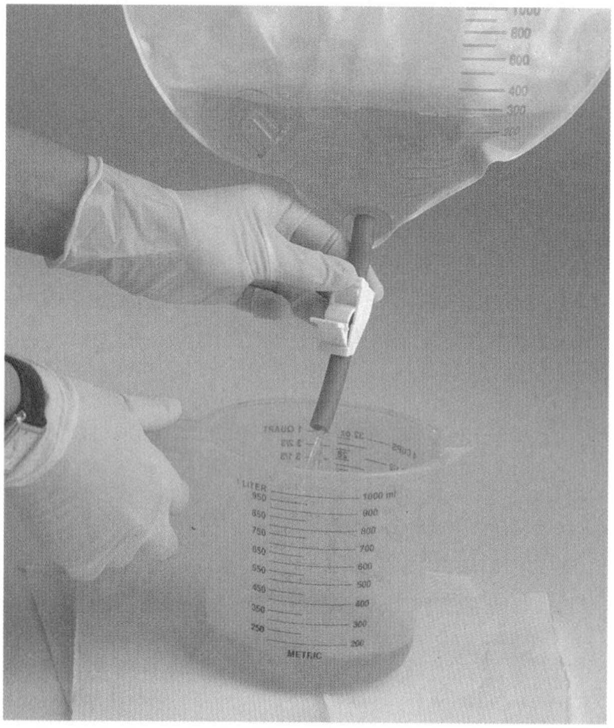

Fig. 14-16.

8. When urine has drained, close spout. Using alcohol wipe, clean the drain spout. Replace the drain in its holder on the bag.
9. Note the amount and the appearance of the urine. Empty into toilet.
10. Clean and store measuring container.
11. Remove gloves.
12. Wash your hands.
13. Document procedure and amount of urine.

Applying a condom catheter

Equipment: condom catheter and collection bag, catheter tape, gloves, plastic bag, bath blanket, supplies for perineal care

1. Wash your hands.
2. Identify yourself by name. Identify the resident by name.
3. Explain procedure to the resident. Speak clearly, slowly, and directly. Maintain face-to-face contact whenever possible.
4. Provide for resident's privacy with curtain, screen, or door.
5. Adjust bed to a safe level, usually waist high. Lock bed wheels.
6. Lower head of bed. Position resident lying flat on his back. Raise the side rail farthest from you.
7. Remove or fold back top bedding. Keep resident covered with bath blanket.
8. Put on gloves.
9. Adjust bath blanket to expose only genital area.
10. If condom catheter is present, gently remove it. Place it in the plastic bag.
11. Help as necessary with perineal care.
12. Attach collection bag to leg.
13. Move pubic hair away from the penis so it does not get rolled into the condom.
14. Hold penis firmly. Place condom at tip of penis. Roll towards base of penis. Leave space between the drainage tip and glans of penis to prevent irritation. If resident is not circumcised, be sure that foreskin is in normal position.
15. Gently secure condom to penis with tape provided (Fig. 14-17).
16. Connect catheter tip to drainage tubing. Make sure tubing is not twisted or kinked.
17. Remove and dispose of your gloves.

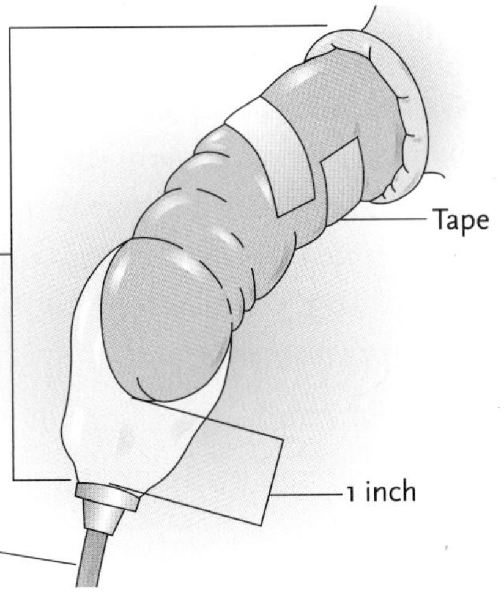

Fig. 14-17.

18. Make resident comfortable. Make sure sheets are free from wrinkles and the bed free from crumbs.
19. Return bed to appropriate position. Remove privacy measures.
20. Before leaving, place call light within resident's reach.
21. Discard plastic bag. Place soiled clothing and linens in proper containers. Clean and store supplies.
22. Wash your hands.
23. Report any changes in resident to the nurse.
24. Document procedure using facility guidelines.

6. Identify types of urine specimens that are collected

You may be asked to collect a specimen from a resident. A **specimen** is a sample. Different types of specimens are used for different tests. Urine specimens may be routine, clean catch (mid-stream), or 24-hour. A **routine urine specimen** is collected anytime the resident voids. The resident will void into a bedpan, urinal, commode, or "hat." The **clean catch specimen** is called "mid-stream." The first and last urine are not included in the sample. Its purpose is to detect the presence of bacteria in the urine. A **24-hour urine specimen** tests for certain chemicals and hormones. This specimen collects all the urine voided by a resident in a 24-hour period. Usually the collection begins at 7 a.m. and runs until 7 a.m. the next day. When beginning a 24-hour urine specimen collection, the resident must void and discard the first urine. The collection begins with an empty bladder. All urine must be collected and stored properly. If any is thrown away or improperly stored, the collection will have to be done over again.

A plastic collection container called a "hat" is sometimes put into a toilet to collect and measure urine or stool (Fig. 14-18). Hats should be labeled. They must be cleaned after each use.

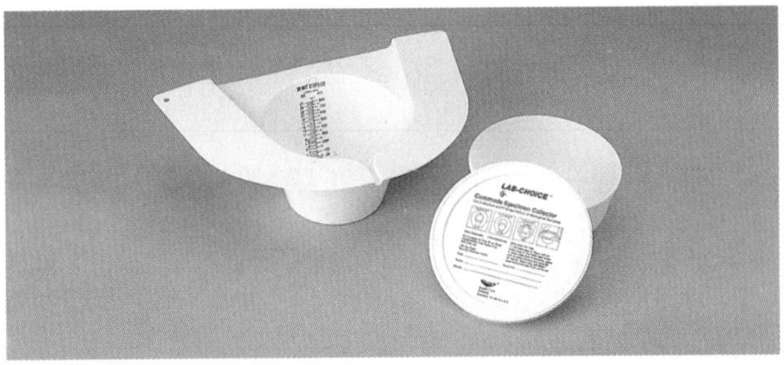

Fig. 14-18. **A "hat" is placed under the toilet seat to collect specimens for residents who use the toilet.**

Some residents will be able to collect their own urine specimens. Others will need your help. Be sure to explain exactly how the specimen must be collected.

Collecting a routine urine specimen

Equipment: urine specimen container and lid, label, gloves, bedpan or urinal (if resident cannot get to the bathroom), "hat" for toilet (if resident can get to the bathroom), 2 plastic bags, washcloth, towel, paper towel, supplies for perineal care

1. Wash your hands.
2. Identify yourself by name. Identify the resident by name.
3. Explain procedure to the resident. Speak clearly, slowly, and directly. Maintain face-to-face contact whenever possible.

4. Provide for resident's privacy with curtain, screen, or door.
5. Put on gloves.
6. Help the resident to the bathroom or commode, or offer the bedpan or urinal.
7. Have resident void into "hat," urinal, or bedpan. Ask the resident not to put toilet paper in with the sample. Provide a plastic bag to discard toilet paper.
8. After urination, help as necessary with perineal care. Help resident wash his or her hands. Make the resident comfortable.
9. Take bedpan, urinal, or commode pail to the bathroom.
10. Pour urine into the specimen container. Specimen container should be at least half full.
11. Cover the urine container with its lid. Do not touch the inside of container. Wipe off the outside with a paper towel.
12. Place the container in a plastic bag.
13. If using a bedpan or urinal, discard extra urine. Rinse and clean equipment. Store.
14. Remove and dispose of gloves. Wash hands. Help resident wash his or her hands.
15. Complete the label for the container. Write the resident's name, room number, the date, and time.
16. Make resident comfortable. Make sure sheets are free from wrinkles and the bed free from crumbs.
17. Return bed to appropriate position if adjusted. Remove privacy measures.
18. Before leaving, place call light within resident's reach.
19. Wash your hands.
20. Report any changes in resident to the nurse.
21. Document procedure using facility guidelines. Note amount and characteristics of urine.

Collecting a clean catch (mid-stream) urine specimen

Equipment: specimen kit with container, label, cleansing solution, gauze or towelettes, gloves, bedpan or urinal if resident cannot use the bathroom, plastic bag, washcloth, paper towel, towel, supplies for perineal care

1. Wash your hands.
2. Identify yourself by name. Identify the resident by name.
3. Explain procedure to the resident. Speak clearly, slowly, and directly. Maintain face-to-face contact whenever possible.
4. Provide for resident's privacy with curtain, screen, or door.
5. Put on gloves.
6. Open the specimen kit. Do not touch the inside of the container or lid.
7. If the resident cannot clean his or her perineal area, you will do it. Using the towelettes or gauze and cleansing solution, clean the area around the urethra. For females, separate the labia. Wipe from front to back along one side. Discard towelette/gauze. With a new towelette or gauze, wipe from front to back along the other side. Using a new towelette or gauze, wipe down the middle.

   For males, clean the head of the penis. Use circular motions with the towelettes or gauze. Clean thoroughly. Change towelettes/gauze after each circular motion. Discard after use. If the man is uncircumcised, pull back the foreskin of the penis before cleaning. Hold it back during urination. Make sure it is pulled back down after collecting the specimen.
8. Ask the resident to urinate into the bedpan, urinal, or toilet, and to stop before urination is complete.
9. Place the container under the urine stream. Have the resident start urinating again. Fill

the container at least half full. Have the resident finish urinating in bedpan, urinal, or toilet.

10. Cover the urine container with its lid. Do not touch the inside of container. Wipe off the outside with a paper towel.
11. Place the container in a plastic bag.
12. If using a bedpan or urinal, discard extra urine. Rinse and clean equipment. Store.
13. Remove and dispose of gloves. Wash hands. Help resident wash his or her hands.
14. Complete the label for the container. Write the resident's name, room number, date, and time.
15. Make resident comfortable. Make sure sheets are free from wrinkles and the bed free from crumbs.
16. Return bed to appropriate position if adjusted. Remove privacy measures.
17. Before leaving, place call light within resident's reach.
18. Wash your hands.
19. Report any changes in resident to the nurse.
20. Document procedure using facility guidelines. Note amount and characteristics of urine.

Collecting a 24-hour urine specimen

Equipment: 24-hour specimen container, label, bedpan or urinal (for residents confined to bed), "hat" for toilet (if resident can get to the bathroom), plastic bag, gloves, washcloth, towel, supplies for perineal care, sign to alert other team members that a 24-hour urine specimen is being collected

1. Wash your hands.
2. Identify yourself by name. Identify the resident by name.
3. Explain procedure to the resident. Speak clearly, slowly, and directly. Maintain face-to-face contact whenever possible. Emphasize that all urine must be saved.
4. Provide for resident's privacy with curtain, screen, or door.
5. Place a sign on the resident's bed to let all care team members know that a 24-hour specimen is being collected. Sign may read "Save all urine for 24-hour specimen."
6. When starting the collection, have the resident completely empty the bladder. Discard the urine. Note the exact time of this voiding. The collection will run until the same time the next day (Fig. 14-19).
7. Label the container. Write resident's name, address, and dates and times the collection period began and ended.
8. Put on gloves each time the resident voids.
9. Pour urine from bedpan, urinal, or toilet attachment into the container. Container may be stored on ice when not used. The ice will keep the specimen cool. Follow facility policy.
10. After each voiding, help as necessary with perineal care. Help the resident wash his or her hands.
11. Clean equipment after each voiding.
12. Remove gloves.
13. Wash your hands.
14. After the last void of the 24-hour period, add the urine to the specimen container. Remove the sign.
15. Place container in plastic bag. Remove and dispose of gloves.
16. Wash your hands.
17. Make resident comfortable. Make sure sheets are free from wrinkles and the bed free from crumbs.
18. Return bed to appropriate position if adjusted. Remove privacy measures.
19. Before leaving, place call light within resident's reach.

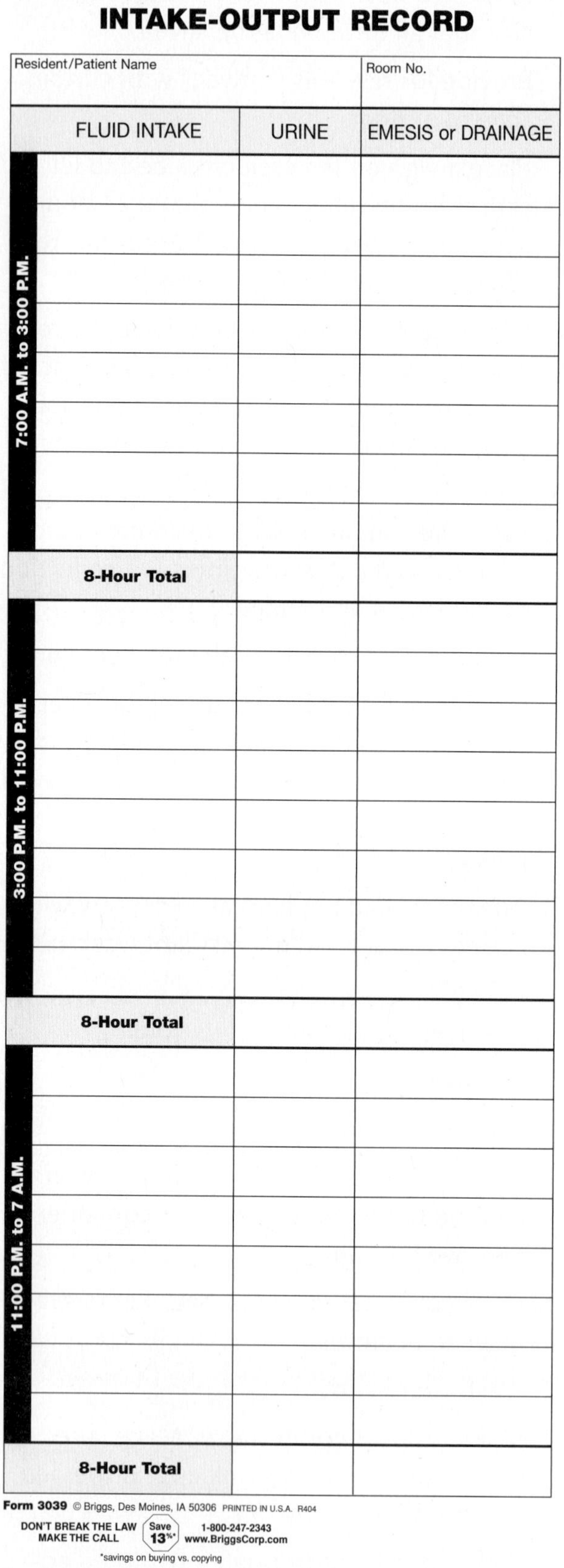

INTAKE-OUTPUT RECORD

Resident/Patient Name			Room No.
	FLUID INTAKE	URINE	EMESIS or DRAINAGE
7:00 A.M. to 3:00 P.M.			
8-Hour Total			
3:00 P.M. to 11:00 P.M.			
8-Hour Total			
11:00 P.M. to 7 A.M.			
8-Hour Total			

Form 3039 © Briggs, Des Moines, IA 50306 PRINTED IN U.S.A. R404
DON'T BREAK THE LAW MAKE THE CALL Save 13%* 1-800-247-2343 www.BriggsCorp.com
*savings on buying vs. copying

Fig. 14-19. **One type of form to record urine output over 24 hours. (Reprinted with permission of Briggs Corporation, 800-247-2343.)**

20. Report any changes in resident to the nurse.
21. Document procedure using facility guidelines.

Urine is strained to detect the presence of **calculi**, or kidney stones, that can develop in the urinary tract. Urine straining is the process of pouring all urine through a fine filter to catch any particles. Kidney stones can be as small as grains of sand or as large as golf balls. If any stones are found, they are saved and then sent to a laboratory for examination.

To strain urine, you will collect a routine urine specimen. In the bathroom, pour it through a strainer or a 4x4-inch piece of gauze into a specimen container. Any stones are wrapped in the filter. They are placed in the specimen container to go to the lab.

7. Explain types of tests performed on urine

Facilities use different methods to test urine. Your facility may use a dip strip that can test for such things as pH level, glucose, ketones, blood, and specific gravity. These strips, called reagent strips, have different sections that change color when they react with urine (Fig. 14-20).

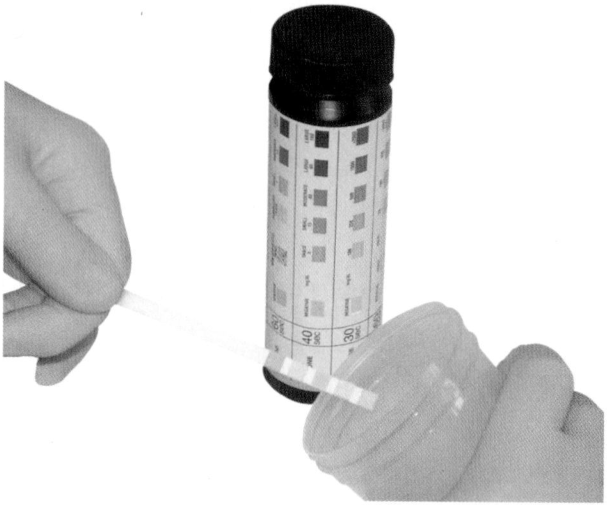

Fig. 14-20. **Reagent strips. (Photo courtesy of LW Scientific, Inc., www.lwscientific.com, 800-726-7345.)**

Testing pH levels: The term "pH" means "parts Hydrogen." The pH scale ranges from 0 to 14. The lower the number, the more acidic the fluid. The higher the number, the more alkaline the fluid. Normal pH range for urine is 4.6–8.0. A disruption of pH may be due to medication, food, or illness.

Testing for glucose and ketones: In diabetes mellitus, commonly called diabetes, the pancreas does not produce enough insulin (see chapter 18). Insulin is the substance the body needs to convert glucose, or natural sugar, into energy. Without insulin to process glucose, these sugars collect in the blood. Some sugar appears in the urine.

Diabetics may also have ketones in the urine. Ketones are produced when the body burns fat for energy or fuel. Ketones are produced when there is not enough insulin to help the body use sugar for energy. Without enough insulin, glucose builds up in the blood. Since the body cannot use glucose for energy, it breaks down fat instead. When this occurs, ketones form in the blood and spill into the urine.

Testing for blood: In normal urine, blood should not be present. Illness and disease can cause blood to appear in urine. Some blood is hidden, or occult. This blood can be detected by testing the urine.

Specific gravity: A specific gravity test is done to test urine density. It can be ordered to make sure the kidneys are functioning properly. Density is how much the substance weighs compared to another substance, which in this case is water. Urine can be very dilute, or close to water. It can also be very dense, or concentrated. This test is done to see how the urine compares to water. Normal values are between 1.002 to 1.028.

The doctor will order which type and how often urine tests should be done. Follow the care plan.

Testing urine with reagent strips

Equipment: urine specimen as ordered, reagent strip, gloves

1. Wash your hands.
2. Put on gloves.
3. Take a strip from the bottle and recap bottle. Close it tightly.
4. Dip the strip into the specimen.
5. Follow manufacturer's instructions for when to remove strip. Remove strip at correct time.
6. Follow manufacturer's instructions for how long to wait after removing strip. After proper time has passed, compare strip with color chart on bottle. Do not touch bottle with strip.
7. Read results.
8. Discard used items. Discard specimen in the toilet.
9. Remove gloves.
10. Wash your hands.
11. Document procedure using facility guidelines.

8. Explain guidelines for assisting with bladder retraining

Injury, illness, or inactivity may cause a loss of normal bladder function. Residents may need help to re-establish a regular bathroom routine. Problems with elimination can be embarrassing or difficult to talk about. Be sensitive. Residents may have incontinence. Always be professional when handling incontinence or helping to establish routines. Never show anger or frustration toward residents who are incontinent.

GUIDELINES
Bladder Retraining

- Ⓖ Follow Standard Precautions. Wear gloves when handling body wastes.

- Explain the bladder training schedule to the resident. Follow the schedule carefully.
- Keep a record of the resident's bladder habits. When you see a pattern of elimination, you can predict when the resident will need a bedpan or a trip to the bathroom.
- Offer a commode or a trip to the bathroom before beginning long procedures (Fig. 14-21).

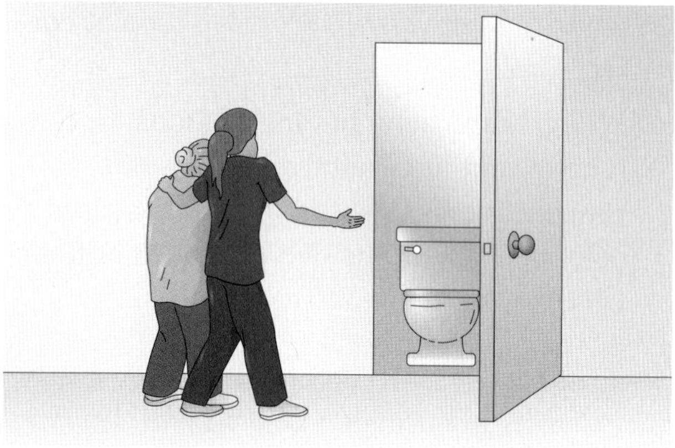

Fig. 14-21. **Offer regular trips to the bathroom.**

- Encourage the resident to drink plenty of fluids. Do this even if urinary incontinence is a problem. About 30 minutes after fluids are taken, offer a trip to the bathroom or a bedpan or urinal.
- Answer call lights promptly. Residents cannot wait long when the urge to go to the bathroom occurs. Leave call lights within reach (Fig. 14-22).

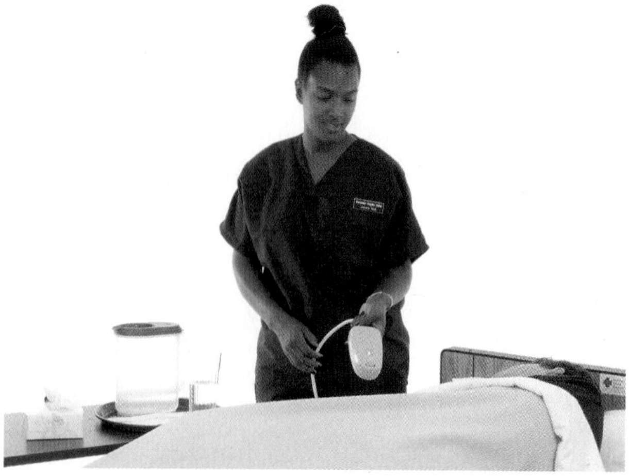

Fig. 14-22. **Answer call lights promptly.**

- Provide privacy for elimination—both in the bed and in the bathroom.
- If a resident has trouble urinating, try running water in the sink. Have him or her lean forward slightly. This puts pressure on the bladder.
- Do not rush the resident.
- Help residents with good perineal care. This prevents skin breakdown and promotes proper hygiene. Carefully observe for skin changes.
- Discard wastes according to facility rules.
- Discard clothing protectors and incontinence briefs properly. Some facilities require double bagging these items. This stops odors from collecting.
- Some facilities use washable bed pads or briefs. Follow Standard Precautions when rinsing before placing these items in the laundry.
- Keep an accurate record of urination. This includes episodes of incontinence.
- Offer positive words for successes, or attempts, to control bladder.
- Never show frustration or anger toward residents who are incontinent. The problem is out of their control. Your negative reactions will only make things worse. Be positive.

Chapter Review

1. What is the normal color of urine?
2. List five signs about urine that should be reported to the nurse.
3. Describe six things that affect urination.
4. In what direction should women be wiped during perineal care?
5. What will women who are unable to get out of bed use for urination? What will men use?

6. What is the best position for women to have normal urination? What is the best position for men?
7. List and define five types of incontinence.
8. Why should you never refer to an incontinence brief as a "diaper?"

True or False. Mark each statement with either a "T" for true or an "F" for false.

9. _____ Incontinence is a normal part of aging.
10. _____ A straight catheter stays inside a person.
11. _____ Catheter tubing should be kept as straight as possible. It should not be kinked.
12. _____ The catheter drainage bag should be kept higher than the hips or bladder.
13. _____ A clean catch specimen does not include the first and last urine in the sample.
14. _____ If any urine is accidentally discarded during a 24-hour collection, the collection will have to be done again another day.
15. _____ Urine is strained to detect calculi.
16. List four things reagent strips can test for in urine.
17. Why do incontinent residents need good perineal care?
18. About how long after fluids are taken should you offer to take a resident to the bathroom?
19. List two ways to promote dignity during bladder retraining.

Chapter 15
Bowel Elimination

1. List qualities of stools and identify signs and symptoms to report about stool

Bowel elimination is the process of emptying the colon, or large intestine, of stool or feces. **Feces**, or **stool**, are solid waste products eliminated by the colon. The frequency of bowel movements varies. They can occur from one to three times a day to two to three times a week. Regular bowel movements keep the gastrointestinal (GI) system healthy.

Stool is brown, soft, and formed (not loose). Foods can change the color of stool. For example, beets can change the color of stool so that it looks bloody. The shape of the stool is tubular, from its passage through the colon. The amount of stool produced per day depends upon the food eaten.

OBSERVING AND REPORTING
Stool

Report any of these to the nurse:

- whitish, black, or red stools
- liquid stools (**diarrhea**)
- **constipation** (inability to have a bowel movement)
- pain when having a bowel movement
- blood, pus, mucous, or discharge in stool
- fecal incontinence (inability to control the muscles of the bowels)

2. List factors affecting bowel elimination

There are many things that affect normal bowel elimination:

Growth and Development: In the elderly, peristalsis slows. Peristalsis refers to the involuntary contractions that move food through the GI system. Proteins, vitamins, and minerals are absorbed less. The elderly have less muscle tone. They may also have tooth loss and less saliva.

Psychological factors: Stress, anger, fear, and depression all affect GI function. Stress, anger, and fear increase peristalsis. Depression decreases it. A lack of privacy can affect elimination, too.

Diet: Fiber improves bowel elimination. Foods high in fiber include fruits, whole grains, and raw vegetables (Fig. 15-1). Some foods cause constipation. These include foods high in animal fats (dairy products, meats, and eggs) or refined sugar but low in fiber. Other foods cause gas, which can help elimination, but can also cause discomfort. These include:

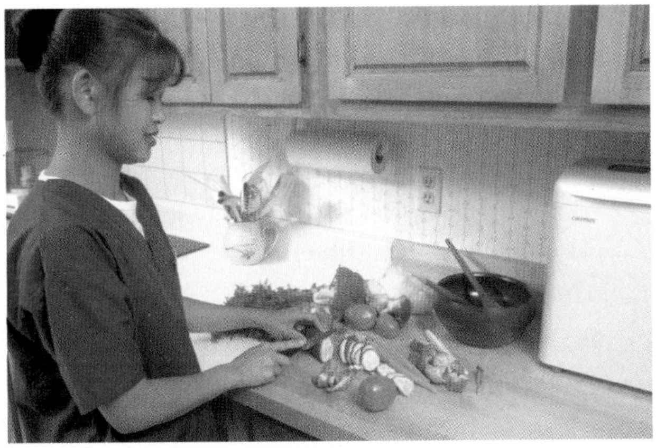

Fig. 15-1. **Raw fruits and vegetables are high in fiber. This helps bowel elimination. Some may cause gas or discomfort.**

- beans
- fruits (e.g., pears, apples, peaches)
- whole grains
- vegetables (e.g., broccoli, cabbage, onions, asparagus)
- dairy products
- carbonated drinks

Fluid intake: Proper fluid intake helps bowel elimination. Generally, a healthy person needs from 64 to 96 ounces (oz.) of fluid each day. Milk can cause constipation. Juices soften stool.

Physical activity: Regular physical activity helps bowel elimination (Fig. 15-2). It strengthens abdominal and pelvic muscles, which helps peristalsis. Immobility weakens these muscles. It may slow elimination.

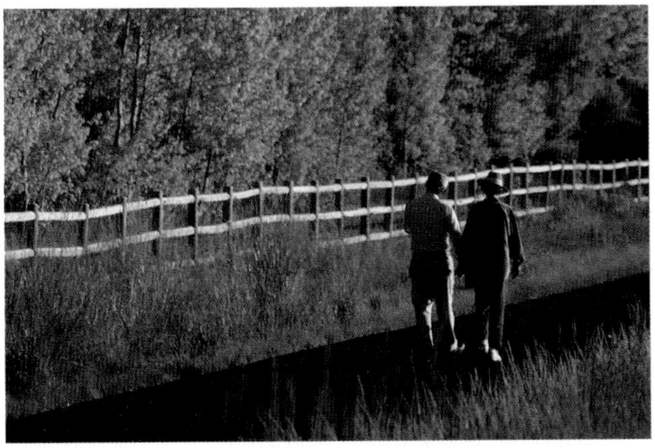

Fig. 15-2. **Regular exercise is important for bowel elimination.**

Personal habits: The time of day of bowel movements varies. Elimination usually occurs after meals. Position affects elimination. A person who is supine (flat on his back) will have the most trouble with bowel elimination. It is impossible to contract muscles in this position. The head of the bed should be raised if possible. The best position for elimination is squatting and leaning forward.

Medications: Medications affect the GI tract. Laxatives help elimination. Other drugs, such as pain relievers, can slow elimination. Antibiotics may cause diarrhea.

Disorders and problems affect bowel elimination. You will learn more about these in the next learning objective.

Process of digestion

Lazzaro Spallanzani [1729-1799] studied digestion. He did experiments with birds called kites. Spallanzani found that gastric juice works to dissolve food in the stomach.

3. Discuss common bowel elimination problems

Constipation is the difficult and often painful elimination of a hard, dry stool. Constipation occurs when the feces move too slowly through the intestine. This can result from decreased fluid intake, poor diet, inactivity, medications, aging, disease, or ignoring the need to eliminate. Signs of constipation include abdominal swelling, gas, irritability, and record of no recent bowel movement.

Treatment often includes increasing the amount of fiber eaten and activity level, and possibly medication. An enema or suppository may be ordered. An **enema** is a specific amount of water flowed into the colon to eliminate stool. A **suppository** is a medication given rectally to cause a bowel movement.

A **fecal impaction** results from unrelieved constipation. It is a hard stool stuck in the rectum. It cannot be expelled. Symptoms include no stool for several days and oozing of liquid stool. Cramping, abdominal swelling, and rectal pain also occur. When an impaction occurs, a healthcare provider will insert one or two gloved fingers into the rectum and break the mass into fragments. Then it can be passed.

Hemorrhoids are enlarged veins in the rectum. They may also be visible outside the anus. Rectal itching, burning, pain, and bleeding are symptoms of hemorrhoids. Treatment may include medications, compresses, and sitz baths (chapter 17). Surgery may be necessary. When cleaning the anus, take care to avoid causing pain and bleeding from hemorrhoids.

Diarrhea is frequent elimination of liquid or semi-liquid feces. Abdominal cramps, urgency, nausea, and vomiting can accompany diarrhea, depending on the cause. Infections, microorganisms, irritating foods, and medications can cause diarrhea. Treatment is usually medication and a change of diet. A diet of bananas, rice, apples, and tea/toast (BRAT diet) is often suggested.

Fecal incontinence is the inability to control the bowels. It causes frequent, loose stools. Common causes are constipation, muscle and nerve damage, loss of storage capacity in the rectum, and diarrhea. Treatment includes a change in diet, medication, bowel training, or surgery.

Gas, also called **flatus** or flatulence, is air in the intestine that is passed through the rectum. Gas can cause cramping or abdominal pain. Gas can be caused by:

- Swallowing air while eating
- Eating high-fiber foods
- Eating foods that a person cannot tolerate. For example, gas can occur when a resident has lactose intolerance and eats dairy products. **Lactose intolerance** is the inability to digest lactose, a type of sugar found in milk and other dairy products. It is caused by a deficiency of lactase enzyme.
- Antibiotics
- **Irritable bowel syndrome** is a chronic form of stomach upset that gets worse from stress.
- **Malabsorption** means that a body cannot absorb or digest a particular nutrient properly. It is often accompanied by diarrhea.

Methods used for the relief of flatus are the rectal tube and the Harris flush. A Harris flush, also called a return-flow enema or a colonic irrigation, is a special type of enema that reduces gas. A rectal tube is placed in the rectum to reduce gas.

4. Describe how to promote normal bowel elimination

There are things you can do to help residents with bowel elimination.

GUIDELINES

Promoting Normal Bowel Elimination

- Follow a toileting schedule.
- Provide plenty of privacy.
- Do not rush or interrupt the person.
- If the person cannot get out of bed, raise the head of the bed. Then the resident does not have to work against gravity. The best position for elimination is squatting and leaning forward.
- Encourage a healthy diet. Encourage residents to drink enough water daily.
- Encourage regular activity. Help as needed.

Promote good hygiene. Help with perineal care as needed. Residents who have fecal incontinence or diarrhea must be kept clean and dry. Give good skin care to avoid skin breakdown. Help resident to wash hands often. Report any changes in appearance or frequency of bowel elimination.

5. Discuss how enemas are given

An enema is given to help eliminate stool from the colon. A specific amount of water flows inside of the colon to help remove stool. Some facilities allow NAs to give enemas. If you are allowed to give enemas, follow your facility's policies. Make sure you are trained to give one. If you have questions or concerns, ask the nurse before beginning.

Doctors will write an enema order. Different types of enemas include:

- **Tap water enema** (TWE): 500-1000 cc of water from a faucet
- **Soapsuds enema** (SSE): 500-1000 cc water with 5 cc of mild castile soap added
- **Saline enema**: 500-1000 cc water with two teaspoons of salt added
- **Commercial enema**: 120 cc solution; may have additives

During an enema, the resident must be in the Sims' position (Fig. 15-3). If the person is positioned on the left side, the water does not have to flow against gravity. Give the enema slowly. Hold the enema tubing in place. Stop immediately if the resident has pain or if you feel resistance. Tell the nurse if this happens.

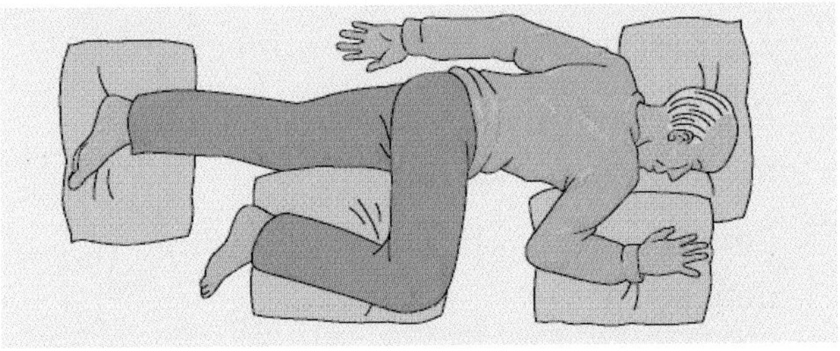

Fig. 15-3. During an enema the resident should be placed in the Sims' position, which is a left side-lying position.

Giving a cleansing enema

Equipment: 2 pair of gloves, bath blanket, IV pole, enema solution, tubing and clamp, bed protector, bedpan, lubricating jelly, bath thermometer, tape measure, toilet paper, two washcloths, robe, non-skid footwear

1. Wash your hands.
2. Identify yourself by name. Identify the resident by name.
3. Explain procedure to the resident. Speak clearly, slowly, and directly. Maintain face-to-face contact whenever possible.
4. Provide for resident's privacy with curtain, screen, or door.
5. Adjust bed to a safe level, usually waist high. Lock bed wheels.
6. Raise side rail on far side of bed. Lower side rail nearest you.
7. Help resident into left-sided Sims' position. Cover with a bath blanket.
8. Place the IV pole beside the bed. Raise the side rail.
9. Clamp the enema tube. Prepare the enema solution. Fill bag with 500-1000 cc of warm water (105° F).
10. Unclamp the tube. Let a small amount of solution run through the tubing. Re-clamp the tube.
11. Hang bag on IV pole. Make sure bottom of enema bag is not more than 12 inches above the resident's anus (Fig. 15-4).

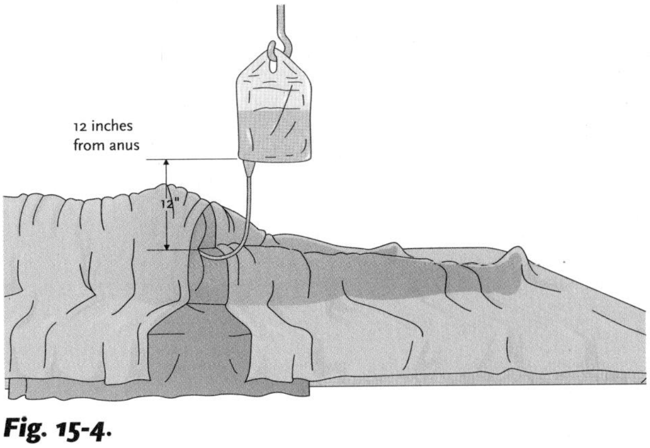

Fig. 15-4.

12. Apply gloves.
13. Lower the side rail. Uncover resident enough to expose anus only.
14. Place bed protector under resident. Place bedpan close to resident's body.

15. Lubricate tip of tubing with lubricating jelly.
16. Ask resident to breathe deeply. This relieves cramps during procedure.
17. Place one hand on the upper buttock. Lift to expose the anus (Fig. 15-5). Ask the resident to take a deep breath and exhale. Using other hand, gently insert the tip of the tubing two to four inches into the rectum. Stop immediately if you feel resistance or if the resident complains of pain. If this happens, clamp the tube. Tell the nurse immediately.

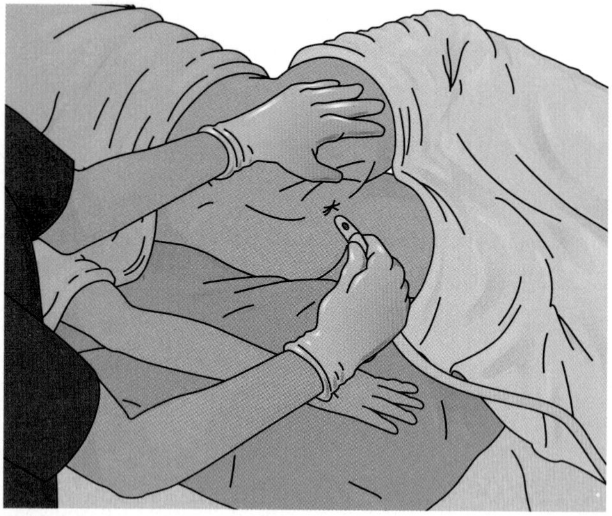

Fig. 15-5.

18. Unclamp the tubing. Allow the solution to flow slowly into the rectum. Ask resident to take slow, deep breaths. If resident complains of cramping, clamp the tubing and stop for a couple of minutes. Encourage him or her to take as much of the solution as possible.
19. Clamp the tubing when the solution is almost gone. Remove the tip from the rectum. Place the tip into the enema bag. Do not contaminate yourself, resident, or bed linens.
20. Ask the resident to hold the solution inside as long as possible.
21. Help resident to use bedpan, commode, or get to the bathroom. If the resident uses a commode or bathroom, apply robe and non-skid footwear. Lower the bed to an appropriate level for the resident before the resident gets up.
22. Place call light and toilet paper within resident's reach. If the resident is using the bathroom, ask him not to flush the toilet when finished.
23. Leave the resident if possible. Ask him to signal when he's finished.
24. Discard disposable equipment. Clean area.
25. Remove gloves. Wash your hands.
26. When resident is done, put on clean gloves. Using washcloths, help with perineal care as needed.
27. Remove bedpan. Remove the bed protector.
28. Empty bedpan. Check for consistency, color, and amount. If resident used toilet, check toilet contents.
29. Rinse bedpan. Pour rinse water into toilet. Use approved disinfectant. Return to proper storage. Dispose of soiled washcloths.
30. Remove gloves. Wash your hands.
31. Help resident wash hands.
32. Remove bath blanket. Make resident comfortable. Make sure sheets are free from wrinkles and the bed free from crumbs.
33. Return bed to appropriate position. Remove privacy measures.
34. Before leaving, place call light within resident's reach.
35. Wash your hands.
36. Report any changes in resident to the nurse.
37. Document procedure using facility guidelines.

Giving a commercial enema

Equipment: 2 pairs of gloves, bath blanket, standard or oil retention commercial enema kit, bed protector, bedpan, lubricating jelly, washcloths or wipes, toilet tissue, robe, non-skid footwear

1. Wash your hands.
2. Identify yourself by name. Identify the resident by name.
3. Explain procedure to the resident. Speak clearly, slowly, and directly. Maintain face-to-face contact whenever possible.
4. Provide for resident's privacy with curtain, screen, or door.
5. Adjust bed to a safe level, usually waist high. Lock bed wheels.
6. Raise side rail on far side of bed. Lower side rail nearest you.
7. Help resident into left-sided Sims' position. Cover with a bath blanket.
8. Apply gloves.
9. Place bed protector under resident. Place bedpan close to resident's body.
10. Uncover resident enough to expose anus only.
11. Lubricate tip of bottle with lubricating jelly.
12. Ask resident to breathe deeply to relieve cramps during procedure.
13. Place one hand on the upper buttock. Lift to expose the anus. Ask the resident to take a deep breath and exhale. Using other hand, gently insert the tip of the tubing about one and a half inches into the rectum. Stop immediately if you feel resistance or if the resident complains of pain.
14. Slowly squeeze and roll the enema container so that the solution runs inside the resident. Only release pressure after removing tip from the rectum.
15. When tip is removed, place bottle inside the box upside down (Fig. 15-6).
16. Ask the resident to hold the solution inside as long as possible.
17. Help resident to use bedpan, commode, or get to the bathroom. If the resident uses a commode or bathroom, apply robe and non-skid footwear. Lower the bed to its lowest position before the resident gets up.

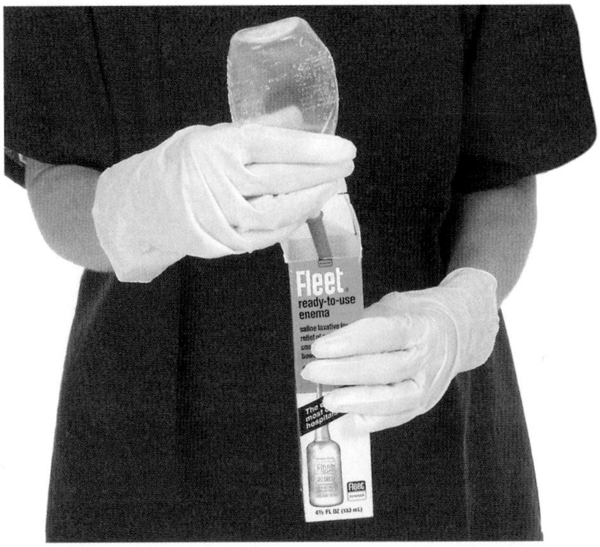

Fig. 15-6.

18. Place call light and toilet paper within resident's reach. If resident is using the bathroom, ask him not to flush the toilet when finished.
19. Leave the resident if possible. Ask him to signal when he's finished.
20. Discard disposable equipment. Clean area.
21. Remove gloves. Wash your hands.
22. When resident is done, put on clean gloves. Using washcloths, help with perineal care as needed.
23. Remove bedpan. Remove the bed protector.
24. Empty bedpan. Check for consistency, color, and amount. If resident used toilet, check the toilet contents.
25. Rinse bedpan. Pour rinse water into toilet. Use approved disinfectant. Return it to proper storage. Dispose of soiled washcloths properly.
26. Remove gloves. Wash your hands.
27. Help resident wash hands.
28. Remove bath blanket. Make resident comfortable. Make sure sheets are free from wrinkles and the bed free from crumbs.

29. Return bed to appropriate position. Remove privacy measures.
30. Before leaving, place call light within resident's reach.
31. Wash your hands.
32. Report any changes in resident to the nurse.
33. Document procedure using facility guidelines.

6. Demonstrate how to collect a stool specimen

Stool is collected and tested for blood, pathogens, and other things. A common test is an ova and parasites test, which can detect worms or amebas. If the specimen is to be examined for ova and parasites, take it to the lab immediately. This examination must be made while the stool is warm.

When collecting a stool specimen, do not get urine or tissue in the sample. Urine and paper can ruin the sample.

Collecting a stool specimen

Equipment: specimen container and lid, 2 tongue blades, 2 pairs of gloves, bedpan (if resident cannot use the bathroom or commode), specimen pan (if resident uses toilet or commode), 2 plastic bags, toilet tissue, laboratory slip, washcloth or towel, supplies for perineal care

Ask the resident to let you know when he can have a bowel movement. Be ready to collect the specimen.

1. Wash your hands.
2. Identify yourself by name. Identify the resident by name.
3. Explain procedure to the resident. Speak clearly, slowly, and directly. Maintain face-to-face contact whenever possible.
4. Provide for resident's privacy with curtain, screen, or door.
5. Put on gloves.
6. When the resident is ready to move bowels, ask him not to urinate at the same time. Ask him not to put toilet paper in with the sample. Provide a plastic bag for toilet paper.
7. Fit specimen pan to toilet or commode, or provide resident with bedpan. Leave the room. Ask the resident to signal when he is finished with the bowel movement. Make sure call light is within reach.
8. After the bowel movement, help with perineal care. Help resident wash his hands. Make the resident comfortable. Remove gloves.
9. Wash hands again.
10. Put on clean gloves.
11. Using the two tongue blades, take about two tablespoons of stool. Put it in the container. Cover it tightly.
12. Wrap the tongue blades in toilet paper and throw them away. Empty the bedpan or container into the toilet. Clean and store the equipment.
13. Label for the container. Write the resident's name, address, the date, and time. Bag the specimen.
14. Remove and dispose of gloves.
15. Make resident comfortable. Make sure sheets are free from wrinkles and the bed free from crumbs.
16. Return bed to appropriate position if adjusted. Remove privacy measures.
17. Before leaving, place call light within resident's reach.
18. Wash your hands.
19. Report any changes in resident to the nurse.
20. Document procedure using facility guidelines. Note amount and characteristics of stool.

7. Explain occult blood testing

Hidden, or **occult**, blood is found in stool with a microscope or a special chemical test. This may be a sign of a serious problem, such as cancer. The Hemoccult test checks for occult blood in stool (Fig. 15-7). In some facilities, staff members do not perform this test. Laboratories do instead.

Testing a stool specimen for occult blood

Equipment: stool specimen, Hemoccult test kit, tongue blade, paper towel, plastic bag, gloves

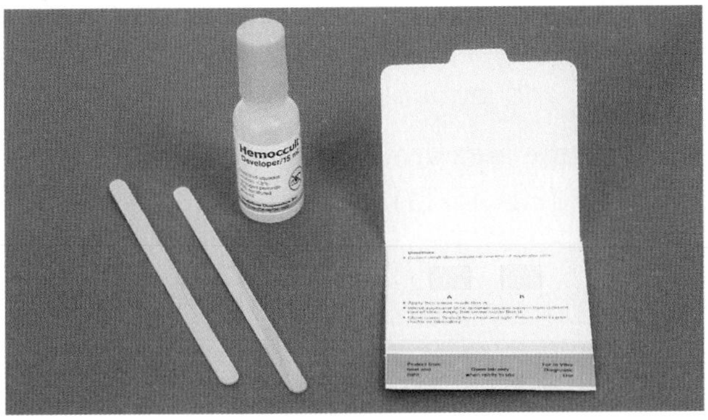

Fig. 15-7.

1. Wash your hands.
2. Put on gloves.
3. Open the test card.
4. Pick up a tongue blade. Get small amount of stool from specimen container.
5. Using tongue blade, smear a small amount of stool onto box A of test card (Fig. 15-8).

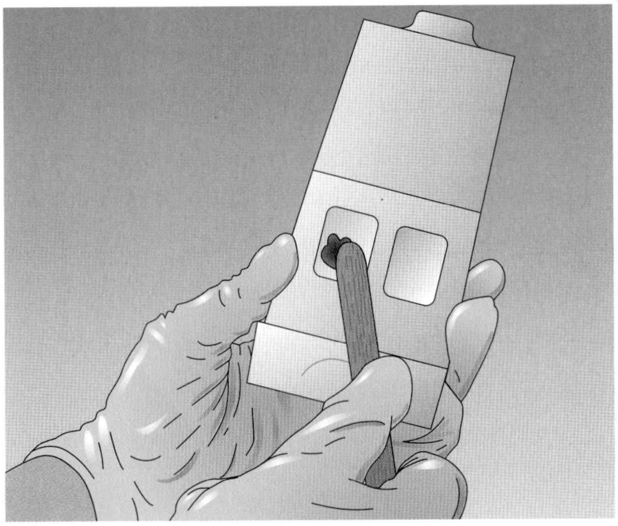

Fig. 15-8.

6. Flip tongue blade. Get some stool from another part of specimen. Smear small amount of stool onto box B of test card.
7. Close the test card. Turn over to other side.
8. Open the flap.
9. Open developer. Apply developer to each box. Follow manufacturer's instructions.
10. Wait the amount of time listed in instructions, usually between 10 and 60 seconds.
11. Watch the squares for any color changes. Record color changes. Follow instructions.
12. Place tongue blade and test packet in disposable bag.
13. Dispose of plastic bag properly.
14. Remove gloves. Wash hands.
15. Document procedure using facility guidelines.

8. Define the term "ostomy" and list care guidelines

An **ostomy** is an operation to create an opening from an area inside the body to the outside. It may be done due to bowel disease, cancer, or trauma. (Information on cancer is found in chapter 18.) In a resident with an ostomy, the end of the intestine is brought out of the body through an opening in the abdomen. This opening is called a **stoma**. Stool, or feces, are eliminated through the ostomy rather than through the anus. (When an ureter is opened to abdomen for urine to be eliminated it is called a **ureterostomy**.)

The terms "**colostomy**" and "**ileostomy**" tell what part of the intestine was removed and the type of stool that will be eliminated (Fig. 15-9). In a colostomy, stool will generally be semi-solid. With an ileostomy, stool may be liquid. It may be irritating to the skin.

Residents who have had an ostomy wear a disposable bag. It fits over the stoma to collect the feces. The bag is attached to the skin by adhesive. A belt may also be used to secure

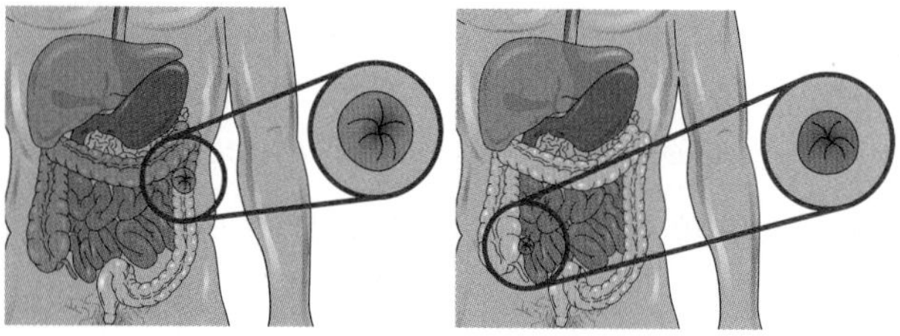

Fig. 15-9. **A colostomy and an ileostomy.**

it (Fig. 15-10). Many people manage the ostomy appliance by themselves. If you are giving ostomy care, make sure the resident receives good skin care and hygiene. Empty and clean or replace the ostomy bag whenever stool is eliminated. Always wear gloves and wash hands carefully. Teach proper handwashing to residents with ostomies.

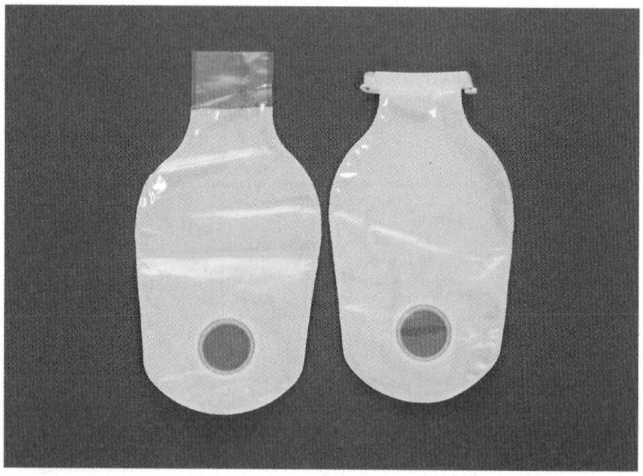

Fig. 15-10. **An open and a closed ostomy bag.**

Many residents with ostomies feel they have lost control of a basic function. They may be embarrassed or angry. Be sensitive and supportive. Always provide privacy for ostomy care.

Ostomy care

Equipment: bedpan, disposable bed protector, bath blanket, clean ostomy bag and belt/appliance, toilet paper, basin of warm water, soap or cleanser, washcloth, skin cream as ordered, two towels, plastic disposable bag, gloves

1. Wash your hands.
2. Identify yourself by name. Identify the resident by name.
3. Explain procedure to the resident. Speak clearly, slowly, and directly. Maintain face-to-face contact whenever possible.
4. Provide for resident's privacy with curtain, screen, or door.
5. Adjust bed to a safe level, usually waist high. Lock bed wheels.
6. Place protective sheet under resident. Cover resident with a bath blanket. Pull down the top sheet and blankets. Only expose ostomy site. Offer a towel to keep clothing dry.
7. Put on gloves.
8. Remove ostomy bag carefully. Place it in plastic bag. Note the color, odor, consistency, and amount of stool in the bag.
9. Wipe the area around the stoma with toilet paper (Fig. 15-11). Discard paper in plastic bag.

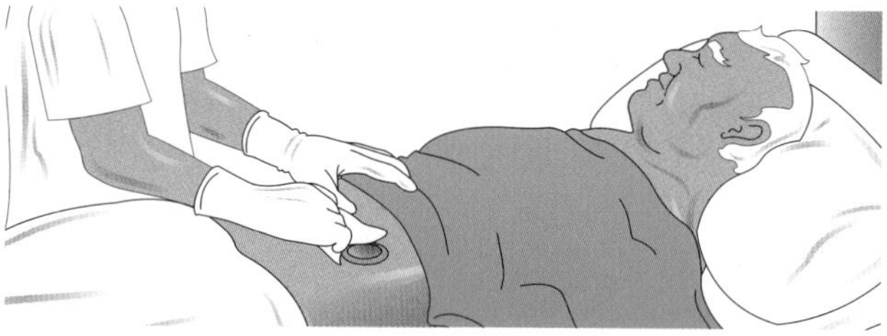

Fig. 15-11.

10. Use a washcloth and warm soapy water. Wash the area in one direction, away from the stoma. Pat dry. Apply cream as ordered.
11. Place the clean ostomy appliance on resident. Make sure the bottom of the bag is clamped.
12. Remove disposable bed protector. Discard. Place soiled linens in proper container.
13. Remove bag and bedpan. Discard bag in proper container. Empty bedpan into toilet.
14. Clean bedpan. Pour rinse water into toilet. Return to proper storage.
15. Remove and dispose of gloves properly.
16. Make resident comfortable. Make sure sheets are free from wrinkles and the bed free from crumbs.
17. Return bed to appropriate position.

Remove privacy measures.

18. Place call light within resident's reach.
19. Wash your hands.
20. Report any changes in resident to the nurse. Report if stoma is very red or blue, or if swelling or bleeding is present.
21. Document procedure using facility guidelines.

9. Explain guidelines for assisting with bowel retraining

Residents who have had a disruption in their bowel routines from illness, injury, or inactivity may need help to re-establish a regular routine and normal function. The doctor may order suppositories, laxatives, stool softeners, or enemas to help.

GUIDELINES
Bowel Retraining

- Follow Standard Precautions. Wear gloves when handling body wastes.
- Explain the training schedule to the resident. Follow it carefully.
- Keep a record of the resident's bowel habits. When you see a pattern, you can predict when the resident will need a bedpan or a trip to the bathroom.
- Encourage the resident to drink plenty of fluids.
- Encourage the resident to eat foods that are high in fiber, as allowed. Chapter 16 has more information on diet and nutrition.
- Answer call lights promptly. Leave call lights within reach.
- Provide privacy—both in the bed and in the bathroom.
- Do not rush the resident.
- Help your resident with good perineal care. This prevents skin breakdown and promotes proper hygiene. Carefully watch for skin changes.
- Discard wastes according to facility rules.
- Discard clothing protectors and incontinence briefs properly. Some facilities require double bagging to stop odors.
- Some facilities use washable bed pads or briefs. Follow Standard Precautions when placing these items in the laundry.
- Keep a record of elimination.
- Praise successes or attempts to control bowels.
- Never show frustration or anger toward residents who are incontinent. The problem is out of their control. Your negative reactions will only make things worse. Be positive.

STOP ***Handling Incontinence***

Be professional when handling incontinence. It is hard enough for residents without having to worry about your reactions. Showing frustration or anger is abusive behavior. Negative reactions only make the problem worse. Be patient when setbacks occur.

Chapter Review

1. List five things you should observe and report about stool.
2. How does regular activity help bowel elimination?
3. What is the best position for bowel elimination?
4. List three possible treatments for constipation.
5. List three causes of diarrhea.
6. List six guidelines for promoting normal bowel elimination.
7. What are four types of enemas?

8. What position must the resident be in for an enema?
9. What should you do if a resident feels pain or if you feel resistance while giving an enema?
10. How far above a resident's anus should the bottom of the enema bag be?
11. How should the bottle be placed in the box after a commercial enema?
12. What should not be included in a stool specimen?
13. How is occult blood found in stool?
14. Why may a resident have an ostomy?
15. How often should an ostomy bag be emptied?
16. List eight guidelines for bowel retraining.

Chapter 16
Nutrition and Hydration

1. Describe the importance of good nutrition

Good nutrition is very important. **Nutrition** is how the body uses food to maintain health. Bodies need a well-balanced diet with nutrients and plenty of fluids. This helps us grow new cells, maintain normal body function, and have energy. Good nutrition in early life helps ensure good health later. For the ill or elderly, a well-balanced diet helps maintain muscles and skin and prevent pressure sores. A good diet promotes healing. It also helps us cope with stress.

2. Identify nutritional problems of the elderly or ill

Aging and illness can lead to emotional and physical problems. They may also affect food intake. For example, people who are lonely or depressed may have little interest in food. Weaker hands and arms due to paralysis or tremors make it hard to eat. People with illnesses that affect their ability to chew and swallow may not want to eat. Care must be taken in meal planning to ensure good nutrition.

Physical changes due to aging that may affect nutrition include the following:

- Metabolism slows. Muscles weaken and lose tone. Body movement slows. Reduced activity or exercise affects appetite.
- Loss of vision may affect the way food looks. This may decrease appetite.
- Weakened sense of smell and taste affect appetite. Medication may impair these senses (Fig. 16-1).
- Less saliva production affects chewing and swallowing.
- Dentures, tooth loss, or poor dental health make chewing difficult.
- Digestion takes longer. It is less efficient.

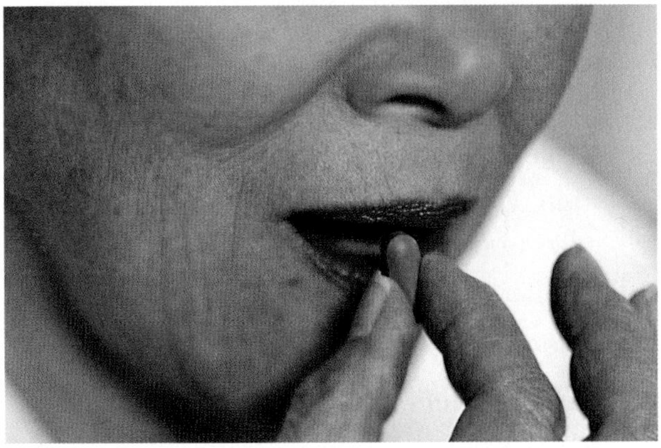

Fig. 16-1. **Many residents take a variety of medications. This can affect the way food smells and tastes.**

Medications or limited activity may cause constipation. Constipation may interfere with appetite. Fiber, fluids, and exercise can help.

Many illnesses require restrictions in fluids, proteins, certain minerals, or calories. In addition, residents who are ill are often tired, nauseated, or in pain. This contributes to poor fluid and food intake. Conditions that make eating or swallowing hard include:

- stroke, or CVA, which can cause weakness and paralysis
- nerve and muscle damage from head and neck cancer
- Multiple Sclerosis
- Parkinson's disease
- Alzheimer's disease

You will learn more about these diseases in chapter 18. If a resident has trouble swallowing, soft foods and thickened liquids will be served. You will learn more about swallowing problems and thickened liquids later in the chapter. A straw or special cup will help make swallowing easier.

Swallowing problems cause a high risk for choking on food or drink. Inhaling food or drink into the lungs is called **aspiration**. Aspiration can cause pneumonia or death. Alert the nurse immediately if any problems occur while feeding.

GUIDELINES
Preventing Aspiration

- Position residents properly when eating. They must sit in a straight, upright position. Do not try to feed residents in a reclining position.
- Offer small pieces of food or small spoons of pureed food.
- Feed resident slowly.
- Place food in the non-paralyzed, or unaffected, side of the mouth.
- Make sure mouth is empty before each bite of food or sip of drink.
- Residents should stay in the upright position for about 30 minutes after eating and drinking.

When a person is completely unable to swallow, he or she may be fed through a tube. A **nasogastric tube** is inserted into the nose and goes to the stomach. A tube can also be placed through the skin directly into the stomach. This is called a **PEG** (Percutaneous Endoscopic Gastrostomy) **tube**. The opening in the stomach and abdomen is called a **gastrostomy** (Fig. 16-2). Tube feedings are used when residents cannot swallow but can digest food. Conditions that may prevent swallowing include coma, cancer, stroke, refusal to eat, or extreme weakness.

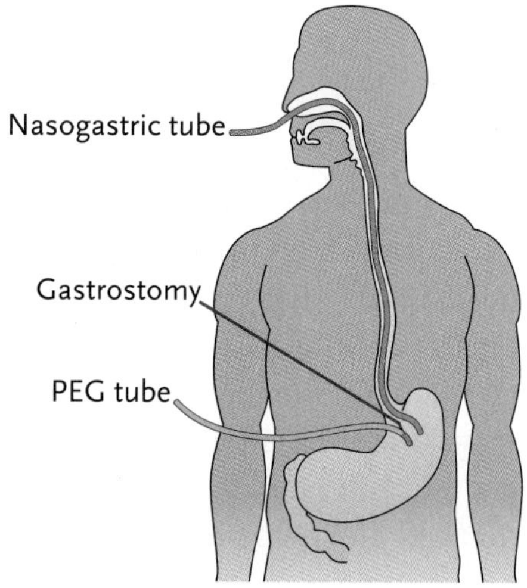

Fig. 16-2.

If a person's digestive system does not function properly, hyperalimentation or **total parenteral nutrition** (**TPN**) may be needed. With TPN, a resident receives nutrients directly into the bloodstream. It bypasses the digestive system.

NAs never insert tubes, do the feeding, or clean the tubes. You may assemble equipment and supplies and hand them to the nurse. You may position the resident. You may also discard used equipment and supplies, clean, or store equipment and supplies.

GUIDELINES
Tube Feedings

- Make sure that the tubing is not kinked or pulled.

- Make sure the resident is not resting on the tubing.
- The resident may have an order for nothing by mouth, or NPO. Be aware of this.
- Give regular and careful mouth and nose care.

OBSERVING AND REPORTING

Tube Feedings

Report any of these to the nurse:

- mouth or nose sores
- shortness of breath
- difficulty breathing
- pale or blue-tinged skin
- nausea
- vomiting
- choking
- abdominal cramping
- the resident pulling on the tube
- redness or drainage near the opening
- feeding pump alarm sounds (report to the nurse immediately)

3. List the six basic nutrients and explain the USDA Food Guide Pyramid

The Six Basic Nutrients

The body needs these nutrients for growth and development:

1. **Protein**. Proteins are part of every body cell. They are needed for tissue growth and repair. Proteins also supply energy for the body. Sources include fish, seafood, poultry, meat, eggs, milk, cheese, nuts, peas, and dried beans (Fig. 16-3).

   Whole grain cereals, pastas, rice, and breads have some proteins of lower quality. These must be combined with more complete proteins. Beans and rice or cereal and milk are some complementary proteins.

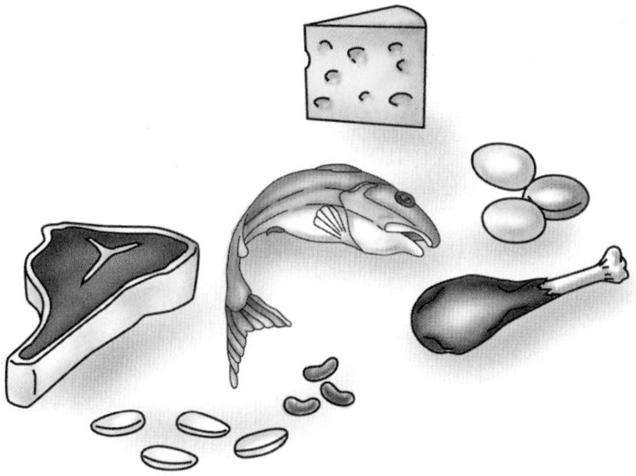

Fig. 16-3. **Sources of protein.**

2. **Carbohydrates**. Carbohydrates supply fuel for energy. They help the body use fat efficiently. Carbohydrates also have fiber, which is necessary for bowel elimination.

   Carbohydrates can be divided into two basic types: complex and simple. Complex carbohydrates are found in bread, cereal, potatoes, rice, pasta, vegetables, and fruits. Simple carbohydrates are found in sugars, sweets, syrups, and jellies. Simple carbohydrates do not have the same nutritional value as complex carbohydrates (Fig. 16-4).

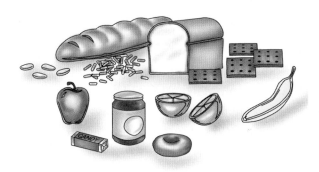

Fig. 16-4. **Sources of carbohydrates.**

   The only value of simple carbohydrates is as energy for people who eat very little. In others, simple carbohydrates are stored as fat.

3. **Fats**. Fat helps the body store energy. Body fat also provides insulation. It protects body organs. Fats help the body absorb vitamins. Fats also add flavor to food. Excess fat in the diet is stored as fat in the body.

Examples of fats are butter, margarine, salad dressings, oils, and animal fats in meats, fowl, and fish (Fig. 16-5). Monounsaturated vegetable fats (including olive oil and canola oil) and polyunsaturated vegetable fats (including corn and safflower oils) are healthier. Saturated fats, including animal fats, are not as healthy. They should be limited.

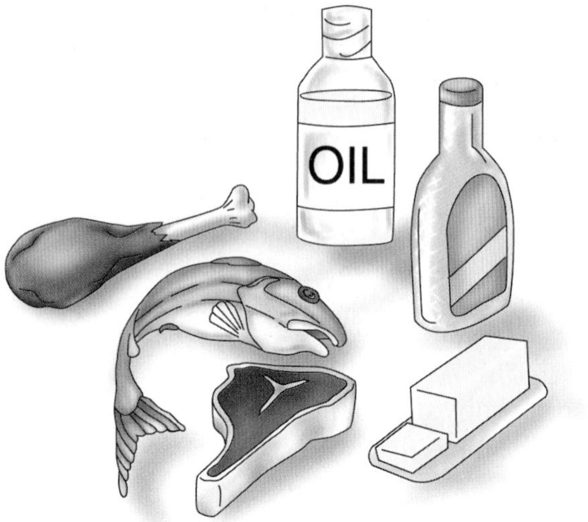

***Fig. 16-5.* Sources of fat.**

4. **Vitamins**. Vitamins are substances the body needs to function. The body cannot make most vitamins. They can only be gotten from food, but they are essential to body functions. Vitamins A, D, E, and K are fat-soluble vitamins. This means they are carried and stored in body fat. Vitamins B and C are water-soluble vitamins. They are broken down by water in our bodies. They cannot be stored. They are eliminated in urine and feces.

5. **Minerals**. Minerals form and maintain cell functions. They give energy and control processes. Zinc, iron, calcium, and magnesium are some minerals. Minerals are found in many foods.

6. **Water**. One-half to two-thirds of our body weight is water. We need about eight glasses, or 64 ounces, of water or other fluids a day. Water is the most essential nutrient for life. Without it, a person can only live a few days. Water helps in the digestion and absorption of food. It helps with waste elimination. Through perspiration, water helps maintain normal body temperature. Keeping enough fluid in our bodies is necessary for good health (Fig. 16-6).

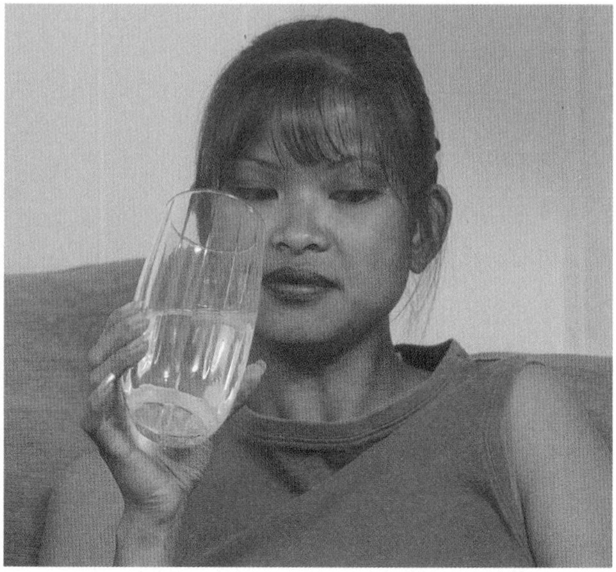

***Fig. 16-6.* Drinking plenty of water is good for you, too.**

Most foods have nutrients. No one food has all the nutrients needed for a healthy body. This is why it is important to eat a daily diet that is well-balanced.

The U.S. Department of Agriculture (USDA) has divided the foods that we eat into six groups. Diets should have some foods from each of the food groups below:

1. Grains, including cereals, bread, rice, and pasta
2. Fruits
3. Vegetables
4. Milk and milk products
5. Meat, poultry, fish, eggs, dry beans, and nuts
6. Fats, oils, and sweets

These six groups make up the **Food Guide Pyramid** (Fig. 16-7). Foods near the bottom of the pyramid should make up most of our diet. Foods closer to the top should be eaten in smaller amounts.

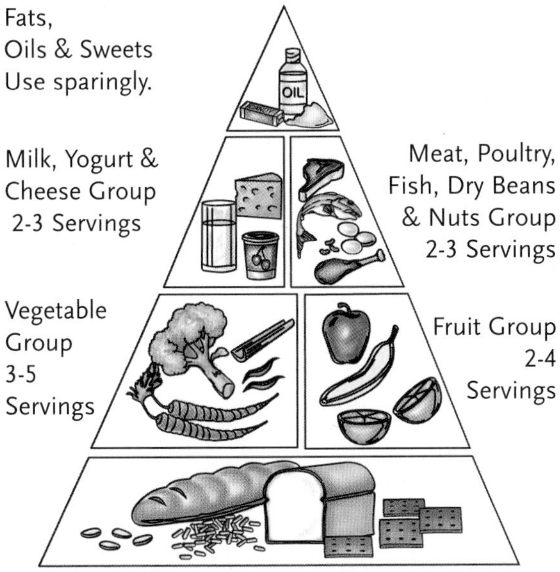

***Fig. 16-7*. The Food Guide Pyramid was created by the U.S. Department of Agriculture. It shows the six food groups. Together, they form a healthy diet.**

Grains. Grains are found in cereal, bread, rice, and pasta. Grains are a great source of carbohydrates. The Food Guide Pyramid recommends six to eleven servings from this group each day. A serving is a single portion or helping of food or drink. Examples of one serving include one slice of bread, one cup of dry cereal, or 1/2 cup of cooked cereal, pasta, or rice. Complex carbohydrates take longer to break down. They provide longer-lasting energy than simple carbohydrates. Whole-grain foods, such as whole-wheat breads, bran cereals, brown rice, and whole-wheat pastas, have more complex carbohydrates than white breads, rice, pastas, and processed cereals. They also have more vitamins, protein, and energy.

Vegetables. Vegetables are excellent sources of vitamins and fiber. Choose from green leafy vegetables, including lettuce, spinach, and kale; tomatoes, green beans, peas, corn, cabbage, cauliflower, broccoli, and other vegetables. Vegetable sources of vitamin C include brussels sprouts, green or red peppers, and broccoli. The Food Guide Pyramid suggests three to five servings from the vegetable group each day. One serving consists of one cup of raw, leafy vegetables, 1/2 cup of other vegetables, cooked or chopped, or 3/4 cup of vegetable juice.

Fruits. Fruits are good sources of complex carbohydrates, vitamins, and fiber. Fruits are one of the best sources of vitamin C, which we should eat each day. Good sources of vitamin C include oranges and orange juice, grapefruit and grapefruit juice, strawberries, mango, papaya, and cantaloupe. The Food Guide Pyramid suggests two to four servings from the fruit group each day. One serving from this group could be one medium-sized apple, orange, or banana; 3/4 cup of fruit juice; or 1/2 cup of chopped, cooked, or canned fruit.

Dairy Products. Milk and milk products, such as cheese and yogurt, are good sources of calcium (Fig. 16-8). We need calcium for healthy bones and teeth. Milk products also have other minerals, protein, and vitamins. Other milk products are buttermilk, evaporated milk, and cottage cheese. Whole milk, cheese, and products made with whole milk have a lot of saturated fat. Most adults should eat low-fat or nonfat milk and milk products. Adults should have two to three servings from the dairy group each day. A serving of milk is one cup. Other serving sizes are one cup of yogurt, one-and-a-half ounces of natural cheese, or two ounces of processed cheese.

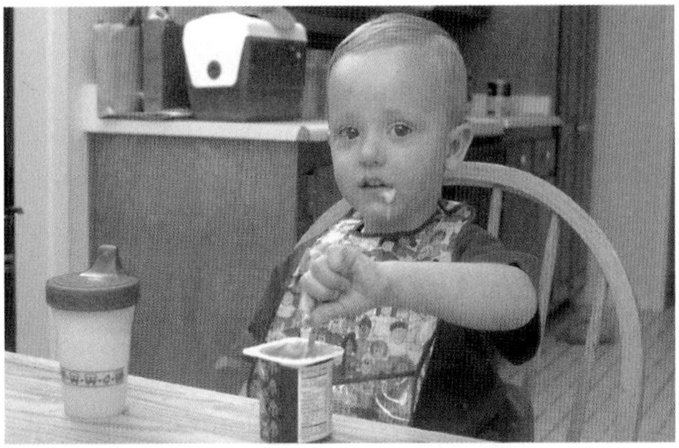

***Fig. 16-8*. Yogurt is a good source of calcium.**

Meat, Poultry, Fish, Dry Beans, Eggs, and Nuts. These foods have protein, minerals, and vitamins. Meat is a good source of iron. Lower-fat choices include most fish, chicken or turkey breast, lean cuts of meat, and dry beans. The Food Guide Pyramid suggests two to three servings from this group each day. One serving is two to three ounces of cooked lean meat, poultry or fish, one egg, 1/2 cup cooked dry beans, or 1/3 cup of nuts.

Fats, Oils, and Sweets. Fats and oils help the body absorb fat-soluble vitamins. They also add flavor and make us feel full. Fats are needed by the body in very small quantities.

Most adults eat more fat than they need. Fats have more than twice as many calories per gram as carbohydrates or proteins. The body stores excess fat as fatty tissue. The best fats to use in a healthy diet are vegetable oils. These include olive, canola, and corn oil (Fig. 16-9).

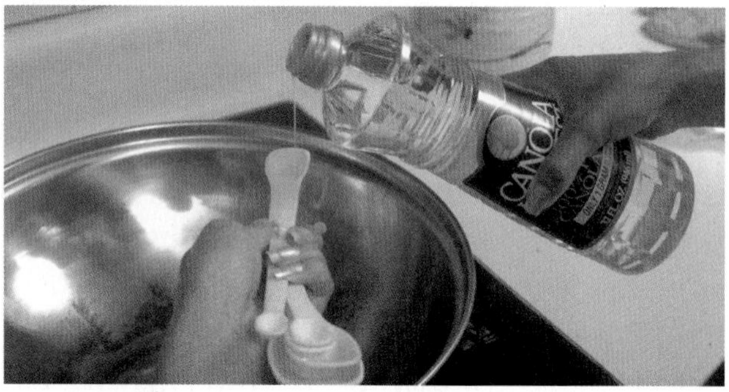

Fig. 16-9. **Olive, canola, and corn oils are the best kind of fats to use in food.**

Sweets, including candy, cookies, cakes, pies, and ice cream, have large amounts of fat and sugar. They should be eaten in much smaller amounts. Most sweets have no nutritional value. Eating too many sweets will cause weight gain. Some residents, particularly those with diabetes, must avoid sweets completely.

Some groups recommend a different Food Guide Pyramid for the elderly. It has a narrower base to reflect a decrease in energy needs. It emphasizes nutrient-dense foods, fiber, and water. Dietary supplements may be appropriate for many older people.

Due to slower metabolism and less activity, the elderly need to eat less to maintain body weight. Although calories can be reduced, daily needs for most vitamins and minerals do not decrease.

Scurvy: The Scourge of the Early Sea Traveler

Scurvy was a terrible problem for people who had to travel by sea for long periods of time. It caused bleeding gums, loose teeth, joint pain, weakness, and hemorrhages from mucous membranes. In 1747, James Lind identified a cure for the dreaded scurvy. He found that citrus juice, such as lime juice, could successfully treat the disease. Vitamin C, also known as ascorbic acid, was the cure.

4. Explain the role of the dietary department

The dietary department plans meals for all residents. Residents have different nutritional needs. When planning meals, the dietary department considers these needs and residents' likes and dislikes. Meals must be balanced and provide proper nutrition for all residents. Food has to be prepared in a way that each resident can manage. Food must also look good to residents. Infection control procedures must always be followed.

The dietary department also makes diet cards. **Diet cards** list the resident's name and information about special diets, allergies, likes and dislikes, and any other instructions.

5. Describe factors that influence food preferences

Culture, ethnicity, income, education, religion, and geography all affect ideas about nutrition. Food preferences may be formed by what you ate as a child, by what tastes good, or by your beliefs about what should be eaten (Fig. 16-10). Some people choose not to eat any animals or animal products, such as steak, chicken, butter, or eggs. These people are vegetarians or vegans.

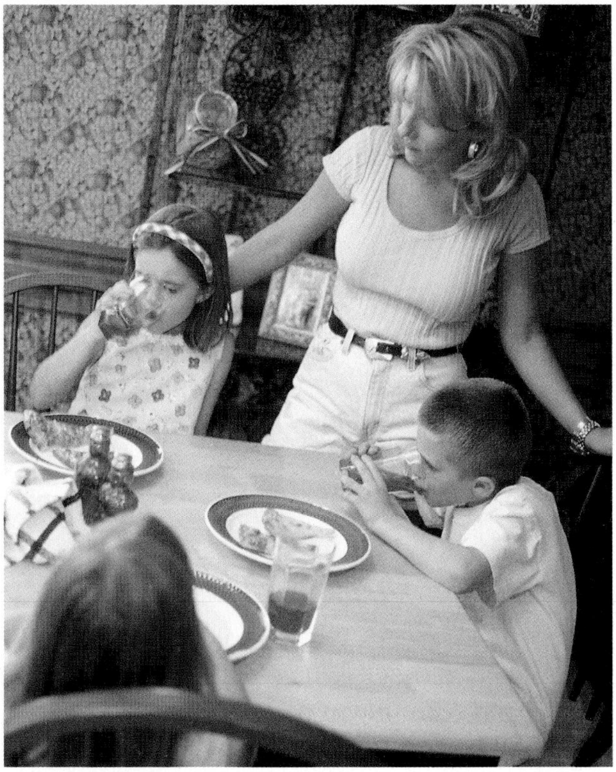

Fig. 16-10. **Food likes and dislikes are influenced by what you ate as a child.**

The region or culture you grow up in often affects your food preference. People from the southwestern US may like spicy foods. "Southern cooking" may include fried foods, like fried chicken or fried okra. Ethnic groups often share common foods. These may be eaten at certain times of the year or all the time. Religious beliefs affect diet, too. Some Muslims and Jewish people do not eat any pork. Some Mormons may not drink alcohol, tea, or coffee.

Food preferences may change while a resident is living at a facility. Just as you may decide that you like some foods for a time and then change your mind, so may residents. Whatever your residents' food preferences may be, respect them. Never make fun of a personal preference. If you notice that certain food is not being eaten—no matter how small the amount—tell the nurse.

STOP ***Food Choices***

Residents' Rights include the right to make choices. You must honor a resident's personal beliefs about specific foods.

6. List ways to identify and prevent dehydration

Most residents should be encouraged to drink at least eight glasses, or 64 ounces, of water or other fluids a day. Water is essential for life. Proper fluid intake is important. It helps prevent constipation and urinary incontinence. Without enough fluid, urine becomes concentrated. More concentrated urine creates a higher risk for infection. Proper fluid intake also helps to dilute wastes and flush out the urinary system. It may even help prevent confusion.

The sense of thirst can lessen as people age. Remind elderly residents to drink fluids often (Fig. 16-11). Some residents will have an order to force fluids (FF) or restrict fluids (RF) because of medical conditions. **Force fluids** means to encourage the resident to drink more fluids. **Restrict fluids** means the person is allowed to drink, but must limit the daily amount to a level set by the doctor. When a resident has a restrict fluids order, NAs cannot give the resident any extra fluids or a water pitcher unless the nurse approves it. Make sure you know which residents have these orders.

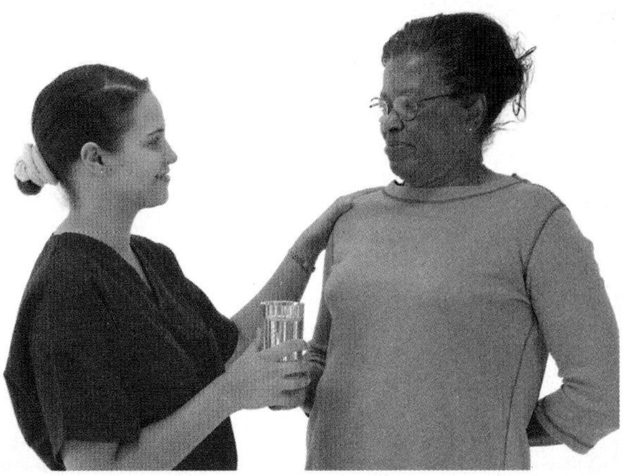

Fig. 16-11. **Encourage residents to drink every time you see them.**

Dehydration occurs when a person does not have enough fluid in the body. Dehydration is a major problem among the elderly, in and out of nursing homes. People can become dehydrated if they do not drink enough or if they have diarrhea or are vomiting. Preventing dehydration is very important. You play an important role.

OBSERVING AND REPORTING
Dehydration

Report any of these immediately:

- resident drinks less than six 8oz glasses of liquid per day
- resident drinks little or no fluids at meals
- resident needs help drinking from a cup or glass
- resident has trouble swallowing liquids
- resident has frequent vomiting, diarrhea, or fever
- resident is easily confused or tired

Report if resident has any of these symptoms:

- dry mouth
- cracked lips
- sunken eyes
- dark urine
- strong-smelling urine

GUIDELINES
Preventing Dehydration

- Report observations and warning signs to the nurse immediately.
- Encourage residents to drink every time you see them.
- Offer fresh water or other fluids often. Be aware that residents have different preferences. Some may like juice; others may want water or milk. Report if the resident tells you he does not like the fluids being served. Offer drinks that the resident enjoys. Some residents will prefer fluids without ice. Honor this.
- Record fluid intake and output.
- Ice chips, frozen flavored ice sticks, and gelatin are also liquids. Offer them often. Do not offer ice chips or sticks if a resident has a swallowing problem.
- If appropriate, offer sips of liquid between bites of food at meals and snacks.
- Make sure pitcher and cup are near enough and light enough for the resident to lift.
- Offer assistance if resident cannot drink without help. Use adaptive cups as needed. See chapter 21 for more information on assistive devices for eating and drinking.

STOP ***A request for a drink must be honored.***

When residents are thirsty, they may ask for water, juice, or some other beverage. Respond promptly to these requests. Ignoring a request for a drink is abuse. The only time you should not honor this request is when a resident is on a fluid restriction or "NPO." NPO stands for "Nothing by Mouth." In this situation, explain why a drink cannot be given. Report the request to the nurse.

Serving fresh water

Equipment: water pitcher, ice scoop, glass, straw, gloves

1. Wash your hands.
2. Identify yourself by name. Identify the resident by name.
3. Put on gloves.
4. Scoop ice into water pitcher. Add fresh water.
5. Use and store ice scoop properly:

   Do not allow ice to touch your hand and fall back into container.

   Place scoop in proper receptacle after each use.

6. Take pitcher to resident.
7. Pour glass of water for resident. Leave pitcher and glass at the bedside.
8. Make sure that pitcher and glass are light enough for resident to lift. Leave a straw if the resident desires.
9. Before leaving, place call light within resident's reach.
10. Remove gloves.
11. Wash your hands.

Handling ice and ice scoop

You must be very careful not to contaminate the ice as you scoop it. Never touch the ice and allow it to fall back into the container. Make sure the scoop is placed in the proper place after each use.

7. Explain intake and output (I&O) and list signs of fluid overload

To maintain health, the body must take in a certain amount of fluid each day. Fluid comes in the form of liquids you drink. It is also found in semi-liquid foods like gelatin, soup, ice cream, pudding, and yogurt. The fluid a person consumes is called **intake**, or **input**. When a person's intake is not in a healthy range, he or she can become dehydrated.

All fluid taken in each day cannot stay in the body. It must be eliminated as **output**. Output includes urine, feces, and vomitus. It also includes perspiration and moisture in the air we exhale. If a person's intake exceeds his or her output, fluid builds up in body tissues. This fluid retention can cause medical problems and discomfort.

Fluid balance is maintaining equal input and output, or taking in and eliminating equal amounts of fluid. Most people do this naturally. Some residents must have their intake and output, or I&O, watched and recorded.

You will need to measure and document all fluids the resident takes by mouth. You will also need to measure and record all urine and vomitus. This is recorded on an Intake/Output (I&O) sheet (Fig. 16-12).

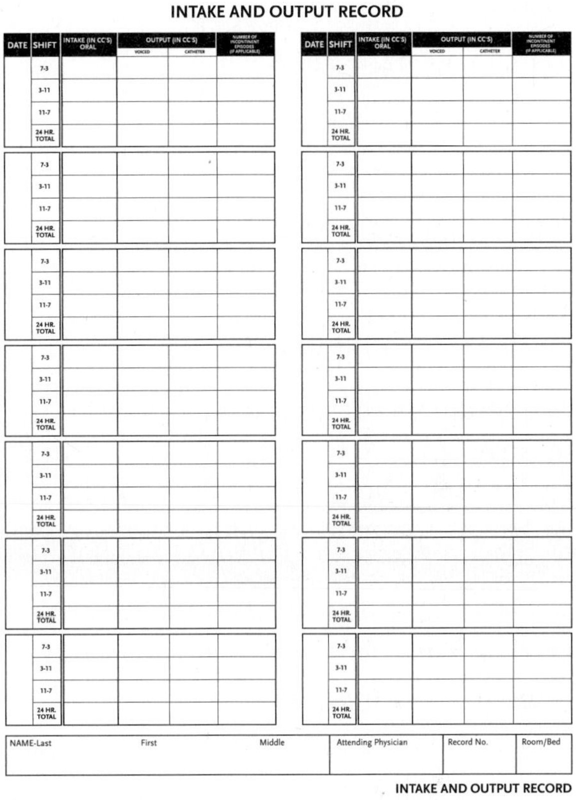
INTAKE AND OUTPUT RECORD

DATE	SHIFT	INTAKE (IN CC'S) ORAL	OUTPUT (IN CC'S) VOICED	OUTPUT (IN CC'S) CATHETER	NUMBER OF INCONTINENT EPISODES (IF APPLICABLE)	DATE	SHIFT	INTAKE (IN CC'S) ORAL	OUTPUT (IN CC'S) VOICED	OUTPUT (IN CC'S) CATHETER	NUMBER OF INCONTINENT EPISODES (IF APPLICABLE)
	7-3						7-3				
	3-11						3-11				
	11-7						11-7				
	24 HR. TOTAL						24 HR. TOTAL				
	7-3						7-3				
	3-11						3-11				
	11-7						11-7				
	24 HR. TOTAL						24 HR. TOTAL				
	7-3						7-3				
	3-11						3-11				
	11-7						11-7				
	24 HR. TOTAL						24 HR. TOTAL				
	7-3						7-3				
	3-11						3-11				
	11-7						11-7				
	24 HR. TOTAL						24 HR. TOTAL				
	7-3						7-3				
	3-11						3-11				
	11-7						11-7				
	24 HR. TOTAL						24 HR. TOTAL				
	7-3						7-3				
	3-11						3-11				
	11-7						11-7				
	24 HR. TOTAL						24 HR. TOTAL				
	7-3						7-3				
	3-11						3-11				
	11-7						11-7				
	24 HR. TOTAL						24 HR. TOTAL				

NAME-Last	First	Middle	Attending Physician	Record No.	Room/Bed

INTAKE AND OUTPUT RECORD

Fig. 16-12. **A sample intake and output form.**

Fluids are usually measured in cubic centimeters (cc). Ounces (oz) are converted to cc. To convert ounces to cubic centimeters, multiply by 30.

Conversions

A cubic centimeter (cc) is a unit of measure equal to one milliliter (ml). Follow your facility's policies on whether to document using "cc" or "ml."

1 oz. = 30 cc or 30 ml

2 oz. = 60 cc

3 oz. = 90 cc

4 oz. = 120 cc

5 oz. = 150 cc

6 oz. = 180 cc

7 oz. = 210 cc

8 oz. = 240 cc

1/4 cup = 2 oz. = 60 cc

1/2 cup = 4 oz. = 120 cc

1 cup = 8 oz. = 240 cc

Example: You serve Mrs. Wyant a glass of milk. You know the glass holds 6 oz. She finishes most but not all of the milk. You guess that she drank 4 oz. What was her input?

To convert ounces to cc, multiply 4 oz by 30. The answer is 120 cc. Document 120 cc milk on your input sheet.

Measuring and recording intake and output

Equipment: I&O sheet, graduate (measuring container), pen and paper to record your findings

1. Wash your hands.
2. Identify yourself by name. Identify the resident by name.
3. Explain procedure to the resident. Speak clearly, slowly, and directly. Maintain face-to-face contact whenever possible.
4. Provide for resident's privacy with curtain, screen, or door.
5. Using a graduate, measure how much fluid a resident is served (Fig. 16-13). Note the amount on paper.
6. When resident has finished a meal or snack, measure any leftover fluids. Note this amount on paper.
7. Subtract the leftover amount from the amount served. If you have measured in ounces, convert to cubic centimeters (cc) by multiplying by 30.
8. Record amount of fluid consumed (in cc) in input column on I&O sheet. Record the time and what fluid was taken.

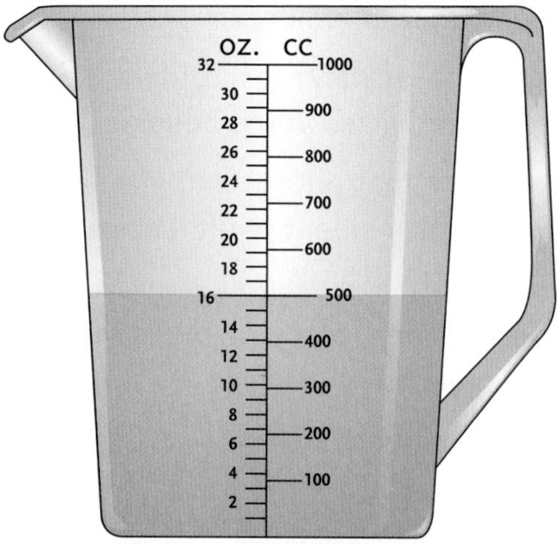

***Fig. 16-13*. A graduate is a measuring container.**

9. Wash your hands.

Measuring output is the other half of monitoring fluid balance.

Equipment: I&O sheet, graduate, gloves, pen and paper to record your findings

1. Wash your hands.
2. Put on gloves before handling bedpan/urinal.
3. Pour the contents of the bedpan or urinal into measuring container. Do not spill or splash any of the urine.
4. Measure the amount of urine. Keep container level.
5. After measuring urine, empty measuring container into toilet. Do not splash.
6. Rinse measuring container. Pour rinse water into toilet. Clean container using facility guidelines.
7. Rinse bedpan/urinal. Pour rinse water into toilet. Use approved disinfectant.
8. Return bedpan/urinal and measuring container to proper storage.
9. Remove and dispose of gloves.
10. Wash hands before recording output.
11. Record contents of container in output column on sheet.
12. Report any changes in resident to the nurse.

Fluid overload occurs when the body cannot handle the fluid consumed. This often affects people with heart or kidney disease.

OBSERVING AND REPORTING
Fluid Overload

- swelling/edema of extremities (ankles, feet, fingers, hands); **edema** is swelling caused by excess fluid in body tissues.
- weight gain (daily weight gain of one to two pounds)
- less urine output
- shortness of breath
- increased heart rate
- skin that appears tight, smooth, and shiny

8. List ways to identify and prevent unintended weight loss

Just like dehydration, unintended weight loss is a serious problem for the elderly. Weight loss can mean that the resident has a serious medical condition. It can lead to skin breakdown. This leads to pressure sores. It is very important to report any weight loss, no matter how small (Fig. 16-14). If a resident has diabetes, chronic obstructive pulmonary disease, cancer, HIV, or other diseases, he is at a greater risk for malnutrition. (See chapter 18 for more information on these diseases.)

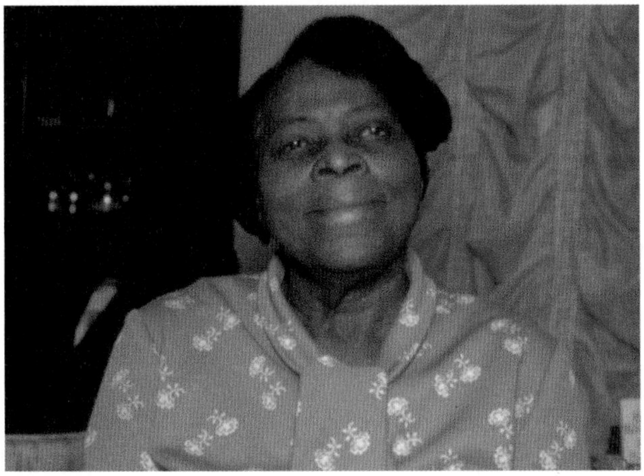

Fig. 16-14. **Observing your residents for weight loss is an important part of your job.**

OBSERVING AND REPORTING
Unintended Weight Loss

Report any of these to the nurse:

- if a resident needs help eating or drinking
- if a resident eats less than 70% of meals/snacks
- if resident has mouth pain
- if a resident has dentures that do not fit
- if resident has any difficulty chewing or swallowing
- if a resident coughs or chokes while eating
- if a resident is sad, has crying spells, or withdraws from others
- if a resident is confused, wanders, or paces

GUIDELINES
Preventing Unintended Weight Loss

- Report observations and warning signs to your supervisor.
- Encourage residents to eat. Talk about food served in a positive tone of voice and with positive words (Fig. 16-15).

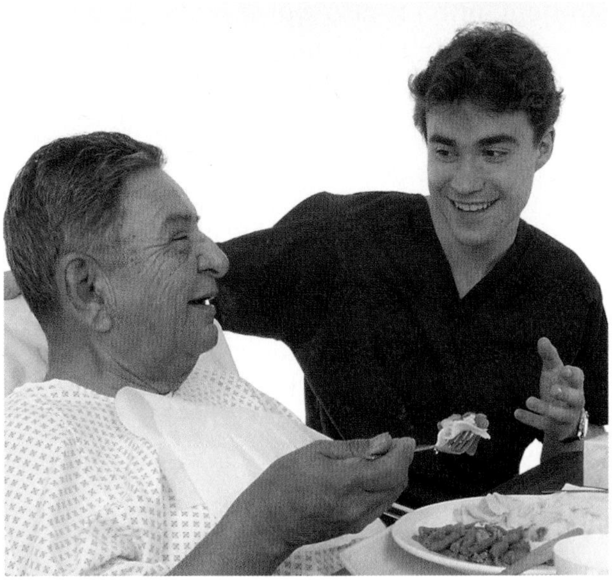

Fig. 16-15. **Be social, friendly, and positive while helping residents with eating. This helps promote appetite and prevent weight loss.**

- Honor residents' food likes and dislikes.
- Offer different kinds of foods and beverages.
- Help residents who have trouble feeding themselves.
- Food should look, taste, and smell good. The person may have a poor sense of taste and smell.
- Season foods to residents' preferences.
- Allow time for residents to finish eating.
- Tell the nurse if residents have trouble using utensils.
- Record the meal/snack intake.
- Give oral care before and after meals.
- Position residents sitting upright for feeding.
- If a resident has had a loss of appetite and/or seems sad, ask about it.

9. Describe how to make dining enjoyable for residents

Meals are an important part of a resident's day. Not only is it the time for getting proper nourishment, but it is also a time for socializing. Weight loss and dehydration are not the only problems residents have. Loneliness and boredom cause other kinds of suffering. You can help the whole person.

Encourage healthy eating. Do all that you can to promote a resident's appetite. Mealtime should be pleasant. Use these tips to help promote appetites and to make dining enjoyable:

GUIDELINES
Promoting Appetites

- Check the environment. The temperature should be comfortable. Address any odors. Keep noise level low. Television sets should be off. Do not shout or raise your voice. Do not bang plates or cups. Some facilities play quiet music while residents are dining (Fig. 16-16).
- Encourage the use of dentures, glasses, and hearing aids. If these are damaged, notify the nurse.

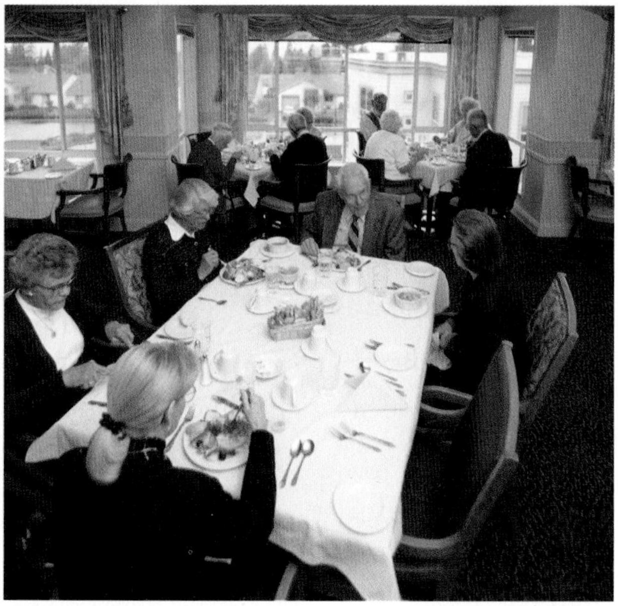

***Fig. 16-16.* A resident's environment is important in promoting appetite. Address odors. Keep noise level low.**

- Residents should be clean and well-groomed for dining.
- Offer a trip to the bathroom or help with toileting before eating.
- Help residents wash hands before eating.
- Give oral care before eating.
- Properly position residents for eating. Usually, the proper position is upright, at a 90-degree angle. This prevents swallowing problems. If residents use a wheelchair, make sure they are sitting at a table that is the right height. Most facilities have adjustable tables for wheelchairs. Residents who use "geri-chairs"—reclining chairs on wheels—should be upright, not reclined, while eating.
- If a resident has poor sitting balance, seat in a regular dining room chair with armrests, rather than in a wheelchair. Proper position in chair means hips at a 90-de-

gree angle, knees flexed, and feet and arms fully supported. Push chair under the table. Place forearms on the table.

- If a resident tends to lean to one side, ask him or her to keep elbows on the table.
- If a resident has poor neck control, a neck brace may be used to stabilize the head. Use assistive devices as needed. If resident is in a geri-chair, a wedge cushion behind the head and shoulders may be used.
- Seat residents next to their friends or people with like interests. Encourage conversation.
- Serve food at the correct temperature.
- Plates and trays should look appetizing.
- Give the resident proper eating tools. Use adaptive utensils if needed (Fig. 16-17).

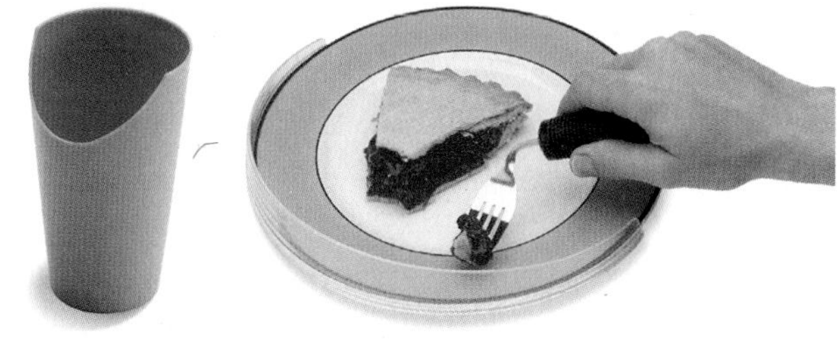

Fig. 16-17. **Sample assistive devices for eating. (Photos courtesy of North Coast Medical, Inc., 800-821-9319, www.ncmedical.com.)**

- Be cheerful, positive, and helpful. Make conversation if the resident wishes.
- Give more food when requested.

Residents' Rights and Eating

Residents have the right to refuse food and drink. Residents also have the right to ask for and receive different food.

10. Explain how to serve meal trays

Food will be served differently in different facilities. Food may be served on trays or carried from the kitchen. You must make sure that food is served at the right temperature. You will have to work quickly. You do not want to make a resident wait for his or her food. Serve all residents who are sitting at one table before serving another table. Residents will then be able to eat together and not have to watch others eat. Before you begin serving or helping residents, wash your hands.

Diet cards list the resident's name and other information. They include special dietary needs, allergies, food likes and dislikes, and any other instructions (Fig. 16-18). Some residents will be on special diet orders or have food allergies. It is very important to identify the resident before serving a meal tray. Feeding a resident the wrong food can cause serious problems, even death.

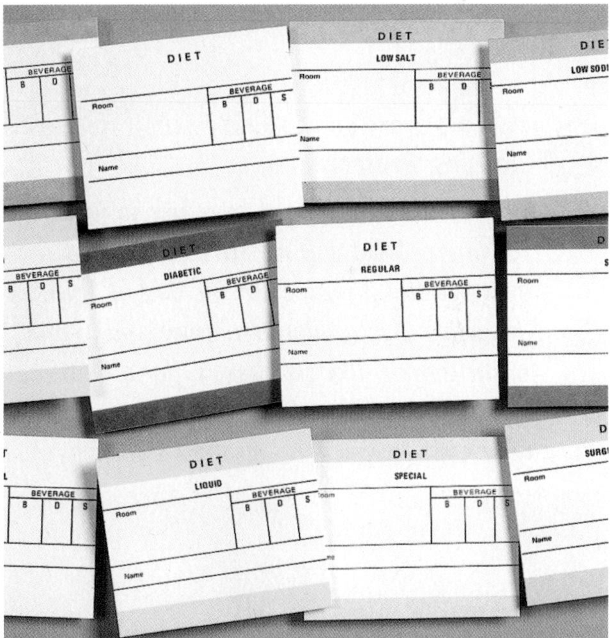

Fig. 16-18. **Sample diet cards. (Reprinted with permission of Briggs Corporation, Des Moines, IA, 800-247-2343.)**

Before helping a resident to eat, prepare the food. Follow these steps. Only do what the resident cannot do for himself.

- Remove the food and drink if it is on a tray. Set it out on the table.
- Cut food into small, bite-sized portions. Only cut meat and vegetables when

necessary. If you know residents need their food cut, cut it before bringing it to the table. This promotes dignity.

- Open milk or juice cartons. Put in straw if resident uses one. Open straws. Place them in the container using the paper wrapper. Do not touch straws directly with your fingers. Some residents may not be able to use straws due to swallowing problems. This should be noted on their diet cards, and no straws should be on the tray. Residents may want you to pour the beverage into a cup. Do so if the resident wishes.
- Butter roll, bread, and vegetables as the resident likes.
- Open any condiment packets. Offer to season food as resident likes, including pureed food.

Clothing Protectors

A resident has the right to refuse to wear a clothing protector (Fig. 16-19). Use the term "clothing protector" instead of "bib." This promotes residents' dignity and avoids treating them like children. Offer a clothing protector, but do not insist that a resident wear one. Respect the resident's wishes.

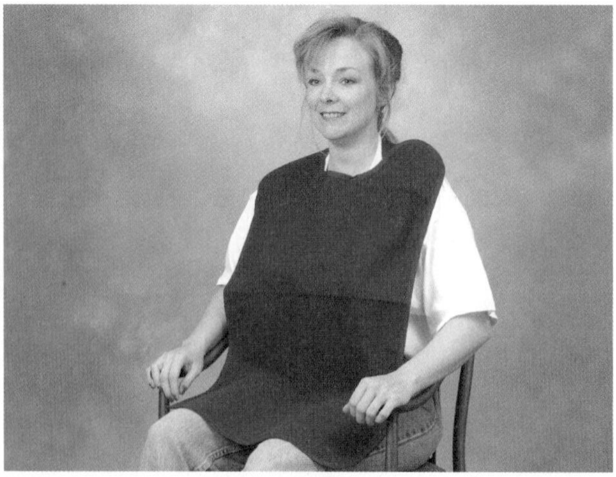

Fig. 16-19. **Residents have the right to choose whether to use a clothing protector. Respect each resident's decision. (Reprinted with permission of Briggs Corporation, Des Moines, IA, 800-247-2343.)**

11. Demonstrate how to assist a resident with eating and drinking

One duty you will have is helping residents with their meals. Residents will need different levels of help. Some residents will not need any help. Some residents will only need help setting up. They may need help opening cartons and cutting and seasoning their food. Once that is done, they can feed themselves. Check in with these residents from time to time to see if they need anything else.

Some residents will need some help. Residents who have had a stroke, who have Parkinson's disease, Alzheimer's disease or other dementias, who have had head trauma, or who are confused or blind may benefit from physical and verbal cues. You will learn more about these diseases in chapters 18 and 19. The hand-over-hand approach is an example of physical cuing. If a resident can help lift the utensils, put your hand over his to help with eating. After the spoon is in the resident's hand, place your hand over the resident's hand. Help the resident in getting some food on the spoon. Steer the spoon from the food to the mouth and back. This promotes independence (Fig. 16-20).

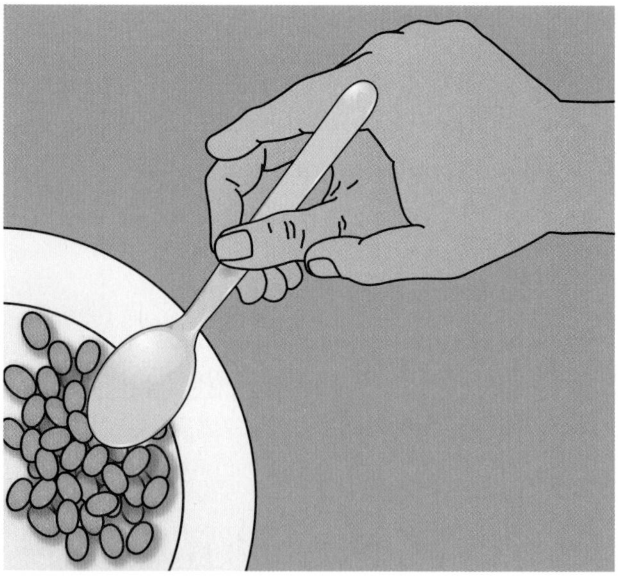

Fig. 16-20. **The hand-over-hand approach is used when a resident can help by lifting utensils.**

Verbal cues must be short and clear. They prompt the resident to do something. Give verbal cues one at a time. Wait until the resident has finished one task before asking him or her to do another. Examples of good verbal cues include:

- "Pick up your spoon."
- "Put some carrots on your spoon."
- "Raise the spoon to your lips."
- "Open your mouth."
- "Place the spoon in your mouth."
- "Close your mouth."
- "Take the spoon out of your mouth."
- "Chew."
- "Swallow."
- "Drink some water."

Other residents will be completely unable to feed themselves. It will be your job to feed them. Residents who must be fed are often embarrassed and depressed about their dependence on another person. Be sensitive to this. Give privacy while the resident is eating. Do not rush him or her.

Encourage residents to do what they can. For example, if a resident can hold and use a napkin, she should. If she can hold and eat finger foods, offer them. There are devices that help residents eat (see Figure 16-17). Cups with lids to avoid spills and utensils with thick handles that are easier to hold are two examples. More adaptive devices are shown in chapter 21.

Here are some other resident behaviors you may encounter while helping with eating:

- **The resident bites down on utensils**. Ask the resident to open his or her mouth. Do not pull the utensil out of the mouth. Wait until the jaw relaxes.
- **The resident pockets food in cheeks**. Ask the resident to chew and swallow the food. Touch the side of the cheek. Ask the resident to use his or her tongue to get the food. Using your fingers on the cheek (near the lower jaw), gently push food toward teeth.
- **The resident holds food in the mouth**. Ask the resident to chew and swallow the food. You may need to trigger swallowing. To do this, gently press down on the tongue when taking the spoon out of the mouth. You can also try to gently press down on the top of his or her head with your hand. Make sure the resident has swallowed the food before offering more.

Mealtime involves more than eating. It is a chance for social interaction. Residents look forward to their interaction with you and with others. It may be the highlight of their day.

To avoid weight loss and dehydration, you must do all that you can to increase food and drink intake. Cheerful company and conversation can greatly increase how much a resident eats and drinks. They also have a positive effect on residents' attitudes. Fewer digestive problems may occur.

The reverse is also true. Negative attitudes and poor communication can decrease how much a resident consumes. Do not make negative comments, such as, "I don't know how you can eat this" or, "This looks awful." Do not judge a resident's food preferences.

When helping a resident, use these tips for positive mealtimes:

- Pay attention to the person you are helping. Do not talk to other staff members while helping residents eat.
- Be polite and friendly.
- Make conversation if the resident wishes. Use appropriate topics, such as the news, weather, the resident's life, things the resident enjoys, and food preferences.
- Say positive things about the food being served, such as "This smells really good," and "The [type of food] looks so fresh."

Social conversation may help raise a resident's self-esteem. It helps prevent loneliness. Your good attitude and attention go a long way in promoting good nutrition for your residents.

GUIDELINES
Assisting a Resident with Eating

- Never treat the resident like a child. This is embarrassing and disrespectful. It is hard for many people to accept help with feeding. Be supportive and encouraging.
- Sit at a resident's eye level. Make eye contact.
- If the resident wishes, allow time for prayer.
- Verify that you have the right resident. Check the diet card against the resident's ID bracelet (Fig. 16-21). Also, check that the diet on the tray is correct.

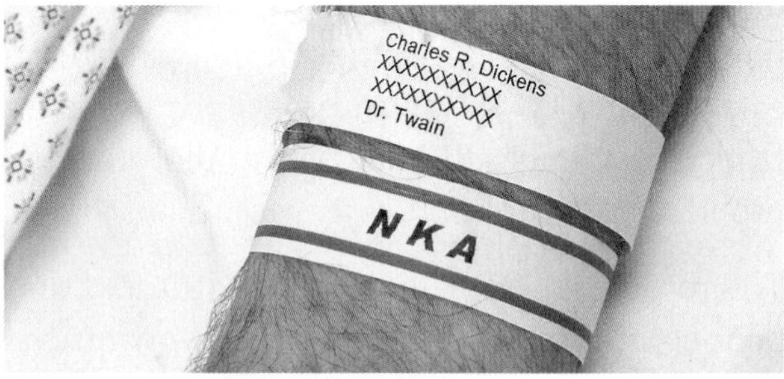

Fig. 16-21. Identify residents before serving meal trays or food.

- Do not touch food to test its temperature. Put your hand over the dish to sense the heat of food. If you think food is too hot, do not blow on it to cool it. Offer other food to give it time to cool. Remove dishes from metal hot plates.
- Cut foods and pour liquids as needed.
- Identify the foods and fluids that are in front of the resident. Call pureed foods by the correct name. For example, ask, "Would you like green beans?" rather than referring to it as "some green stuff."
- Ask the resident what he wants to eat first. Allow him to make the choice, even if he wants dessert first.
- Do not mix foods unless the resident prefers it.
- Do not rush the meal. Allow time for the resident to chew and swallow each bite. Be relaxed.
- Make conversation. Use appropriate topics as listed earlier. Be positive.
- Give the resident your full attention.
- Alternate food and drink. Alternating cold and hot foods or bland foods and sweets can help increase appetite.
- If the resident wants a different food from what is being served, honor this request. Tell the dietitian so that an alternative may be offered.

Feeding a resident who cannot feed self

Equipment: meal tray, clothing protector, 1-2 washcloths

1. Wash your hands.
2. Identify yourself by name. Identify the resident by name.
3. Explain procedure to the resident. Speak clearly, slowly, and directly. Maintain face-to-face contact whenever possible.
4. Help resident to wash hands if resident cannot do it on her own.
5. Adjust bed height to where you will be to able to sit at resident's eye level. Lock bed wheels.
6. Raise the head of the bed. Make sure resident is in an upright sitting position (at a 90 degree angle).
7. Pick up diet card. Verify that resident has received the right tray.
8. Help resident to put on clothing protector, if desired.
9. Sit at resident's eye level (Fig. 16-22). Sit on the stronger side if the resident has one-sided weakness.

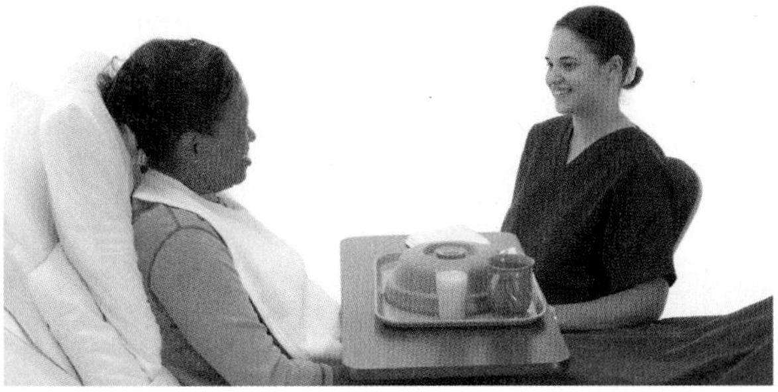

Fig. 16-22.

10. Offer drink of beverage. Alternate types of food, allowing for resident's preferences. (Do not feed all of one type before offering another type.)
11. Offer the food in bite-sized pieces. Report any swallowing problems to the nurse immediately (Fig. 16-23).

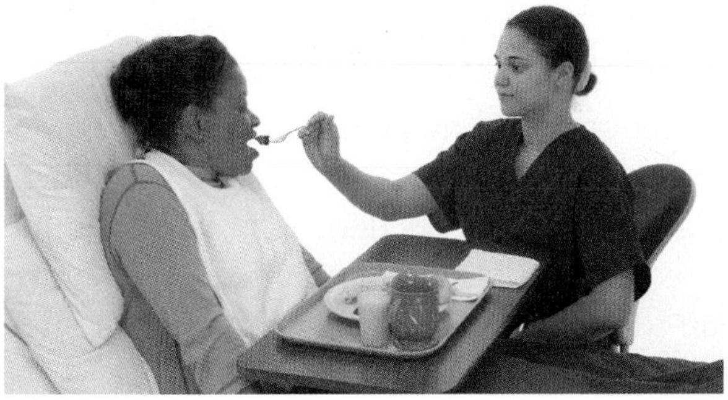

Fig. 16-23.

12. Make sure resident's mouth is empty before next bite or sip.
13. Offer beverage to resident throughout the meal.
14. Talk with resident during meal.
15. Use washcloths to wipe food from resident's mouth and hands as needed during the meal. Wipe again at the end of the meal (Fig. 16-24).

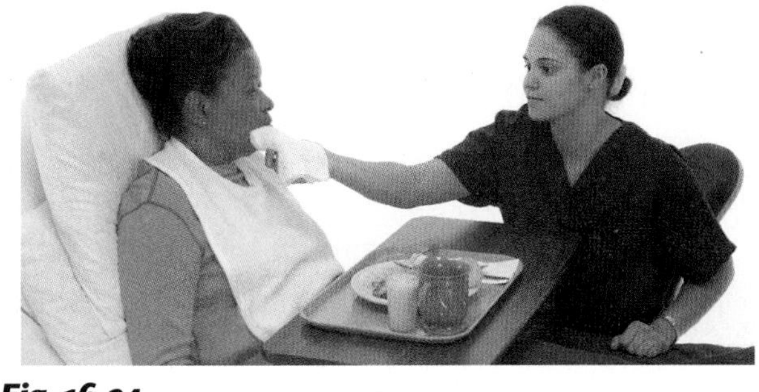

Fig. 16-24.

16. Remove clothing protector if used. Dispose of in proper container.
17. Remove food tray. Check for eyeglasses, dentures, or any personal items before removing tray.
18. Make resident comfortable. Make sure sheets are free from wrinkles and the bed free from crumbs.
19. Return bed to appropriate position. Remove privacy measures.
20. Before leaving, place call light within resident's reach.
21. Wash your hands.
22. Report any changes in resident to the nurse.
23. Document procedure using facility guidelines.

Helping with Eating

You must offer fluid to the resident throughout the meal. You must raise the head of the bed to help prevent aspiration.

12. Define "dysphagia" and identify signs and symptoms of swallowing problems

Dysphagia means difficulty in swallowing. You need to be able to recognize and report signs that a resident has a swallowing problem. Signs and symptoms of swallowing problems include:

- coughing during or after meals
- choking during meals
- dribbling saliva, food, or fluid from the mouth
- food residue inside the mouth or cheeks during and after meals
- gurgling sound in voice during or after meals or loss of voice
- slow eating

- avoidance of eating
- spitting out pieces of food
- several swallows needed per mouthful
- frequent throat clearing during and after meals
- watering eyes when eating or drinking
- food or fluid coming up into the nose
- visible effort to swallow
- shorter or more rapid breathing while eating or drinking
- difficulty chewing food
- difficulty swallowing medications

If you notice any signs of swallowing problems, notify the nurse immediately.

13. Explain special diets

A doctor sometimes places residents who are ill on special diets (Fig. 16-25). These diets are known as **therapeutic**, **modified**, or **special diets**. After a doctor prescribes a special diet, the dietitian plans the diet. Some nutrients or fluids may be restricted or eliminated. Some medications may interact with certain foods. These must be restricted. Doctors may order supplementary diets for residents who do not eat enough. Diets are also used for weight control and food allergies. Examples of therapeutic diets are listed below:

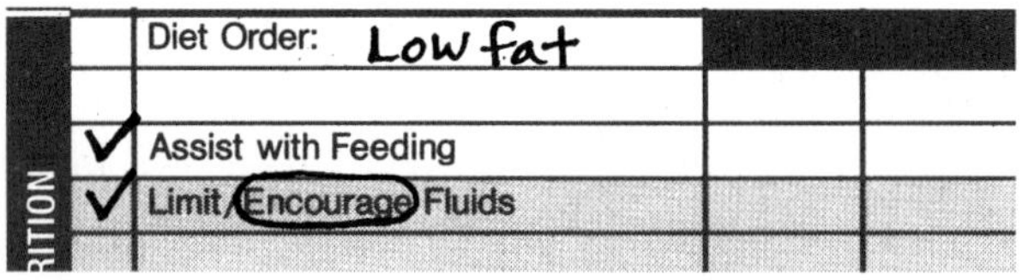

Fig. 16-25. **The care plan specifies special diets or dietary restrictions.**

Low-Sodium Diet. Residents with heart disease, kidney disease, or fluid retention may be placed on a low-sodium diet. Many foods have sodium, but people are most familiar with it as an ingredient in table salt. Salt is the first food to be restricted in a low-sodium diet because it is high in sodium. For residents on a low-sodium diet, salt will not be used. Salt shakers or packets will not be on the diet tray. Common abbreviations for this diet found on diet cards are "Low Na," which means low sodium or "NAS," which stands for "No Added Salt."

Fluid-Restricted Diets. The fluid taken through food and fluids must equal the fluid that leaves the body through perspiration, stool, urine, and expiration. This is fluid balance. When fluid intake is greater than fluid output, body tissues become swollen with fluid. People with severe heart disease and kidney disease may have trouble processing fluid. To prevent further damage, doctors may restrict fluid intake. For residents on fluid restriction, you will need to measure and document exact amounts of fluid intake and report excesses to the nurse.

Do not offer additional fluids or foods that count as fluids, such as ice cream, puddings, gelatin, etc. If the resident complains of thirst or requests fluids, tell the nurse. The abbreviation for this diet is "RF." This stands for "Restrict Fluids."

Low-Protein Diet. People who have kidney disease may be on low-protein diets. Protein is restricted because it breaks down into compounds that may further damage the kidneys. The extent of the restrictions depends on the stage of the disease and if the resident is on dialysis.

Low-Fat/Low-Cholesterol Diet. People who have high levels of cholesterol are at risk for heart attacks and heart disease. People with gallbladder disease, diseases that interfere with fat digestion, and liver disease are also placed on low-fat/low-cholesterol diets.

Low-fat/low-cholesterol diets permit skim milk, low-fat cottage cheese, fish, white meat of turkey and chicken, veal, and vegetable fats (especially monounsaturated fats such as olive, canola, and peanut oils) (Fig. 16-26).

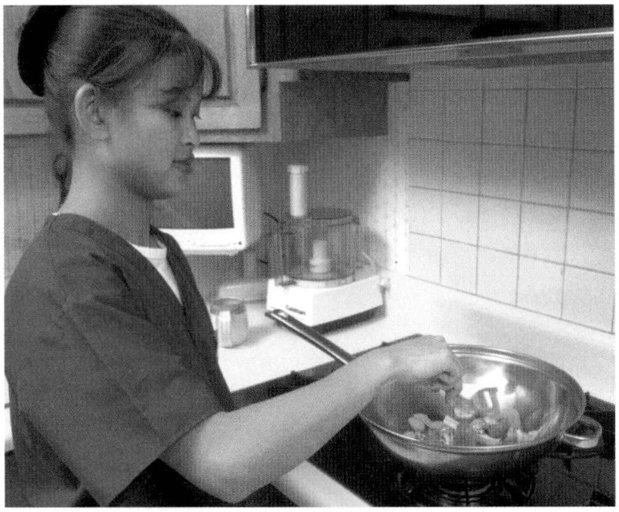

Fig. 16-26. **Vegetables are an important part of a low-fat/low-cholesterol diet.**

People who have gallbladder disease or other digestive problems may be placed on a diet that restricts all fats. A common abbreviation for this diet is "Low-Fat/Low-Chol."

Modified Calorie Diet for Weight Management. Some residents may need to reduce calories to lose weight or prevent weight gain. Other residents may need to increase calories because of malnutrition, surgery, illness, or fever. A common abbreviation for this diet is "Low-Cal" or "High-Cal."

Dietary Management of Diabetes. People with diabetes must be very careful about what they eat (Fig. 16-27). Calories and carbohydrates are carefully controlled in the diets of diabetic residents. Protein and fats are also regulated. The foods and the amounts are determined by nutritional and energy needs. See chapter 21 for more information on diabetes.

A dietitian and the resident will make up a meal plan. It will include all the right types and amounts of food for each day. The resident uses exchange lists, or lists of similar foods that can substitute for one another, to make up a menu. Using meal plans and exchange lists, a person with diabetes can control his diet while still making food choices. See the following list.

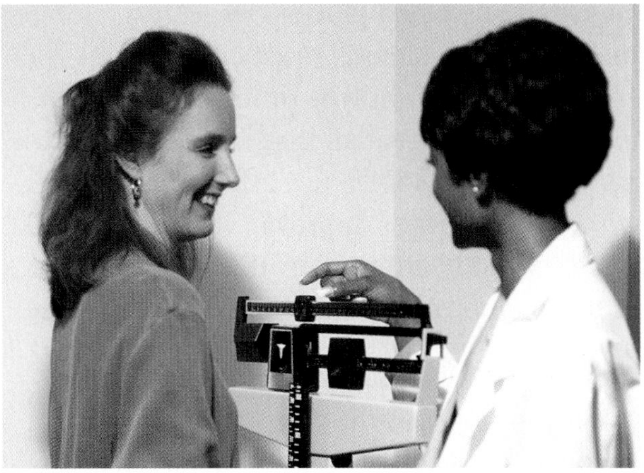

Fig. 16-27. **Diabetics must be very careful about what they eat. They should also keep their weight in a healthy range. Dietitians will help diabetics manage their illness.**

Sample Exchange List

Following the meal plan, the person chooses specific foods and determines serving sizes using the exchange lists.

Exchange List Sample Items

Starch list: 1 slice of bread, ½ bagel, ½ cup cereal, ½ cup pasta, ½ cup rice, 1 baked potato, 3 cups popcorn, 15-20 fat-free potato chips

Milk list: 1 cup milk (skim, 1%, 2%, or whole, depending on other dietary guidelines), ¾ cup yogurt

Fruit list: ½ cup unsweetened applesauce, 1 small banana, ½ cup orange juice, 2 tablespoons raisins, 1 small orange, ½ cup canned pears

Vegetable list: ½ cup cooked vegetables or vegetable juice, 1 cup raw vegetables (not included are corn, potatoes, and peas, which are on the starch exchange list instead)

Meat list: 1 oz. meat, fish, poultry, or cheese, 1 egg, or ½ cup dried beans

Fat list: 1 tsp margarine or butter, 2 tsp peanut butter, 2 tbsp sour cream, 1 tsp mayonnaise, 10 peanuts

To keep their blood glucose levels near normal, diabetic residents must eat the right amount of the right type of food at the right time. They must eat all that is served. Encourage them to do so. Do not offer other foods without the nurse's approval. If a resident will not eat what is directed, or if you think that he or she is not following the diet, tell the nurse.

A diabetic's meal tray may have artificial sweetener, low-calorie jelly, and maple syrup. When serving coffee or tea to a diabetic resident, use artificial sweeteners rather than sugar. The common abbreviations for this diet on a diet card are "NCS," which stands for "No Concentrated Sweets" or the amount of calories followed by the abbreviation "ADA," which stands for American Diabetic Association.

Diets may also be modified in consistency:

Liquid Diets. A liquid diet is made up of foods that are liquid at body temperature. Liquid diets are usually ordered as "clear" or "full." A clear liquid diet includes clear juices, broth, gelatin, and popsicles. A full liquid diet includes clear liquids with the addition of cream soups, milk, and ice cream. A liquid diet is usually ordered for a short time. It may be ordered due to a medical condition or before or after a test or surgery.

Soft Diet. The soft diet is soft in texture. It consists of soft or chopped foods that are easier to chew and swallow. Doctors order this diet for residents who have chewing and swallowing problems due to dental problems or other medical conditions.

Pureed Diet. To **puree** a food means to chop, blend, or grind it into a thick paste of baby food consistency. The food should be thick enough to hold its form in the mouth. This diet does not need to be chewed. A pureed diet is often used for people who have trouble chewing and/or swallowing more textured foods.

The abbreviation "**NPO**" stands for "Nothing by Mouth." This means that a resident is not allowed to have anything to eat or drink. Some residents have such a severe problem with swallowing that it is unsafe to give them anything by mouth. These types of residents will receive nutrition through a feeding tube or intravenously.

Some residents may be NPO for a short time before a medical test or surgery. You need to know this abbreviation. Never offer any food or drink to a resident with this order.

Some special diets are based on a person's religious, moral, or other beliefs:

- Many Jewish people eat kosher foods. They do not eat pork or shellfish, and do not eat meat products at the same meal with dairy products. **Kosher** food is food prepared according to Jewish dietary laws.
- Many Muslims do not eat pork or shellfish. They may not drink alcohol. Muslims may have regular periods of fasting. Fasting means not eating food or eating very little food.
- Some Catholics do not eat meat on Fridays.
- Some people are vegetarians. **Vegetarians** do not eat meat, fish, and poultry. They may or may not eat eggs and dairy products. **Vegans** are vegetarians who do not eat or use any animal products, including milk, cheese, other dairy items, eggs, wool, silk, and leather. Reasons for being a vegetarian include:
  - health
  - religious issues
  - dislike of meat
  - compassion for animals
  - belief in non-violence
  - financial issues

Honor your residents' dietary restrictions. Respect their wishes. Do not make judgments about what a person does or does not eat. Do not change food from one resident's tray to another. Report requests for diet substitutions to the nurse.

Ask before you pass.

Ask nurses before you pass meal trays to residents on a unit. Always find out any special diet orders and names of residents who are NPO.

14. Explain thickened liquids and identify three basic thickened consistencies

Residents with dysphagia or swallowing problems may be restricted to consuming only thickened liquids.

Thickening improves the ability to control fluid in the mouth and throat. A doctor orders the necessary thickness after the resident has been evaluated by a speech therapist.

Special products are used for thickening. Some beverages arrive already thickened from the dietary department. In other facilities, the thickening agent is added on the nursing unit before serving. If thickening is ordered, it must be used with all liquids. You need to know what thickened liquids mean. Do not offer these residents regular liquids. Never offer a water pitcher to a resident who must have thickened liquids. Follow the directions for each resident as ordered.

Three basic thickened consistencies are:

1. **Nectar Thick**: This consistency is thicker than water. It is the thickness of a thick juice, such as a pear nectar or tomato juice. A resident can drink this from a cup.
2. **Honey Thick**: This consistency has the thickness of honey. It will pour very slowly. A resident will usually use a spoon to consume it.
3. **Pudding Thick**: With this consistency, the liquids have become semi-solid, much like pudding. A spoon should stand up straight in the glass when put into the middle of the drink. A resident must consume these liquids with a spoon.

15. Understand the importance of observing and reporting a resident's diet

You have learned that it is important to always identify residents before placing meal trays or helping with feeding. Not doing so can cause serious problems. Before you deliver trays or plates, check them closely. Make sure that you have the correct resident and the correct food and beverages for that person. Trays and plates should also be closely checked for added sugar and salt packets (Fig. 16-28).

Be aware of residents who are diabetic or have heart conditions. They will be on special diets. Their families may not know or understand about food restrictions. Family often bring treats into the facility for their loved ones. Watch for foods in residents' rooms or in the dining room that are not permitted by their doctors. Report any problems to the nurse.

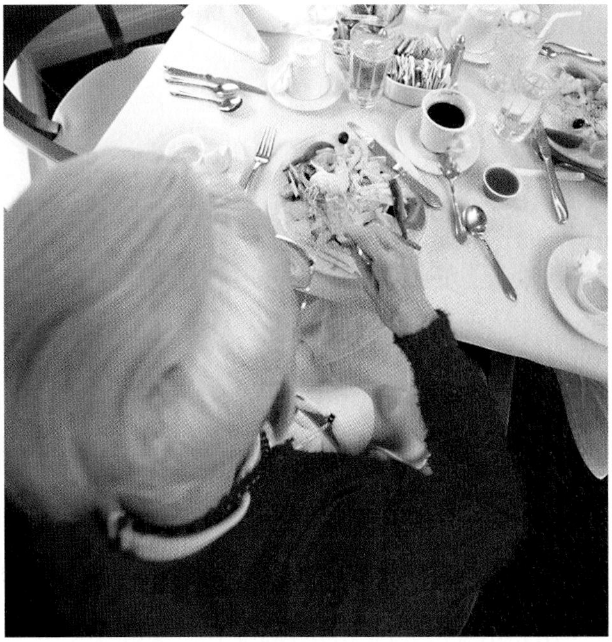

Fig. 16-28. **Observe residents' plates for any restricted food.**

Food trays and plates should also be observed after the meal. It is important to observe what and how much the resident is eating. This helps to identify residents with poor appetites. It may also signal illness, a problem, such as dentures that do not fit properly, or a change in food preferences.

All facilities keep track of how much food and liquid a resident consumes. The method varies. Some facilities use a percentage method. Below is one example of a percentage method:

"R"Refused = 0% No food eaten

"P" Poor = 25% Very little food eaten

"F" Fair = 50% Half of the food eaten

"G"Good = 75% Most of the food is eaten

"A" All = 100% Entire meal is eaten

Other facilities may document the percentage of specific foods eaten—protein, carbohydrates, fats, etc. Your instructor will explain your facility's documentation. Follow your facility's policy. Document food intake very carefully. Accuracy is important. Report to the charge nurse if a resident eats less than 70% of his or her meal.

16. Describe how to assist residents with special needs

Many devices can help people who are recovering from or adapting to a physical condition to feed themselves. These devices are called adaptive equipment or assistive devices. These include special plates, cups, and utensils. Examples are shown in Figure 16-17.

In addition to the cues you learned about earlier, residents may use other special dining techniques.

For visually-impaired residents, use the face of an imaginary clock to explain the position of what is in front of them (Fig. 16-29).

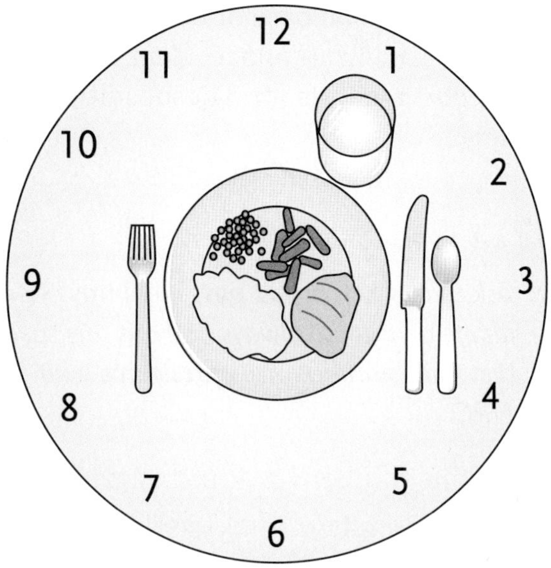

Fig. 16-29. **Use the face of an imaginary clock to explain the position of food to residents.**

For residents who have had a stroke:

- Place food in the resident's field of vision (Fig. 16-30). A resident may have "blind spots." The nurse will determine a resident's field of vision.

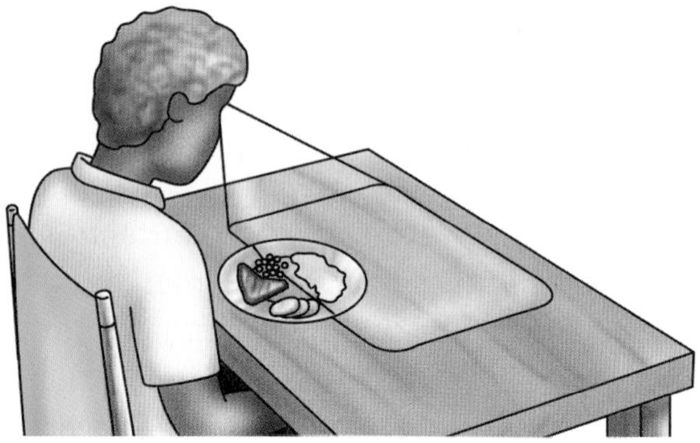

Fig. 16-30. **A resident who has had a stroke may have a limited field of vision. Make sure the resident can see what you place in front of him.**

- Use assistive devices such as utensils with built-up handle grips, plate guards, and drinking cups. These are ordered for specific residents. They should already be on the tray.
- Watch for signs of choking.
- Always place food in the unaffected, or non-paralyzed, side of the mouth.
- Make sure the resident swallows the food before offering more bites.

Another resident who may have special needs is a resident with Parkinson's disease. **Parkinson's disease** is a progressive disease. It causes the brain to degenerate. **Progressive** and **degenerative** mean the disease gets worse. It causes greater and greater loss of health and abilities. Parkinson's affects the muscles, causing them to become stiff. It causes stooped posture and a shuffling **gait**, or walk. Tremors or shaking make it very difficult for a person to eat. For residents who have Parkinson's disease:

- Help them as needed if tremors make it hard for them to eat.
- Place food and drinks close so that the resident can easily reach them.
- Use assistive devices. These promote independence.

Chapter Review

1. How does a well-balanced diet help the ill and the elderly?
2. List four physical changes due to aging that may affect nutrition.
3. How should residents be positioned when eating to prevent aspiration?
4. List three conditions that make eating or swallowing difficult.
5. List the six basic nutrients. Which nutrient is most essential for life?
6. According to the Food Guide Pyramid, Figure 16-7, which foods should be eaten least?
7. What does the dietary department consider when planning meals?
8. List three factors that influence food preferences.
9. How many ounces of water should a healthy resident be encouraged to drink every day?
10. List six ways to prevent dehydration.
11. What is fluid balance?
12. How many cubic centimeters (cc) equal one ounce?
13. List four symptoms of fluid overload.
14. List seven guidelines to prevent unintended weight loss.
15. List eight guidelines to promote appetites.
16. What information do diet cards contain?
17. What is important to do before you serve a resident a meal tray?
18. Should you insist that a resident wear a clothing protector if he does not want to?
19. In addition to eating, what does mealtime involve?
20. If you are cheerful and positive while a resident eats, how can that affect the amount a resident consumes?
21. How should you sense the heat of food properly?
22. If a resident requests a different food from what is being served, what should you do?
23. Look at the guidelines for helping a resident with eating. List four that help promote residents' dignity.
24. What is the first food to be restricted in a low-sodium diet?
25. What does the abbreviation "NPO" stand for?
26. Why might a resident be placed on a low-fat/low-cholesterol diet?
27. When might a liquid diet be ordered for a resident?
28. List four reasons that a person may become a vegetarian.

29. Which type of resident may have an order for thickened liquids?

30. Why is it important for staff to observe what and how much the resident is eating?

31. How can you explain the position of food and drink to visually-impaired residents?

32. List three ways you can help a resident who has had a stroke with eating.

Chapter 17
Basic Nursing Skills

1. Explain the importance of monitoring vital signs

You will monitor, document, and report your residents' vital signs. **Vital signs** are important. They show how well the vital organs of the body, such as the heart and lungs, are working. They consist of:

- taking the temperature
- counting the pulse
- counting the rate of respirations
- taking the blood pressure
- observing and reporting the level of pain

Watching for changes in vital signs is very important. Changes can indicate a resident's condition is worsening. You should always notify the nurse if:

- the resident has a fever (temperature is above average for the resident or outside the normal range)
- the resident has a respiratory or pulse rate that is too rapid or too slow
- the resident's blood pressure changes
- the resident's pain is worse or is not relieved by pain management

Normal Ranges for Adult Vital Signs

Temperature	**Fahrenheit**	**Celsius**
Oral	97.6° - 99.6°	36.5° - 37.5°
Rectal	98.6° - 100.6°	37.0° - 38.1°
Axillary	96.6° - 98.6°	36.0° - 37.0°

Pulse: 60 - 90 beats per minute

Respirations: 12 - 20 respirations per minute

Blood Pressure

Normal:

Systolic 100 - 119

Diastolic 60 - 79

Prehypertension:

Systolic 120 - 139

Diastolic 80 - 89

High:

140/90 or above *

** Millions of people whose blood pressure was considered normal (120/80) now fall into the "prehypertension" range. Prehypertension means that the person does not have high blood pressure now but is likely to have it in the future. This is based on the new, more aggressive high blood pressure guidelines from* *the Seventh Report of the Joint National Committee (JNC 7) on Prevention, Detection, Evaluation, and Treatment of High Blood Pressure (2003).*

2. List guidelines for taking body temperature

Body temperature is normally very close to 98.6°F (Fahrenheit) or 37°C (Celsius). Body temperature is a balance between the heat created by our bodies and the heat lost to the environment. Many factors affect temperature. Age, illness, stress, environment, exercise, and the circadian rhythm can all cause changes in body temperature.

The **circadian rhythm** is the 24-hour day-night cycle. Average temperature readings change throughout the day. People tend to have lower temperatures in the morning.

Increases in body temperature may indicate an infection or disease. There are four sites for taking body temperature:

1. the mouth (oral)
2. the rectum (rectal)
3. the armpit (axillary)
4. the ear (tympanic)

The different sites require different thermometers. Temperatures are most often taken orally. Do not take an oral temperature on a person who:

- is unconscious
- is using oxygen
- is confused or disoriented
- is paralyzed from stroke
- has facial trauma
- is likely to have a seizure
- has a nasogastric tube (chapter 16)
- is younger than six years old
- has sores, redness, swelling, or pain in her mouth
- has an injury to the face or neck

A rectal temperature is the most accurate. However, taking a rectal temperature on an uncooperative person can be dangerous. An axillary temperature is the least accurate.

Using glass bulb or mercury thermometers to take oral or rectal temperatures used to be common (Fig. 17-1). Because mercury is dangerous, many healthcare facilities now discourage the use of mercury. Many states have passed laws to ban the sale of mercury thermometers.

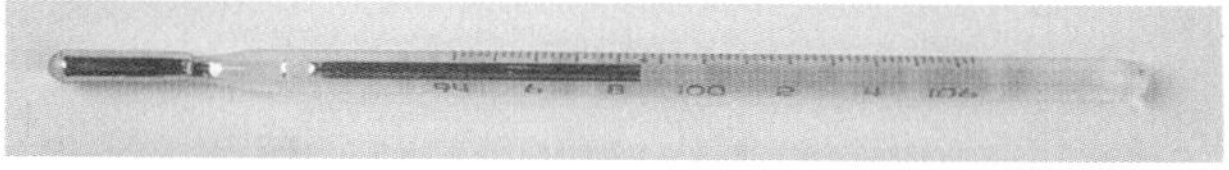

Fig. 17-1. **A mercury glass thermometer.**

Mercury-free thermometers are becoming more common (Fig. 17-2). They can be used to take an oral or rectal temperature. They are considered much safer.

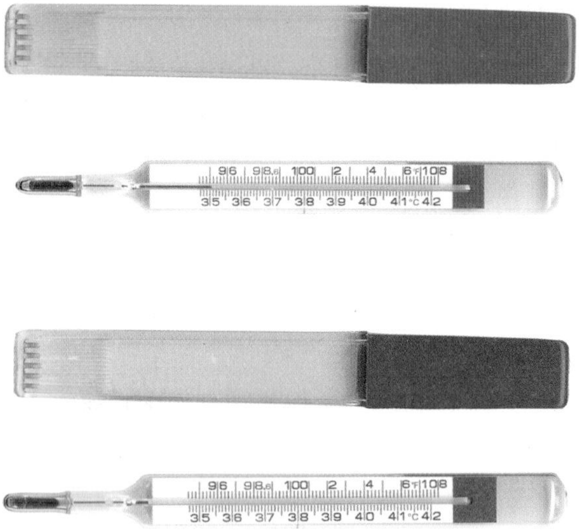

Fig. 17-2. **A mercury-free oral thermometer and a mercury-free rectal thermometer. (Photos courtesy of RG Medical Diagnostics of Southfield, MI.)**

If you must use a mercury thermometer, be careful. If you break one, never touch the mercury or broken glass. Tell the nurse immediately. Specific policies must be followed to clean and dispose of mercury safely.

Mercury-free thermometers are slightly larger than glass bulb thermometers. They operate identically. Numbers on the thermometer let you read the temperature after it registers. Most thermometers show the temperature in degrees Fahrenheit (F). Each long line represents one degree. Each short line represents two-tenths of a degree. Some thermometers show the temperature in degrees Celsius (C). The long lines represent one degree. The short lines represent one-tenth of a degree. The small arrow points to the normal temperature: 98.6°F and 37°C (Fig. 17-3).

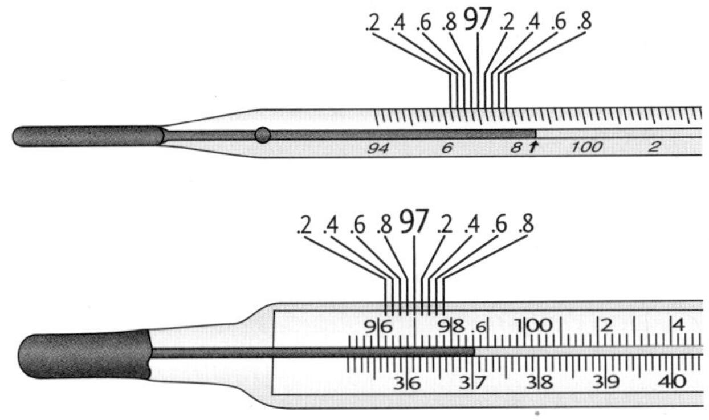

Fig. 17-3. You read a mercury glass and a mercury-free thermometer the same way.

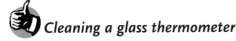

Cleaning a glass thermometer

When cleaning a mercury glass thermometer, wipe it with tissues first. Use lukewarm or cool water. Never use hot water. Hot water can heat the mercury and break the thermometer.

Battery-powered, digital, or electronic thermometers are other types of thermometers (Fig. 17-4). These thermometers display the results digitally. They register the temperature more quickly than mercury-free or glass bulb thermometers. Digital thermometers usually take two to sixty seconds to register the temperature. The thermometer will beep or flash when the temperature has registered. Digital thermometers may be used to take oral, rectal, or axillary temperatures. Follow the manufacturer's guide for proper use of these thermometers.

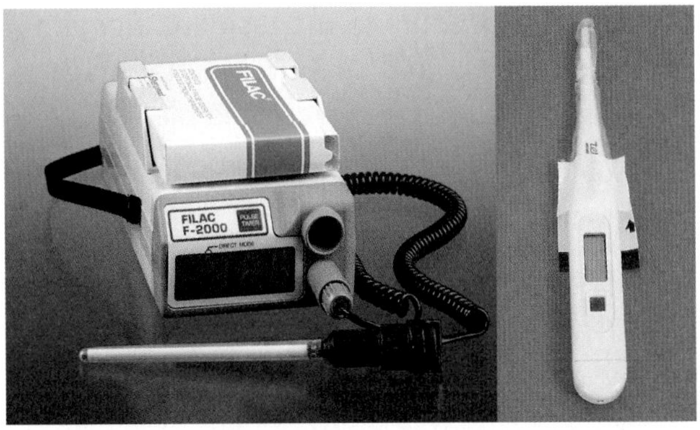

Fig. 17-4. a) An electronic thermometer. b) A digital thermometer.

The tympanic thermometer, or ear thermometer, also registers a temperature quickly (Fig. 17-5). These thermometers may not be as common. They also require more practice to be able to take accurate temperatures.

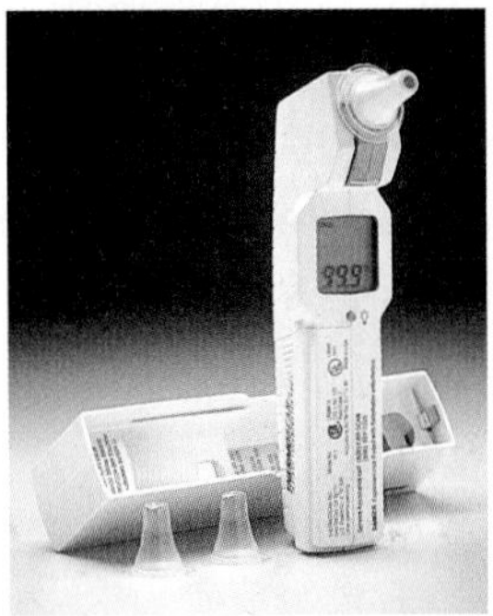

Fig. 17-5. A tympanic thermometer.

There is a range of normal temperatures. Some people's temperatures normally run low. Other people in good health will run slightly higher temperatures. Normal temperature readings also vary by the method used to take the temperature.

Taking and recording an oral temperature

Do not take an oral temperature on a resident who has smoked, eaten or drunk fluids, or exercised in the last 10-20 minutes.

Equipment: mercury-free, glass, digital, or electronic thermometer, disposable plastic sheath/cover for thermometer, tissues, pen and paper

1. Wash your hands.
2. Identify yourself by name. Identify the resident by name.

3. Explain procedure to the resident. Speak clearly, slowly, and directly. Maintain face-to-face contact whenever possible.
4. Provide for resident's privacy with curtain, screen, or door.
5. If the bed is adjustable, adjust to a safe level, usually waist high. If the bed is movable, lock bed wheels.

Using a mercury-free thermometer or glass thermometer:

6. Hold the thermometer by the stem.
7. Before inserting thermometer in resident's mouth, shake thermometer down to below the lowest number (at least below 96°F or 35°C). To shake thermometer down, hold it at the side opposite the bulb with the thumb and two fingers. With a snapping motion of the wrist, shake the thermometer (Fig. 17-6). Stand away from furniture and walls while doing so.

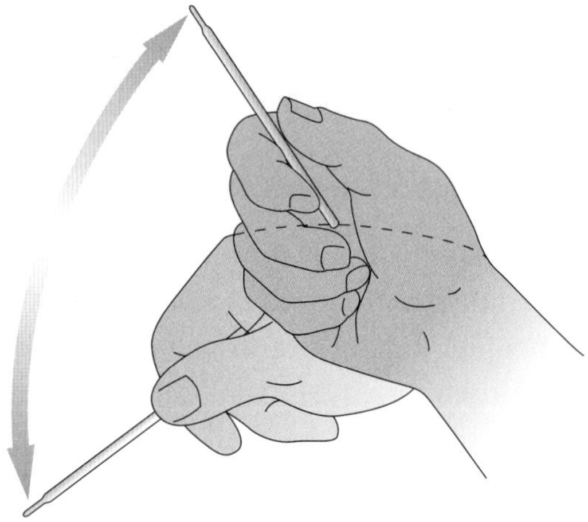

Fig. 17-6.

8. Put a disposable sheath on thermometer, if applicable. Insert bulb end of thermometer into resident's mouth. Place under tongue and to one side (Fig. 17-7). Resident should breathe through his or her nose.
9. Tell resident to hold oral thermometer in mouth with lips closed. Help as necessary. Ask the resident not to bite down or to talk.
10. Leave thermometer in place for at least three minutes.

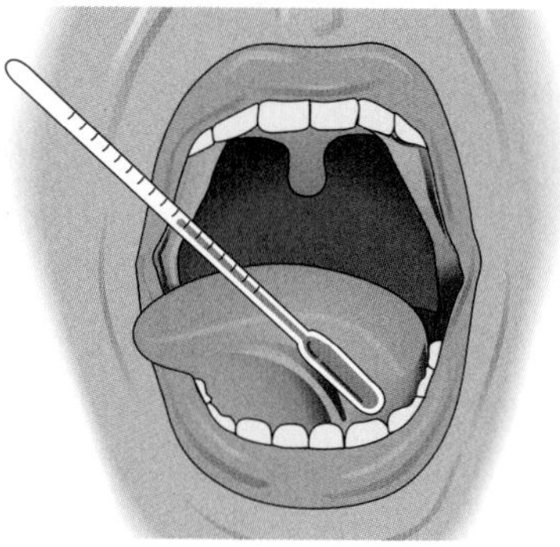

Fig. 17-7.

11. Remove the thermometer. Wipe with tissue from stem to bulb or remove sheath. Dispose of tissue or sheath.
12. Hold thermometer at eye level. Rotate until line appears. Roll the thermometer between your thumb and forefinger. Read temperature. Record temperature, date, time, and method used (oral).
13. Rinse the thermometer in lukewarm water. Dry. Return it to plastic case or container. If using a mercury/glass thermometer, store it away from a heat source.

Using a digital thermometer:

6. Put a disposable sheath on thermometer.
7. Turn on thermometer. Wait until "ready" sign appears.
8. Insert end of digital thermometer into resident's mouth. Place under tongue and to one side.
9. Leave in place until thermometer blinks or beeps.
10. Remove the thermometer.
11. Read temperature on display screen. Record the temperature, date, time, and method used (oral).
12. Using a tissue, remove and dispose of sheath.
13. Replace thermometer in case.

Using an electronic thermometer:

6. Remove probe from base unit.
7. Put probe cover on thermometer.

8. Insert end of electronic thermometer into resident's mouth. Place under tongue and to one side.
9. Leave in place until you hear a tone or see a flashing or steady light.
10. Read the temperature on the display screen.
11. Remove the probe. Press the eject button to discard the cover (Fig. 17-8).

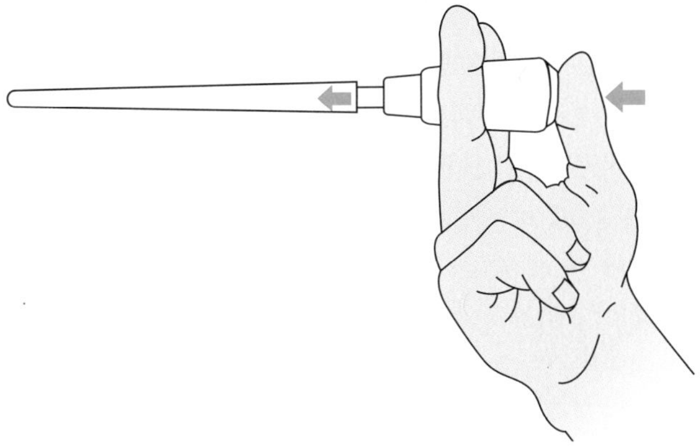

Fig. 17-8.

12. Record temperature, date, time, and method used (oral).
13. Return the probe to the holder.

Final steps:

14. Make resident comfortable. Make sure sheets are free from wrinkles and the bed free from crumbs.
15. Return bed to appropriate position. Remove privacy measures.
16. Before leaving, place call light within resident's reach.
17. Wash your hands.
18. Report any changes in resident to the nurse.
19. Document procedure using facility guidelines.

You may need to take a rectal temperature. You can use a mercury-free, digital, or glass thermometer. Rectal temperatures can be necessary for unconscious residents, residents who have seizures, residents with poorly-fitted dentures or missing teeth, and anyone having trouble breathing through the nose. Always explain what you will do before starting this procedure. You need the resident's cooperation to take a rectal temperature. Ask the resident to hold still. Reassure him or her that the task will only take a few minutes. Hold onto the thermometer at all times.

Taking and recording a rectal temperature

Equipment: rectal mercury-free, glass, or digital thermometer, lubricant, gloves, tissue, disposable sheath/cover, pen and paper

1. Wash your hands.
2. Identify yourself by name. Identify the resident by name.
3. Explain procedure to the resident. Speak clearly, slowly, and directly. Maintain face-to-face contact whenever possible.
4. Provide for resident's privacy with curtain, screen, or door.
5. If the bed is adjustable, adjust to a safe level, usually waist high. If the bed is movable, lock bed wheels.
6. Help the resident to the left-lying (Sims') position (Fig. 17-9).

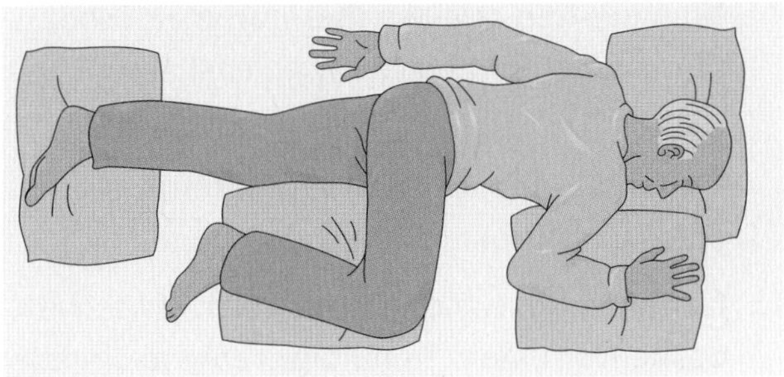

Fig. 17-9.

7. Fold back linens to expose only the rectal area.
8. Put on gloves.
9. **Mercury-free or glass thermometer**: Hold thermometer by stem.

   Digital thermometer: Apply probe cover.

10. **Mercury-free or glass thermometer**: Shake the thermometer down to below the lowest number.
11. Apply small amount of lubricant to tip of bulb or probe cover (or apply pre-lubricated cover).
12. Separate the buttocks. Gently insert thermometer one inch into rectum (Fig. 17-10). Stop if you meet resistance. Do not force the thermometer in the rectum.

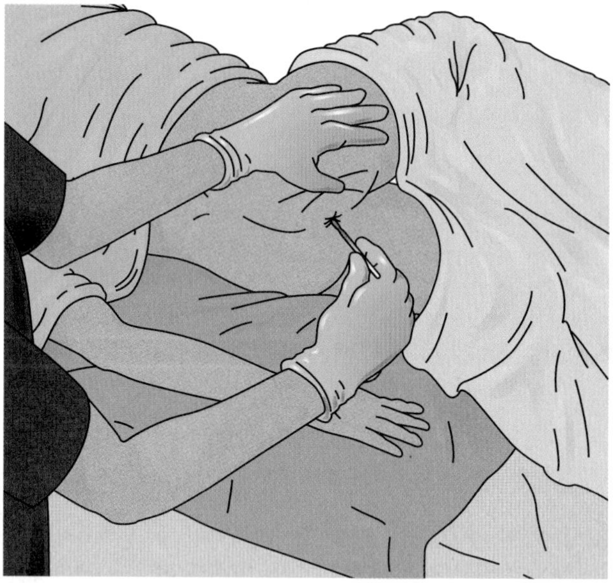

Fig. 17-10.

13. Replace sheet over buttocks. Hold onto the thermometer at all times.
14. **Mercury-free or glass thermometer**: Hold thermometer in place for at least three minutes.

    Digital thermometer: Hold thermometer in place until it blinks or beeps.
15. Gently remove the thermometer. Wipe with tissue from stem to bulb or remove sheath. Dispose of tissue or sheath.
16. Read the thermometer at eye level as you would for an oral temperature. Record temperature, date, time, and method used (rectal).
17. **Mercury-free or glass thermometer**: Rinse the thermometer in lukewarm water. Dry it. Return it to plastic case or container. If using a mercury/glass thermometer, store it away from a heat source.

    Digital thermometer: Throw away probe cover. Return thermometer to storage area.
18. Remove and dispose of gloves.
19. Make resident comfortable. Make sure sheets are free from wrinkles and the bed free from crumbs.
20. Return bed to appropriate position. Remove privacy measures.
21. Before leaving, place call light within resident's reach.
22. Wash your hands.
23. Report any changes in resident to the nurse.
24. Document procedure using facility guidelines.

Tympanic thermometers can take fast and accurate temperature readings. As always, explain what you will do before beginning the procedure. Tell the resident that you will be placing a thermometer in the ear canal. Reassure the resident that this is painless. The short tip of the thermometer will only go into the ear one-quarter to one-half inch. Thermometer models vary. Follow the manufacturer's instructions.

Taking and recording a tympanic temperature

Equipment: tympanic thermometer, disposable probe sheath/cover, pen and paper to record your findings

1. Wash your hands.
2. Identify yourself by name. Identify the resident by name.
3. Explain procedure to the resident. Speak clearly, slowly, and directly. Maintain face-to-face contact whenever possible.
4. Provide for resident's privacy with curtain, screen, or door.

5. If the bed is adjustable, adjust to a safe level, usually waist high. If the bed is movable, lock bed wheels.
6. Put a disposable sheath over earpiece of the thermometer.
7. Position the resident's head so that the ear is in front of you. Straighten the ear canal by pulling up and back on the outside edge of the ear (Fig. 17-11). Insert the covered probe into the ear canal. Press the button.

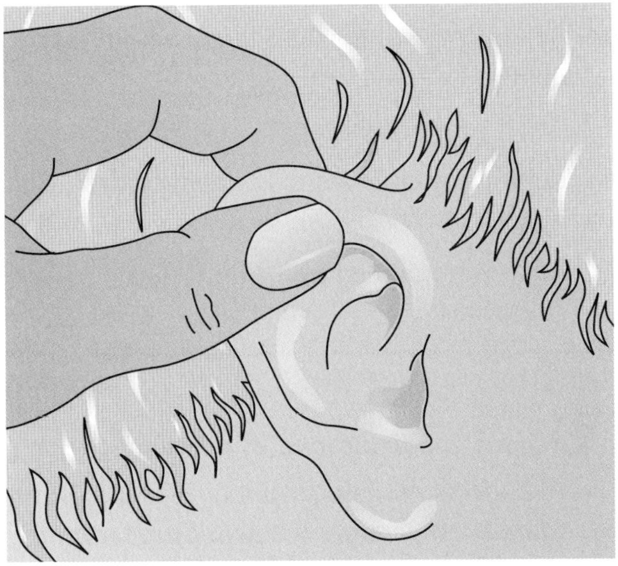

Fig. 17-11.

8. Hold thermometer in place until thermometer blinks or beeps.
9. Read temperature. Record temperature, date, time, and method used (tympanic).
10. Dispose of sheath. Return the thermometer to storage or to the battery charger if thermometer is rechargeable.
11. Make resident comfortable. Make sure sheets are free from wrinkles and the bed free from crumbs.
12. Return bed to appropriate position. Remove privacy measures.
13. Before leaving, place call light within resident's reach.
14. Wash your hands.
15. Report any changes in resident to the nurse.
16. Document procedure using facility guidelines.

Axillary temperatures are much less reliable than temperatures taken at other sites. The axillary site is usually used as a last resort.

Taking and recording an axillary temperature

Equipment: mercury-free, glass, digital, or electronic thermometer, tissues, disposable sheath/cover, pen and paper

1. Wash your hands.
2. Identify yourself by name. Identify the resident by name.
3. Explain procedure to the resident. Speak clearly, slowly, and directly. Maintain face-to-face contact whenever possible.
4. Provide for resident's privacy with curtain, screen, or door.
5. If the bed is adjustable, adjust to a safe level, usually waist high. If the bed is movable, lock bed wheels.
6. Remove resident's arm from sleeve of gown. Wipe axillary area with tissues.

Using a mercury-free thermometer or glass thermometer:

7. Hold thermometer at stem end. Shake down to below the lowest number.
8. Put disposable sheath on thermometer, if applicable.
9. Place bulb end of thermometer in center of armpit. Fold resident's arm over chest.
10. Hold in place, with the arm close against the side, for 10 minutes (Fig. 17-12).
11. Remove the thermometer. Wipe with tissue from stem to bulb or remove sheath. Dispose of tissue or sheath.
12. Hold thermometer at eye level. Rotate until line appears. Read temperature. Record temperature, date, time, and method used (axillary).

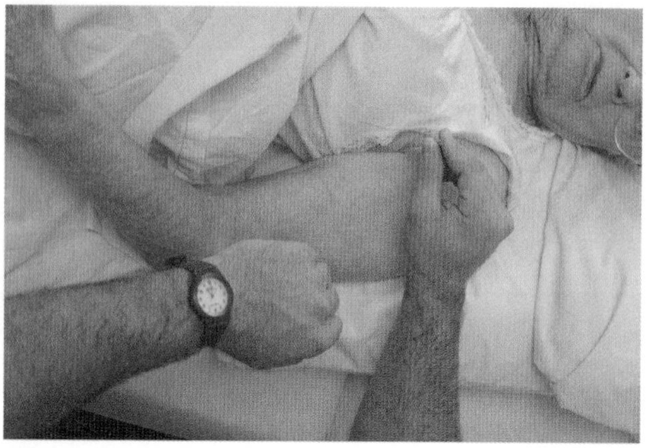

Fig. 17-12.

13. Clean thermometer and/or return it to container for used thermometers.

Using a digital thermometer:

7. Put on disposable sheath. Turn on thermometer. Wait until "ready" sign appears.
8. Position end of digital thermometer in center of armpit. Fold resident's arm over chest.
9. Hold in place until thermometer blinks or beeps.
10. Remove the thermometer.
11. Read temperature on display screen. Record the temperature, date, time, and method used (axillary).
12. Using a tissue, remove and dispose of sheath.
13. Replace thermometer in case.

Using an electronic thermometer:

7. Remove probe from base unit. Put on probe cover.
8. Position end of electronic thermometer in center of armpit. Fold resident's arm over chest.
9. Leave in place until you hear a tone or see a flashing or steady light.
10. Read the temperature on the display screen.
11. Remove the probe. Press the eject button to discard the cover.
12. Record temperature, date, time, and method used (axillary).
13. Return the probe to the holder.

Final steps:

14. Put resident's arm back into sleeve of gown. Make resident comfortable. Make sure sheets are free from wrinkles and the bed free from crumbs.
15. Return bed to appropriate position. Remove privacy measures.
16. Before leaving, place call light within resident's reach.
17. Wash your hands.
18. Report any changes in resident to the nurse.
19. Document procedure using facility guidelines.

Signs and Symptoms of a Fever

Residents may show symptoms of a fever before a temperature is taken. Symptoms include headaches, fatigue, muscle aches, and chills. The skin may feel hot to the touch and look flushed. If you notice any of these symptoms, notify the nurse. You may be asked to take a temperature right away.

3. List guidelines for taking pulse and respirations

The pulse is the number of heartbeats per minute. The beat that you feel at certain pulse points in the body represents the wave of blood moving. This is a result of the heart pumping. The most common site for taking the pulse is on the inside of the wrist, where the radial artery runs just beneath the skin. This is called the **radial pulse**. The procedure for taking this pulse is located later in this chapter.

The **brachial pulse** is the pulse inside of the elbow. It is about one to one and a half inches above the elbow. The radial and brachial pulse are used in taking blood pressure. Blood pressure is explained later in this chapter. Other common pulse sites are shown in Fig. 17-13.

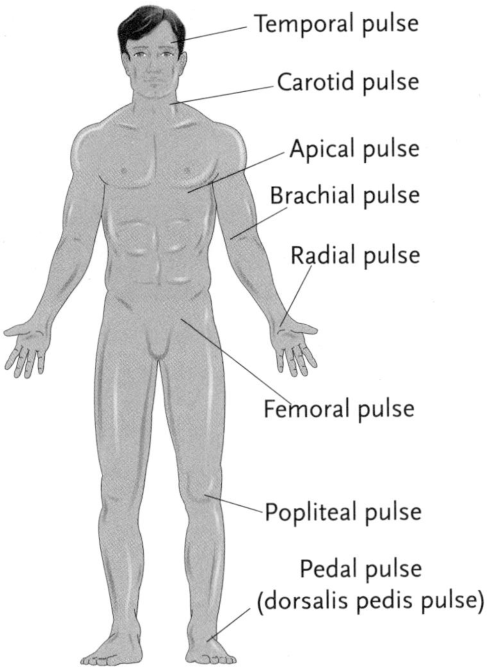

Fig. 17-13. **Common pulse sites.**

For adults, the normal pulse rate is 60–90 beats per minute. Small children have faster pulses, in the range of 100–120 beats per minute. A newborn baby's pulse may be as high as 120–140 beats per minute. Many things can affect the pulse rate. Some are exercise, fear, anger, anxiety, heat, medications, and pain. An unusually high or low rate may not indicate disease, but sometimes the pulse rate can be a signal of serious illness. A rapid pulse may result from fever, infection, or heart failure. A slow or weak pulse may indicate dehydration, infection, or shock.

The **apical pulse** is heard by listening directly over the heart with a stethoscope. A **stethoscope** is an instrument for listening to sounds within the body, such as the heartbeat or air in the lungs (Fig. 17-14).

The apical pulse is on the left side of the chest, just below the nipple. This is often the easiest way to measure the pulse in infants and small children. Their pulse points are harder to find. For residents, the apical pulse may be taken when the person has heart disease or takes drugs that affect the heart. It may also be taken on residents who have a weak radial pulse or an irregular pulse.

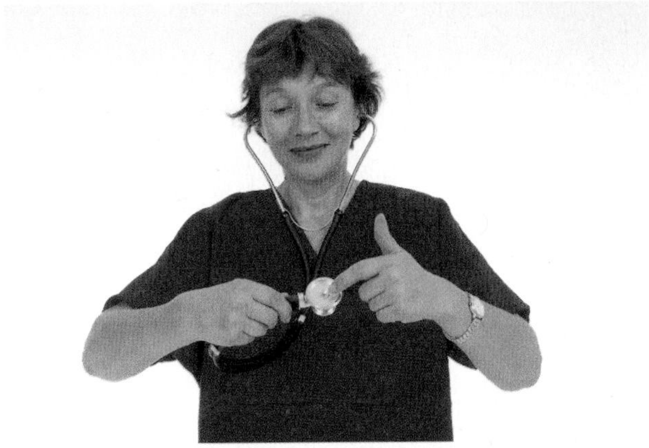

Fig. 17-14. **Use the diaphragm side of the stethoscope to hear a pulse and to take blood pressure. The diaphragm is the larger, round side of the stethoscope.**

Taking and recording apical pulse

Equipment: stethoscope, watch with second hand, alcohol wipes, pen and paper to record your findings

1. Wash hands.
2. Identify yourself by name. Identify the resident by name.
3. Explain procedure to the resident. Speak clearly, slowly, and directly. Maintain face-to-face contact whenever possible.
4. Provide for resident's privacy with curtain, screen, or door.
5. If the bed is adjustable, adjust to a safe level, usually waist high. If the bed is movable, lock bed wheels.
6. Fit the earpieces of the stethoscope snugly in your ears. Place the flat metal diaphragm on the left side of the chest, just below the nipple (Fig. 17-15). Listen for the heartbeat.
7. Use the second hand of your watch. Count beats for one full minute. Each "lubdub" that you hear is counted as one beat. A nor-

mal heartbeat is rhythmical. Leave the stethoscope in place to count respirations (see procedure later in chapter).

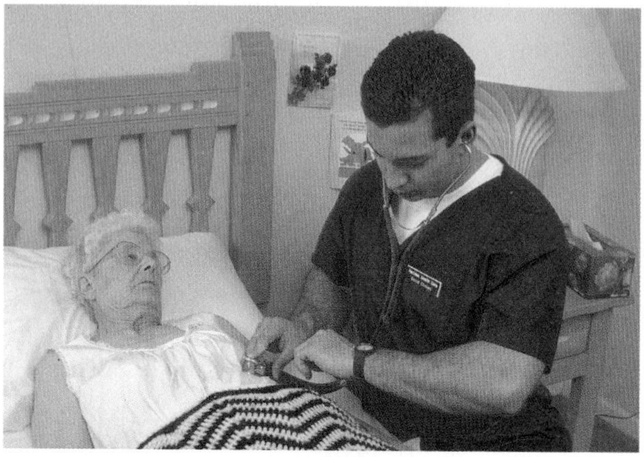

Fig. 17-15.

8. Record pulse rate, date, time, and method used (apical). Note any differences in the rhythm.
9. Clean earpieces and diaphragm of stethoscope with alcohol wipes. Store stethoscope.
10. Make resident comfortable. Make sure sheets are free from wrinkles and the bed free from crumbs.
11. Return bed to appropriate position. Remove privacy measures.
12. Before leaving, place call light within resident's reach.
13. Wash your hands.
14. Report any changes in resident to the nurse.
15. Document procedure using facility guidelines.

Respiration is the process of breathing air into the lungs, or **inspiration**, and exhaling air out of the lungs, or **expiration**. Each respiration has an inspiration and an expiration. The chest rises during inspiration and falls during expiration.

The normal respiration rate for adults ranges from 12–20 breaths per minute. Infants and children have a faster respiratory rate. Infants normally breathe at a rate of 30–40 respirations per minute. People may breathe more quickly if they know they are being observed. Count respirations immediately after taking the pulse. Keep your fingers on a resident's wrist or on the stethoscope over the heart. Do not make it obvious that you are watching the resident's breathing.

Taking and recording radial pulse and counting and recording respirations

Equipment: watch with a second hand, pen and paper to record your findings

1. Wash your hands.
2. Identify yourself by name. Identify the resident by name.
3. Explain procedure to the resident. Speak clearly, slowly, and directly. Maintain face-to-face contact whenever possible.
4. Provide for resident's privacy with curtain, screen, or door.
5. If the bed is adjustable, adjust to a safe level, usually waist high. If the bed is movable, lock bed wheels.
6. Place fingertips on the thumb side of resident's wrist. Locate pulse (Fig. 17-16).

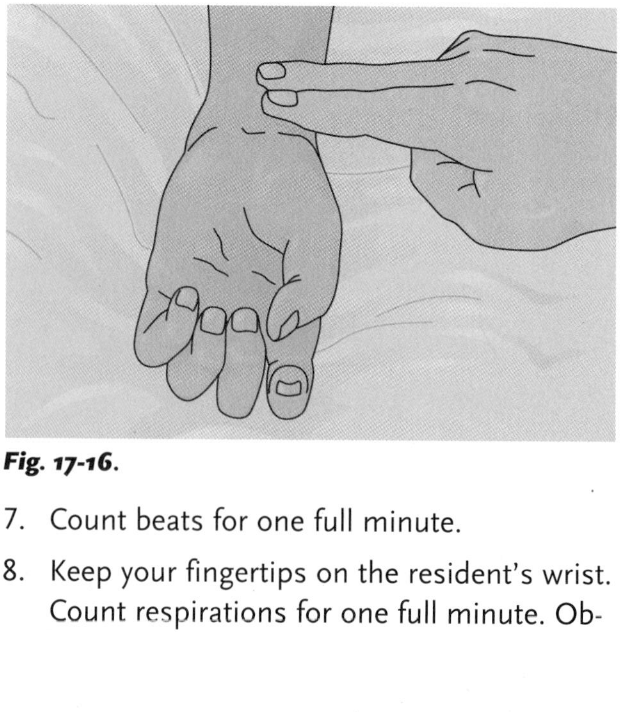

Fig. 17-16.

7. Count beats for one full minute.
8. Keep your fingertips on the resident's wrist. Count respirations for one full minute. Ob-

serve for the pattern and character of the resident's breathing. Normal breathing is smooth and quiet. If you see signs of troubled breathing, shallow breathing, or noisy breathing, such as wheezing, report it.

9. Record pulse rate, date, time, and method used (radial). Record the respiratory rate and the pattern or character of breathing.
10. Make resident comfortable. Make sure sheets are free from wrinkles and the bed free from crumbs.
11. Return bed to appropriate position. Remove privacy measures.
12. Before leaving, place call light within resident's reach.
13. Wash your hands.
14. Report any changes in resident to the nurse.
15. Document procedure according to facility guidelines.

4. Explain guidelines for taking blood pressure

Blood pressure is an important measure of health. Blood pressure is measured in millimeters of mercury (mmHg). The measurement shows how well the heart is working. There are two parts of blood pressure. They are the systolic measurement and the diastolic measurement.

In the **systolic** phase, the heart is at work. It contracts and pushes the blood from the left ventricle of the heart. The reading shows the pressure on the walls of arteries as blood is pumped through the body. The normal range for systolic blood pressure is 100–119 mmHg.

The second measurement reflects the **diastolic** phase. This is when the heart relaxes. The diastolic measurement is always lower than the systolic measurement. It shows the pressure in the arteries when the heart is at rest. The normal range for adults is 60–79 mmHg.

People with high blood pressure, or **hypertension**, have elevated systolic and/or diastolic blood pressures. A blood pressure level of 140/90 mmHg or higher is considered high.

However, if blood pressure is between 120/80 mmHg and 139/89 mmHg, it is called prehypertension. This person does not have high blood pressure now but is likely to have it in the future. Report to the nurse if a resident's blood pressure is 140/90 or above.

Many factors can increase blood pressure. These include aging, exercise, stress, pain, medications, and the volume of blood in circulation. Loss of blood will lead to abnormally low blood pressure, or **hypotension**. Hypotension can be life-threatening.

Blood pressure is taken with a stethoscope and a blood pressure cuff, or **sphygmomanometer** (Fig. 17-17). Inside the cuff is an inflatable balloon. It expands when air is pumped into the cuff. Two pieces of tubing are connected to the cuff. One leads to a rubber bulb that pumps air into the cuff. A pressure control button lets you control the release of air from the cuff. The other piece of tubing is connected to a pressure gauge with numbers. The gauge is either a mercury column or a round dial.

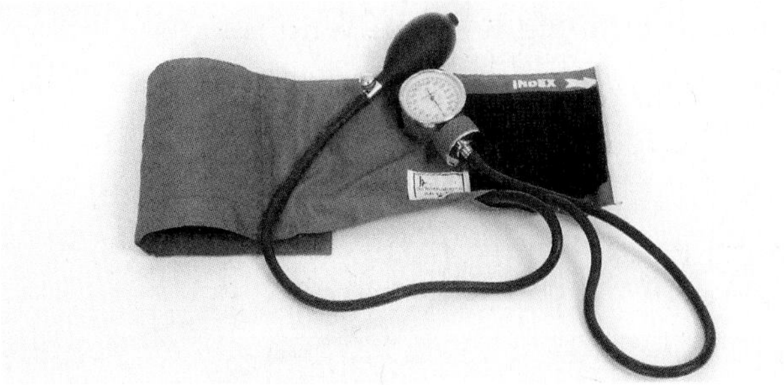

Fig. 17-17. **A sphygmomanometer.**

There may be an electronic sphygmomanometer available (Fig. 17-18). The systolic and diastolic pressure readings and pulse are displayed digitally. Some units automatically inflate and deflate. You do not need a stethoscope with an electronic sphygmomanometer. Ask for instructions on the proper use of the equipment.

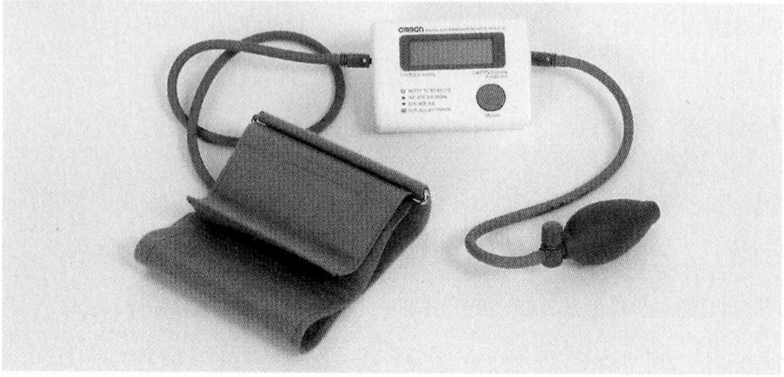

Fig. 17-18. **An electronic sphygmomanometer.**

When taking blood pressure, the first clear sound you will hear is the systolic pressure (top number). When the sound changes to a soft muffled thump or disappears, this is the diastolic pressure (bottom number). Blood pressure is recorded as a fraction. The systolic reading is on top. The diastolic reading is on the bottom (for example: 120/80).

Never measure blood pressure on an arm that has an IV or any medical equipment. Avoid a side that has a cast, recent trauma, paralysis from a stroke, burn(s), or breast surgery (mastectomy).

This textbook includes two methods for taking blood pressure. They are the one-step method and the two-step method. In the two-step method, you will get an estimate of the systolic blood pressure before you start. After getting an estimated systolic reading, you will deflate the cuff and begin again. With the one-step method, you will not get an estimated systolic reading before getting the blood pressure reading. Your state may require that you know one or both of these methods. Follow your facility's policy on which method to use.

Taking and recording blood pressure (one-step method)

Equipment: sphygmomanometer (blood pressure cuff), stethoscope, alcohol wipes, pen and paper to record your findings

1. Wash your hands.
2. Identify yourself by name. Identify the resident by name.
3. Explain procedure to the resident. Speak clearly, slowly, and directly. Maintain face-to-face contact whenever possible.
4. Provide for resident's privacy with curtain, screen, or door.
5. If the bed is adjustable, adjust to a safe level, usually waist high. If the bed is movable, lock bed wheels.
6. Position resident's arm with palm up. The arm should be level with the heart.
7. With the valve open, squeeze the cuff. Make sure it is completely deflated.
8. Place blood pressure cuff snugly on resident's upper arm. The center of the cuff is placed over the brachial artery (1-1½ inches above the elbow toward inside of elbow) (Fig. 17-19).

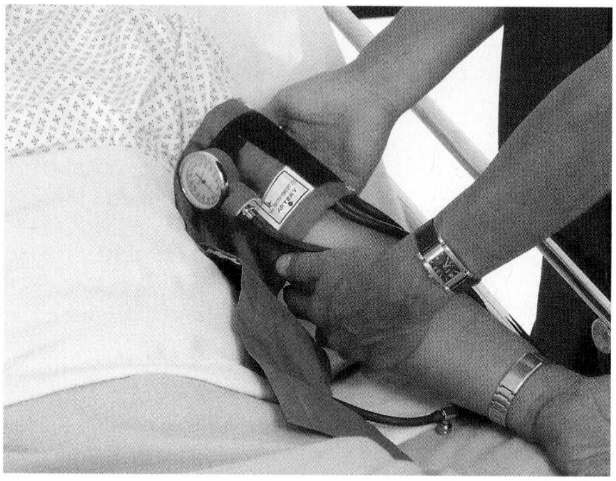

Fig. 17-19.

9. Before using stethoscope, wipe diaphragm and earpieces with alcohol wipes.
10. Locate brachial pulse with fingertips.
11. Place diaphragm of stethoscope over brachial artery.
12. Place earpieces of stethoscope in ears.
13. Close the valve (clockwise) until it stops. Do not tighten it (Fig. 17-20).

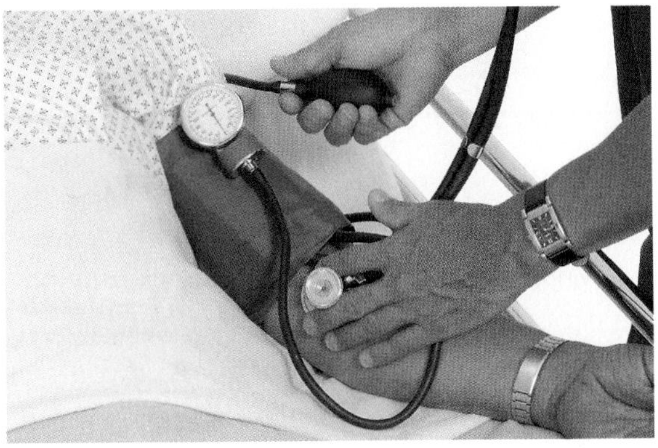

Fig. 17-20.

14. Inflate cuff to 30 mmHg above the point at which the pulse is last heard or felt.
15. Open the valve slightly with thumb and index finger. Deflate cuff slowly.
16. Watch gauge. Listen for sound of pulse.
17. Remember the reading at which the first clear pulse sound is heard. This is the systolic pressure.
18. Continue listening for a change or muffling of pulse sound. The point of a change or the point the sound disappears is the diastolic pressure. Remember this reading.
19. Open the valve. Deflate cuff completely. Remove cuff.
20. Record both the systolic and diastolic pressures.
21. Wipe diaphragm and earpieces of stethoscope with alcohol. Store equipment.
22. Make resident comfortable. Make sure sheets are free from wrinkles and the bed free from crumbs.
23. Return bed to appropriate position. Remove privacy measures.
24. Before leaving, place call light within resident's reach.
25. Wash your hands.
26. Report any changes in resident to the nurse.
27. Document procedure using facility guidelines.

Taking and recording blood pressure (two-step method)

Equipment: sphygmomanometer (blood pressure cuff), stethoscope, alcohol wipes, pen and paper to record your findings

1. Wash your hands.
2. Identify yourself by name. Identify the resident by name.
3. Explain procedure to the resident. Speak clearly, slowly, and directly. Maintain face-to-face contact whenever possible.
4. Provide for resident's privacy during procedure with curtain, screen, or door.
5. If the bed is adjustable, adjust to a safe level, usually waist high. If the bed is movable, lock bed wheels.
6. Position resident's arm with palm up. The arm should be level with the heart.
7. With the valve open, squeeze the cuff to make sure it is completely deflated.
8. Place blood pressure cuff snugly on resident's upper arm. The center of cuff is placed over the brachial artery (1-1½ inches above the elbow toward inside of elbow).
9. Locate the radial (wrist) pulse with fingertips.
10. Close the valve (clockwise) until it stops. Inflate cuff, watching gauge.
11. Stop inflating when you can no longer feel the pulse. Note the reading. The number is an estimate of the systolic pressure.
12. Open the valve. Deflate cuff completely.
13. Write down the systolic reading.
14. Before using stethoscope, wipe diaphragm and earpieces of stethoscope with alcohol wipes.
15. Locate brachial pulse with fingertips.
16. Place diaphragm of stethoscope over brachial artery.
17. Place earpieces of stethoscope in ears.

18. Close the valve (clockwise) until it stops. Do not tighten it (Fig. 17-21).

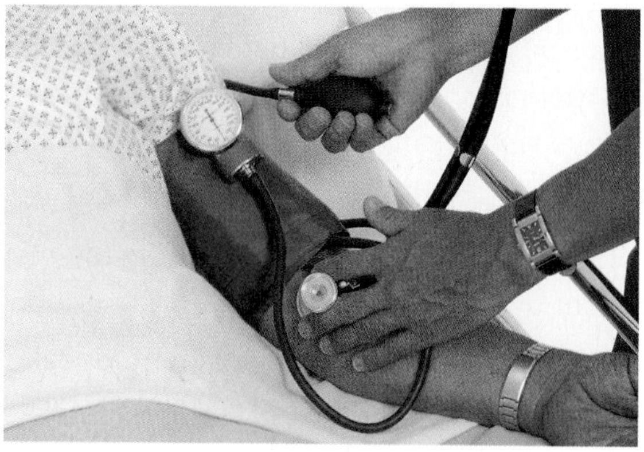

Fig. 17-21.

19. Inflate cuff to 30 mmHg above your estimated systolic pressure.
20. Open the valve slightly with thumb and index finger. Deflate cuff slowly.
21. Watch gauge. Listen for sound of pulse.
22. Remember the reading at which the first clear pulse sound is heard. This is the systolic pressure.
23. Continue listening for a change or muffling of pulse sound. The point of a change or the point the sound disappears is the diastolic pressure. Remember this reading.
24. Open the valve. Deflate cuff completely. Remove cuff.
25. Record both systolic and diastolic pressures.
26. Wipe diaphragm and earpieces of stethoscope with alcohol. Store equipment.
27. Make resident comfortable. Make sure sheets are free from wrinkles and the bed free from crumbs.
28. Return bed to appropriate position. Remove privacy measures.
29. Before leaving, place call light within resident's reach.
30. Wash your hands.
31. Report any changes in resident to the nurse.
32. Document procedure using facility guidelines.

STOP ***Never guess.***

When taking vital signs, readings may be difficult to get on some residents. If you cannot get a reading, do not guess. If you record a guess, it is illegal. It may put a resident's life in danger. Nurses and doctors make care decisions based on your reports. If you cannot obtain a proper reading, tell the nurse. Always be truthful and accurate in your reporting.

5. Describe guidelines for pain management

It is important to observe and report on a resident's pain. Pain is called the "fifth vital sign" because it is so important to monitor.

Pain is uncomfortable. It is also a personal experience. It is different for each person. What one person thinks is painful is not for another. You spend the most time with residents. You play an important role in pain monitoring and prevention. Care plans are made based on your reports.

Treat residents' complaints of pain seriously. Take action to help them (Fig. 17-22). If a resident complains of pain, ask these questions to get the most accurate information. Immediately report the information to the nurse.

- Where is the pain?
- When did the pain start?
- Is the pain mild, moderate, or severe? To help find out, ask the resident to rate the pain on a scale of 1 to 10. Ten is the worst.
- Ask the resident to describe the pain. Make notes if you need to. Use the resident's words when reporting to the nurse.
- Ask the resident what he or she was doing before the pain started.

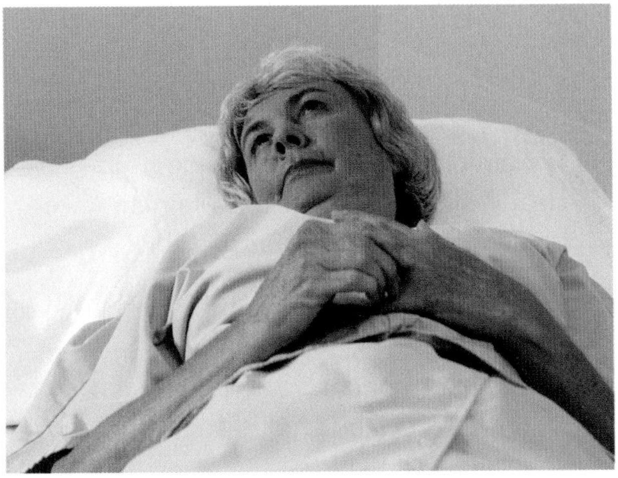

Fig. 17-22. **Believe residents when they complain of pain. Being in pain is unpleasant. Help them by asking questions and reporting your observations.**

Understand that some people do not feel comfortable saying that they are in pain. A person's culture affects how he or she responds to pain. Some cultures believe that it is best not to react to pain. Other cultures believe in expressing pain freely. Watch for body language or other messages that residents may be in pain. Signs and symptoms of pain to observe and report are:

OBSERVING AND REPORTING
Pain

Report any of these to the nurse:

- increased pulse, respirations, blood pressure
- sweating
- nausea
- vomiting
- tightening the jaw
- squeezing eyes shut
- holding a body part tightly
- frowning
- grinding teeth
- increased restlessness
- agitation
- change in behavior
- crying
- sighing
- groaning
- breathing heavily

Measures to reduce pain are:

- Report complaints of pain or unrelieved pain promptly to the nurse.
- Gently position the body in good alignment. Use pillows for support. Help in changes of position if the resident wishes.
- Give back rubs.
- Offer warm baths or showers.
- Help the resident to the bathroom or commode or offer the bedpan or urinal.
- Encourage slow, deep breaths when the resident has trouble breathing.
- Provide a calm and quiet environment. Use soft music to distract the resident.
- Be patient, caring, gentle, and sympathetic.

6. Explain the benefits of warm and cold applications

Applying heat or cold to injured areas can have several good effects. Heat relieves pain and muscular tension. It decreases swelling, elevates the temperature in the tissues, and increases blood flow. Increased blood flow brings more oxygen and nutrients to the tissues for healing.

Cold can help stop bleeding. It prevents swelling and reduces pain. Cold helps brings down high fevers.

Warm and cold applications may be dry or moist. Moisture strengthens the effect of heat and cold. This means that moist applications are more likely to cause injury. Be careful when using these applications. Know how long it should be performed. Use the correct temperature as given in the care plan. Check on the application as directed.

Types of dry applications are:

- Aquamatic K-pad ® (warm or cold)
- Electric heating pad (warm)
- Disposable warm pack (warm)
- Ice bag (cold)
- Disposable cold pack (cold)

Types of moist applications are:

- Compresses (warm or cold)
- Soaks (warm or cold)
- Tub baths (warm)
- Sitz baths (warm)
- Ice packs (cold)

Some states allow nursing assistants to prepare and apply warm and cold applications. Never perform a procedure you are not trained or allowed to do. Only perform procedures that are assigned to you.

OBSERVING AND REPORTING

Warm and Cold Applications

Report these to the nurse:

- excessive redness
- pain
- blisters
- numbness

If you observe these signs, the application may be causing tissue damage.

Hot opens; cold closes.

When using hot and cold applications, it helps to remember what happens with each. The following tip may help you remember the response to hot and cold:

Hot opens (blood vessels) and cold closes (blood vessels).

Applying warm compresses

Equipment: washcloth or compress, plastic wrap, towel, basin, bath thermometer

1. Wash your hands.
2. Identify yourself by name. Identify the resident by name.
3. Explain procedure to the resident. Speak clearly, slowly, and directly. Maintain face-to-face contact whenever possible.
4. Provide for the resident's privacy with curtain, screen, or door.
5. If the bed is adjustable, adjust to a safe level, usually waist high. If the bed is movable, lock bed wheels.
6. Fill basin one-half to two-thirds with hot water. Test water temperature with thermometer or your wrist. Ensure it is safe. Water temperature should be 105° to 110°F. Have resident check water temperature. Adjust if necessary.
7. Soak the washcloth in the water. Wring it out. Immediately apply it to the area needing a warm compress. Note the time. Quickly cover the washcloth with plastic wrap and the towel to keep it warm (Fig. 17-23).

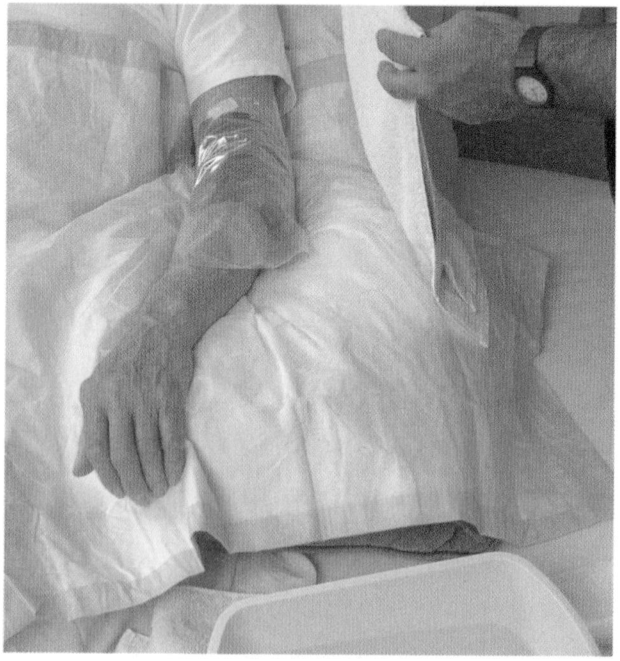

Fig. 17-23.

8. Check the area every five minutes. Remove the compress if the area is red or numb or

if the resident has pain or discomfort. Change the compress if cooling occurs. Remove the compress after 20 minutes.

9. Commercial warm compresses are also available. If you are using these, follow the package directions and the nurse's instructions.
10. Place soiled clothing and linens in appropriate containers.
11. Empty, rinse, and wipe basin. Return to proper storage. Discard plastic wrap.
12. Make resident comfortable. Make sure sheets are free from wrinkles and the bed free from crumbs.
13. Return bed to appropriate position. Remove privacy measures.
14. Before leaving, place call light within resident's reach.
15. Wash your hands.
16. Report any changes in resident to the nurse.
17. Document procedure using facility guidelines.

Administering warm soaks

Equipment: towel, basin, bath thermometer, bath blanket

1. Wash your hands.
2. Identify yourself by name. Identify the resident by name.
3. Explain procedure to the resident. Speak clearly, slowly, and directly. Maintain face-to-face contact whenever possible.
4. Provide for the resident's privacy with curtain, screen, or door.
5. If the bed is adjustable, adjust to a safe level, usually waist high. If the bed is movable, lock bed wheels.
6. Fill the basin half full of hot water. Test water temperature with thermometer or your wrist. Ensure it is safe. Water temperature should be 105° to 110°F. Have resident check water temperature. Adjust if necessary.
7. Immerse the body part in the basin. Pad the edge of the basin with a towel if needed (Fig. 17-24). Use a bath blanket to cover the resident if needed for extra warmth.

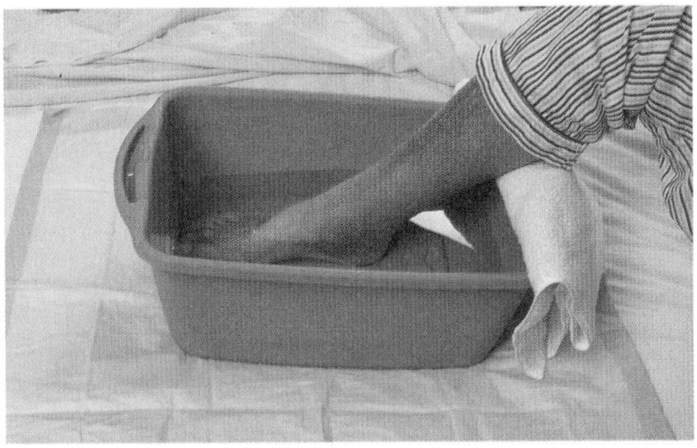

Fig. 17-24.

8. Check water temperature every five minutes. Add hot water as needed to maintain the temperature. Never add water hotter than 110°F. To prevent burns, tell the resident not to add hot water. Observe the area for redness. Discontinue the soak if the resident has pain or discomfort.
9. Soak for 15-20 minutes, or as ordered.
10. Remove basin. Use the towel to dry resident.
11. Place soiled clothing and linens in appropriate containers.
12. Empty, rinse, and wipe basin. Return to proper storage.
13. Make resident comfortable. Make sure sheets are free from wrinkles and the bed free from crumbs.
14. Return bed to appropriate position. Remove privacy measures.
15. Before leaving, place call light within resident's reach.
16. Wash your hands.
17. Report any changes in resident to the nurse.

18. Document procedure using facility guidelines.

Applying an Aquamatic K-Pad ®

Equipment: K-Pad ® and control unit (Fig. 17-25), covering for pad, distilled water

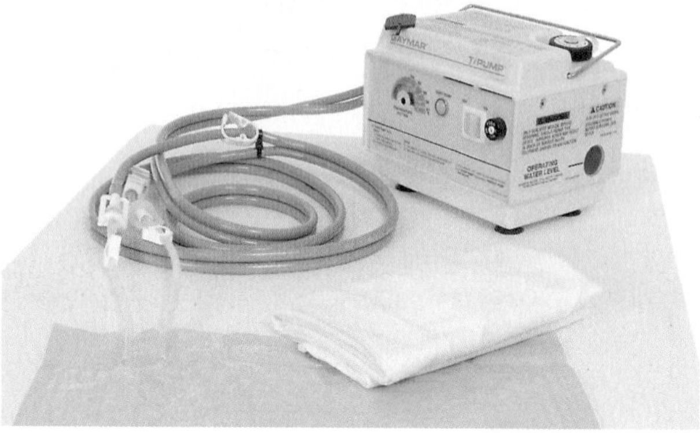

Fig. 17-25.

1. Wash your hands.
2. Identify yourself by name. Identify the resident by name.
3. Explain procedure to the resident. Speak clearly, slowly, and directly. Maintain face-to-face contact whenever possible.
4. Provide for the resident's privacy during procedure with curtain, screen, or door.
5. If the bed is adjustable, adjust to a safe level, usually waist high. If the bed is movable, lock bed wheels.
6. Place the control unit on the bedside table. Make sure cords are not frayed or damaged. Check that tubing between pad and unit is intact.
7. Remove cover of control unit to check level of water. If it is low, fill it with distilled water to the fill line.
8. Put the cover of control unit back in place.
9. Plug unit in. Turn pad on. Temperature should have been pre-set. If it was not, check with the nurse for proper temperature.
10. Place the pad in the cover. Do not pin the pad to the cover.
11. Uncover area to be treated. Place the covered pad. Note the time. Make sure the tubing is not hanging below the bed. It should be coiled on the bed.
12. Return and check area every five minutes. Remove the pad if the area is red or numb or if the resident reports pain or discomfort.
13. Check water level. Refill with distilled water to the fill line when necessary.
14. Remove pad after 20 minutes.
15. Clean and store supplies.
16. Make resident comfortable. Make sure sheets are free from wrinkles and the bed free from crumbs.
17. Return bed to appropriate position. Remove privacy measures.
18. Before leaving, place call light within resident's reach.
19. Wash your hands.
20. Report any changes in resident to the nurse.
21. Document procedure using facility guidelines.

Another type of heat application is a **sitz bath**. This is a warm soak of the perineal area. Sitz baths clean perineal wounds and reduce inflammation and pain. Circulation is increased. Voiding may be stimulated by a sitz bath. Residents with perineal swelling (such as hemorrhoids) may be ordered to take sitz baths. Because the sitz bath causes increased blood flow to the pelvic area, blood flow to other parts of the body decreases. Residents may feel weak, faint, or dizzy after a sitz bath. Always wear gloves when helping with a sitz bath.

Assisting with a sitz bath

A disposable sitz bath fits on the toilet seat. It is attached to a rubber bag containing warm water (Fig. 17-26).

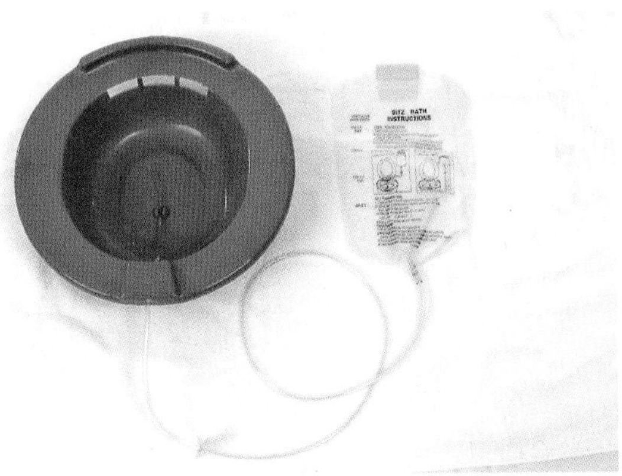

Fig. 17-26.

Equipment: disposable sitz bath, bath thermometer, towels, gloves

1. Wash your hands.
2. Identify yourself by name. Identify the resident by name.
3. Explain procedure to the resident. Speak clearly, slowly, and directly. Maintain face-to-face contact whenever possible.
4. Provide for the resident's privacy with curtain, screen, or door.
5. Put on gloves.
6. Fill the sitz bath two-thirds full with hot water. Place the disposable sitz bath on the toilet seat. If the sitz bath is prescribed for cleaning the perineal area, the temperature should be 100°F-104°F. For pain and to stimulate circulation, the water temperature should be 105°F-110°F. Check the water temperature using the bath thermometer.
7. Help the resident undress and get seated on the sitz bath. A valve on the tubing connected to the bag allows the resident or you to fill the sitz bath again with hot water.
8. You may be required to stay with the resident during the bath for safety reasons. If you leave the room, check on the resident every five minutes to make sure he or she is not dizzy or weak.
9. Help the resident out of the sitz bath in 20 minutes. Provide towels. Help with dressing if needed.
10. Clean and store supplies.
11. Remove gloves.
12. Make sure resident is comfortable.
13. Before leaving, place call light within resident's reach.
14. Wash your hands.
15. Report any changes in resident to the nurse.
16. Document procedure using facility guidelines.

Applying ice packs

Equipment: ice pack or sealable plastic bag and crushed ice, towel to cover pack or bag

1. Wash your hands.
2. Identify yourself by name. Identify the resident by name.
3. Explain procedure to the resident. Speak clearly, slowly, and directly. Maintain face-to-face contact whenever possible.
4. Provide for the resident's privacy with curtain, screen, or door.
5. If the bed is adjustable, adjust to a safe level, usually waist high. If the bed is movable, lock bed wheels.
6. Fill plastic bag or ice pack one-half to two-thirds full with crushed ice. Seal bag. Remove excess air. Cover bag or ice pack with towel (Fig. 17-27).

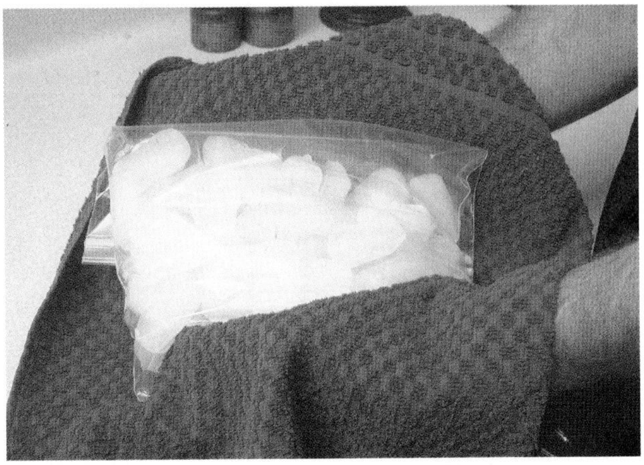

Fig. 17-27.

7. Apply bag to the area as ordered. Note the time. Use another towel to cover bag if it is too cold.
8. Check the area after ten minutes for blisters or pale, white, or gray skin. Stop treatment if resident reports numbness or pain.
9. Remove ice after 20 minutes or as ordered.
10. Store ice pack.
11. Make resident comfortable. Make sure sheets are free from wrinkles and the bed free from crumbs.
12. Return bed to appropriate position. Remove privacy measures.
13. Before leaving, place call light within resident's reach.
14. Wash your hands.
15. Report any changes in resident to the nurse.
16. Document procedure using facility guidelines.

The 20-minute Rule

Warm and cold applications should not be applied for too long. When they are on for too long, the opposite effect of what is intended occurs. This means that if you leave an ice bag on for longer than 20 minutes, blood vessels may start to open again. This could increase bleeding and swelling at the site. Remember to limit warm or cold applications to 20 minutes.

7. Explain how to apply non-sterile dressings

Sterile dressings cover open or draining wounds. A nurse changes these dressings. Non-sterile dressings are applied to dry wounds that have less chance of infection. Nursing assistants may help with non-sterile dressing changes.

Changing a dry dressing using non-sterile technique

Equipment: package of square gauze dressings, adhesive tape, scissors, 2 pairs of gloves

1. Wash your hands.
2. Identify yourself by name. Identify the resident by name.
3. Explain procedure to the resident. Speak clearly, slowly, and directly. Maintain face-to-face contact whenever possible.
4. Provide for resident's privacy with curtain, screen, or door.
5. If the bed is adjustable, adjust to a safe level, usually waist high. If the bed is movable, lock bed wheels.
6. Cut pieces of tape long enough to secure the dressing. Hang tape on the edge of a table within reach. Open four-inch gauze square package without touching gauze. Place the open package on a flat surface.
7. Put on gloves.
8. Remove soiled dressing by gently peeling tape toward the wound. Lift dressing off the wound. Do not drag it over wound. Observe dressing for any odor. Notice color and size of the wound. Dispose of used dressing in proper container. Remove and dispose of gloves.
9. Put on new gloves. Touching only outer edges of new four-inch gauze, remove it from package. Apply it to wound. Tape gauze in place. Secure it firmly (Fig. 17-28).

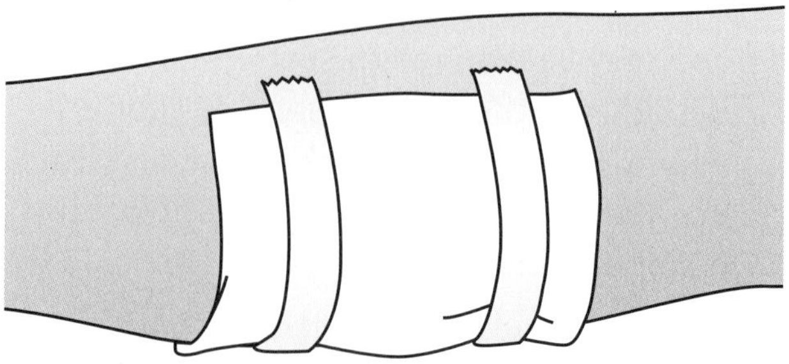

Fig. 17-28.

10. Remove and dispose of gloves properly.
11. Make resident comfortable. Make sure sheets are free from wrinkles and the bed free from crumbs.
12. Return bed to appropriate position. Remove privacy measures.
13. Before leaving, place call light within resident's reach.
14. Wash your hands.
15. Report any changes in resident to the nurse.
16. Document procedure using facility guidelines.

The History of the Rubber Glove

William Halsted developed rubber gloves to protect his nurse's (and future wife's) hands in the early 20th century. A student suggested that surgeons adopt them. The gloves were very thick, though. Many surgeons would not wear them. Some surgeons wore cloth gloves over the rubber. Gradually, rubber gloves became thinner and easier to wear. Today's gloves are made of different materials, such as latex.

8. Discuss guidelines for non-sterile bandages

Non-sterile or elastic bandages are used to hold dressing in place, secure splints, and support and protect body parts. In addition, these bandages may decrease swelling that occurs with an injury.

When using non-sterile bandages, they should be applied snug enough to control bleeding and to prevent movement of dressings. However, it is important that the bandage is not wrapped too tightly. Wrapping a bandage too tightly can decrease circulation. A resident with a non-sterile bandage should be checked 15 minutes after the bandage is first applied.

Signs and symptoms of poor circulation include:

- swelling
- bluish, or cyanotic, skin
- numbness
- tingling
- skin cold to touch
- pain or discomfort

Loosen the bandage if you note any signs of poor circulation. Tell the nurse immediately.

9. List care guidelines for a resident who is on an IV

IV stands for **intravenous**, or into a vein. A resident with an IV receives medication, nutrition, or fluids through a vein. When a doctor prescribes an IV, a nurse inserts a needle or tube into a vein. This gives direct access to the bloodstream. Medication, nutrition, or fluids either drip from a bag suspended on a pole or are pumped by a portable pump through a tube and into the vein (Fig. 17-29). Some residents with chronic conditions have a permanent opening for IVs. It has been surgically created to allow easy access for IV fluids. Nursing assistants never insert or remove IV lines. You will not be responsible for care of the IV site. Your only responsibility for IV care is to report and document any observations of changes or problems with the IV.

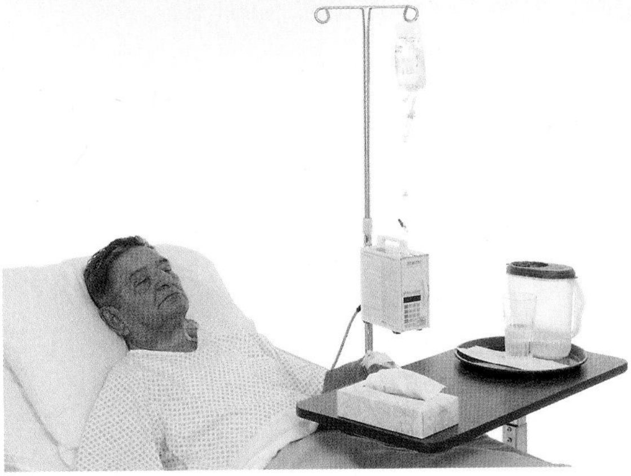

Fig. 17-29. A resident with an IV.

OBSERVING AND REPORTING
IVs

- O&R The tube/needle falls out or is removed.
- O&R The tubing disconnects.
- O&R The dressing around the IV site is loose or not intact.
- O&R Blood is in the tubing or around the site of the IV.
- O&R The site is swollen or discolored.
- O&R The resident reports pain.
- O&R The bag is broken, or the level of fluid does not seem to decrease.
- O&R The IV fluid is not dripping.
- O&R The IV fluid is nearly gone.
- O&R The pump beeps, indicating a problem.

Do not do any of these when caring for a resident with an IV:

- take a blood pressure in an arm with an IV
- get the IV site wet
- pull on or catch the tubing in anything, such as clothing
- leave the tubing kinked
- lower the IV bag below the IV site
- touch the clamp
- disconnect IV from pump or turn off alarm

Chapter Review

1. List five vital signs that must be monitored.
2. What temperature site is considered to be the most accurate?
3. Under what conditions should you not take an oral temperature?
4. What is the most common site for monitoring the pulse? Where is it located?
5. List the normal pulse rate for adults.
6. Where is the apical pulse located?
7. What are the two parts of measuring blood pressure?
8. Under what conditions should you not measure blood pressure on an arm?
9. List five measures to reduce pain.
10. List five questions you can ask if a resident reports pain.
11. What are some benefits of applying heat? What are some benefits of applying cold?
12. What signs should you watch for at the site of a heat or cold application?
13. When are non-sterile dressings usually used?
14. List six signs that a non-sterile bandage is causing decreased circulation.
15. What is an NA's responsibility with IV care?
16. List seven things to observe and report about an IV.

Chapter 18 Common Chronic and Acute Conditions

Residents in long-term care may have many different diseases and conditions. Diseases and conditions are either acute or chronic. **Acute** means an illness has severe symptoms. An acute illness is short-term. **Chronic** means the disease or condition is long-term or long-lasting. Symptoms are managed. Chronic conditions are usually less severe from day to day. Chronic conditions may have short periods of severity. The person may be hospitalized to stabilize the disease. This book describes diseases or conditions according to the body system in which they are located. Pressure sores, a common disorder of the integumentary system, are covered in chapter 13.

1. Describe common diseases and disorders of the musculoskeletal system

Arthritis

Arthritis is a general term. It refers to **inflammation**, or swelling, of the joints. It causes stiffness, pain, and decreased mobility. Arthritis may be the result of aging, injury, or an autoimmune illness. With an autoimmune illness, the body's immune system attacks normal tissue in the body. There are several types of arthritis.

Osteoarthritis is a common type of arthritis in the elderly. It may occur with aging or as the result of joint injury. Hips and knees, which are weight-bearing joints, are usually affected. Joints of the fingers, thumbs, and spine can also be affected. Pain and stiffness seem to increase in cold or damp weather.

Rheumatoid arthritis can affect people of all ages. Joints become red, swollen, and very painful (Fig. 18-1). Movement is restricted. Fever, fatigue, and weight loss are also symptoms. Rheumatoid arthritis usually affects the smaller joints first. It then progresses to larger ones. Other parts of the body that may be affected are the heart, lungs, eyes, kidneys, and skin.

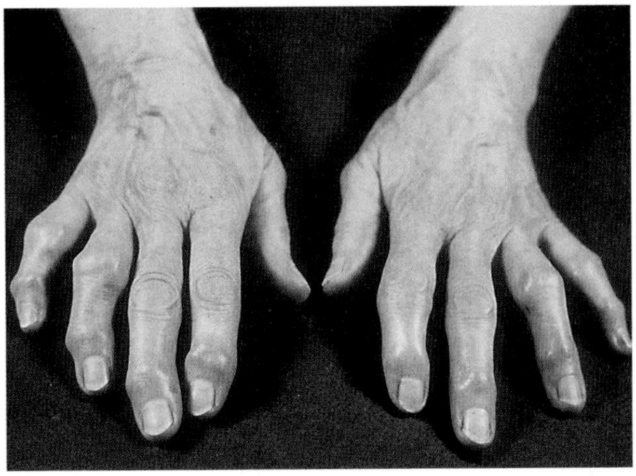

Fig. 18-1. **Rheumatoid arthritis. (Photo courtesy Frederick Miller, MD.)**

Arthritis is generally treated with some or all of these:

- anti-inflammatory medications such as aspirin or ibuprofen
- local applications of heat to reduce swelling and pain
- range of motion exercises (chapter 21)
- regular exercise and/or activity routines
- diet to reduce weight or maintain strength

GUIDELINES

Caring for Residents with Arthritis

- Watch for stomach irritation or heartburn from aspirin or ibuprofen. Some residents cannot take these medications. Report signs of stomach irritation immediately.
- Encourage activity. Gentle activity can help reduce the effects of arthritis. Follow care plan instructions carefully. Use canes or other walking aids as needed.
- Adapt activities of daily living (ADLs) to allow independence. Many devices are available to help residents to bathe, dress, and feed themselves even when they have arthritis (chapter 21).
- Choose clothing that is easy to put on and fasten. Encourage use of handrails and safety bars in the bathroom.
- Special utensils make it easier for residents to feed themselves (Fig. 18-2).

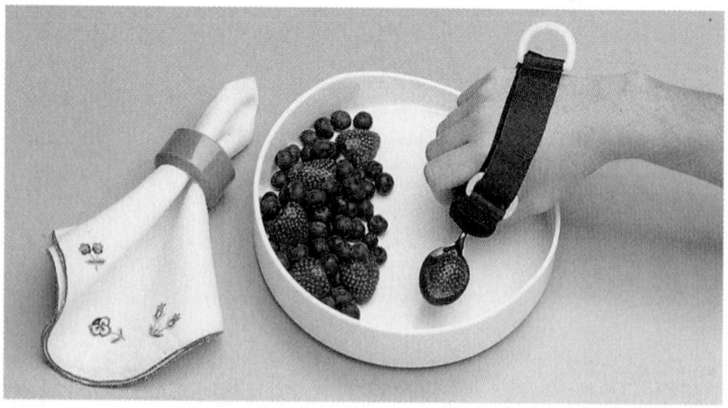

Fig. 18-2. **Special equipment can help a person with arthritis be independent. (Photo courtesy of North Coast Medical, Inc., www.ncmedical.com, 800-821-9319.)**

- Treat each resident as an individual. Arthritis is very common among elderly residents. Do not assume that each resident has the same symptoms and needs the same care.
- Help resident's self-esteem. Encourage self-care. Have a positive attitude. Listen to the resident's feelings. You can help him or her be independent for as long as possible.

Osteoporosis

Osteoporosis causes bones to become brittle. Brittle bones can break easily. Weakness in the bones may be due to age, lack of hormones, not enough calcium in bones, alcohol, or lack of exercise. NAs must move residents with osteoporosis very carefully.

Osteoporosis is more common in women after menopause. **Menopause** is the stopping of menstrual periods. Extra calcium and regular exercise can help prevent osteoporosis. Medication, calcium, and fluoride supplements are used to treat osteoporosis.

Signs and symptoms of osteoporosis include:

- low back pain
- loss of height
- stooped posture (Fig. 18-3)

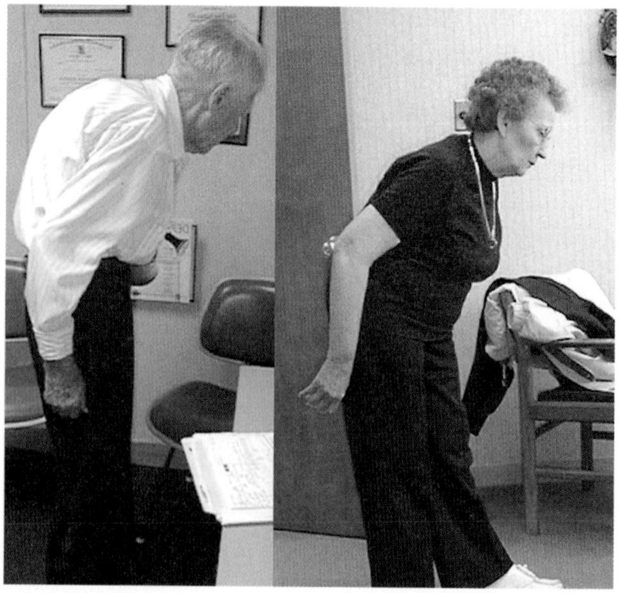

Fig. 18-3. **Stooped posture, or "dowager's hump" is a common sign of osteoporosis. (Photos courtesy of Jeffrey T. Behr, MD.)**

Fractures

Fractures are broken bones. They are caused by accidents or by osteoporosis. Preventing falls, which can lead to fractures, is very important. Fractures of arms, elbows, legs, and hips are the most common. Signs and symptoms of a fracture are pain, swelling, bruising, changes in skin color at the site, and limited movement.

When bones are fractured, they must be placed in alignment to heal. The body grows new bone tissue and fuses the sections of fractured bone together. The bone must be unable to move for this healing to occur. This is often accomplished by a cast.

Two common types of casts are made of plaster and fiberglass. Plaster casts take longer to dry, up to one to two days. Fiberglass casts dry quickly. A cast must be completely dry before a person can bear weight on it. As a cast dries, it gives off heat. This heat must escape or it will burn the skin. Never cover a cast until it has completely dried.

GUIDELINES
Cast Care

- Do not cover a cast until it is dry. Follow instructions with position changes. Help the resident change positions as ordered. This allows the cast to dry evenly. Do not place the cast on a hard surface. Place it on pillows. A hard surface alters the shape of the cast. Use the palms of the hands to lift the cast. Fingers will dent it. Dents will cause pressure on the resident's skin.
- Tell the nurse prior to moving/exercising if pain medication is needed. Help with range of motion exercises as ordered (chapter 21). Allow plenty of time for movement.
- Elevate the extremity that is in a cast. This helps stop swelling (Fig. 18-4).
- Observe the affected extremity for redness, pale or blue-tinged skin, cast tightness or pressure, swelling, sores, skin that feels hot or cold, pain, burning, numbness or tingling, drainage, bleeding, or odor. Compare to the extremity that does not have a cast. Report any of these to the nurse, along with any signs of infection, such as fever or chills.
- Protect the skin from the rough edges of the cast. The stocking that lines the inside of the cast can be pulled up and over the edges and secured with tape. Tell the nurse if cast edges irritate the resident's skin.
- Keep the cast dry. Wet casts lose their shape. Keep the cast clean.
- Do not insert, or allow the resident to insert, anything inside the cast, even when skin itches. Pointed or blunt objects may injure dry and fragile skin. Skin can become infected under the cast.
- Assist resident with cane, walker, or crutches as needed (chapter 21).
- Use bed cradles as needed.

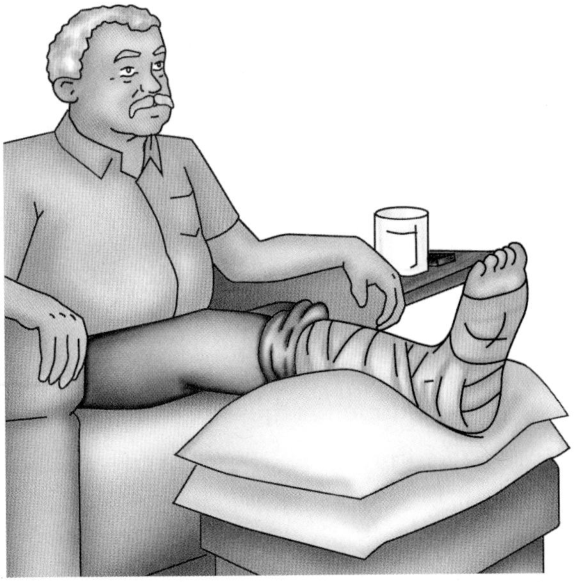

Fig. 18-4. **To stop swelling, elevate the extremity that is in a cast.**

Fragile bones mean fragile residents.

When a person has osteoporosis, bones are weak and fragile. Bones can break with a simple movement. It is important to understand this. Movements that you take for granted, such as turning in bed, sitting down, or standing can cause fragile bones to break. Be very careful when moving residents.

Hip Fractures

Weakened bones make hip fractures more common (Fig. 18-5). A sudden fall can result in a fractured hip. These take months to heal. Preventing falls is very important. Hip fractures can also occur when weakened bones fracture and cause a fall. A hip fracture is a serious condition. The elderly heal slowly. They are also at risk for secondary illnesses and disabilities.

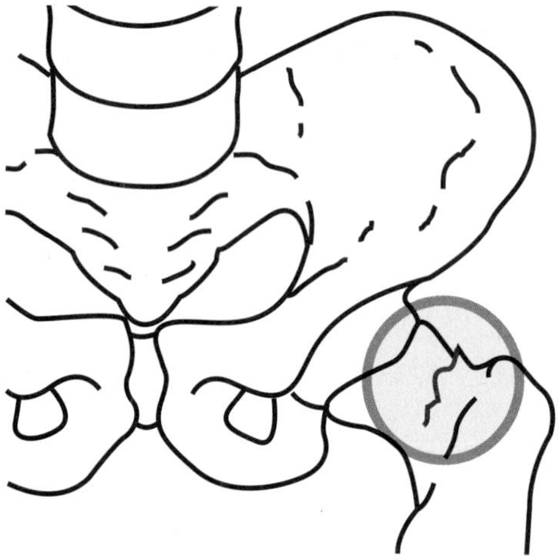

Fig. 18-5. **A fractured hip.**

Most fractured hips need surgery. Total hip replacement is surgery that replaces the head of the long bone of the leg (femur) where it joins the hip. This is done for these reasons:

- Fractured hip from an injury or fall which does not heal properly.
- Weakened hip due to aging.
- Hip is painful and stiff because the joint is weak. The bones are no longer strong enough to bear the person's weight.

The surgery is done through a cut at the hip. An artificial ball and socket joint replaces the hip. After the surgery, the resident cannot stand on that leg while the hip heals. A physical therapist will help after surgery. The goals of care include slowly strengthening the hip muscles and getting the resident walking on that leg.

Be familiar with the resident's care plan. It will state when the resident may begin putting weight on the hip. It will also tell how much the resident is able to do. It is important to help with personal care and using assistive devices, such as walkers or canes.

GUIDELINES
Hip Replacement Care

- Keep often-used items, such as medications, telephone, tissues, call light, and water, within easy reach. Avoid placing items in high places.
- Dress the affected side first.
- Never rush the resident. Use praise and encouragement often. Do this even for small tasks.
- Ask the nurse to give pain medication prior to moving and positioning if needed.
- Have the resident sit to do tasks if allowed. This saves energy.
- Follow the care plan exactly, even if the resident wants to do more. Follow orders for weight-bearing. An order may be written as partial weight bearing (PWB) or non-weight bearing (NWB). **Partial weight bearing** means the resident is able to support some weight on one or both legs. **Non-weight bearing** means the resident is unable to support any weight on one or both legs. Assist resident as needed with cane, walker, or crutches (chapter 21).
- Never perform range of motion exercises on a leg on the side of a hip replacement unless directed by the nurse.

- Caution the resident not to cross legs or turn toes inward. The hip cannot be bent more than 90-degrees. The hip cannot be turned inward (Fig. 18-6). Sometimes an order will limit the operated hip from being turned outward.

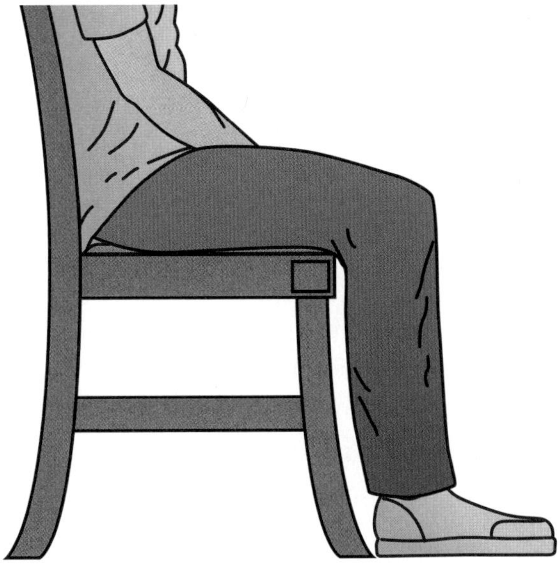

***Fig. 18-6.* The hip must maintain a 90-degree angle in the sitting position.**

OBSERVING AND REPORTING
Hip Replacement

Report any of these to the nurse:

- if the incision is red, draining, bleeding, or warm to the touch
- an increase in pain
- numbness or tingling
- abnormal vital signs, especially change in temperature
- if the resident cannot use equipment properly and safely
- if the resident is not following doctor's orders for activity and exercise
- any problems with appetite

Knee Replacement

Knee replacement is the surgical insertion of a prosthetic knee. Some reasons why it is performed are:

- to relieve severe pain
- to restore motion to a knee damaged by injury or arthritis
- to help stabilize a knee that buckles or gives out repeatedly

Care is similar to that for the hip replacement. However, the recovery time is much shorter. These residents have more ability to care for themselves. Keep these guidelines in mind:

GUIDELINES
Knee Replacement

- To prevent blood clots, apply special stockings as ordered. One type is a compression stocking. It is a plastic, air-filled, sleeve-like device that is applied to the legs and hooked to a machine. This machine inflates and deflates on its own. It acts in the same way that the muscles usually do under normal activity circumstances. The sleeves are normally applied after surgery while the resident is in bed.

  Anti-embolic stockings are another type of special stocking. They aid circulation. See later in the chapter for more information on this type of stocking.
- Perform ankle pumps as ordered. These are simple exercises that promote circulation to the legs. Ankle pumps are done by raising the toes and feet toward the ceiling and lowering them again.
- Encourage fluids, especially cranberry and orange juice, which contain Vitamin C, to prevent urinary tract infections (UTIs).
- Assist with deep breathing exercises as ordered.
- Ask the nurse to give pain medication prior to moving and positioning if needed.

Report to the nurse if you notice redness, swelling, heat, or deep tenderness in one or both calves.

Traction

A cast or traction may also be used to immobilize fractured hips. Traction is also used for other types of broken bones. Traction may be used to reduce pressure and pain due to injury or to relieve muscle spasms (Fig. 18-7).

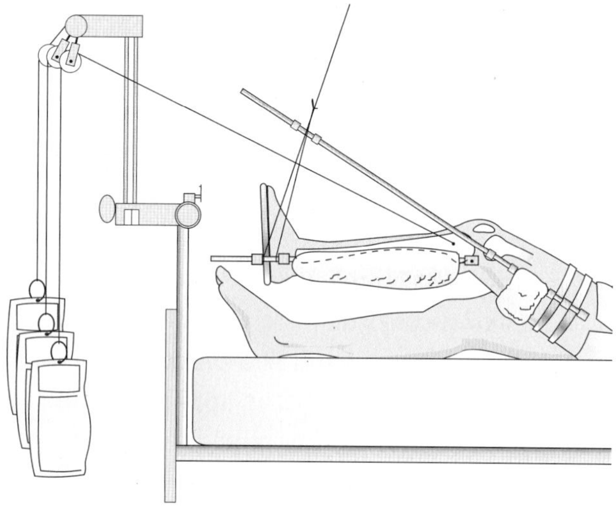

Fig. 18-7. **NAs must never disconnect a traction assembly. The weights must be kept off the floor.**

A resident in traction will need special care. The traction assembly must never be disconnected. Keep the weights off the floor. Do not add or remove weights for any reason.

Keep the resident in good alignment. Good skin care is essential. Position the resident as directed by the nurse. Skin will rapidly deteriorate over pressure points. Perform range of motion exercises as directed (chapter 21).

OBSERVING AND REPORTING
Traction

Report these to the nurse:

- redness, drainage, bleeding, or sores
- wetness on sling
- odor around the sling or boot
- numbness or tingling
- pain, burning, pressure, swelling
- changes in skin temperature
- resident sliding down in bed
- weights touching floor

Muscular Dystrophy (MD)

MD refers to several progressive diseases that cause various disabilities. MD is an inherited disease. It causes a gradual wasting of muscle and weakness and deformity. The muscles of the hands are impaired. There may be twitching of the hand and arm muscles. Legs may be weak and stiff. The person may be in a wheelchair.

Most forms of MD are present at birth or during childhood. Many forms of MD are very slow to progress. Often people with MD can live to middle or even late adulthood.

In the early stages of this disease, help with ADLs or range of motion exercises. In the more advanced stages, help with skin care and positioning. Do ADLs for the resident.

Amputations

Amputation is the removal of some or all of a body part. It is usually a foot, hand, arm or leg. Amputation may be the result of an injury or disease.

After amputation, some people feel that the limb is still there. They may feel pain in the part that has been amputated. This is called **phantom sensation**. It may last for a short time or for years. The pain or sensation is caused by remaining nerve endings. It is real. It should not be ignored or made fun of.

A **prosthesis** is an artificial body part. It replaces a missing body part, such as an eye, arm, hand, foot, or leg. The prosthesis will be custom-fitted to the resident (Fig. 18-8). When a body part has been amputated, day-to-day activities may be limited. A resident will need special care to help him adjust to these changes. When the condition is new and a prosthesis has been ordered, a physical and/ or occupational therapist may work with the resident.

You will help with ADLs and ambulation. You must know how to care for the limb and how to use a prosthesis. Prostheses are expensive. Take great care with them.

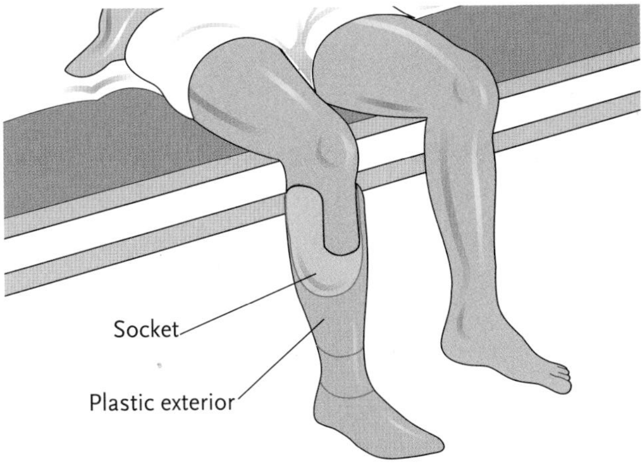

Fig. 18-8. **Prostheses are specially fitted, expensive pieces of equipment.**

GUIDELINES
Amputation and Prosthesis Care

- Residents who have had a body part amputated must make many physical, psychological, social, and occupational adjustments to their disability. Be supportive.
- Help residents with ADLs.
- Follow the care plan for care of the prosthesis and the limb.
- A nurse or therapist will demonstrate application of a prosthesis. Follow instructions to apply and remove the prosthesis. Follow the manufacturer's care directions.
- Keep a prosthesis and the skin under it dry and clean.
- If ordered, apply a stump sock before putting on the prosthesis.
- Observe the skin on stump. Watch for signs of skin breakdown caused by pressure and abrasion.
- Report any redness or open areas.
- Check with the nurse prior to exercising to see if pain medication is needed.
- Phantom sensation is real pain and should be treated that way.
- Never try to fix a prosthesis. Report any problems to the nurse.
- Do not show negative feelings about the stump during care.
- Again, take care when handling a prosthesis. They are very expensive (an artificial leg may cost from $10,000 to $20,000).

An Early Method of Amputation

Fabricus Hildanus [1560-1624] performed an early form of amputation. Hildanus used a knife that had been heated red-hot. He developed the method of cutting above the gangrene in a leg. This improved the survival rate for people with these injuries.

Artificial Eyes

Artificial eyes are needed for people who have lost an eye to cancer, disease, or injury. An artificial eye is a type of prosthesis. Some artificial eyes will be surgically implanted into the eye socket. It will not be removed for cleaning. Others are removed for cleaning and storage. Regular removal of the eye at night is not always recommended unless there are special problems, such as discomfort. The resident will usually be taught how to remove, clean, and insert the eye.

Artificial eyes are made of glass or plastic. They must be handled very carefully. Never clean or soak the eye in alcohol. It will crack the plastic and destroy it. If the eye must be removed, store it in water or saline. This will keep deposits from drying on the surface.

Artificial eyes are held in by suction. They will come out quickly when pressure is applied below the lower eyelid. It can be reinserted by placing it far under the upper eyelid. Pull down on lower eyelid. The eye should slide into place.

Follow directions exactly for cleaning an artificial eye. It may be washed in mild soap and warm water. Do not use abrasives, such as cleaners or tooth polish, or other agents, such as alcohol, Lysol™, or iodine. You may rub it with moist gauze to remove surface secretions. Be sure you rinse it well.

If the eye is to be removed and not reinserted, line an eye cup or basin with a soft cloth or a piece of 4 x 4 gauze. This prevents scratches and damage. Fill with water or saline solution. Place the eye in the container. Close the container. Label the container with the resident's name and room number.

If the eye is removed, wash the eye socket with warm water or saline. Use a clean gauze square to clean it. Clean the eyelid. Wipe gently from inner corner (canthus) outward. Use a clean cotton ball for each eye.

2. Describe common diseases and disorders of the nervous system

Chapter 19 has information on dementia and Alzheimer's disease. Dementia and Alzheimer's disease are common disorders of the nervous system.

Stroke

The medical term for a stroke is a **cerebral vascular accident** (CVA). CVA, or **stroke**, is caused when the blood supply to the brain is cut off suddenly by a clot or a ruptured blood vessel (Fig. 18-9).

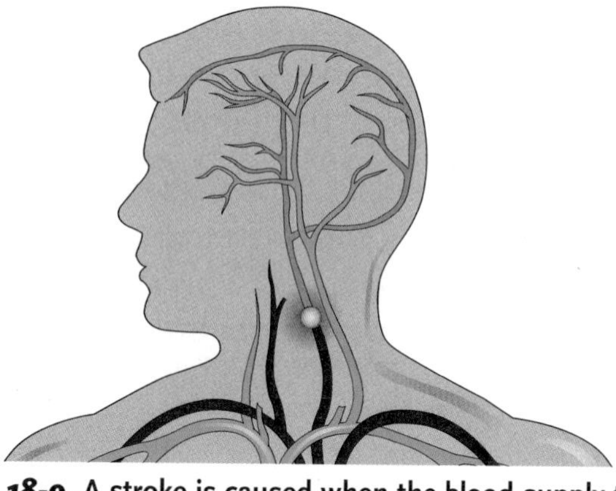

Fig. 18-9. **A stroke is caused when the blood supply to the brain is cut off suddenly by a clot or ruptured blood vessel.**

Without blood, part of the brain gets no oxygen. Brain cells die. Brain tissue is further damaged by leaking blood, clots, and swelling. They cause pressure on surrounding areas of healthy tissue.

A **transient ischemic attack**, or TIA, is a warning sign of a CVA. It is the result of a temporary lack of oxygen in the brain. Symptoms may last up to 24 hours. They include tingling, weakness, confusion, or some loss of movement in an extremity. These symptoms should not be ignored. Report any of these symptoms to the nurse immediately.

A stroke may be preceded by symptoms. They include dizziness, ringing in the ears, headache, nausea, vomiting, slurring of words, and loss of memory. These should be reported immediately. Signs that a stroke is occurring include the following: loss of consciousness; redness in the face; noisy breathing; seizures; loss of bowel and bladder control; hemiplegia; hemiparesis; aphasia; use of inappropriate words; high blood pressure; and slow pulse rate. **Hemiplegia** is paralysis on one side of the body. **Hemiparesis** is weakness on one side of the body. **Aphasia** is the inability to speak or to speak clearly.

The two sides of the brain control different functions. Symptoms depend on which side of the brain the stroke affected. Weaknesses on the right side show that the left side of the brain was affected. Weaknesses on the left side show that the right side of the brain was affected.

Strokes can be mild or severe. Afterward, a resident may experience any of these problems:

- hemiparesis
- hemiplegia
- tendency to ignore a weak or paralyzed side of the body
- aphasia

- inability to express needs to others through speech or writing, called expressive aphasia
- trouble understanding spoken or written words
- loss of sensations, such as temperature or touch
- loss of bowel or bladder control
- confusion
- laughing or crying without any reason, or when it is inappropriate, called **emotional lability**
- poor judgment
- memory loss
- loss of thinking and learning abilities
- trouble swallowing, called **dysphagia**

If the stroke was mild, the resident may experience few, if any, of these complications. Physical therapy may help regain physical abilities. Speech and occupational therapy can also help a person learn to communicate and perform ADLs again.

GUIDELINES

Residents Recovering from Stroke

A resident with paralysis, weakness, or loss of movement will usually have physical or occupational therapy. Residents may also perform leg exercises to aid circulation. Safety is always important when residents are exercising.

- Adapt procedures when caring for residents with one-sided paralysis or weakness. Carefully assist with shaving, grooming, and bathing. Diminished sensation or paralysis causes lack of awareness about such things as water temperature and sharpness of razors. Take care so that injury does not occur.
- When helping with transfers or walking, stand on the weaker side. Support the weaker side. Lead with the stronger side (Fig. 18-10). Always use a gait belt for safety.

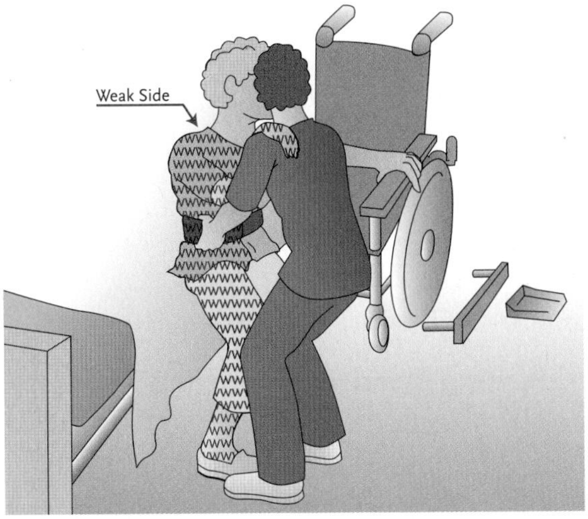

Fig. 18-10. **When helping a resident transfer, support the weak side. Lead with the stronger side.**

- Never refer to the weaker side as the "bad side." Do not talk about the "bad" leg or arm. Use the terms "weaker" or "involved" to refer to the side with paralysis.
- If residents have a loss of touch or sensation, check for potentially harmful situations (for example, heat and sharp objects). If residents are unable to sense or move part of body, check and change positioning to prevent pressure sores.
- Residents with speech loss or communication problems may have speech therapy. You may be asked to help. This may include helping residents recognize written words or spoken words. Speech therapists will also evaluate a resident's swallowing ability. They will decide if therapy or thickened liquids are needed.
- Confusion and memory loss are upsetting. Residents often cry for no reason after suffering a stroke. Be very patient and understanding. Keep a routine of care. This helps residents feel more secure.

Here are ways to help residents recovering from stroke:

- Encourage independence and self-esteem. Let the resident do things for herself whenever possible even if you could do a better or faster job.

- Make tasks less difficult for the resident.
- Notice and praise residents' efforts to do things for themselves even when they are unsuccessful.
- Praise even the smallest successes. This builds confidence.

Parkinson's Disease

Parkinson's disease is a progressive disease. It causes a section of the brain to degenerate. It affects the muscles, causing them to become stiff. It causes stooped posture and a shuffling gait, or walk. It can also cause pill-rolling. This is moving the thumb and first finger together like rolling a pill. Tremors or shaking make it hard for a person to perform ADLs such as eating and bathing. A person with Parkinson's may have a mask-like facial expression.

GUIDELINES
Parkinson's Disease

- Residents are at a high risk for falls. Protect residents from any unsafe areas and conditions.
- Help with ADLs as needed.
- Assist with range of motion exercises exactly as ordered to prevent contractures and to strengthen muscles.
- Encourage self-care. Be patient with self-care and communication. Allow the resident time to do and say things. Listen.

Multiple Sclerosis (MS)

Multiple sclerosis is a progressive disease. It affects the central nervous system. When a person has MS, the protective covering for the nerves, spinal cord, and white matter of the brain breaks down over time. Without this covering, or sheath, nerves cannot send messages to and from the brain in a normal way.

Residents with MS have varying abilities (Fig. 18-11). MS is usually diagnosed when a person is in his or her early twenties to thirties. It progresses slowly and unpredictably. Symptoms include blurred vision, fatigue, tremors, poor balance, and trouble walking. Weakness, numbness, tingling, incontinence, and behavior changes are also symptoms. MS can cause blindness, contractures, and loss of function in the arms and legs.

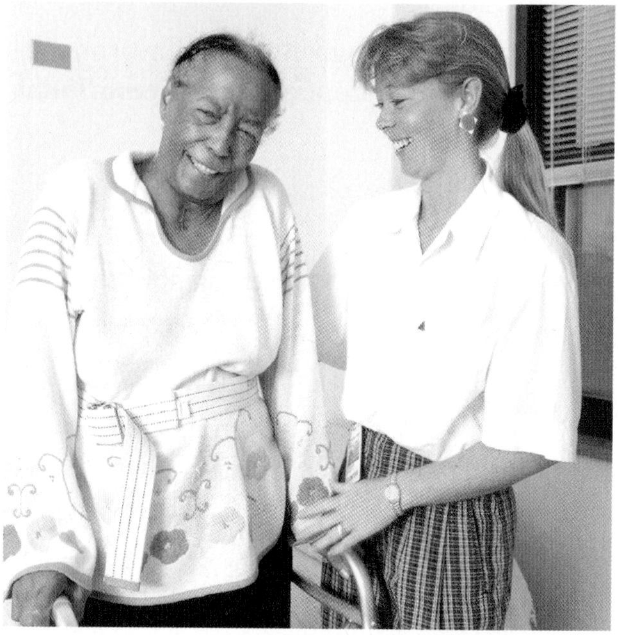

Fig. 18-11. **MS can cause a range of problems. These include fatigue, poor balance, and trouble walking.**

GUIDELINES
Multiple Sclerosis

- Help with ADLs.
- Be patient with self-care and movement.
- Allow enough time for tasks. Offer rest periods as necessary.
- Give a resident plenty of time to communicate. People with MS may have trouble forming their thoughts. Be patient while he or she is thinking. Do not rush him or her.
- Prevent falls due to a lack of coordination, fatigue, or vision problems.
- Stress can worsen the effects of MS. Be calm. Listen to residents when they want to talk.
- Encourage proper diet. Offer plenty of fluids.

- Give excellent skin care to prevent pressure sores.
- Assist with range of motion exercises exactly as ordered to prevent contractures and to strengthen muscles.

Head and Spinal Cord Injuries

Diving, sports injuries, falls, car and motorcycle accidents, industrial accidents, war, and criminal violence are common causes of injuries. Problems from these injuries range from mild confusion or memory loss to coma, paralysis, and death.

Head injuries can cause permanent brain damage. Residents who have had a head injury may have these problems: mental retardation, personality changes, trouble breathing, seizures, coma, memory loss, loss of consciousness, paresis, and paralysis. **Paresis** is paralysis, or loss of ability, of only part of the body. Often, paresis describes a weakness or loss of ability on one side of the body.

The effects of spinal cord injuries vary. They depend on the force of impact and where the spine is injured. The higher the injury, the greater the loss of function. People with head and spinal cord injuries may have **paraplegia**. This is a loss of function of lower body and legs. These injuries may also cause **quadriplegia**. The person is then unable to use his legs, trunk, and arms (Fig. 18-12).

Rehabilitation is needed for residents with spinal cord injuries. It will help them keep muscle function and live as independently as possible. Residents will need emotional support as they adjust. Their specific needs will vary.

GUIDELINES
Head or Spinal Cord Injury

- Give emotional support, as well as physical help. Frustration and anger may surface as they deal with the reality of their lives. Do not take it personally.

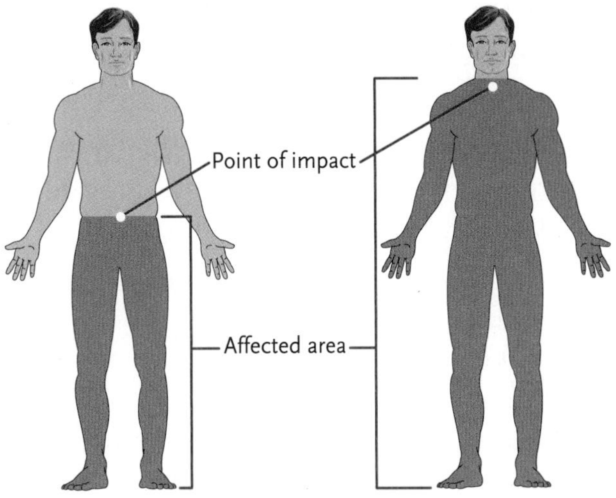

Fig. 18-12.

- Be patient with all care.
- Safety is very important. Be very careful that residents do not fall or burn themselves. Because these residents have no sensation, they cannot feel a burn.
- Give good skin care. It is needed to prevent pressure sores when mobility is limited.
- Assist residents to change positions at least every two hours to prevent pressure sores. Be gentle when turning and repositioning.
- Perform passive range of motion exercises exactly as ordered to prevent contractures and to strengthen muscles.
- Allow as much independence as possible with ADLs.
- Immobility leads to constipation. Encourage fluids and proper diet—high in fiber, if ordered.
- Loss of control of urination leads to the need of a catheter. Urinary tract infections are common. Encourage a high intake of fluids and give extra catheter care as needed.
- Lack of activity leads to poor circulation and fatigue. You may be directed to use special stockings to help increase circulation. Offer rest periods as necessary.

- Difficulty coughing and shallow breathing can lead to pneumonia. Encourage deep breathing exercises as ordered.
- Male residents may have involuntary erections. These are not deliberate. Provide for privacy and be sensitive to this.
- Assist with bowel and bladder training if needed.

Epilepsy

Epilepsy is an illness of the brain that causes seizures. Epileptic seizures can be mild tremors or brief blackouts. They may be violent convulsions lasting several minutes. The cause of most cases of epilepsy is unknown. Excessive alcohol use, substance abuse, brain tumors, or injuries can sometimes cause it.

During a seizure, the main goal is to make the resident safe. Move furniture away to prevent injury. If a pillow is nearby, place it under his or her head. Do not try to restrain the person. Do not force anything between the person's teeth. Do not place your hands in his or her mouth for any reason. You could be bitten. Do not give liquids. Notice the time it begins so that you can report the length of the seizure.

Vision Impairment

As you learned in chapter 4, vision impairment can affect people of all ages. Some vision impairment creates the need for people to wear corrective lenses. These can be contact lenses or eyeglasses (Fig. 18-13). **Farsightedness** is the ability to see distant objects better than objects nearby. It develops in most people as they age. **Nearsightedness** is the ability to see things near but not far. It may occur in younger persons.

Some people need eyeglasses all the time. Others only need them to read or for things such as driving that require seeing distant objects. People over the age of 40 are at risk for certain serious vision problems. These include

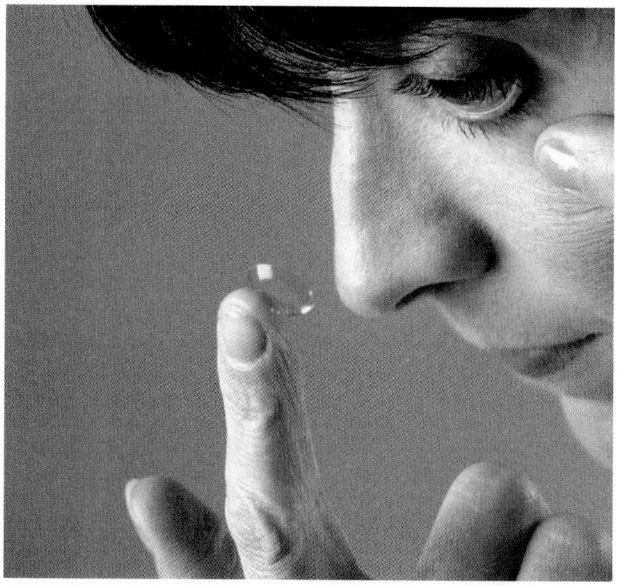

Fig. 18-13. **Contact lenses are made of many types of plastic. Some can be worn and disposed of daily. Others are worn for longer periods.**

cataracts and glaucoma. They can cause blindness. When a **cataract** develops, the lens of the eye becomes cloudy. This prevents light from entering the eye (Fig. 18-14). Vision blurs and dims initially. All vision is eventually lost. This can occur in one or both eyes. It is corrected with surgery. A permanent lens is usually implanted.

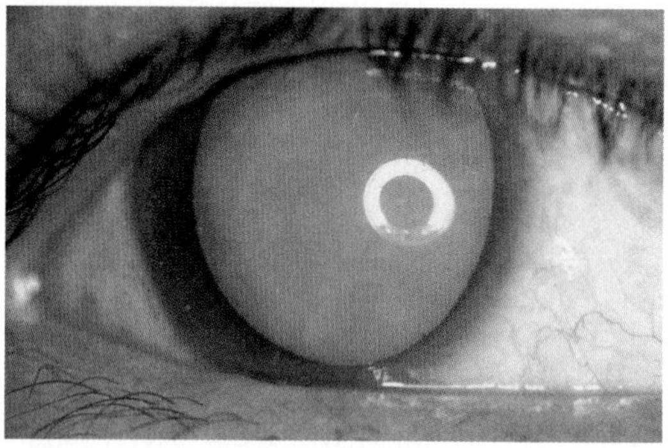

Fig. 18-14. **When a cataract develops, the lens of the eye becomes cloudy. This keeps light from entering the eye.**

Glaucoma causes the pressure in the eye to increase. This damages the optic nerve. It causes blindness. Glaucoma can occur suddenly, causing severe pain, nausea, and vomiting. It can also occur gradually. Symptoms include blurred vision, tunnel vision, and blue-green halos around lights. Glaucoma is treated with medication or surgery.

GUIDELINES
Vision Impairment

- Identify yourself as soon as you enter the room. Do not touch the resident until you do so.
- Do not leave a room without telling your resident that you are going.
- Do not move furniture and other objects.
- Provide good lighting at all times.
- When you enter a new room with the resident, show him or her where things are.
- Keep doors entirely open or entirely shut, never partly open.
- Use the face of an imaginary clock as a guide to explain the position of things in the room.
- If your resident needs help getting around, walk slightly ahead. Let the resident touch or grasp your arm lightly.
- Some residents may need help with completing menus, cutting food, and opening containers.
- Books on tape, large-print books, and Braille books are available. Reading Braille, however, takes a long time and takes special training (Fig. 18-15).

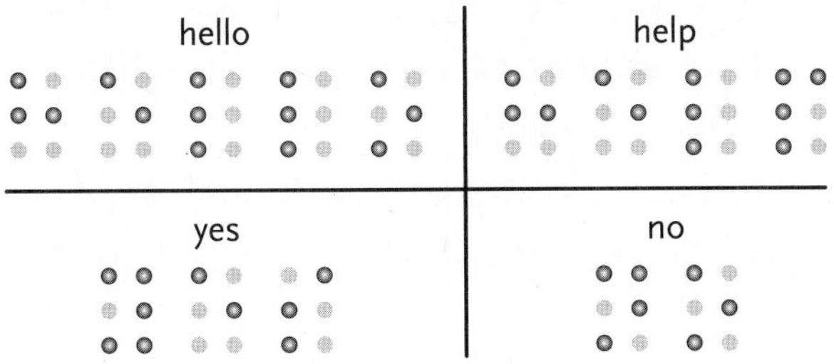

Fig. 18-15. **Examples of phrases in Braille.**

- If the resident has glasses, make sure they are clean and that he or she wears them. Clean glass lenses with water and soft tissue. Clean plastic lenses with cleaning fluid and a lens cloth. Also, make sure that glasses are in good condition and fit well. If they do not, tell the nurse.

Hearing Impairment

People who have impaired hearing or are deaf may have lost their hearing gradually. They also may have been born deaf. If they have a gradual hearing loss, they may not be aware of it. Signs of hearing loss include:

- speaking loudly
- leaning forward when a person is speaking
- cupping the ear to hear better
- responding inappropriately
- asking the speaker to repeat things
- speaking in a monotone
- avoiding social gatherings or acting irritable around people who are talking
- suspecting others of talking about them or of deliberately speaking softly

People who have hearing impairment may use a hearing aid. They may read lips, or use sign language. A **hearing aid** is a battery-operated device that amplifies sound. People with impaired hearing also closely observe the facial expressions and body language of others. This adds to their knowledge of what is being said.

GUIDELINES
Hearing Impairment

- If the person has a hearing aid, make sure he or she wears it and that it is on. Make sure hearing aid is positioned correctly and in the correct ear.
- There are many types of hearing aids. Follow manufacturer's directions for cleaning the hearing aid. In general, wash the external ear piece daily with soap and water. Put a little soap and water on a cloth, cotton swab, or pipe cleaner. Dry it thoroughly. Do not put it in water. Handle the hearing aid carefully. Do not drop it. Always keep it in the same safe place when it is not worn. Turn if off when it is not in use.

- Reduce or eliminate any background noise, such as televisions, radios, and loud speech. Close doors.
- Get the resident's attention before speaking. Do not startle residents from behind. Walk in front of them or touch them lightly on the arm to let them know you are near.
- Speak clearly and slowly. Do not shout. Communicate in good lighting. Directly face the person. He or she may be able to read lips.
- Lower the pitch of your voice.
- If your resident hears better out of one ear, speak to that side.
- Use short sentences and simple words. Repeat words or rephrase sentences and ideas. Write out instructions if needed.
- Avoid long, tiring conversations.
- Be supportive.

Some hearing-impaired residents have speech problems. They may be hard to understand. Do not pretend you understand if you do not. Ask your resident to repeat what was said. Watch the lips, face, and body language. Then tell your resident what you think you heard. You can also ask the resident to write down words.

3. Describe common diseases and disorders of the circulatory system

High Blood Pressure or Hypertension

When blood pressure is consistently 140/90 or higher, a person is diagnosed as having **hypertension**, or high blood pressure. If blood pressure is between 120/80 and 139/89 mmHg, it is called **prehypertension**. The person does not have high blood pressure now but is likely to develop it in the future.

A hardening and narrowing of the blood vessels causes high blood pressure (Fig. 18-16). It can also result from kidney disease, tumors of the adrenal gland, and pregnancy. High blood pressure can develop in persons of any age.

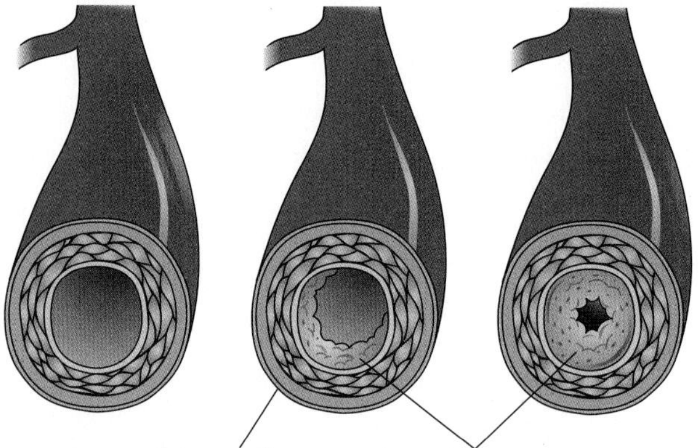

Fig. 18-16. **Arteries may harden or narrow because of a build-up of plaque. Hardened arteries cause high blood pressure.**

Signs and symptoms of high blood pressure are not always obvious. This is especially true in the early stages. Often it is only found when blood pressure is taken. People may complain of headaches, blurred vision, and dizziness.

GUIDELINES

High Blood Pressure

- High blood pressure can lead to serious conditions such as CVA, heart attack, kidney disease, or blindness. Treatment to control it is vital. Residents may take diuretics or medication that lowers cholesterol. **Diuretics** are drugs that reduce fluid in the body.
- Residents may also have a prescribed exercise program or be on a low-fat, low-sodium diet. You may need to take blood pressure often. You can also help by encouraging residents to follow their diet and exercise programs.

Coronary Artery Disease (CAD)

Coronary artery disease occurs when the blood vessels in the coronary arteries narrow. This lowers the supply of blood to the heart muscle and deprives it of oxygen and nutrients. Over time, as fatty deposits block the artery, the muscle that was supplied by the blood vessel dies. CAD can lead to heart attack or stroke.

The heart muscle that is not getting enough oxygen causes chest pain, or **angina pectoris**. The heart needs more oxygen during exercise, stress, excitement, or a heavy meal. In CAD, narrow blood vessels keep the extra blood with oxygen from getting to the heart (Fig. 18-17).

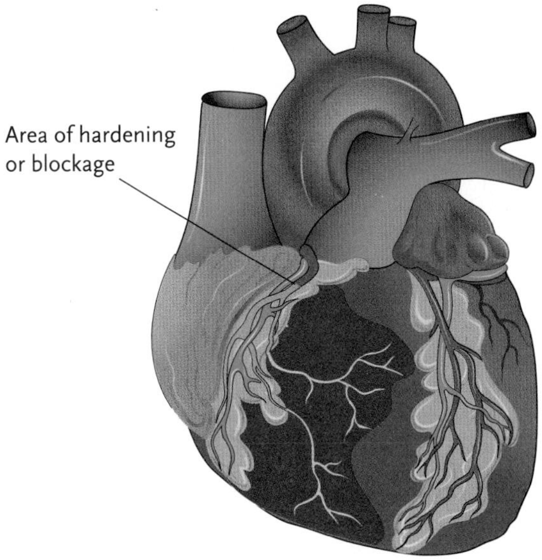

Fig. 18-17. **Angina pectoris results from the heart not getting enough oxygen.**

The pain of angina pectoris is usually described as pressure or tightness. It occurs in the left side or the center of the chest behind the sternum or breastbone. Some people have pain moving down the inside of the left arm or to the neck and left side of the jaw. A person suffering from angina pectoris may sweat or look pale. The person may feel dizzy and have trouble breathing.

GUIDELINES
Angina Pectoris

- Rest is extremely important. Rest reduces the heart's need for extra oxygen. It helps the blood flow return to normal, often within three to fifteen minutes.
- Medication is also needed to relax the walls of the coronary arteries. This lets them open and get more blood to the heart. This medication, **nitroglycerin**, is a small tablet that the resident places under the tongue. There it dissolves and is rapidly absorbed. Residents with angina pectoris should keep nitroglycerin on hand to use as soon as symptoms arise. NAs are not allowed to give any medication unless they have had special training. Tell the nurse if a resident needs help taking the medication. Nitroglycerin is also available as a patch. Do not remove the patch. Tell the nurse immediately if the patch comes off.
- Residents may also need to avoid heavy meals, overeating, intense exercise, and cold or hot and humid weather.

Heart Attack or Myocardial Infarction

When blood flow to the heart muscle is completely blocked, oxygen and nutrients fail to reach these cells (Fig. 18-18). Waste products are not removed. The muscle cells die. This is called a **heart attack** or **myocardial infarction** (MI). See chapter 7 for warning signs of a heart attack.

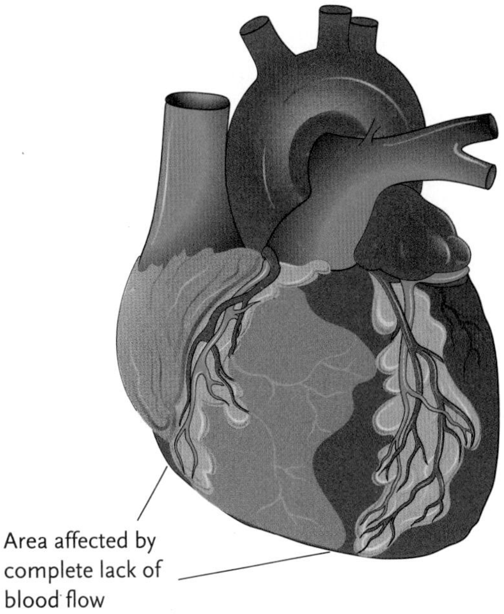

Fig. 18-18. **A heart attack occurs when blood flow to the heart or a part of the heart is cut off completely.**

GUIDELINES
Heart Attack

- Most residents will be placed on a regular exercise program.
- Residents may be on a diet that is low in fat and cholesterol and/or a low-sodium diet.
- Medications may be used to regulate heart rate and blood pressure.
- Quitting smoking will be encouraged.
- A stress management program may be started to help reduce stress levels.
- Residents recovering from a heart attack may need to avoid cold temperatures.

Congestive Heart Failure (CHF)

Coronary artery disease, heart attack, high blood pressure, or other disorders may harm the heart. When the heart muscle has been severely damaged, it fails to pump effectively. Blood backs up into the heart instead of circulating. This is called **congestive heart failure**, or CHF. It can occur on one or both sides of the heart.

Signs and symptoms of congestive heart failure are:

- trouble breathing; coughing or gurgling with breathing
- dizziness, confusion, and fainting
- pale or blue skin
- low blood pressure
- swelling of the feet and ankles (**edema**)
- bulging veins in the neck
- weight gain

GUIDELINES
CHF

- Although CHF is a serious illness, it can be treated and controlled. Medications can strengthen the heart muscle and improve its pumping.
- Medications help remove excess fluids. This means more trips to the bathroom. Answer call lights promptly.
- A low-sodium diet or a fluid restriction may be prescribed.
- A weakened heart pump may make it hard for residents to walk, carry items, or climb stairs. Limited activity or bedrest may be prescribed.
- Intake and output of fluids may need to be measured (see chapter 16).
- Resident may be weighed daily at the same time to note weight gain from fluid retention.
- Elastic leg stockings may be used to reduce swelling in feet and ankles (see procedure below).
- Range of motion exercises improve muscle tone when activity and exercise are limited (Fig. 18-19). See chapter 21 for range of motion information.
- Extra pillows may help residents who have trouble breathing.
- Help with personal care and ADLs as needed.

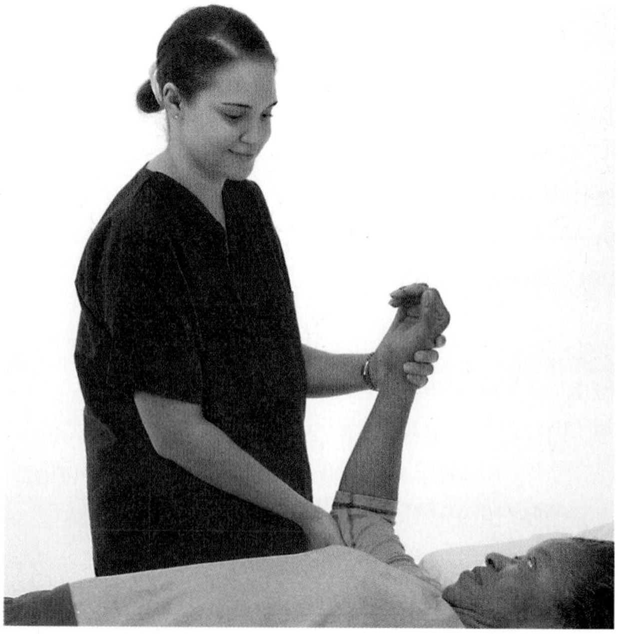

Fig. 18-19. **Range of motion exercises improve muscle tone.**

A common side effect of medications for CHF is dizziness. This may result from a lack of potassium. High-potassium foods and drinks such as bananas or raisins, orange juice, or other citrus juices can help. Follow the instructions in the care plan.

Peripheral Vascular Disease (PVD)

Peripheral vascular disease is a condition in which the legs, feet, arms, or hands do not have enough blood circulation. This is due to fatty deposits in the blood vessels that harden over time. Signs and symptoms include:

- cool or cold arms and legs
- swelling in hands or feet
- pale or bluish hands or feet (cyanosis)
- bluish nail beds
- ulcers of legs or feet

Some changes in health may lead to inactivity. A lack of mobility may contribute to PVD. For some cases of poor circulation to legs and feet, elastic stockings are ordered. These stockings help prevent swelling and blood clots. They aid circulation. These stockings are called anti-embolic hose. They need to be put on before the resident gets out of bed. Follow manufacturer's instructions and illustrations on how to put them on.

Putting a knee-high elastic stocking on a resident

Equipment: elastic stockings

1. Wash your hands.
2. Identify yourself by name. Identify resident by name.
3. Explain procedure to resident. Speak clearly, slowly, and directly. Maintain face-to-face contact whenever possible.
4. Provide for resident's privacy with curtain, screen, or door.
5. Turn stocking inside-out at least to heel area (Fig. 18-20).

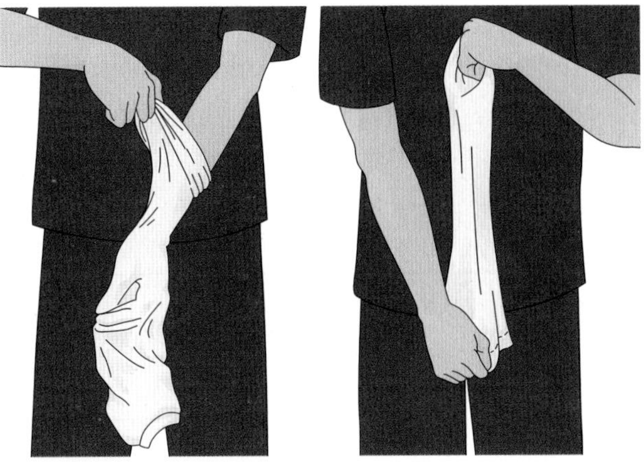

Fig. 18-20.

6. Gently place foot of stocking over toes, foot, and heel (Fig. 18-21).

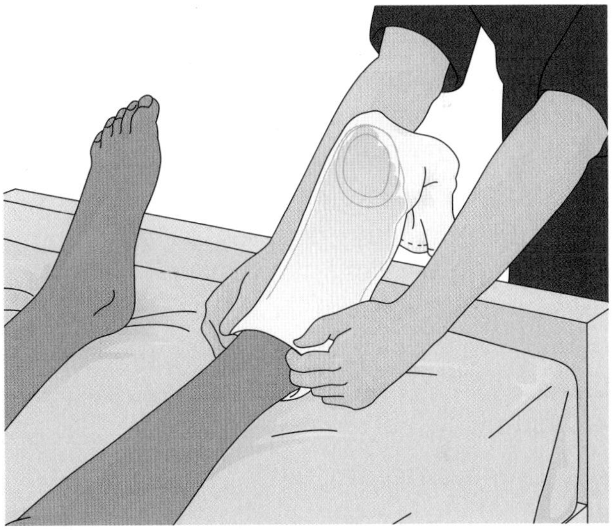

Fig. 18-21.

7. Gently pull top of stocking over foot, heel, and leg (Fig. 18-22).

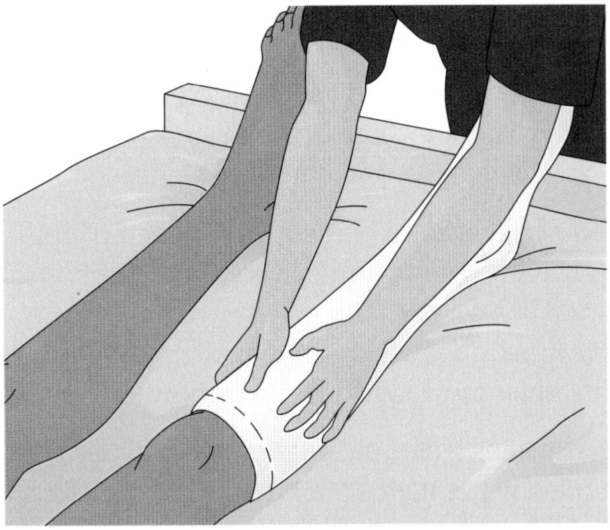

Fig. 18-22.

8. Make sure there are no twists or wrinkles in stocking after it is on. It must fit smoothly.
9. Before leaving, place call light within resident's reach.
10. Wash your hands.
11. Report any changes in resident to nurse.
12. Document procedure using facility guidelines.

4. Describe common diseases and disorders of the respiratory system

COPD

Chronic obstructive pulmonary disease (COPD) is a chronic disease. The resident may live for years with it but never be cured. Residents with COPD have trouble breathing, especially in getting air out of the lungs. There are four chronic lung diseases that are grouped under COPD:

- Chronic bronchitis
- Pulmonary emphysema
- Asthma
- Chronic bronchiectasis

Bronchitis is an irritation and inflammation of the lining of the bronchi. Acute bronchitis is usually caused by infection. It starts with an upper respiratory infection that spreads to the lungs. Mucus, dead cells, and other fluid produce a discharge. This results in a productive cough. Airborne irritants cause chronic bronchitis. These include cigarette smoke, car exhaust, allergens, and other pollutants.

Emphysema is a chronic disease of the lungs. It usually results from chronic bronchitis and smoking. People with emphysema have trouble breathing. Other symptoms are coughing, breathlessness, and a fast heartbeat.

Asthma is a chronic inflammatory disease. It occurs when the respiratory system reacts quickly and strongly to irritants, infection, cold air, or to allergens such as pollen and dust. Exercise and stress can also cause asthma attacks. The bronchi become irritated. They constrict, making it hard to breathe. As a response, the mucous membrane produces thick mucus. This further inhibits respiration. Air is trapped in the lungs, causing coughing and wheezing.

Bronchiectasis is a condition in which the tubes (bronchi) of the lungs are opened out too wide. A person may be born with it or may acquire it later in life as a result of chronic infections. This abnormal state is permanent. It causes coughing and shortness of breath.

Over time, a resident with any of these lung disorders becomes chronically ill and weakened. There is a high risk for acute lung infections, such as pneumonia. **Pneumonia** can be caused by a bacterial, viral, or fungal infection. Acute inflammation occurs in lung tissue. The affected person develops a high fever, chills, cough, chest pains, and rapid pulse. In the later stages, a thick discharge is produced by the mucous membrane. Recovery may take longer for older adults and persons with chronic illnesses.

Sometimes medications for lung conditions are given directly into the lungs with sprays or inhalers (Fig. 18-23).

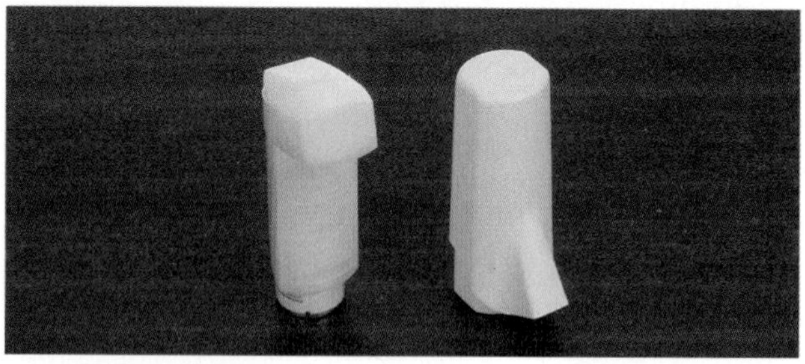

Fig. 18-23. **An inhaler.**

When the lungs and brain do not get enough oxygen, all body systems are affected. Residents may have a constant fear of not being able to breathe. This can cause them to sit upright to improve their ability to expand the lungs. These residents can have poor appetites. They usually do not get enough sleep. All of this can add to feelings of weakness and poor health. They may feel they have lost control of their bodies, and particularly their breathing. They may fear suffocation.

Residents with COPD may have these symptoms:

- chronic cough or wheeze
- trouble breathing, especially when inhaling and exhaling deeply
- shortness of breath, especially during physical effort
- pale or blue skin (cyanosis) or reddish-purple skin
- confusion
- general state of weakness
- trouble completing meals due to shortness of breath
- fear and anxiety

GUIDELINES
COPD

- Colds or viruses can make residents very ill quickly. Always observe and report signs of symptoms getting worse.
- Help residents sit upright or lean forward. Offer pillows for support (Fig. 18-24).

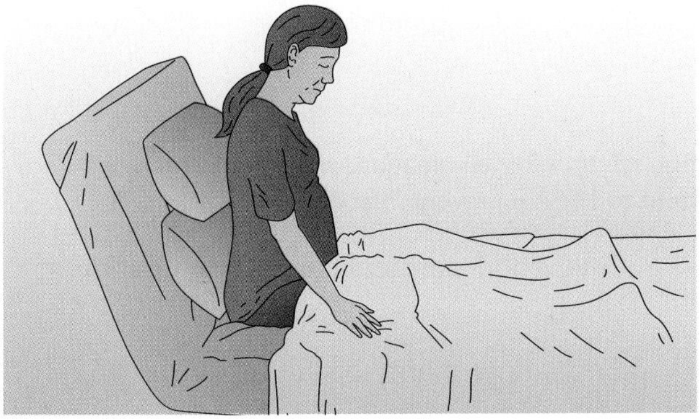

Fig. 18-24. **It helps residents with COPD to sit upright and lean forward slightly.**

- Offer plenty of fluids and small frequent meals.
- Encourage a well-balanced diet.
- Keep oxygen supply available as ordered.
- Be calm and supportive. Being unable to breathe or fearing suffocation is very frightening.
- Use good infection control. Encourage handwashing and the disposal of used tissues.
- Encourage as much independence with ADLs as possible.
- Remind residents to avoid exposure to infections, especially colds and the flu. Ensure that residents always have help ready, especially in case of a breathing crisis.
- Encourage pursed-lip breathing. Pursed-lip breathing is placing the lips as if kissing and taking controlled breaths. A nurse should teach residents how to do this type of breathing.
- Encourage residents to save energy for important tasks. Encourage residents to rest.

OBSERVING AND REPORTING
COPD

Report any of these to the nurse:

- temperature over 101°F
- changes in breathing patterns, including shortness of breath
- changes in color or consistency of lung secretions
- changes in mental state or personality
- refusal to take medications
- excessive weight loss
- increasing dependence upon caregivers and family

Tuberculosis (TB)

Tuberculosis (TB) is a highly contagious lung disease. You learned about TB in chapter 5. For residents with TB, you may need to collect a sputum specimen. **Sputum** is mucus coughed up from the lungs. Early morning is the best time to collect sputum.

Collecting a sputum specimen

Equipment: specimen container with cover, label, tissues, plastic bag, gloves, mask

1. Wash your hands.
2. Identify yourself by name. Identify resident by name.
3. Explain procedure to resident. Speak clearly, slowly, and directly. Maintain face-to-face contact whenever possible.
4. Provide for resident's privacy with curtain, screen, or door.
5. Put on mask and gloves. If the resident has known or suspected TB or another infectious disease, wear a mask when collecting a sputum specimen.
6. Ask the resident to cough deeply, so that sputum comes up from the lungs. To prevent the spread of infectious material, give the resident tissues to cover his or her mouth. Ask the resident to spit the sputum into the container.
7. When you have obtained a good sample (about two tablespoons of sputum), cover the container tightly. Wipe any sputum off the outside of the container with tissues. Discard the tissues. Put the container in the plastic bag, and seal the bag.
8. Remove and dispose of gloves and mask.
9. Complete the label for the container. Write the resident's name, room number, the date, and time.
10. Before leaving, place call light within resident's reach.
11. Wash your hands.
12. Report any changes in resident to the nurse.
13. Document procedure using facility guidelines.

5. Describe common diseases and disorders of the urinary system

Urinary Tract Infection (UTI)

Urinary tract infection (UTI) causes inflammation of the bladder and the ureters. This causes burning during urination. It also causes a frequent feeling of needing to urinate. UTI or **cystitis**, also inflammation of the bladder, may be caused by bacterial infection. Being bedbound can cause urine to stay in the bladder too long. This helps bacteria to grow.

Cystitis is more common in women. The urethra is much shorter in women (three to four inches) than in men (seven to eight inches). Bacteria can reach a woman's bladder more easily.

GUIDELINES
Preventing UTIs

- Encourage female residents to wipe from front to back after elimination (Fig. 18-25). When you give perineal care, make sure you do this as well.

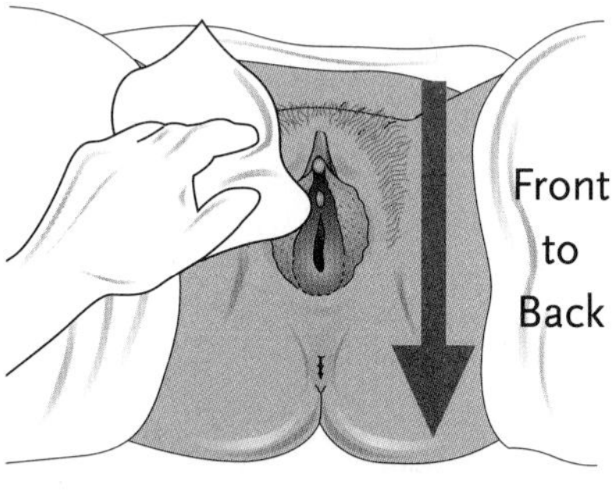

Fig. 18-25. **After elimination, women need to wipe from front to back to prevent infection.**

- Give good perineal care when changing briefs.
- Encourage plenty of fluids. Drinking 2-3 glasses of cranberry or blueberry juice daily acidifies urine. This helps to prevent infection. Vitamin C also has this effect.
- Offer bedpan or a trip to the toilet at least every two hours. Answer call lights promptly.

- Taking showers, rather than baths, helps prevent UTIs.
- Report cloudy, dark, or foul-smelling urine, or if a resident urinates often and in small amounts.

Chronic Kidney Failure

Chronic kidney failure occurs when the kidneys cannot eliminate certain waste products from the body. This disease can be the result of chronic urinary tract infections, nephritis, or diabetes. Excessive salt in the diet can also damage the kidneys. Over time, the disease becomes worse.

Kidney **dialysis** is an artificial means of removing the body's waste products. It can improve and extend life for several years. Residents will be on fluid restrictions of different degrees. Some residents may have a kidney transplant.

6. Describe common diseases and disorders of the gastrointestinal system

Constipation, diarrhea, and hemorrhoids, all GI disorders, are discussed in chapter 15. Information on hepatitis is in chapter 5.

Heartburn

Heartburn is the result of a weakening of the sphincter muscle which joins the esophagus and the stomach. When healthy, this muscle prevents the leaking of stomach acid and other contents back into the esophagus. Stomach acid causes a burning feeling, commonly called heartburn, in the esophagus. If heartburn occurs often and is untreated, it can cause scarring.

Gastroesophageal Reflux Disease (GERD)

Gastroesophageal reflux disease, commonly referred to as GERD, is a chronic condition in which the liquid contents of the stomach back up into the esophagus. The liquid can inflame and damage the lining of the esophagus. It can cause bleeding or ulcers. In addition, scars from tissue damage can narrow the esophagus and make swallowing difficult.

Heartburn is the most common symptom of GERD. Heartburn and GERD must be reported. These conditions are usually treated with medications. Serving the evening meal three to four hours before bedtime may increase comfort. Give an extra pillow so the body is more upright during sleep. Ask the resident not to lay down until at least 2–3 hours after eating. Serving the largest meal of the day at lunchtime, serving several small meals throughout the day, and reducing fast foods, fatty foods, and spicy foods may help. Stopping smoking, not drinking alcohol, and wearing loose-fitting clothes may also help.

Peptic Ulcers

Peptic ulcers are raw sores in the stomach or the small intestine. A dull or gnawing pain occurs one to three hours after eating, accompanied by belching or vomiting. Food, antacids, and medications temporarily relieve the pain. Ulcers are caused by excessive acid. Residents with peptic ulcers should avoid smoking and drinking too much alcohol and caffeine. These increase the production of gastric acid. Peptic ulcers may cause bleeding. Stool may appear black and tarry from the bleeding.

Ulcerative Colitis

Ulcerative colitis is a chronic inflammatory disease of the large intestine. Symptoms include cramping, diarrhea, pain on one side of the lower abdomen, rectal bleeding, and loss of appetite. Ulcerative colitis is a serious illness. It can cause intestinal bleeding and death if not treated. Medications can ease symptoms, but cannot cure ulcerative colitis. Surgical treatment may include a colostomy. See chapter 15 for more information on colostomies.

7. Describe common diseases and disorders of the endocrine system

Diabetes

Diabetes mellitus is commonly called **diabetes**. It is a condition in which the pancreas does not produce enough insulin. Insulin converts **glucose**, or natural sugar, into energy for the body. Without insulin to process glucose, these sugars collect in the blood. This causes problems with circulation and can damage vital organs. Diabetes is common in people with a family history of the illness, in the elderly, and people who are obese.

Currently there are about 18.2 million people in the United States who have diabetes. While millions have been diagnosed, many are unaware that they have the disease.

Two major types of diabetes are:

1. Type 1 diabetes is usually diagnosed in children and young adults. It was formerly known as juvenile diabetes. It most often appears before age twenty. In type 1 diabetes, the body does not produce insulin. The condition will continue throughout a person's life. A person can develop type 1 diabetes up to age 40. Type 1 diabetes is treated with insulin and diet.
2. Type 2 diabetes is the most common form of diabetes. In type 2 diabetes, either the body does not produce enough insulin or the body fails to properly use insulin. This is known as "insulin resistance." It can usually be controlled with diet and/or oral medications. It is also called adult-onset diabetes. Type 2 diabetes usually develops slowly. It is the milder form of diabetes. It typically develops after age 35. The risk of getting it increases with age. However, the number of children with type 2 diabetes is growing rapidly. Type 2 diabetes often occurs in obese people or those with a family history of the disease.

Pre-diabetes occurs when a person's blood glucose levels are above normal but not high enough for a diagnosis of type 2 diabetes. In 2004 the American Diabetes Association estimates that at least 20.1 million Americans between the ages of 40 and 74 have pre-diabetes. This is in addition to the 18.2 million with diabetes.

People with diabetes mellitus may have these signs and symptoms (Fig. 18-26):

- excessive thirst
- extreme hunger
- weight loss
- high levels of blood sugar
- sugar in the urine
- frequent urination
- sudden vision changes
- tingling or numbness in hands or feet
- feeling very tired much of the time
- very dry skin
- sores that are slow to heal
- more infections than usual

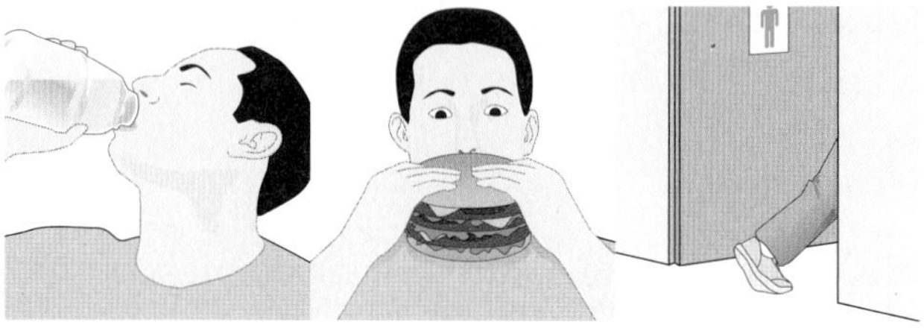

Fig. 18-26. **Increased thirst, hunger, and urination are all symptoms of diabetes.**

Diabetes can lead to further complications:

- Changes in the circulatory system can cause heart attack and stroke, reduced circulation, poor wound healing, and kidney and nerve damage.
- Damage to the eyes can cause vision loss and blindness.
- Poor circulation and impaired wound healing may cause leg and foot ulcers, infected wounds, and gangrene. Gangrene can lead to amputation.

- Insulin shock and diabetic coma can be life-threatening (chapter 7).

Diabetes must be carefully controlled to prevent complications and severe illness. When working with people with diabetes, follow care plan instructions carefully.

GUIDELINES
Diabetes

- As discussed in chapter 16, a person with diabetes must follow diet instructions exactly. The intake of carbohydrates, including breads, potatoes, grains, pasta, and sugars, must be monitored. Meals must be eaten at the same time each day. The resident must eat all that is served. If a resident will not eat what is served, or if you suspect that he or she is not following the diet, tell the nurse.
- Encourage the right portions of healthy foods. This includes foods that have less salt and fat.
- Encourage the person to exercise (Fig. 18-27). A regular exercise program is important. This may include 30 to 60 minutes of activity on most days of the week. Exercise affects how quickly bodies use food. Exercise also improves circulation. Exercise may include walking or other activities. It may also include active range of motion exercises. Help with exercises as necessary. Try to make it fun. A walk can be a chore or it can be the highlight of the day.

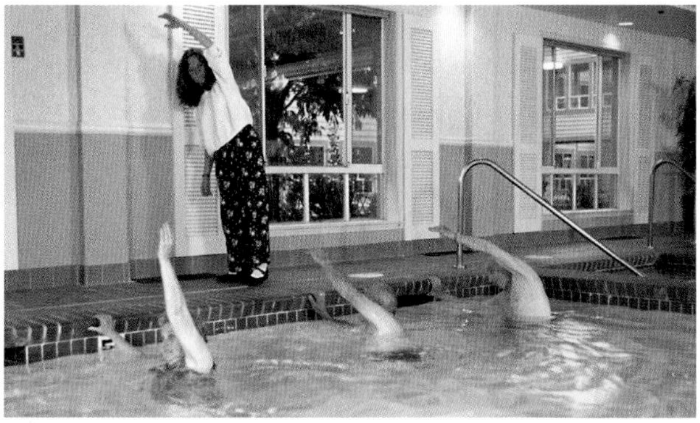

Fig. 18-27. **Exercise programs are very important for diabetic residents.**

- Observe the resident's management of insulin. Doses are calculated exactly. They are given at the same time each day. NAs should know when residents take insulin and when their meals should be served. There must be a balance between the insulin level and food intake. Unless you have had special training, you will not inject insulin.
- Perform urine and blood tests only as directed (Fig. 18-28). Sometimes the care plan will specify a daily blood or urine test for sugar or insulin levels. Not all states allow you to do this. Know your state's rules. Your facility will train you if you need to do these tests. Perform tests only as directed and allowed.

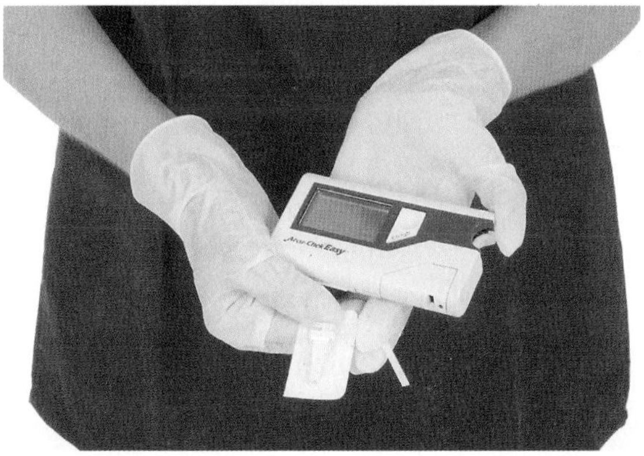

Fig. 18-28. **Blood glucose monitoring equipment.**

- Give foot care as directed. Poor circulation occurs in diabetics. Even a small sore on the leg or foot can grow into a large wound. It can require amputation. Careful foot care, including regular, daily inspection, is vital. The goals of diabetic foot care are to check for irritation or sores, to promote blood circulation, and to prevent infection.
- Encourage diabetics to wear comfortable, well-fitting leather shoes that do not hurt their feet. Leather shoes breathe and help to prevent build-up of moisture. To avoid injuries to the feet, diabetics should never go barefoot. White cotton socks are best to absorb sweat. You should never trim or

clip any resident's toenails, but especially not a diabetic's toenails. Only a nurse or doctor should do this.

OBSERVING AND REPORTING
Diabetes

Report any of these to the nurse:

- skin breakdown
- change in appetite (person overeating or not eating enough)
- increased thirst
- nausea or vomiting
- weight change
- change in mental status
- irritability
- nervousness or anxiety
- feeling faint or dizzy
- change in urine output
- change in vision
- change in mobility
- change in sensation
- sweet or fruity breath
- numbness or tingling in arms or legs

8. Describe common diseases and disorders of the reproductive system

Sexually Transmitted Diseases (STDs)

Sexually transmitted diseases, or venereal diseases, are passed through sexual contact. This includes sexual intercourse, contact of the mouth with the genitals or anus, and contact of the hands to the genitals. Using latex condoms can reduce the chances of being infected with or passing on some STDs. The human immunodeficiency virus (HIV), acquired immune deficiency syndrome (AIDS), and some kinds of hepatitis can be sexually transmitted. (HIV/AIDS is discussed in detail in the next learning objective.) STDs are very common. They can cause serious health problems. Residents may be unaware of or embarrassed by symptoms of an STD.

Chlamydia infection is caused by organisms in the mucous membranes of the reproductive tract. Chlamydia can cause serious infection. It can cause pelvic inflammatory disease (PID) in women. PID can cause sterility. Signs of chlamydia infection are yellow or white discharge from the penis or vagina and burning with urination. It is treated with antibiotics.

Syphilis can be treated effectively in the early stages. If left untreated, it can cause brain damage, mental illness, and even death. Babies born to mothers with syphilis may be born blind or with other serious birth defects. Syphilis is easier to detect in men than in women. This is due to open sores called chancres that form on the penis soon after infection. The chancres are painless and can go unnoticed. If untreated, the infection spreads to the heart, brain, and other vital organs. Common symptoms at this stage include rash, sore throat, or fever. When detected, syphilis can be treated with penicillin or other antibiotics. The sooner it is treated, the better the chances of preventing long-term damages and avoiding infection of others.

Gonorrhea, like syphilis, can be treated with antibiotics. It is easier to detect in men than in women. If untreated, gonorrhea can cause sterility. Most women with gonorrhea show no early symptoms. This makes it easy for women to spread the disease. Men with gonorrhea will often show a greenish or yellowish discharge from the penis within a week after infection. Burning with urination is another common symptom in men.

Herpes simplex II, unlike the other STDs discussed here, is caused by a virus. It cannot be treated with antibiotics. Once infected with the herpes virus, a person cannot be cured. The person may have repeated outbreaks of the disease for the rest of his or her life. A herpes outbreak includes burning, painful, red sores on the genitals. These heal in about two weeks. The sores are infectious. A person with herpes virus can also spread the infection when sores are not present. Some people infected with herpes never have repeated outbreaks. The later episodes may not be as painful as the first outbreak. Antiviral drugs can help people stay symptom-free longer.

Vaginitis

Vaginitis is an infection of the vagina. It may be caused by a bacteria, protozoa (one-celled animals), or fungus (yeast). It may also be caused by hormonal changes after menopause. Women who have vaginitis have a white vaginal discharge. This is accompanied by itching and burning. Report these symptoms to the nurse.

Benign Prostatic Hypertrophy

Benign prostatic hypertrophy is a disorder that occurs in men as they age. The prostate becomes enlarged. This causes pressure on the urethra. The pressure leads to problems urinating and/or emptying the bladder. Benign prostatic hypertrophy is treated with medications or surgery. A test is available to screen for cancer of the prostate. As men age, they are at increased risk for prostate cancer. Prostate cancer is usually slow-growing. It is responsive to treatment if caught early.

9. Describe common diseases and disorders of the immune and lymphatic systems

HIV and AIDS

Acquired immune deficiency syndrome (**AIDS**) is caused by the **human immunodeficiency virus** (**HIV**). HIV attacks the body's immune system and gradually disables it. The HIV-infected person has less resistance to other infections. Death results from these infections. However, medications help people live longer. HIV is a sexually transmitted disease. It is also spread through blood, infected needles, or to the fetus from its mother.

In general, HIV affects the body in stages. The first stage shows symptoms like the flu, with fever, muscle aches, cough, and fatigue. These are signs of the immune system fighting the infection. As the infection worsens, the immune system overreacts. It attacks not only the virus, but also normal tissue.

When the virus weakens the immune system in later stages, a group of problems may appear. These include infections, tumors, and central nervous system symptoms. These would not occur if the immune system were healthy. This stage of the disease is known as AIDS.

In the late stages of AIDS, damage to the central nervous system may cause memory loss, poor coordination, paralysis, and confusion. These symptoms together are known as **AIDS dementia complex**.

These are the signs and symptoms of HIV infection and AIDS:

- appetite loss
- involuntary weight loss of ten pounds or more
- vague, flu-like symptoms, including fever, cough, weakness, and severe or constant fatigue
- night sweats
- swollen lymph nodes in the neck, underarms, or groin
- severe diarrhea
- dry cough
- skin rashes
- painful white spots in the mouth or on the tongue

- cold sores or fever blisters on the lips and flat, white ulcers on a reddened base in the mouth
- cauliflower-like warts on the skin and in the mouth
- inflamed and bleeding gums
- bruising that does not go away
- low resistance to infection, particularly pneumonia, but also tuberculosis, herpes, bacterial infections, and hepatitis
- Kaposi's sarcoma, a form of skin cancer that appears as purple or red skin lesions (Fig. 18-29)
- AIDS dementia complex

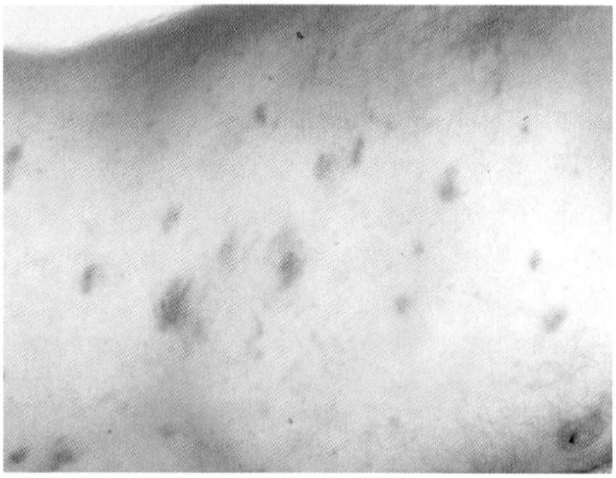

Fig. 18-29. **A purple or red skin lesion called Kaposi's sarcoma can be a sign of AIDS.**

Infections, such as pneumonia, tuberculosis, or hepatitis, invade the body when the immune system is weak and cannot defend itself. These illnesses worsen AIDS. They further weaken the immune system. It is hard to treat these infections. Generally, over time, a person develops a resistance to some antibiotics. These infections often cause death in people with AIDS.

People with HIV are treated with drugs that slow the progress of the disease. They do not cure it. The medicines must be taken at precise times. They have many unpleasant side effects. For some people, the medications work less well than for others. Other aspects of HIV treatment are relief of symptoms and prevention and treatment of infection.

Behaviors that put people at high risk for HIV/AIDS infection include:

- Sharing drug needles
- Having unprotected sex (not using latex condoms during sexual contact)
- Sexual contact with many partners
- Any sexual activity that involves exchange of body fluids with a partner who has not tested negative for HIV or who has had many sexual partners. Be aware that it may take six months after contact with the virus for an HIV test to show positive results.

Ways to protect against the spread of HIV and AIDS:

- Never share needles for injections of any type of drug.
- Practice safer sex. Use latex condoms during sexual contact.
- Stay in a monogamous relationship with a partner who has tested negative for HIV. Being monogamous means having only one sexual partner.
- Practice abstinence. Abstinence means not having sexual contact with anyone.
- Get tested if you think you may have been infected with HIV. It can take up to six months from the time you are infected for the antibodies to be detected in your blood. Get re-tested periodically if necessary. It is especially important that pregnant women get tested.
- Follow Standard Precautions at work to protect yourself.

GUIDELINES
HIV/AIDS

- Involuntary weight loss occurs in almost all people who develop AIDS. High-protein and high-calorie meals can help maintain a healthy weight.

- People with poor immune systems are more sensitive to infections. Wash your hands often. Keep everything clean.
- Residents with infections of the mouth may need food that is low in acid and neither cold nor hot. Spicy seasonings should be removed. Soft or pureed foods may be easier to swallow. Liquid meals and fortified drinks may help ease the pain of chewing. Warm salt water or other rinses may eases sores of the mouth. Good mouth care is vital.
- A person with nausea or vomiting should eat small frequent meals, if possible. The person should eat slowly. Encourage fluids in between meals. These residents must maintain intake of fluids to balance lost fluids.
- Residents with mild diarrhea may need frequent small meals that are low in fat, fiber, and milk products. If diarrhea is severe, the doctor may order a "BRAT" diet (a diet of bananas, rice, apples, and toast). This is helpful for short-term use.
- Numbness, tingling, and pain in the feet and legs is usually treated with medication. Going barefoot or wearing loose, soft slippers may be helpful. If blankets cause pain, a bed cradle can keep sheets and blankets from resting on legs and feet (Fig. 18-30).

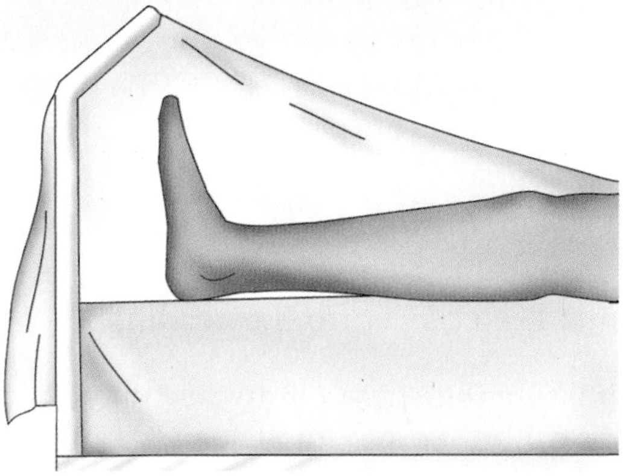

Fig. 18-30. **A bed cradle keeps bed covers from pushing down on a resident's feet.**

- Residents with HIV/AIDS may have anxiety and depression. They often suffer the judgments of family, friends, and society. Some people blame them for their illness. People with HIV/AIDS may have tremendous stress. They may feel uncertainty about their illness, health care, and finances. They may also have lost people in their social support network of friends and family.
- Residents with HIV/AIDS need support from others. This may come from family, friends, religious and community groups, and support groups, as well as the healthcare team. Treat all your residents with respect. Help give the emotional support they need.
- Withdrawal, avoidance of tasks, and mental slowness are symptoms early in HIV infection. Medications may also cause side effects of this type. AIDS dementia complex may cause further mental symptoms. There may also be muscle weakness and loss of muscle control, making falls a risk. Residents will need a safe environment and close supervision in their ADLs.

The right to confidentiality is especially important to people with HIV/AIDS. Others may pass judgment on people with this disease. A person with HIV/AIDS cannot be fired because of the disease. A healthcare worker with HIV/AIDS may be reassigned to job duties with less risk of transmitting the disease.

HIV testing requires consent. No one can test you for HIV unless you agree. HIV test results are confidential. They cannot be shared with a person's family, friends, or employer without his or her consent. If you are HIV-positive, you might want to tell your supervisor. Your tasks can be adjusted to avoid putting you at high risk for exposure to other infections. Everyone has a right to privacy about their health status. Never discuss a resident's status with anyone.

Don't be stingy with handshakes and hugs.

Understanding the facts about HIV/AIDS is important. This will help you not to feel afraid of a person with this disease. A handshake or a hug cannot spread the AIDS virus. The disease cannot be transmitted by telephones, doorknobs, tables, chairs, toilets, mosquitoes, or by breathing the same air as an infected person. Spend time with residents who have HIV/AIDS. They need the same thoughtful, personal attention you give to all your residents.

10. Describe cancer and list care guidelines

Cancer is a general term used to describe many types of malignant tumors. A **tumor** is a group of abnormally growing cells. **Benign** tumors grow slowly in local areas. They are considered non-cancerous. **Malignant** tumors grow rapidly. They invade surrounding tissues.

Cancer invades local tissue. It can spread to other parts of the body. Cancer can spread from the site where it first appeared and affect other body systems. In general, treatment is harder and cancer is more deadly after this has occurred. Cancer often appears first in the breast, colon, rectum, uterus, prostate, lungs, or skin. There is no known cure for cancer. However, some treatments are effective. They are discussed later.

Risk factors that appear to contribute to cancer are:

- tobacco use (Fig. 18-31)
- exposure to sunlight
- excessive alcohol intake
- exposure to some chemicals and industrial agents
- some food additives
- radiation
- poor nutrition
- lack of physical activity

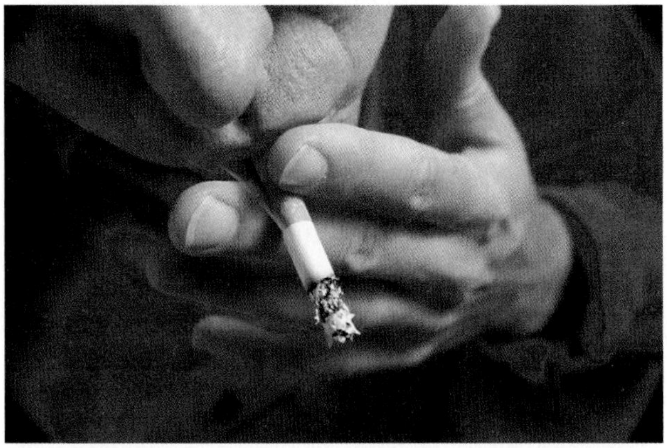

Fig. 18-31. **Tobacco use is considered a risk for cancer.**

When diagnosed early, cancer can often be treated and controlled. The American Cancer Society has identified seven warning signs of cancer:

1. **C**hange in bowel or bladder habits
2. **A** sore that does not heal
3. **U**nusual bleeding or discharge
4. **T**hickening or lump
5. **I**ndigestion or trouble swallowing
6. **O**bvious change in a wart or mole
7. **N**agging cough or persistent hoarseness

People with cancer may live longer and can sometimes recover if they are treated early. There are three common types of treatment for cancer. Often these treatments are combined:

Surgery is the first line of defense against most forms of cancer. It is the key treatment for malignant tumors of the skin, breast, bladder, colon, rectum, stomach, and muscle. Surgeons remove as much of the tumor as they can to keep cancer from spreading.

Chemotherapy refers to medications given to fight cancer. Some drugs destroy cancer cells and limit the rate of cell growth. Many of these drugs are toxic to the body. They kill healthy cells as well as cancer cells. Chemotherapy can have severe side effects, including nausea, vomiting, diarrhea, hair loss, and decreased resistance to infection.

Radiation therapy directs radiation to a limited area to kill cancer cells. Other normal or healthy cells in its path are also destroyed (Fig. 18-32). By controlling cell growth, radiation can reduce pain. Radiation can cause the same side effects as chemotherapy. The skin of the area may become sore, irritated, and sometimes burned.

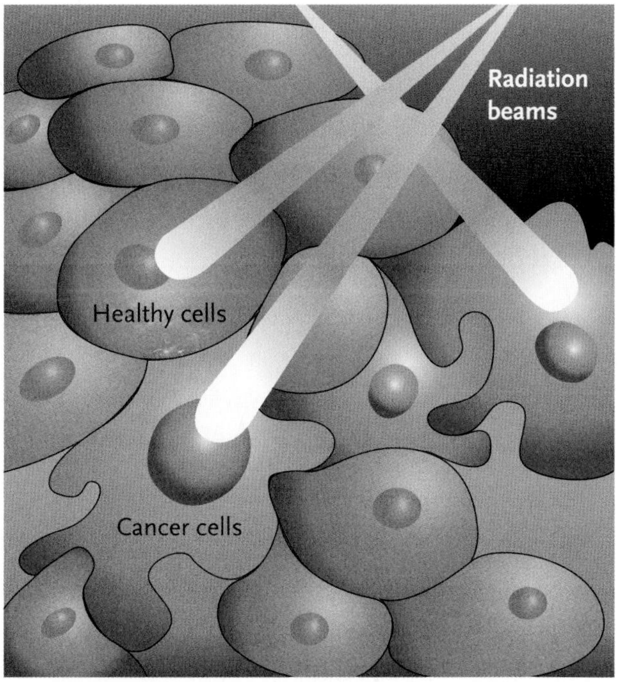

Fig. 18-32. **Radiation is targeted at cancer cells. It also kills some healthy cells in its path.**

GUIDELINES
Cancer

- **Each case is different**. Cancer is a general term. It refers to many separate situations. Residents may live many years or only several months. Treatment affects each person differently. Do not make assumptions about a resident's condition.
- **Communication**. Residents may want to talk or may avoid talking. Respect their needs. Be honest. Never say, "everything will be okay." Be sensitive. Remember that cancer is a disease. We do not know its cause. Have a good attitude. Focus on concrete details, for example, that a resident seems stronger, or that the sun is shining outside.
- **Nutrition**. Good nutrition is important for residents with cancer. Follow the care plan carefully. Use plastic utensils for a resident receiving chemotherapy. It makes food taste better. Silver utensils cause a bitter taste. Residents often have poor appetites. Encourage a variety of food. Liquid nutrition supplements may be used along with, not in place of, meals.
- **Pain control**. Cancer can cause great pain, especially in the late stages. Watch for signs of pain. Report them to the nurse. Help with comfort measures, such as repositioning and providing conversation, music, or reading materials (Fig. 18-33). Report if pain seems to be uncontrolled.

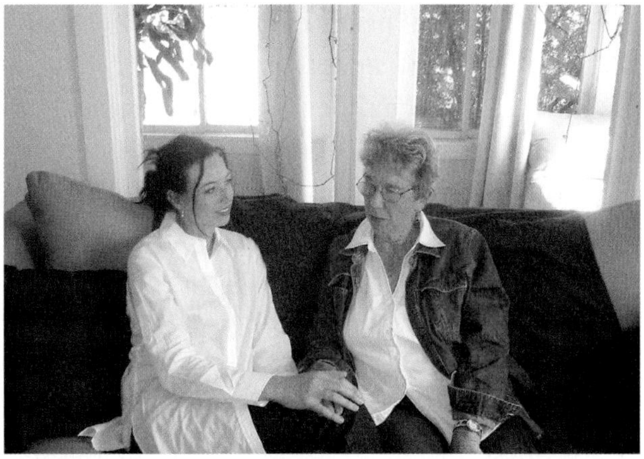

Fig. 18-33. **Distractions such as conversation can help a resident with cancer deal with pain.**

- **Skin care**. Use lotion on dry or delicate skin. Do not apply lotion to areas receiving radiation therapy. Do not remove any markings that are used in radiation therapy. Give back rubs for comfort and to increase circulation. For residents who spend many hours in bed, egg crate mattress covers or sheepskins may be more comfortable. Moving to a chair may improve comfort as well. Residents who are very weak or immobile need to be repositioned every two hours. Follow any special skin care orders (for example: no hot or cold packs, no soap or cosmetics, no tight stockings).

- **Oral care**. Help residents brush and floss teeth regularly. Medications, nausea, vomiting, or mouth infections may cause a bad taste in the mouth. You can help ease discomfort by using a soft-bristled toothbrush, rinsing with baking soda and water, or using a prescribed rinse. Do not use a commercial mouthwash. Alcohol can further irritate a resident's mouth.
- **Self-image**. People with cancer may have a low self-image because they are weak and their appearance has changed. For example, hair loss is a common side effect of chemotherapy. Be sensitive. Provide help with grooming if it is desired. Your concern and interest can help self-image.
- **Psychosocial needs**. If visitors help cheer your resident, encourage them. Do not intrude. If some times of day are better, suggest this. Support groups exist for people with cancer and their families. Check with the nurse for groups in your area. It may help a person with cancer to think of something else for a while. Pursue other topics. Get to know what interests your residents have.
- **Family assistance**. Having a family member with cancer can be very difficult. Be alert to needs that are not being met or stresses created by the illness.

Many services and support groups exist for people with cancer and their families or caregivers. Hospitals, hospice programs, and religious organizations have many resources. These include meal services, transportation to doctors' offices, counseling, and support groups. Check the local yellow pages under "cancer," or call the American Cancer Society.

OBSERVING AND REPORTING
Cancer

Report any of these to the nurse:

- increased weakness or fatigue
- weight loss
- nausea, vomiting, diarrhea
- changes in appetite
- fainting
- signs of depression (see chapter 20 for a discussion of these signs)
- confusion
- blood in stool or urine
- change in mental status
- changes in skin
- new lumps, sores, or rashes
- increase in pain, or pain unrelieved by current measures

11. Explain developmental disabilities and list care guidelines

Developmental disabilities are present at birth or emerge during childhood. A developmental disability is a chronic condition. It restricts physical or mental ability. These disabilities prevent a child from developing at a "normal" rate. NAs help teach residents self-care and help with ADLs.

Mental Retardation

According to the CDC, **mental retardation** is the most common developmental disorder. Approximately 1% of the population has mental retardation. There are different degrees of mental retardation. It is not a disease or a psychiatric illness. People with mental retardation develop at a below-average rate. They have below-average mental functioning. They have difficulty in learning and may have problems adjusting socially. Along with their special needs, residents who are mentally retarded have the same emotional and physical needs as others (Fig. 18-34).

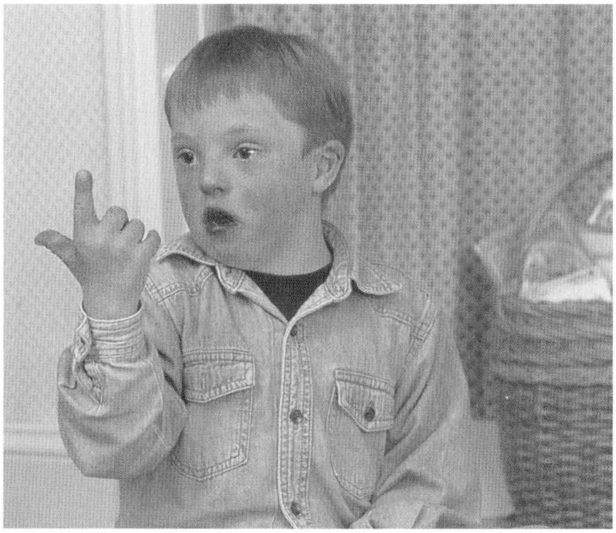

Fig. 18-34. **People who are mentally retarded have the same emotional and physical needs as others.**

For residents who are mentally retarded, the main goal of care is to help them have as normal a life as possible. This means recognizing their individuality, basic human rights, and physical and emotional needs, as well as special needs.

GUIDELINES
Mental Retardation

- Treat adult residents as adults, regardless of their behavior.
- Praise and encourage often, especially positive behavior.
- Help teach ADLs by dividing a task into smaller units.
- Promote independence. Assist residents with activities and motor functions that are difficult.
- Encourage social interaction.
- Repeat words to make sure they understand.
- Be patient.

Down Syndrome

People who are born with **Down syndrome** have different degrees of mental retardation, along with physical symptoms. A person with Down syndrome typically has a small skull, a flattened nose, short fingers, and a wider space between the first two fingers and the first two toes. A person with Down syndrome can become fairly independent.

GUIDELINES
Down Syndrome

- Give the same type of care and instruction for a Down syndrome resident as for any other person with mental retardation.
- Praise and encourage often, especially positive behavior.
- Help teach ADLs by dividing a task into smaller units.

Cerebral Palsy

People with **cerebral palsy** have suffered brain damage while in the uterus or during birth. They may have both physical and mental disabilities. Damage to the brain may stop the development of the child. It can cause disorganized or abnormal development. Muscle coordination and nerves are affected. People with cerebral palsy may lack control of the head, and have trouble using the arms and hands. They can have poor balance or posture. They may be either stiff and spastic or limp and flaccid. They may have speech impairment. Intelligence may also be affected.

GUIDELINES
Cerebral Palsy

- Allow the resident to move slowly. People with cerebral palsy take longer to adjust their body position. They may repeat movements several times.
- Keep the resident's body in as normal an alignment as possible.
- Talk to the resident, even if he or she cannot speak. Be patient and listen.
- Use touch as a form of communication.
- Avoid activities that are tiring or frustrating.

- Be gentle when handling parts of the body that may be painful (Fig. 18-35).
- Promote independence. Encourage socialization.

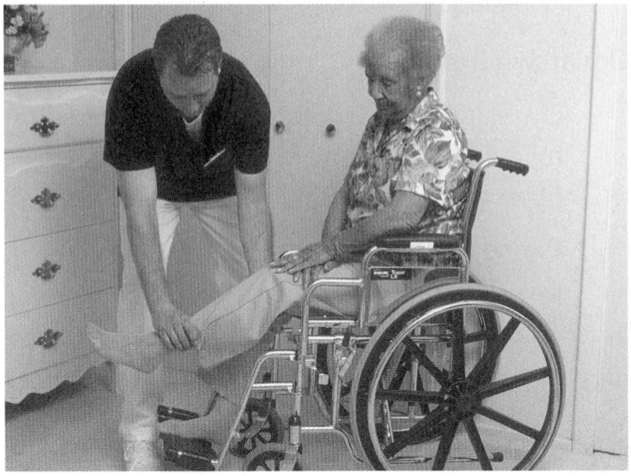

Fig. 18-35. **Be gentle when moving body parts of a resident who has cerebral palsy.**

Spina Bifida

Spina bifida literally means "split spine." When part of the backbone is not well-developed at birth, the spinal cord may bulge out of the back. Spina bifida can cause a range of disabilities. Some babies born with spina bifida will be able to walk and will have no lasting disabilities. Others may be in a wheelchair. They may have little or no bladder or bowel control. Complications of spina bifida may cause brain damage.

When caring for a resident with spina bifida, help with range of motion exercises and ADLs. Be a positive role model for the resident in learning to deal with his or her disabilities.

Chapter Review

1. What are the causes of arthritis?
2. What type of medication might a resident with arthritis take?
3. What health problems can anti-inflammatory medications cause?
4. What can happen to bones when they are brittle?
5. What type of surface can a cast be placed on?
6. What should you do to an extremity in a cast?
7. Why is a hip fracture a serious condition for an elderly person?
8. A person recovering from a hip replacement should not sit at an angle less than how many degrees?
9. What is traction used for?
10. List three physical problems that muscular dystrophy can cause.
11. What is phantom sensation? Is it real?
12. List five care guidelines for amputations and prostheses.
13. What causes a CVA (stroke)?
14. What does "TIA" stand for?
15. What are some symptoms that may signal a stroke is coming?
16. List five effects a resident may experience after a stroke.
17. How should you refer to the weaker side of a person who has had a stroke?
18. When helping a person who has had a stroke with transfers or walking, on which side should you stand? Which side should you lead with?
19. Why may people with Parkinson's disease have trouble eating and bathing themselves?
20. List five care guidelines for a person with multiple sclerosis.
21. List four care guidelines for a person with a head or spinal cord injury.
22. What are three things you should NOT do when a resident is having a seizure?

23. List eight care guidelines for a person with a vision impairment.
24. List eight care guidelines for a person with a hearing impairment.
25. What is hypertension? What does prehypertension mean?
26. List two care guidelines for a resident who has high blood pressure.
27. List three care guidelines for a resident with angina pectoris.
28. List two care guidelines for a resident recovering from a heart attack.
29. List six care guidelines for a resident who has congestive heart failure.
30. What can an elastic stocking help prevent?
31. What are some effects of having chronic obstructive pulmonary disease?
32. List four care guidelines for a resident who has chronic obstructive pulmonary disease.
33. What is sputum?
34. List five guidelines for preventing urinary tract infections.
35. Reducing intake of what type of foods may help with gastric reflux?
36. Briefly describe the two major types of diabetes.
37. Why is good foot care especially important for a resident with diabetes?
38. List six signs or symptoms of diabetes that you need to report.
39. If a diabetic resident refuses to eat what is served, or if you suspect that he or she is not following the diet, what should you do?
40. Why should a diabetic person not walk barefoot?
41. What are three types of sexual contact that can transmit STDs?
42. Why are antibiotics not used to treat Herpes simplex II?
43. How is HIV spread?
44. List seven care guidelines for a resident who has AIDS.
45. List four ways to protect against the spread of HIV and AIDS.
46. Is it possible to get AIDS by breathing the same air as an infected person?
47. What is a tumor?
48. List the seven warning signs for cancer.
49. What are the side effects of chemotherapy and radiation?
50. How can you show sensitivity to a resident who has cancer?
51. What are developmental disabilities?
52. What is the most common developmental disorder?

Chapter 19
Confusion, Dementia, and Alzheimer's Disease

1. Define "confusion" and "delirium"

Confusion is the inability to think clearly. A confused person has trouble focusing his attention and may feel disoriented. Confusion interferes with the ability to make decisions. Personality may change. The person may not know his name, the date, other people, or where he is. A confused person may be angry, depressed, or irritable.

Confusion may come on suddenly or gradually. It can be temporary or permanent. Confusion is more common in the elderly. It may occur when a person is in the hospital. Some causes are:

- low blood sugar
- head trauma or head injury
- dehydration
- nutritional problems
- fever
- sudden drop in body temperature
- lack of oxygen
- medications
- infections
- brain tumor
- illness
- loss of sleep
- seizures

GUIDELINES
Confusion

- Do not leave a confused resident alone.
- Stay calm. Provide a quiet environment.
- Speak in a lower tone of voice. Speak clearly and slowly.
- Introduce yourself each time you see the resident.
- Remind the resident of his or her location, name, and the date. A calendar can help.
- Explain what you are going to do. Use simple instructions.
- Do not rush the resident.
- Talk to confused residents about plans for the day.
- Encourage the use of glasses and hearing aids. Make sure they are clean and are not damaged.
- Keep a routine.
- Promote self-care and independence.
- Follow the care plan.
- Report observations to the nurse.

Delirium is a state of severe confusion. It is usually temporary and occurs suddenly. Some causes are infections, disease, fluid imbalances, and poor nutrition. Drugs and alcohol are other causes. Symptoms include:

- agitation
- anger
- depression
- irritability
- disorientation
- trouble focusing
- problems with speech
- changes in sensation and perception
- changes in consciousness
- decrease in short-term memory

Report these signs to the nurse. The goal of treatment is to control or reverse the cause. Emergency care may be needed, as well as a stay in a hospital.

2. Describe dementia and define related terms

As we age, we may lose some of our ability to think logically and quickly. This ability is called **cognition**. Loss of some of this ability is called cognitive impairment. Cognitive impairment affects focus and memory. Elderly residents may lose their memories of recent events. This can be frustrating for them. You can help. Encourage them to make lists of things to remember. Write down names and phone numbers. Other normal changes of aging in the brain are slower reaction time, trouble finding or using words, and less sleep.

Dementia is a more serious loss of mental abilities. It affects thinking, remembering, reasoning, and communicating. As dementia advances, these losses make it hard to perform ADLs such as eating, bathing, dressing, and toileting. **Dementia is not a normal part of aging** (Fig. 19-1).

Here are some related terms:

Progressive: Once they begin, **progressive** diseases advance. They tend to spread to other parts of the body. They affect many body functions.

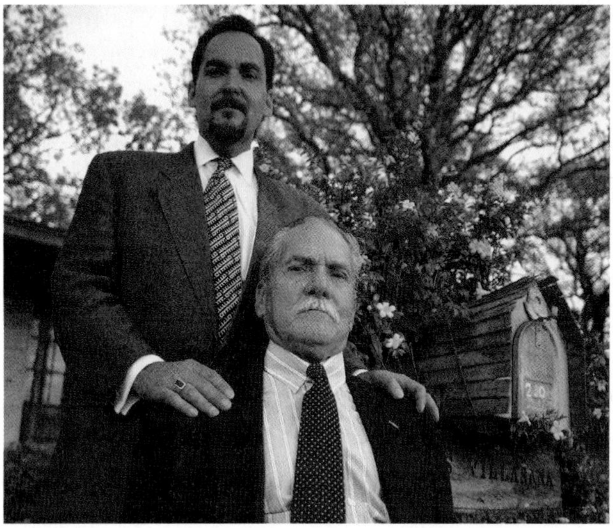

Fig. 19-1. **Some of our ability to think quickly is lost as we age. However, dementia is not a normal change of aging.**

Degenerative: **Degenerative** diseases get continually worse. They eventually cause a breakdown of body systems. Degenerative diseases can cause death. They cause lower and lower levels of mental and physical health.

Onset: The **onset** of a disease is the time the signs and symptoms begin.

Irreversible: An **irreversible** disease or condition cannot be cured. Someone with irreversible dementia (like Alzheimer's) will either die from the disease or die with the disease.

Causes of dementia include:

- Alzheimer's disease
- Multi-infarct or vascular dementia (a series of strokes that damage the brain)
- Lewy body disease (also called Lewy body dementia)
- Parkinson's disease
- Huntington's disease

3. Describe Alzheimer's disease and identify its stages

Alzheimer's disease (AD) is the most common cause of dementia in the elderly. The disease usually occurs after age 65. It can strike younger people. Almost 50% of people over age 85 may have AD. The National Center for Health Statistics estimates that over half of the people in nursing homes have AD or a related disorder. The risk of getting AD increases with age, but it is not a normal part of aging.

Alzheimer's disease is progressive, degenerative, and irreversible. Tangled nerve fibers and protein deposits form in the brain. They eventually cause dementia. There is no known cause of AD. There is no cure. Diagnosis is difficult. It involves many physical and mental tests to rule out other causes. One type of brain scan—the positron emission topography (PET) scan—can help diagnose AD. However, the only sure way to determine AD at this time is by autopsy. The time it takes AD to progress from onset to death varies greatly. It may take from three to 20 years.

Symptoms of AD appear gradually. It begins with memory loss. As AD progresses the symptoms get worse. People with AD may get disoriented. They may be confused about time and place. They can have communication problems. They may lose their ability to read, write, speak, or understand. Mood and behavior changes. Aggressiveness, wandering, and withdrawal are all part of AD.

Those with Alzheimer's will show different signs at different times. For example, one resident with Alzheimer's may be able to read, but cannot use the phone or recall her address. Another may have lost the ability to read, but is still able to do simple math. Skills a person has used often over a lifetime are usually kept longer. Thus some people with Alzheimer's can play an instrument with help long after losing much of their memory (Fig. 19-2).

Though the disease progresses at different rates, eventually all AD victims need constant care. The only current treatments ease some of the symptoms of the disease. They make life more comfortable and care more manageable.

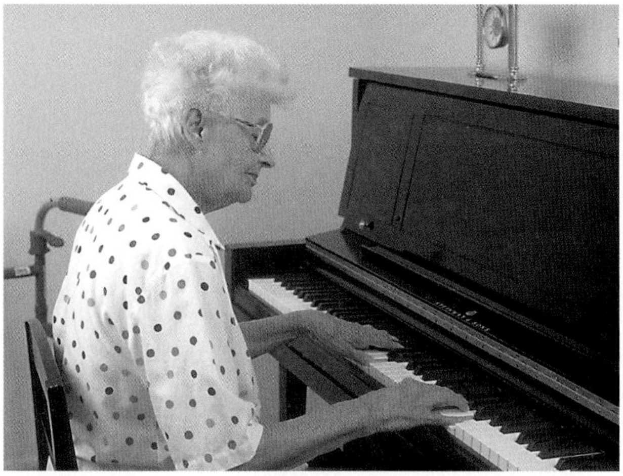

Fig 19-2. **Even when a person loses much of her memory, she may still keep skills she has used her whole life.**

Encourage residents with AD to do ADLs. Help them keep their minds and bodies as active as possible. Working, socializing, reading, problem solving, and exercising should all be encouraged (Fig. 19-3). Having them do as much as possible for themselves may even help slow the disease. Look for tasks that are challenging but not frustrating. Help your residents succeed in doing them.

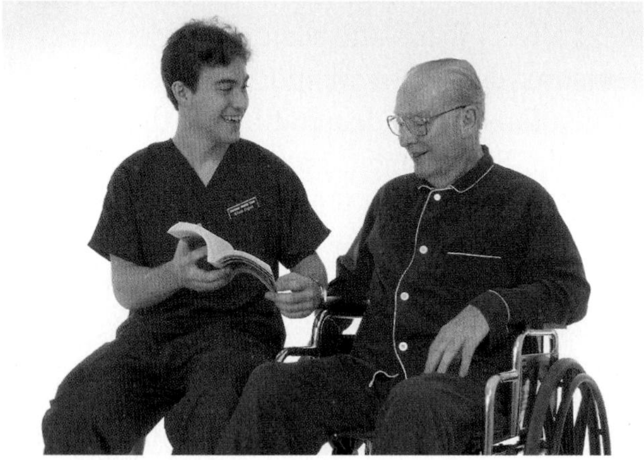

Fig. 19-3. **Encourage reading and thinking activities for residents with AD.**

Alzheimer's disease generally progresses in three stages:

Stage I

- recent (short-term) memory loss
- disorientation to time
- lack of interest in doing things, including work, dressing, recreation

- inability to concentrate
- mood swings
- irritability
- petulance: bad-tempered, ill-humored, rude behavior
- tendency to blame others
- carelessness in personal care
- poor judgment

Stage II

- increased memory loss, may forget family and friends
- slurred speech
- trouble finding words, finishing thoughts, or following directions
- tendency to make illogical statements
- inability to read, write, or do math
- inability to care for self or do ADLs without help
- incontinence
- dulled senses (for example, cannot tell hot from cold)
- restlessness, wandering, and/or agitation (increase of these in the evening is called "sundowning")
- sleep problems
- poor impulse control (for example: swears excessively or is sexually aggressive or rude)
- obsessive repetition of movements, actions, or words
- temper tantrums
- hallucinations or delusions

Stage III

- total disorientation to time, place, and person
- apathy
- total dependence on others for care
- total incontinence
- inability to speak or communicate, except for grunting, groaning, or screaming
- total immobility/confined to bed
- inability to recognize family or self
- increased sleep disturbances
- trouble swallowing, causing risk of choking
- seizures
- coma
- death

4. List strategies for better communication for residents with Alzheimer's disease

Some good communication tips include:

- Always approach from the front. Do not startle the resident.
- Determine how close the resident wants you to be.
- If possible, communicate in a calm place. Reduce noise or distraction.
- Always identify yourself. Use the resident's name.
- Speak slowly. Use a lower voice than normal. This is calming and easier to understand.

These are good communication techniques to use with people who have AD:

If the resident is frightened or anxious:

- Try to keep him or her calm.
- Speak in a low, calm voice. Find a room with little background noise and distraction. Get rid of noise and distractions, such as televisions or radios (Fig. 19-4).
- Move and speak slowly.
- Try to see and hear yourself as they might. Always describe what you are going to do.
- Use simple words and short sentences. If doing a procedure or helping with self-care, list steps one at a time.

- Check your body language. Make sure you are not tense or hurried.

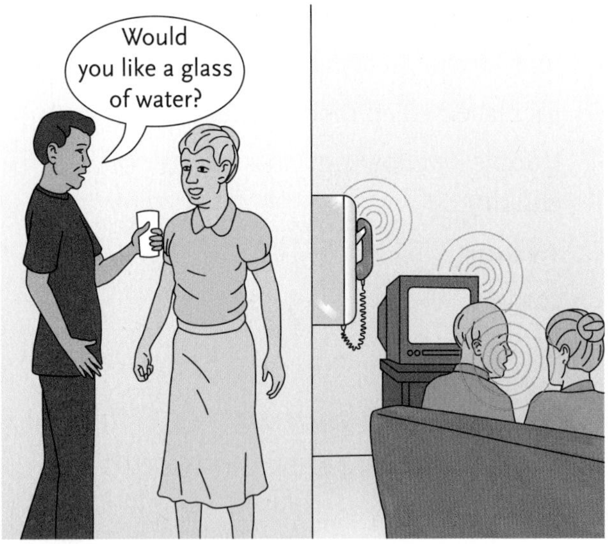

Fig. 19-4. **Reduce noise and distractions when communicating with residents who have AD.**

If the resident forgets or shows memory loss:

- Repeat yourself. Use the same words if you need to repeat an instruction or question. However, you may be using a word the resident does not understand, such as "tired." Try other words like "nap," "lie down," "rest," etc.
- Repetition can also be soothing for a resident with Alzheimer's. Many residents with AD will repeat words, phrases, questions, or actions. This is called **perseveration**. If your resident perseverates, do not try to stop him. Answer his questions, using the same words each time, until he stops.
- Keep messages simple.
- Break complex tasks into smaller, simpler ones.

If the resident has trouble finding words or names:

- Suggest a word that sounds correct. If this upsets the resident, learn from it. Try not to correct a resident who uses an incorrect word. As words (written and spoken) become more difficult, smiling, touching, and hugging can help show love and concern. But remember some people find touch frightening or unwelcome.

If the resident seems not to understand basic instructions or questions:

- Ask the resident to repeat your words.
- Use short words and sentences. Allow time to answer.
- Note the communication methods that are effective. Use them.
- Watch for nonverbal cues as the ability to talk lessens. Observe body language—eyes, hands, and face.
- Use signs, pictures, gestures, or written words. Use pictures, such as a drawing of a toilet on the bathroom door. Use gestures, such as holding up a shirt when you want to help your resident dress. Combine verbal and nonverbal communication. For example, saying "Let's get dressed now," as you hold up clothes.

If the resident wants to say something but cannot:

- Ask him or her to point, gesture, or act it out.
- If the resident is upset but cannot explain why, offer comfort with a hug or a smile, or try to distract. Verbal communication may be frustrating.

If the resident does not remember how to perform basic tasks:

- Break each activity into simple steps. For instance, "Let's go for a walk. Stand up. Put on your sweater. First the right arm..." Always encourage people to do what they can.

If the resident insists on doing something that is unsafe or not allowed:

- Try to limit the times you say "don't." Instead, redirect activities toward something else.

If the resident hallucinates (sees or hears things that are not really happening), is paranoid or accusing:

- Do not take it personally.
- Try to redirect behavior or ignore it. Attention span is limited. This behavior often passes quickly.

If the resident is depressed or lonely:

- Take time, one-on-one, to ask how he or she is feeling. Really listen.
- Try to involve the resident in activities.
- Always report depression to the nurse. You will learn more about depression in chapter 21.

If the resident is verbally abusive, or uses bad language:

- Remember it is the dementia speaking and not the person.
- Try to ignore the language. Redirect attention to something else (Fig. 19-5).

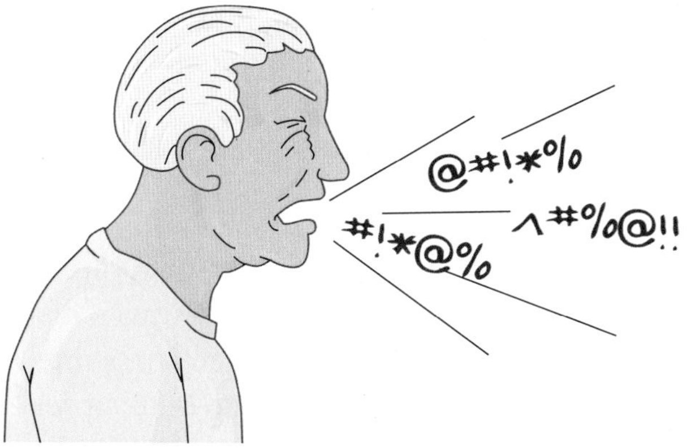

Fig. 19-5. **If a resident with AD says something abusive or uses bad language, try to ignore it. Remember that it is the disease talking.**

If the resident has lost most verbal skills:

- Use nonverbal skills. As speaking abilities decline, people with AD will still understand touch, smiles, and laughter for much longer. Remember that some people do not like to be touched. Approach touching slowly. Be gentle. Softly touch the hand or place your arm around the resident. A hug or a kiss on the hand or cheek can show affection and caring. A smile can say you want to help.
- Even after verbal skills are lost, signs, labels, and gestures can reach people with dementia.
- Assume people with AD can understand more than they can express. Never talk about them as though they were not there.

5. Identify personal attitudes helpful in caring for residents with Alzheimer's disease

These attitudes will help you give the best care to your residents with AD:

Do not take it personally. Alzheimer's disease is a devastating mental and physical disorder. It affects everyone who surrounds and cares for the one with AD. People with AD do not have control over their words and actions. They may not be aware of what they say or do. If a resident with Alzheimer's does not know you, does not do what you say, ignores you, accuses you, or insults you, remember that it is the disease. It is not the person.

Put yourself in their shoes. Think about what it would be like to have Alzheimer's disease. Imagine being unable to do ADLs. Assume that people with AD have insight and are aware of the changes in their abilities. Treat residents with AD with dignity and respect. Give security and comfort.

Work with the symptoms and behaviors you see. Each person with Alzheimer's disease is an individual. People with AD will not all show the same signs at the same times (Fig. 19-6). Each resident will do some things that others will never do. The best plan is to work with what you see today. For example, an Alzheimer's resident may want to go for a walk today. Yesterday he did not seem able to get to the bathroom without help. If allowed, try to go for a walk with him. Notice change in behavior, mood, and independence. Report your observations to the nurse.

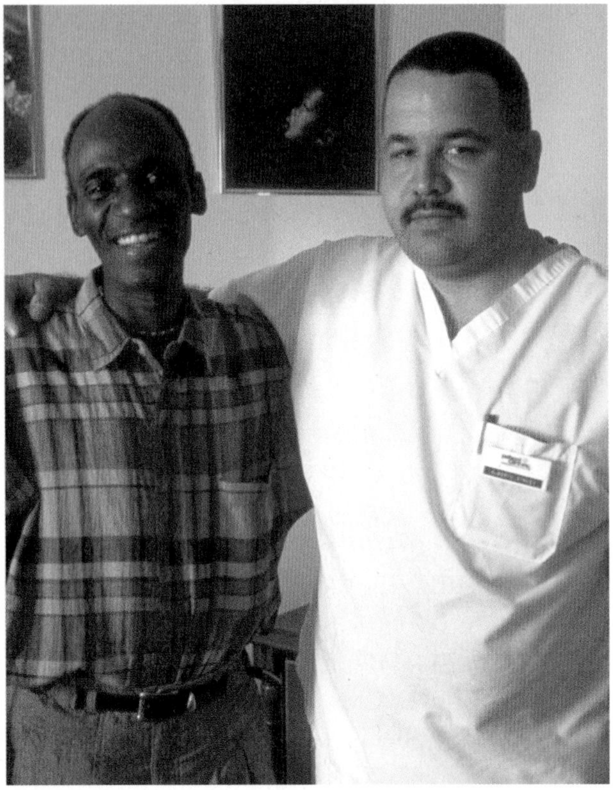

Fig. 19-6. **Treat each resident with AD as an individual. They will not have the same symptoms at the same time.**

Work as a team. Always report and document your observations. Symptoms and behavior change daily. You are in a great position to give details about your residents. Being with residents often lets you be the expert on each case. Make the most of this chance. You will be helping to give the best care. Residents with AD may not recognize aides, nurses, or administrators. Be prepared to help when needed.

Take care of yourself. Caring for someone with dementia can be both physically and emotionally exhausting. Take care of yourself to continue giving the best care (Fig. 19-7). Be aware of your body's signals to slow down, rest, or eat better. Your feelings are real. You have a right to them. Use your mistakes as learning experiences.

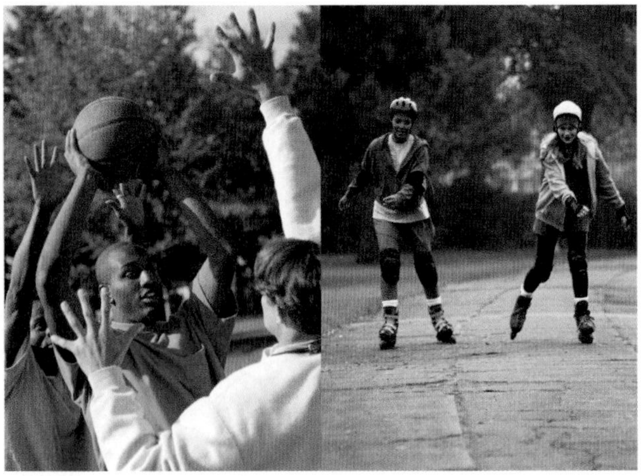

Fig. 19-7. **Regular exercise is an important part of taking care of yourself.**

Work with family members. Family members can be a great resource. They can help you learn more about your resident. They also give stability and comfort to the resident with Alzheimer's. Build relationships with family members. Keep the lines of communication open.

Remember the goals of the care plan. Along with practical tasks, the care plan will also call for maintaining residents' dignity and self-esteem. Help them to be independent.

6. Explain general principles that will help assist residents with personal care

Use the same procedures for personal care and ADLs for residents with Alzheimer's disease as with other residents. There are some guidelines to keep in mind when helping residents with AD. Three general principles will help you give the best care:

1. Make a routine. Stick to it. Being consistent is important for residents who are confused and easily upset.
2. Promote self-care. Help your residents to care for themselves as much as possible. This will help them cope.
3. Take good care of yourself, both mentally and physically. This will help you give the best care.

7. List and describe interventions for problems with common activities of daily living (ADLs)

As Alzheimer's disease worsens, residents will have trouble doing their ADLs. By knowing interventions, you can provide better care. An **intervention** means a way to change an action or development.

Problems with Incontinence

- Be sure the resident is drinking enough fluids. If you notice the resident is not drinking fluids, tell the nurse.
- Follow schedules for drinking fluids.
- Note when the resident is incontinent over two to three days. Check him or her every 30 minutes. This can help determine "bathroom times."
- Take the resident to the bathroom just before his or her "bathroom time."
- Take the resident to the bathroom before and after meals and just before bed.
- Make sure he or she urinates before getting off the toilet.
- Mark the restroom with a sign or a picture. This is a reminder of where it is and to use it.
- Family or friends may be upset by their loved one's incontinence. Be matter-of-fact about cleaning. Do not show any disgust or irritation.
- For incontinence during the night, observe toilet patterns for two to three nights. You may have to take the resident to the bathroom just before his or her "bathroom time."
- Make sure there is enough light in the bathroom and on the way there.
- Put lids on trash cans, waste baskets, or other containers if the resident urinates in them.
- Encourage fluids. Never withhold or discourage fluids because a resident is incontinent.

Problems with Bathing

- Schedule bathing when the resident is least agitated.
- Prepare the resident before bathing. Hand him or her the supplies (washcloth, soap, shampoo, towels). This serves as a visual aid.
- Take a walk with the resident down the hall. Stop at the tub or shower room, rather than asking directly about the bath.
- Be organized so the bath can be quick. Give sponge baths if the resident resists a shower or tub bath.
- Make sure the bathroom is well-lit.
- Keep the temperature comfortable.
- Give privacy.
- Be calm and quiet when bathing.
- Keep the process simple.
- Be sensitive when talking to your resident about bathing (Fig. 19-8).

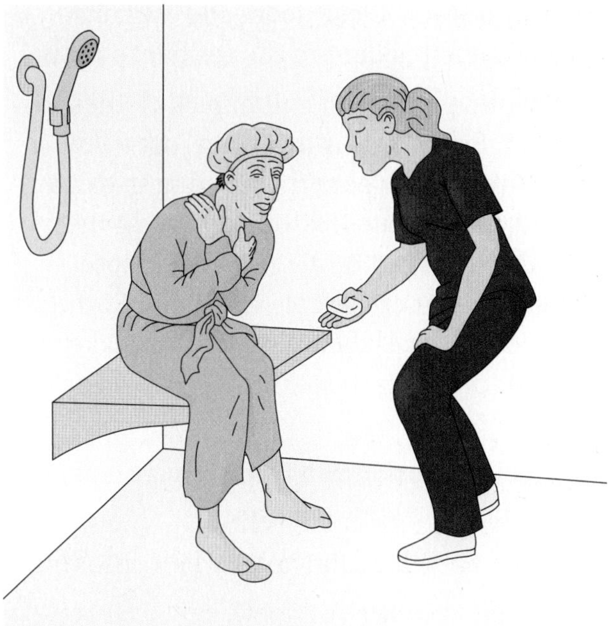

Fig. 19-8. **When a resident has AD, she may be frightened or not understand what you are trying to do. Stay calm. Gently explain what you are trying to do.**

- Give the resident a washcloth to hold. This can distract him or her while you finish the bath.
- Be safe. Always follow safety precautions. Ensure safety by using nonslip mats, tub seats, and hand-holds.
- Be flexible about when you bathe. Your resident may not always be in the mood.
- Be relaxed. Allow the resident to enjoy the bath.
- Be encouraging. Offer praise and support.
- Let the resident do as much as possible.
- Check the skin regularly for signs of irritation.
- Be aware that not everyone bathes with the same frequency. Understand if your resident does not want to bathe.

Problems with Dressing

- Show the resident what he or she is going to wear. This brings up the idea of dressing.
- Avoid delays or interruptions while dressing.
- Give privacy. Close doors and curtains. Dress the resident in the resident's room.
- Encourage the resident to pick clothes to wear. Simplify this by giving just a few choices. Make sure the clothing is clean and appropriate. Lay out clothes in the order to be put on (Fig. 19-9). Choose clothes that are simple to put on. Some people with Alzheimer's disease make a habit of layering clothing regardless of the weather.
- Break the task down into simple steps. Introduce one step at a time.
- Use a friendly, calm voice when speaking.
- Do not rush the resident.
- Praise and encourage the resident at each step.

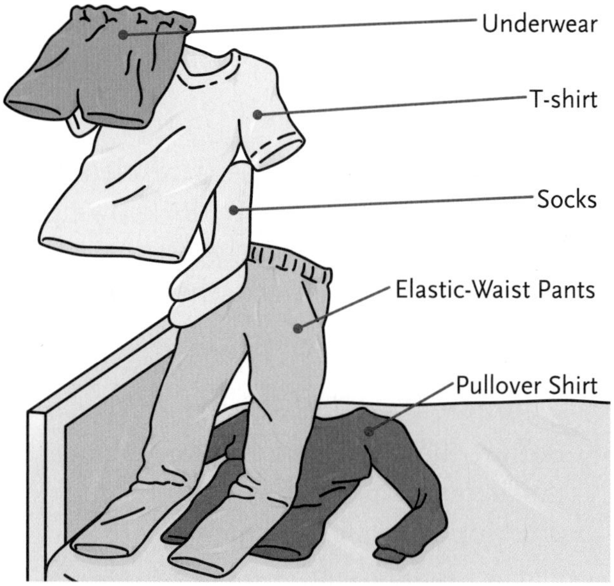

Fig. 19-9. **Lay out clothes in the order to be put on.**

Problems with Eating

Food may not interest a resident with AD at all. It may be of great interest, but a resident may only want to eat a few types of food. In both cases, a resident with AD is at risk for malnutrition. Nutritious food intake should be encouraged. Here are some ideas for improving eating habits:

- Have meals at regular, consistent times each day.
- Foods should look and smell good.
- Make sure there is good lighting.
- Keep noise and distractions low during meals.
- You may need to remind the resident that it is mealtime.
- Keep the task of eating simple.
- Finger foods are easier to eat. They allow residents to choose the food they want to eat. Finger food is food that is easy to pick up with the fingers. Examples are sandwiches cut into fourths, chicken nuggets or small pieces of cooked boneless chicken, fish sticks, cheese cubes, halved hard-boiled eggs, and fresh fruit and soft vegetables cut into bite-sized pieces (Fig. 19-10).

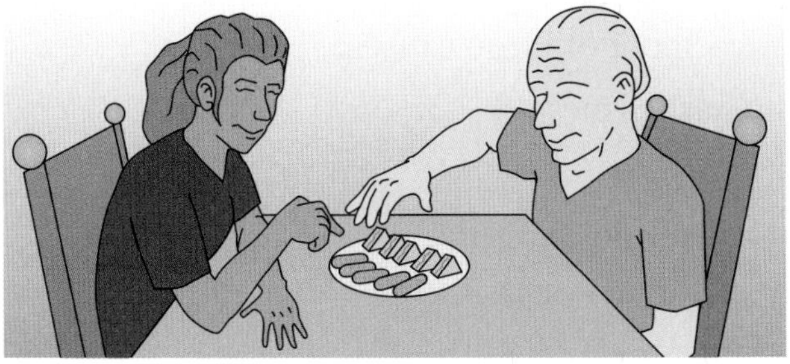

Fig. 19-10. **Finger foods are often easier to eat and promote independence for residents who have AD.**

- Do not serve steaming or very hot foods or drinks.
- Use dishes without a pattern. White usually works best. Use a simple place setting with a single eating utensil. Remove other items from the table (Fig. 19-11).

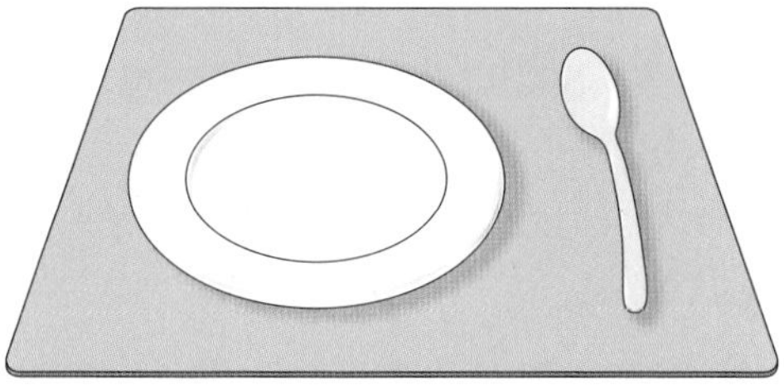

Fig. 19-11. **Use white plates or bowls with a placemat in a solid color. This may help avoid confusion and distraction.**

- Put only one item of food on the plate at a time. The food tray may be overwhelming.
- Help him or her taste a sample of the meal first.
- Place a spoon to the lips. This will encourage the resident to open his or her mouth.
- Ask the resident to open his or her mouth.
- Guide the resident through the meal. Provide simple instructions.
- Offer regular drinks of water, juice, and other fluids to avoid dehydration.
- Use adaptive equipment, such as special spoons and bowls, as needed.
- If a resident needs to be fed, do so slowly. Give small pieces of food.
- Make mealtimes simple and relaxed. Allow time for eating. Give the resident time to swallow before each bite or drink.
- Seat residents with AD with others at small tables. This encourages socializing.
- Observe for eating or swallowing problems. Report them to the nurse as soon as possible.
- Residents with AD may not understand how to eat or use utensils. Give simple, clear instructions.
- Observe and report changes or problems in eating habits.

Additional tips for caring for residents with AD include:

- Help with grooming. Help the people in your care feel attractive and dignified.
- Prevent infections. Follow Standard Precautions.
- Observe the resident's physical health. Report any potential problems. People with dementia may not notice their own health problems.
- Maintain a daily exercise routine.
- Maintain self-esteem. Encourage independence in ADLs.
- Share in fun activities, looking at pictures, talking, and reminiscing.
- Reward positive and independent behavior. Give smiles, hugs, warm touches, and thank yous (Fig. 19-12).

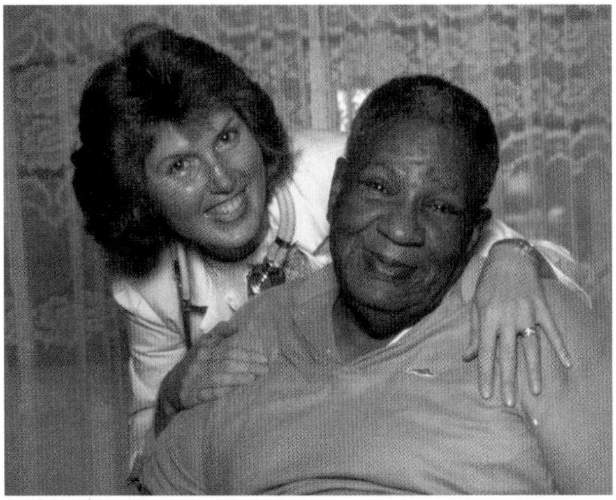

Fig. 19-12. **Reward positive behavior with warm touches, smiles, and thank yous.**

8. List and describe interventions for common difficult behaviors related to Alzheimer's disease

Below are some common difficult behaviors that you may face with Alzheimer's residents. Each resident is different. Work with each as an individual. Report behavior in detail to the nurse.

Agitation. A resident who is excited, restless, or troubled is said to be **agitated** (Fig. 19-13). A situation that leads to agitation is a **trigger**. Triggers may be a change of routine or caregiver, new or frustrating experiences, or even television. Responses that may help calm a resident who is agitated are:

- Try to remove triggers. Keep routine constant. Avoid frustration.
- Focus on a soothing, familiar activity. Try sorting things or looking at pictures.
- Stay calm. Use a low, soothing voice to speak to and reassure the resident.
- An arm around the shoulder, patting, or stroking may soothe some residents.

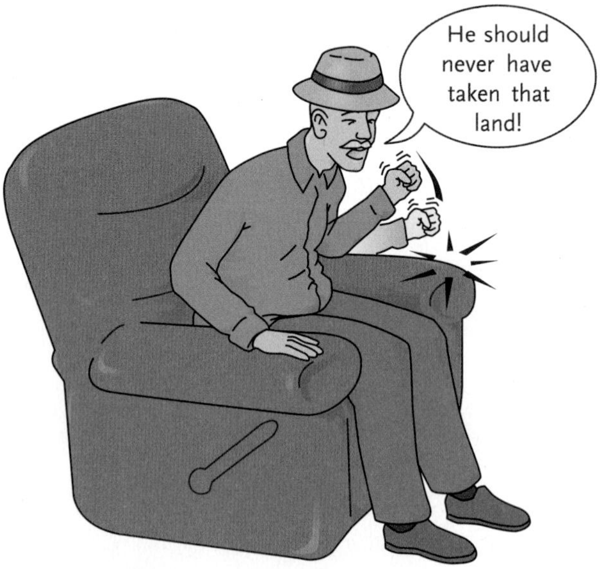

Fig. 19-13. **Take steps early to calm a resident who is agitated. Stay calm. Do not argue with him.**

Pacing and Wandering. A resident who walks back and forth in the same area is **pacing**. A resident who walks aimlessly around the facility is **wandering**. Pacing and wandering may have some of these causes:

- restlessness
- hunger
- disorientation
- need for toileting
- constipation
- pain
- forgetting how or where to sit down
- too much daytime napping
- need for exercise

Remove causes when you can. Give nutritious snacks. Encourage an exercise routine. Maintain a toileting schedule.

Responses to pacing and wandering include:

- Let residents pace or wander in a safe and secure (locked) area. Keep an eye on them (Fig. 19-14).
- Suggest another activity, such as going for a walk together.

If a resident wanders away, follow the facility's policies and procedures for missing residents. Tell the nurse immediately when a resident is missing.

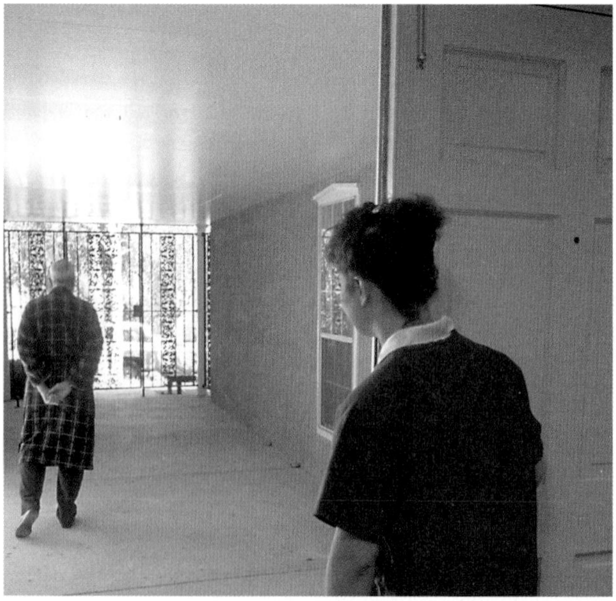

Fig. 19-14. **Make sure a resident is in a safe area if he paces or wanders.**

Hallucinations or Delusions. A resident who sees things that are not there is having **hallucinations** (Fig 19-15). A resident who believes things that are not true is having **delusions** (Fig. 19-16). You can respond to hallucinations and delusions in these ways:

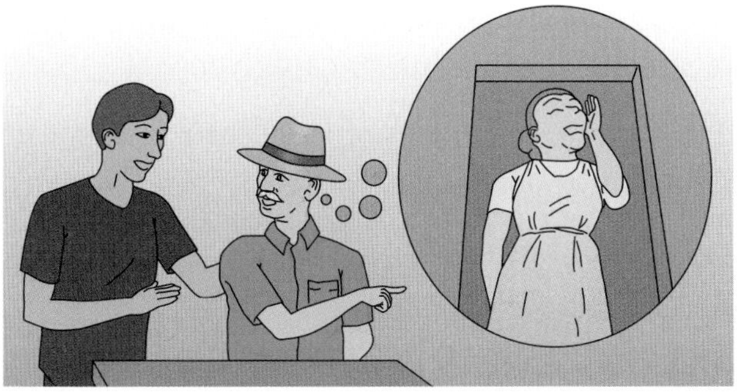

Fig. 19-15. **Hallucinating is seeing or hearing things that are not really there. For example, a resident may think he is hearing his mother calling him to dinner. You know that his mother died twenty years ago, but to him this is very real.**

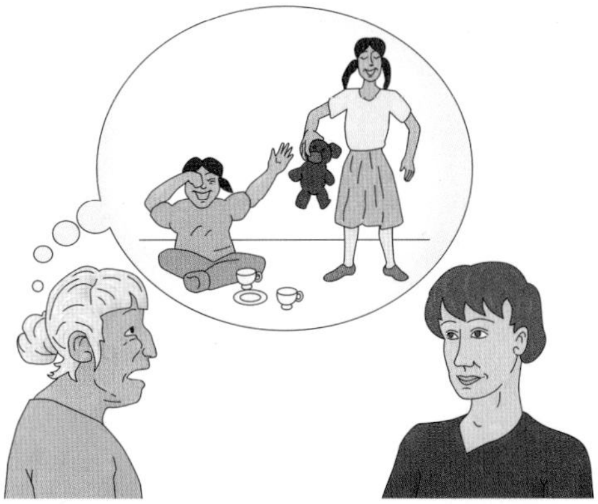

Fig. 19-16. **A delusion is a belief in something that is not true, or is out of touch with reality. For example, a resident thinks that her long-deceased sister is stealing from her room, like she did when they were young.**

- Ignore harmless hallucinations and delusions.
- Reassure a resident who seems upset or worried.
- Do not argue with a resident who is imagining things. The feelings are real to him or her. Do not tell the resident that you can see or hear his or her hallucinations. Redirect resident to other activities or thoughts.
- Be calm. Reassure resident that you are there to help.

Sundowning. When a person gets restless and agitated in the late afternoon, evening, or night, it is called **sundowning**. Sundowning may be caused by hunger or fatigue, a change in routine or caregiver, or any new or frustrating situation. Some effective responses are:

- Remove triggers. Give snacks or encourage rest.
- Avoid stressful situations during this time. Limit activities, appointments, trips, and visits.
- Play soft music.
- Set a bedtime routine and keep it.
- Recognize when sundowning occurs. Plan a calming activity just before.
- Remove caffeine from the diet.
- Give a soothing back massage.
- Distract the resident with a simple, calm activity like looking at a magazine.
- Have a daily exercise routine.

Catastrophic Reactions. When a person with AD overreacts to something in an unreasonable way it is called a **catastrophic reaction** (Fig. 19-17). It may be triggered by:

- fatigue
- change of routine, environment, or caregiver
- overstimulation (too much noise or activity)
- difficult choices or tasks
- physical pain
- hunger
- need for toileting

Respond to catastrophic reactions as you would to agitation or sundowning. For example, remove triggers. Help the resident focus on a soothing activity.

Depression. When residents become withdrawn, lack energy, do not eat or do things they used to enjoy, they may be **depressed**. Chapter 20 has more information on depression and its symptoms.

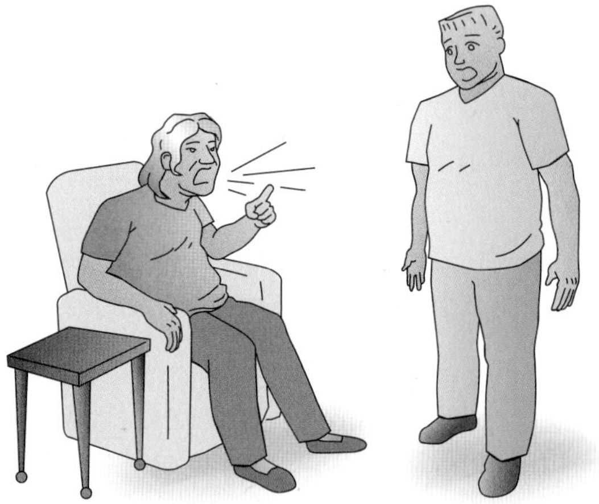

Fig. 19-17. **Nonverbal clues, such as facial expressions or body language, can warn you of increasing agitation. Take steps early to calm down a resident who is becoming agitated.**

Depression may have many causes:

- loss of independence
- inability to cope
- feelings of failure, fear
- facing a progressive, incurable illness
- chemical imbalance

You can respond to depression in a number of ways:

- Report signs of depression to the nurse immediately. It can be treated with medication.
- Encourage independence, self-care, and activity.
- Talk about moods and feelings if the resident wishes. Be a good listener.
- Encourage social interaction.

Perseveration or Repetitive Phrasing. A resident who repeats a word, phrase, question, or activity over and over is perseverating. Repeating a word or phrase is also called **repetitive phrasing**.

This may be caused by several factors. These include disorientation or confusion. Respond with patience. Do not try to silence or stop the resident. Answer questions each time they are asked. Use the same words each time.

Violent Behavior. A resident who attacks, hits, or threatens someone is **violent**. Violence may be triggered by many situations. These include frustration, overstimulation, or a change in routine, environment, or caregiver.

Appropriate responses to violent residents are:

- Block blows but never hit back (Fig. 19-18).
- Step out of reach.
- Call for help if needed.
- Do not leave resident in the home alone.
- Try to remove triggers.
- Calm resident as you would for agitation or sundowning.

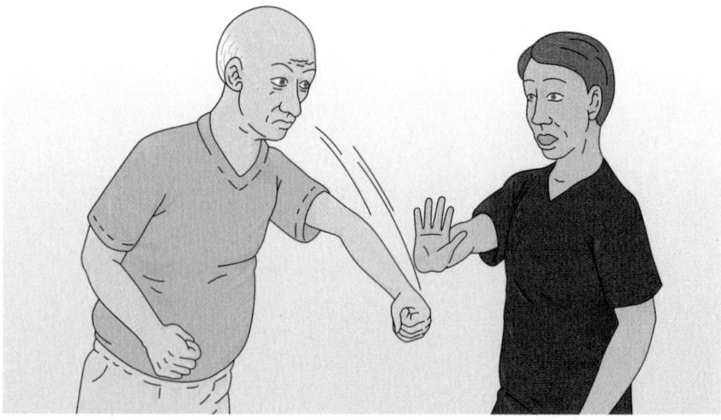

Fig. 19-18. **Block blows or step out of the way. Never hit back.**

Disruptiveness. Disruptive behavior is anything that disturbs others, such as yelling, banging on furniture, slamming doors, etc. (Fig. 19-19). Often this behavior is triggered by a wish for attention, by pain or constipation, or by frustration.

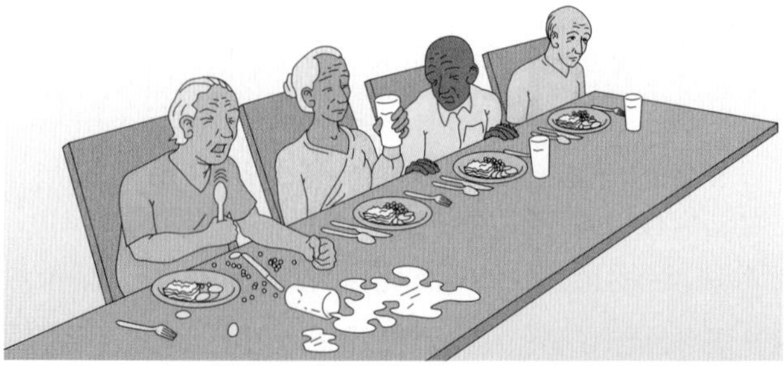

Fig. 19-19. **Be calm and friendly when a resident is disruptive. Try to find out why the behavior is occurring.**

Gain the resident's attention. Be calm and friendly. Gently direct the resident to a more private area, if possible. Find out why the behavior is occurring. Ask the resident about it, if possible. There may be a physical reason, such as pain or discomfort.

Notice and praise improvements in behavior. Be tactful and sensitive when you do this. Avoid treating the resident like a child. Tell the resident any changes in schedules, routines, or the environment in advance. Involve the resident in developing routine activities and schedules, if possible. Encourage the resident to join in independent activities that are safe (for example, folding towels). This helps the resident feel in charge. It can prevent feelings of powerlessness. Independence is power. Help the resident find ways to cope. Focus on positive activities he or she may still be able to do, such as knitting, crocheting, crafts, etc. This can provide a diversion.

Inappropriate Social Behavior. Inappropriate social behavior may be cursing, name calling, or other behavior. As with violent or disruptive behavior, there may be many reasons why a resident is behaving in this manner. Try not to take it personally. The resident may only be reacting to frustration or other stress, not to you.

Stay calm. Be reassuring. Try to find out what caused the behavior (for example, too much noise, too many people, too much stress, pain, or discomfort). If possible, gently direct the resident to a private area if he or she is disturbing others. Respond positively to any appropriate behavior. Report any physical abuse or serious verbal abuse to the nurse.

Inappropriate Sexual Behavior. Inappropriate sexual behavior, such as removing clothes or touching one's own genitals, can embarrass those who see it. Responses include:

- Be matter-of-fact when dealing with such behavior. Do not over-react. This may reinforce the behavior.
- Be sensitive to the nature of the problem. Is the behavior actually intentional? Is it excessive or consistent? Try to distract the resident. If this does not work, gently direct him or her to a private area. Tell the nurse.

A resident may be reacting to a need for physical stimulation or affection. Consider other ways to provide physical stimulation. Try backrubs, a soft doll or stuffed animal to cuddle, comforting blankets, pieces of cloth, or physical touch that is appropriate.

Pillaging and Hoarding. **Pillaging** is taking things that belong to someone else. A person with dementia may honestly think something belongs to him, even when it clearly does not. **Hoarding** is collecting and putting things away in a guarded way.

Pillaging and hoarding should not be considered stealing (Fig. 19-20). A person with Alzheimer's disease cannot and does not steal. Stealing is planned. It requires a conscious effort. In most cases, the person with AD is only collecting something that catches his or her attention.

It is common for those with AD to wander in and out of rooms collecting things. They may carry these objects around for a while, and then leave them in other places. This is not intentional. People with AD will often take their own things and leave them in another room, not knowing what they are doing.

You can help lessen problems by doing the following:

- Label all personal belongings with the resident's name and room number. This way there is no confusion about what belongs to whom.
- Place a label, symbol, or object on the resident's door. This helps the resident find his or her own room.
- Do not tell family that their loved one is "stealing" from others.

- Prepare the family so they are not upset when they find items that do not belong to their family member.
- Ask the family to tell staff if they notice strange items in the room.
- Provide a rummage drawer—a drawer with items that are okay and safe for the resident to take with him or her.

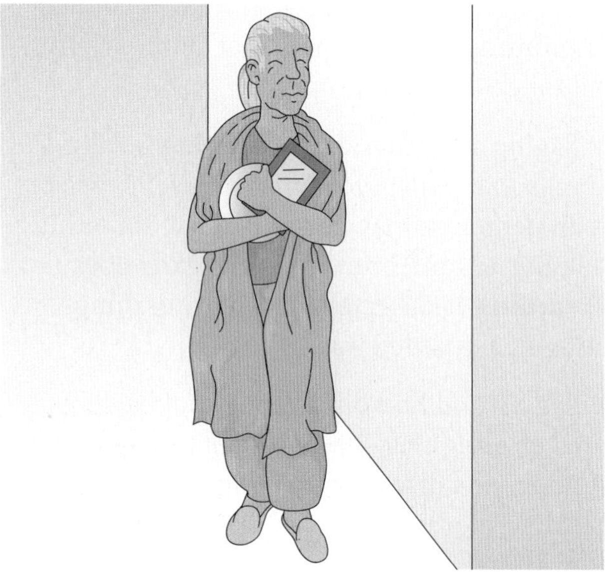

Fig. 19-20. **When a person with dementia takes something that belongs to someone else, it is not considered stealing.**

9. Describe creative therapies for residents with Alzheimer's disease

Although AD cannot be cured, there are many ways to improve life for residents with AD.

Reality Orientation is using calendars, clocks, signs, and lists to help residents remember who and where they are. It is useful in early stages of AD, when residents are confused but not totally disoriented. In later stages, reality orientation may frustrate residents.

Example: Each day when you go into Mrs. Elkin's room, you show her the calendar. You point out what day of the week it is. On the calendar or another piece of paper, you list all the things you will do today. For example, take a shower, eat lunch, and go for a walk. When you speak to her, you call her by her name, Mrs. Elkin. When helping with tasks, you explain why you do things as you do: "We use a shower chair in the shower so you don't have to stand up for so long, Mrs. Elkin."

Validation Therapy is letting residents believe they live in the past or in imaginary circumstances. **Validating** means giving value to or approving. Make no attempt to reorient the resident to actual circumstances. Explore the resident's beliefs. Do not argue. Validating can give comfort and reduce agitation. It is useful in cases of moderate to severe disorientation.

Example: Mr. Baldwin tells you he does not want to eat lunch today. He is going out to a restaurant with his wife. You know his wife has been dead for many years and that Mr. Baldwin can no longer eat out. Instead of telling him that he is not going out to eat, you ask what restaurant he is going to and what he will have. You suggest that he eat a good lunch now because sometimes the service is slow in restaurants (Fig. 19-21).

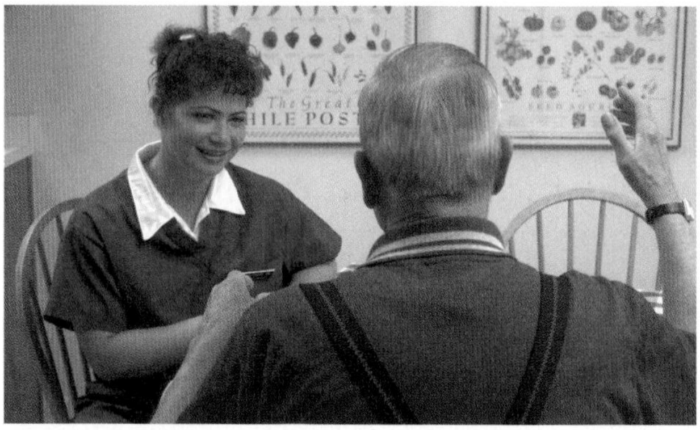

Fig. 19-21. **Validation therapy accepts a resident's fantasies. There is no attempt to reorient him to reality. By "playing along" with a resident's fantasies, you let him know that you take him seriously. You do not think of him as child who does not know what is happening in his own life. You also learn more about your residents.**

Reminiscence Therapy is encouraging residents to remember and talk about the past. Explore memories. Ask about details. Focus on a time of life that was pleasant. Work through feelings about a hard time in the past. It is useful in many stages of AD, but especially with moderate to severe confusion.

Example: Mr. Benton, an 82-year-old man with Alzheimer's, fought in World War II. In his room are many mementos of the war. He has pictures of his war buddies, a medal he was given, and more. You ask him to tell you where he was sent in the war. He tells you about being in the Pacific. You ask him more detailed questions. Eventually he tells you a lot: the friends he made in the service, why he was given the medal, times he was scared, and how much he missed his wife (Fig. 19-22).

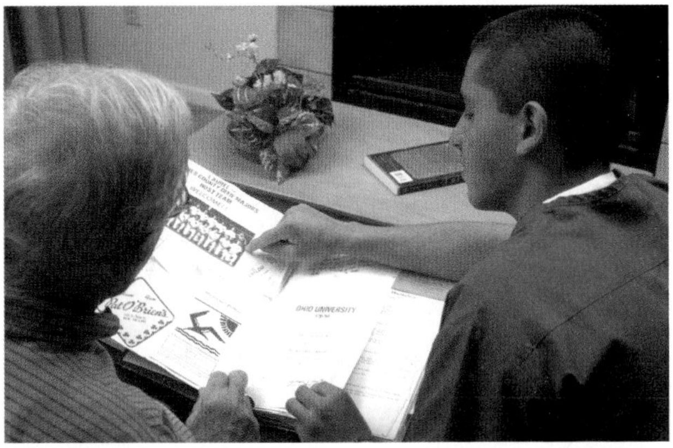

Fig. 19-22. **Reminiscence therapy encourages a resident to remember and talk about his past. It helps you show an interest in him as a person, not just as a resident. You let him show you that he is a person who was competent, social, responsible, and brave. This boosts his self-esteem.**

Activity Therapy uses things the resident enjoys to prevent boredom and frustration. These activities also aid self-esteem. Help the resident take walks, listen to music, read, or do other things he or she enjoys (Fig. 19-23). It is useful in most stages of AD.

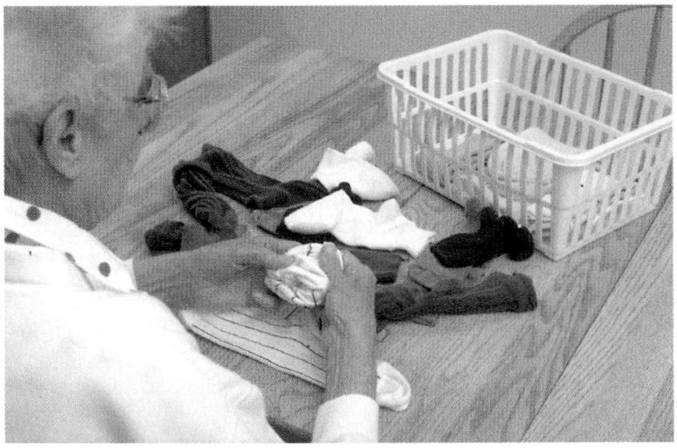

Fig. 19-23. **Activities that are not frustrating can help residents with AD. They promote mental exercise.**

Example: Mrs. Hoebel, a 70-year-old woman with AD, was a librarian for almost 45 years. She loves books and reading, but she cannot read much anymore. You bring in books that are filled with pictures. She sits with the books, turning pages and looking at pictures.

Chapter Review

1. What is confusion?
2. What is delirium?
3. What is dementia?
4. Alzheimer's disease is a progressive, degenerative, and irreversible disease. In your own words, what does this mean?
5. What type of skills does a person with Alzheimer's disease usually retain?
6. What can you encourage residents to do that may help slow the progression of AD?
7. Possible communication challenges for residents with AD are listed in learning objective 4. They include challenges with a resident who may:

- be frightened or anxious
- forget or show memory loss
- have trouble finding words or names
- seem not to understand basic instructions or questions
- want to say something but cannot
- not remember how to perform basic tasks
- insist on doing something that is unsafe or not allowed
- hallucinate, or be paranoid or accusing
- be verbally abusive, or use bad language
- have lost most verbal skills

For each communication challenge, list one tip that may help.

8. Helpful personal attitudes when working with residents who have AD are in learning objective 5. They include the following:

- Do not take it personally.
- Put yourself in their shoes.
- Work with the symptoms and behaviors you see.
- Work as a team.
- Take care of yourself.
- Work with family members.
- Remember the goals of the care plan.

For each attitude, list one example of what you can do to express that attitude.

9. List four interventions for each of the following problems: incontinence, bathing, dressing, and eating.

Matching. Match each definition below with the correct key term from the list.

a. agitation
b. catastrophic reaction
c. delusions
d. depression
e. hallucinations
f. hoarding
g. pacing
h. perseverating
i. pillaging
j. sundowning
k. violent behavior
l. wandering

10. _____ Repeating a word, phrase, question, or activity over and over.
11. _____ Attacking, hitting, or threatening someone.
12. _____ Moving from one area to another aimlessly.
13. _____ Collecting and putting things away in a guarded manner.
14. _____ Overreacting to something in an unreasonable way.
15. _____ Being excited, restless, or troubled.
16. _____ Becoming withdrawn and having no energy or interest in doing things.
17. _____ Taking things that belong to someone else.
18. _____ Walking back and forth in the same area.
19. _____ Seeing things that are not there.
20. _____ Believing things that are not true.
21. _____ Becoming restless and agitated in the late afternoon, evening, or night.
22. Describe each of the four creative therapies for AD.

Chapter 20
Mental Health and Mental Illness

1. Identify seven characteristics of mental health

Mental health is the normal function of emotional and intellectual abilities (Fig. 20-1). Traits of a person who is mentally healthy include the ability to:

- get along with others
- adapt to change
- care for self and others
- give and accept love
- deal with situations that cause stress, disappointment, and frustration
- take responsibility for decisions, feelings, and actions
- control and meet desires and impulses appropriately

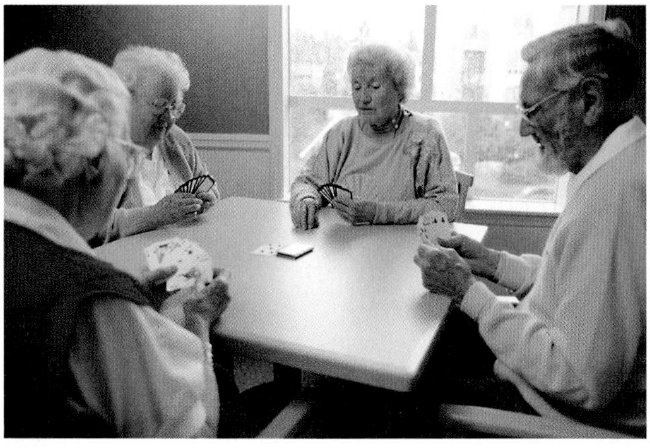

Fig. 20-1. **Interacting well with others is a trait of mental health.**

2. Identify four causes of mental illness

While it involves the emotions and mental functions, **mental illness** is a disease. It is like any physical disease. It produces signs and symptoms. It affects the body's ability to function. It responds to proper treatment and care. Mental illness disrupts a person's ability to function at a normal level in the family, home, or community. It often causes inappropriate behavior. Some signs and symptoms of mental illness are confusion, disorientation, agitation, and anxiety.

However, signs and symptoms like those of mental illness can occur when mental illness is not present. A crisis, temporary physical changes in the brain, side effects or interactions from medications, and severe change in the environment may cause a situation response. In a **situation response**, the signs and symptoms are temporary.

Mental illness can be caused or made worse by these conditions:

1. **Physical factors**. Illness, disability, or aging can cause stress. This may lead to mental illness. Substance abuse or a chemical imbalance can also cause mental illness. Self-respect and self-worth are the building blocks of mental health. They are challenged when ill or disabled people have

trouble with their ADLs. They may fear the future. They may worry about their dependency on others.

2. **Environmental factors**. Weak interpersonal or family relationships, or trauma early in life (such as being abused as a child) can lead to mental illness.
3. **Heredity**. Mental illness can occur repeatedly in some families. This may be due to inherited traits or family influence.
4. **Stress**. People can bear different levels of stress. People have different ways of handling stress. When stress is too great, a person may not cope with it. Mental illness may then arise.

3. Distinguish between fact and fallacy concerning mental illness

A **fallacy** is a false belief. The greatest fallacy about mental illness is that people who are mentally ill can control it. Mentally ill people cannot simply choose to be well. Mental illness is a disease. It is like any other physical illness. Mentally healthy people are able to control their emotions and actions. Mentally ill people may not have this control. Knowing it is a disease helps you work with mentally ill residents.

Fact and Fallacy

Fact: Mental illness is a disease like any physical illness. People with mental illness cannot control their illness.

Fallacy: People with mental illness can control their illness. They can choose to be well.

4. Explain the connection between mental and physical wellness

Mental health is important to physical health. The ability to reduce stress can help prevent some physical illnesses (Fig. 20-2). It can help people cope if illness or disability occur. Mental health can help protect and improve physical health. The reverse is also true. Physical illness or disability can cause or worsen mental illness. The stress these things cause takes a toll on mental health.

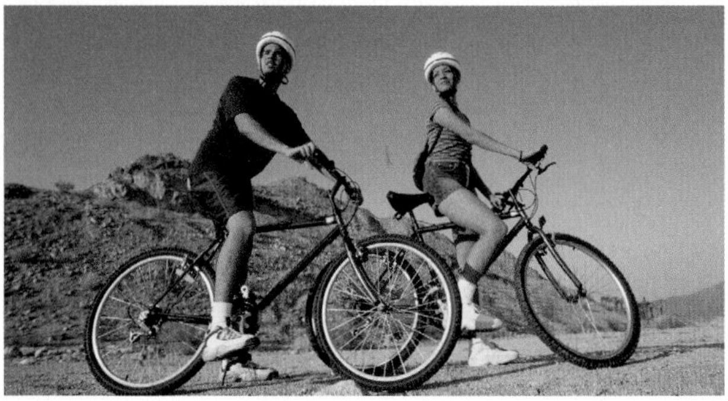

Fig. 20-2. **Regular exercise can promote mental and physical health.**

5. List guidelines for communicating with mentally ill residents

Different types of mental illness will affect how well residents communicate. Treat each as an individual. Tailor your approach to the situation. Use these tips to communicate with residents who are mentally ill (Fig. 20-3).

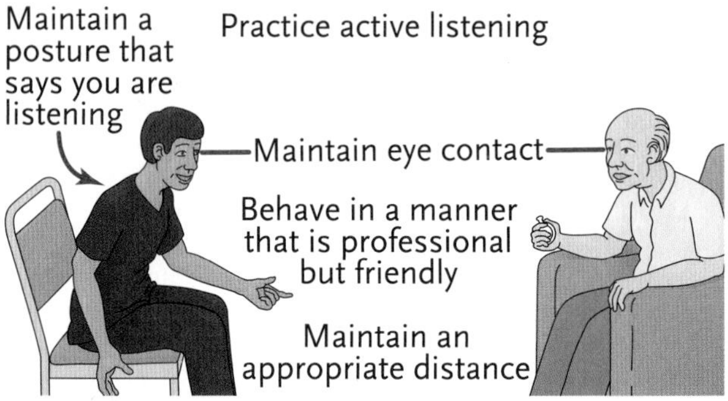
Maintain a posture that says you are listening
Practice active listening
Maintain eye contact
Behave in a manner that is professional but friendly
Maintain an appropriate distance

Fig. 20-3. **Practice good communication skills with mentally ill residents.**

GUIDELINES
Mental Illness

- Do not talk to adults like children.
- Use simple, clear statements. Use a normal tone of voice.
- Be sure that what you say and how you speak show respect and concern.
- Sit or stand at a normal distance from the resident. Be aware of your body language.

- Be honest and direct, as with any resident.
- Avoid arguments.
- Maintain eye contact.
- Listen carefully.

6. Identify and define common defense mechanisms

Defense mechanisms are unconscious behaviors. They are used to release tension or cope with stress. They help to block uncomfortable or threatening feelings. All people use them at times. People who are mentally ill use them more. Overuse of these mechanisms keeps a person from understanding their emotional problems and actions. If a person cannot recognize problems, he or she will not solve them. They may get worse. Common defense mechanisms are:

Denial: Rejecting the thought or feeling—"I'm not upset with you!"

Projection: Seeing feelings in others that are really one's own—"My teacher hates me."

Displacement: Transferring a strong negative feeling to a safer place. For example, an unhappy employee cannot yell at his boss for fear of losing his job. He later yells at his wife.

Rationalization: Making excuses to justify a situation—After stealing something, saying "Everybody does it."

Repression: Blocking painful thoughts or feelings from the mind—For example, forgetting sexual abuse.

Regression: Going back to an old, usually immature behavior—For example, throwing a temper tantrum as an adult.

7. Describe the symptoms of anxiety, depression, and schizophrenia

There are many degrees of mental illness. It ranges from mild to severe. A person with severe mental illness may lose touch with reality and become unable to communicate or make decisions. Some people with mild mental illness seem to function normally. They may sometimes become overwhelmed by stress or overly emotional. Many signs of mental illness are simply extreme behaviors most people sometimes experience. Being able to recognize such behavior may make it easier to understand the mentally ill.

Anxiety-related Disorders. Anxiety is uneasiness or fear, often about a situation or condition. When a mentally healthy person feels anxiety, he or she usually knows the cause. The anxiety fades once the cause is removed. A mentally ill person may feel anxiety all the time. He or she may not know the reason why. Physical signs of anxiety-related disorders include shakiness, muscle aches, sweating, cold and clammy hands, dizziness, fatigue, racing heart, cold or hot flashes, a choking or smothering sensation, or a dry mouth (Fig. 20-4).

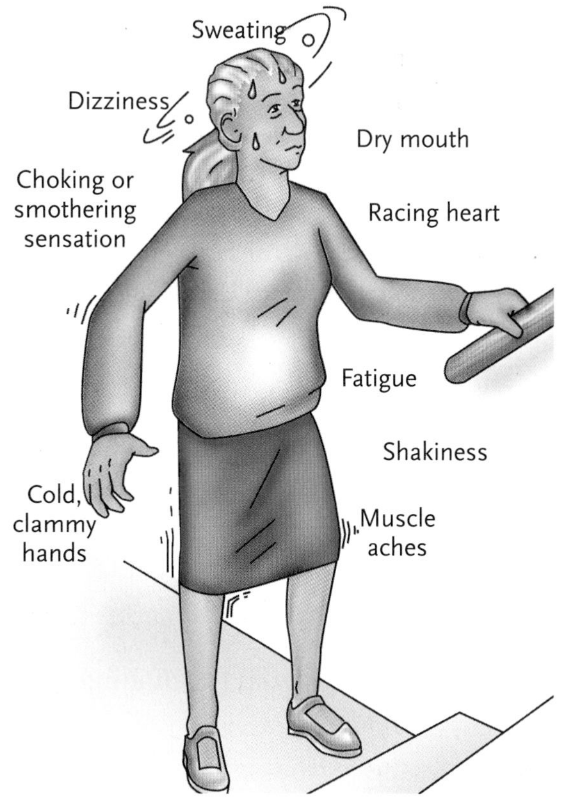

Fig. 20-4. **Common symptoms of anxiety.**

Phobias are an intense form of anxiety. Many people are very afraid of some things or situations. Examples are fear of dogs or of flying. For a mentally ill person, a phobia is a disabling terror. It keeps the person from doing normal things. For example, the fear of being in a confined space, **claustrophobia**, may make using an elevator a terrifying task.

Other anxiety-related disorders include **panic disorder**, in which a person is terrified for no known reason. **Obsessive compulsive disorder** is obsessive behavior a person uses to cope with anxiety. For example, a person may wash his hands over and over as a way of dealing with anxiety. Anxiety-related disorders may also be caused by a traumatic experience. This is known as **post-traumatic stress disorder**.

Depression. Clinical depression is a serious mental illness. It may cause deep mental, emotional, and physical pain and disability. It makes other illnesses worse. If untreated, it may result in suicide. The National Institute of Mental Health lists depression as one of the most common links with suicide in older adults.

Clinical depression is not a normal reaction to stress. Sadness is only one sign of this illness. Not all people who have depression report sadness or appear sad. Other common symptoms of clinical depression include (Fig. 20-5):

- pain, including headaches, stomach pain, and other body aches
- low energy or fatigue
- **apathy**, or lack of interest
- irritability
- anxiety
- loss of appetite
- problems with sexual functioning and desire
- sleeplessness, trouble sleeping, or excessive sleeping
- guilt
- trouble concentrating
- frequent thoughts of suicide and death

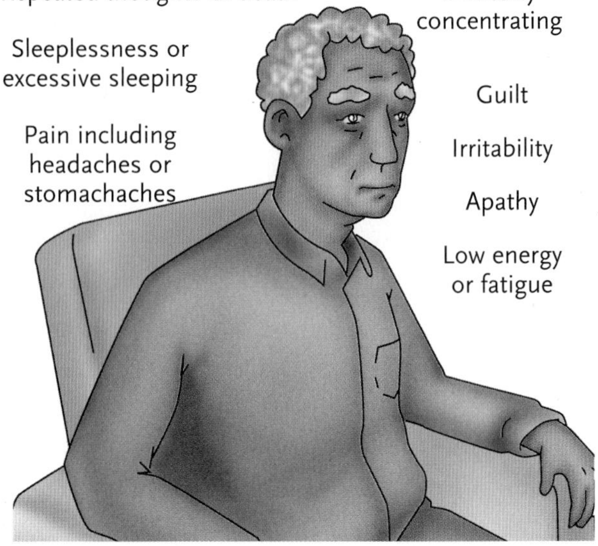

Fig. 20-5. **Common symptoms of clinical depression.**

Depression can occur along with other illnesses. Examples are cancer, HIV or AIDS, Alzheimer's disease, diabetes, and after a heart attack. Depression due to having one or more of these illnesses is common among the elderly.

There are different types and degrees of depression. **Major depression** may cause a person to lose interest in everything he once cared about. **Manic depression**, or **bipolar disorder**, causes a person to swing from deep depression to extreme activity. These episodes include high energy, little sleep, big speeches, rapidly changing moods, high self-esteem, overspending, and poor judgment.

People cannot overcome depression through sheer will. It is an illness like any other illness. It can be treated successfully. People who suffer from depression need compassion and support. Know the symptoms. Recognize the beginning or worsening of depression. Any suicide threat should be taken seriously. Report it immediately. It should not be regarded as an attempt to get attention.

Schizophrenia. Despite popular belief, schizophrenia does not mean "split personality." **Schizophrenia** is a brain disorder. It affects a person's ability to think and communicate clearly. It also affects the ability to manage emotions, make decisions, and understand reality. It affects a person's ability to interact with other people. Treatment allows many people to lead relatively normal lives. Some of the signs of schizophrenia are easy to see (Fig. 20-6). **Paranoid schizophrenia** centers mainly on hallucinations and delusions. You learned about hallucinations and delusions in chapter 19. Not all hallucinations or delusions are caused by schizophrenia.

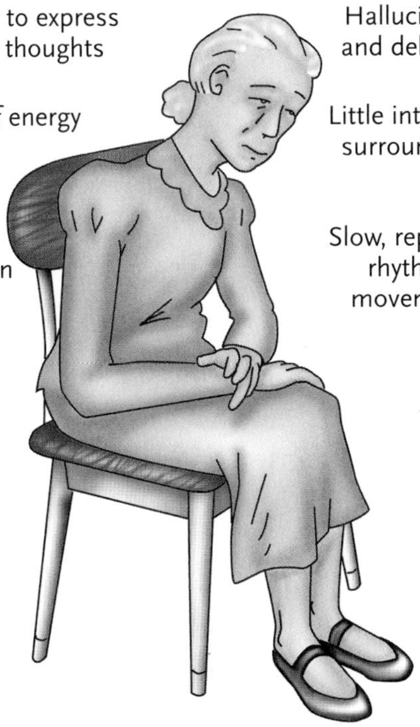

Fig. 20-6. **Common symptoms of schizophrenia.**

Other signs of schizophrenia include disorganized thinking and speech. This makes a person unable to express logical thoughts. Disorganized behavior is another sign. This means a person moves slowly, repeating gestures or movements. People with schizophrenia may also show less emotion. They may have less interest in the things around them. They may lack energy.

8. Explain your role in caring for residents who are mentally ill

Care of residents who are mentally ill is like care of any resident. The care plan and your assignment sheet will tell you what to do. You will also have some special responsibilities, including:

GUIDELINES

Mentally Ill Residents

- Observe residents carefully for changes in condition or abilities. Document and report your observations.
- Support the resident and his or her family and friends. Mental illness can be very frustrating. Your positive, professional attitude encourages the resident and the family. If you need help coping with stress, speak to the nurse.
- Encourage residents to do as much as possible for themselves. Progress may be very slow. Be patient, supportive, and positive.
- Mental illness can be treated. Medication and psychotherapy are common methods. Medication can have a very positive effect. It may let mentally ill people function more completely. Drugs must be taken properly to promote benefits and reduce side effects. You may be assigned to observe residents taking their medications.

Abilities vary among the mentally ill. Residents should do as much as possible for themselves.

9. Identify important observations that should be made and reported

Carefully observe your residents. Do not draw conclusions about the cause of the behavior. Report the facts of your observations. Include what you saw or heard, how long it lasted, and how often it occurred.

OBSERVING AND REPORTING

Mentally Ill Residents

- changes in ability
- positive or negative mood changes, especially withdrawal (Fig. 20-7)
- behavior changes, including changes in personality, extreme behavior, and behavior that does not seem to fit the situation
- comments, including jokes, about hurting self or others
- failure to take medicine or improper use of medicine
- real or imagined physical symptoms
- events, situations, or people that upset or excite residents

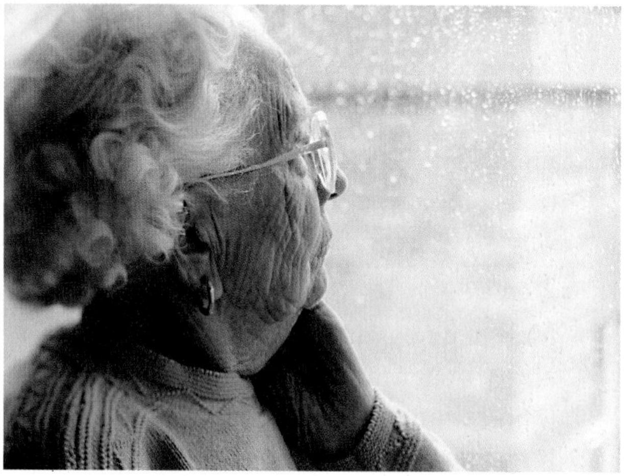

Fig. 20-7. **Withdrawal is an important change to report.**

10. List the signs of substance abuse

Substance abuse is the use of legal or illegal drugs, cigarettes, or alcohol in a way that is harmful to oneself or others. A substance need not be illegal for it to be abused (Fig. 20-8). Alcohol and cigarettes are legal for adults, but are often abused. Over-the-counter medications, including diet aids and decongestants, can be addictive and harmful. Even substances such as paint or glue are abused. They may cause injury and death.

You may observe the signs of substance abuse in your residents. Report these signs to the nurse. You can report your observations without accusing anyone. Simply report what you see, not what you think the cause may be.

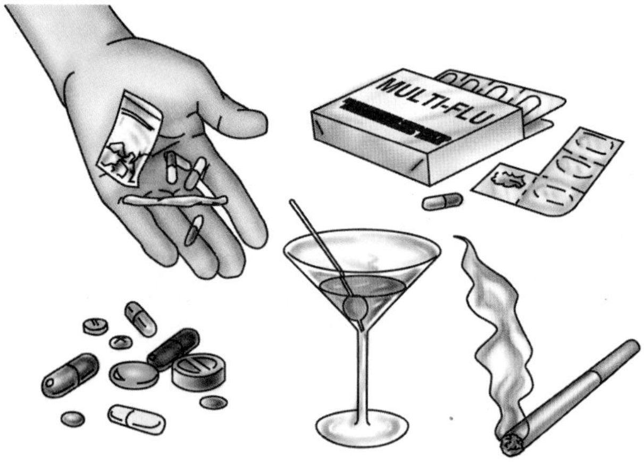

Fig. 20-8. **Illegal drugs are not the only substances that are abused.**

OBSERVING AND REPORTING

Substance Abuse

- changes in personality, moodiness, strange behavior, disruption of routines
- irritability
- changes in appearance (red eyes, dilated pupils, weight loss)
- smell of cigarettes, liquor, or other substances on breath or clothes
- reduced sense of smell
- unexplained changes in vital signs
- loss of appetite
- inability to function normally
- need for money
- confusion/forgetfulness
- blackouts or memory loss
- frequent accidents
- problems with family/friends

Chapter Review

1. For each of the seven characteristics of mental health, give one example of behavior that shows the characteristic.
2. What are four possible causes of mental illness?

3. What is the most common fallacy about mental illness?
4. Why might a physical illness cause or worsen a mental illness?
5. List six guidelines for communicating with a resident who is mentally ill.
6. Briefly define each of these common defense mechanisms: denial, projection, displacement, rationalization, repression, and regression.
7. List three symptoms of each of these mental illnesses: anxiety, depression, and schizophrenia.
8. What are the most common treatments for mental illness?
9. List three care guidelines for mentally ill residents.
10. List five important observations to make about mentally ill residents.
11. List four legal substances than can be abused.

Chapter 21
Rehabilitation and Restorative Care

1. Discuss rehabilitation and restorative care

When a resident loses some ability to function due to illness or injury, rehabilitation may be ordered. **Rehabilitation** is managed by professionals. It helps to restore a person to the highest possible level of functioning. These professionals include physical, occupational, and speech therapists.

Rehabilitation involves all parts of the person's disability. This includes psychological effects.

The therapy used and progress made are based on:

- the type of illness or injury and how serious it is
- the person's overall health
- motivation of the resident and the rehabilitation team
- when rehabilitation began

Goals of rehabilitation include:

- helping a resident regain function or recover from illness
- developing a resident's independence
- helping a resident to control his or her life
- helping a resident adapt to the limitations of a disability

Restorative services usually follow rehabilitation. The goal is to keep the resident at the level achieved by rehabilitation. Restorative services also take a team approach (Fig. 21-1). Staff create a care plan. It includes the goals of restorative care. You will be an important member of this team.

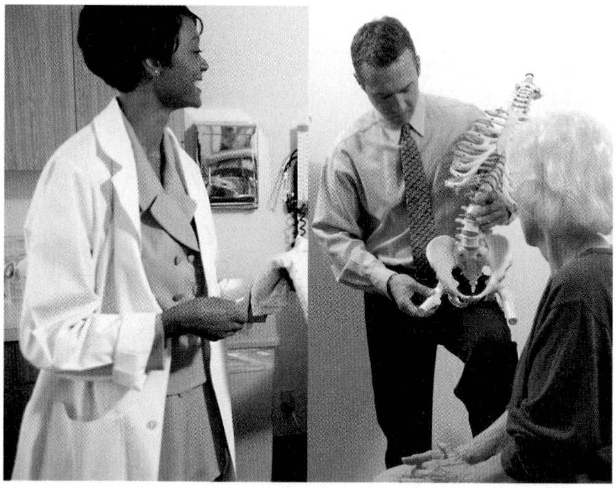

Fig. 21-1. **When you work with residents in restorative care, you will be part of a team. The team may include doctors, nurses, physical and occupational therapists, speech therapists, and social workers or other counselors.**

Nursing assistants spend more time with residents than other team members. You play a critical role in recovery and independence. Along with required tasks, remember to:

Be patient. Progress may be slow. It will seem slower to you and your residents if you are impatient. Your residents must do as much as possible for themselves. Encourage self-care, regardless of how long it takes or how poorly they are able to do it. The more patient you are, the easier it will be for them to regain abilities and confidence.

Be positive and supportive. A positive attitude can set the tone for success. Family, friends, and residents will take cues from you. Be supportive and positive. You will help create the atmosphere for successful rehabilitation.

Focus on small tasks and small accomplishments. For example, getting dressed may seem overwhelming to some residents. Break the task down into smaller steps. Today's goal might be putting on a shirt without buttoning it. Next week the goal could be buttoning the shirt if that seems manageable. When the resident can put the shirt on without help, congratulate him. Take things one step at a time.

Recognize that setbacks occur. Progress occurs at different rates. Sometimes a resident can do something one day but cannot do it the next. Reassure residents that setbacks are normal. Document any decline in a resident's abilities.

Be sensitive to the resident's needs. Some residents may need more encouragement than others. Some may be embarrassed by encouragement. Get to know your residents. Understand what motivates them. Adapt your encouragement to each personality.

Encourage independence. A resident's independence may help his or her ability to be active in the process of rehabilitation. Independence improves self-image and attitude. It also helps speed recovery.

OBSERVING AND REPORTING
Restorative Care

- O&R any increase or decrease in abilities (For example, "Yesterday Mr. Martinez used the portable commode without help. Today he asked for the bedpan.")
- O&R any change in attitude or motivation, positive or negative
- O&R any change in general health, such as changes in skin condition, appetite, energy level, or general appearance
- O&R signs of depression or mood changes

Enjoy seeing residents move toward independence or recovery. Take pride in your role in their improving health.

2. Describe the importance of promoting independence and list ways exercise improves health

Maintaining independence is vital during and after rehabilitation and restorative services. When an active and independent person is dependent, physical and mental problems may result. The body becomes less mobile. The mind is less focused. Studies show that the more active a person is, the better the mind and body work.

The staff's job is to keep residents as active as possible—physically and mentally. **Ambulation** is walking. A resident who is ambulatory can get out of bed and walk. Residents should ambulate to maintain independence and prevent problems. Lack of mobility may cause a loss of:

- independence
- self-esteem
- ability to move without help
- muscle strength, leading to contractures
- circulation of blood

Regular ambulation and exercise help improve:

- quality and health of the skin
- circulation
- strength
- sleep and relaxation
- appetite
- elimination

- blood flow
- oxygen level

Promoting social interactions and thinking abilities is important, too. Most facilities have activities geared to residents' ages and abilities.

Social involvement should be encouraged. When possible, NAs should join in activities with residents. This promotes independence. It also gives NAs a chance to observe residents' abilities.

3. Describe assistive devices and equipment

Many devices help people who are recovering from or adapting to a physical condition. Examples are shown below in Figure 21-2.

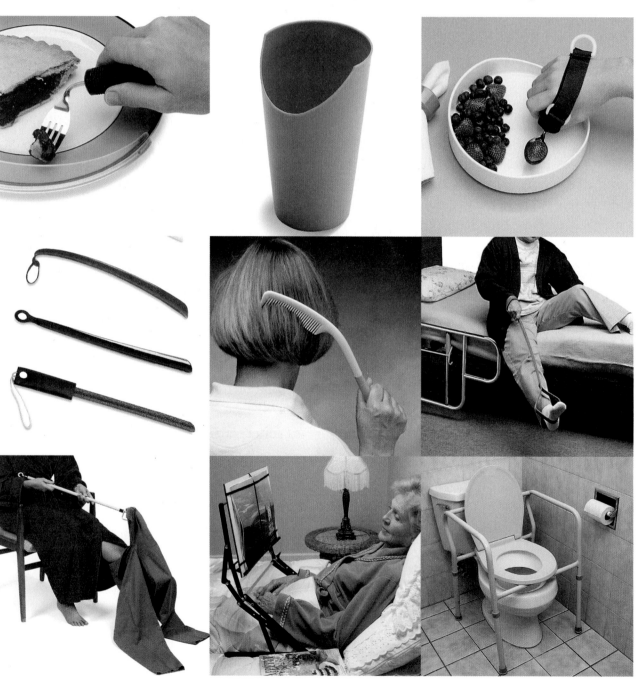

Fig. 21-2. **Many adaptive items are available. They help make it easier for residents to adapt to physical changes. (Photos courtesy of North Coast Medical, Inc.,www.ncmedical.com, 800-821-9319.)**

You first learned about adaptive, or assistive, equipment in chapter 2. Adaptive equipment helps residents do ADLs. Each adaptive device is made to support a particular disability.

- Personal care equipment includes long-handled brushes and combs.
- Supportive devices are used when ambulating. Canes, walkers, and crutches are examples.
- Safety devices, such as shower chairs and gait or transfer belts (Fig. 21-3), prevent accidents.

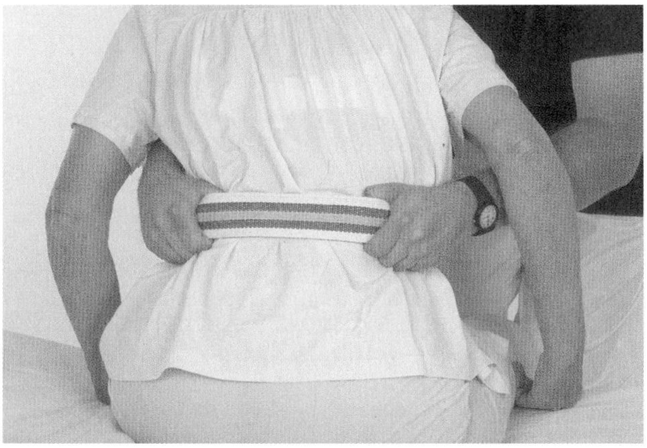

Fig. 21-3. **A transfer belt, or gait belt, is used to help residents who can walk but are weak or unsteady. The belt is made of canvas or other heavy material.**

Residents who have trouble walking may use canes, walkers, or crutches to help themselves (Fig. 21-4). Knowing the purpose of each will help you know how to use it properly.

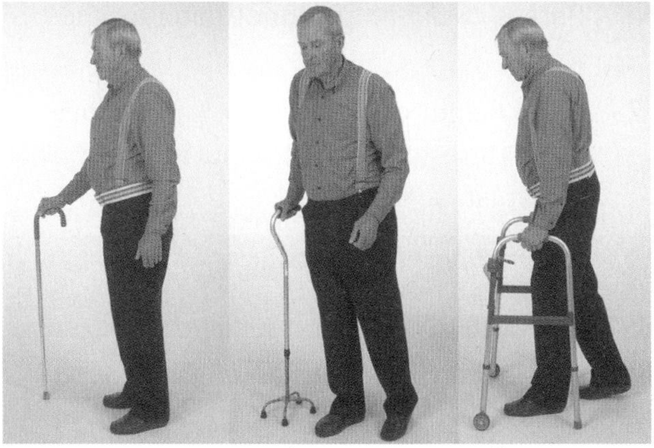

Cane Quad cane Walker

Fig. 21-4. **Residents who have trouble walking may use canes, walkers, or crutches to help themselves.**

A cane helps with balance. A **straight cane** is not designed to bear weight. A **quad cane**, with four rubber-tipped feet, can bear a little weight. Residents using canes should be able to bear weight on both legs. If one leg is weaker, the cane should be held on the strong side.

A **walker** is used when the resident can bear some weight on the legs. The walker gives stability for residents who are unsteady or lack balance. The metal frame may have rubber-tipped feet and/or wheels.

Crutches are used for residents who can bear no weight or limited weight on one leg. Some people use one crutch. Some use two. Your role is to ensure safety. Stay near the resident. Stay on the weak side. Make sure the equipment is in good condition. It must be sturdy. It must have rubber tips on the bottom.

Check the care plan before helping a resident ambulate. Discuss the resident's abilities and disabilities with the nurse. Know the resident's limitations. Know the goals for restoring and maintaining function. Any time you help a resident, communicate what you would like to do. Let him do what he can. The two of you will have to work together, especially during transfers.

Assisting a resident to ambulate

Equipment: transfer belt, non-skid shoes for the resident

1. Wash your hands.
2. Identify yourself by name. Identify the resident by name.
3. Explain procedure to resident. Speak clearly, slowly, and directly. Maintain face-to-face contact whenever possible.
4. Provide for resident's privacy with curtain, screen, or door.
5. Before ambulating, put and properly fasten non-skid footwear on the resident.

6. Adjust bed to a safe level, usually waist high. Lock bed wheels.
7. Stand in front of and face the resident.
8. Brace the resident's lower extremities. Bend your knees. Place one foot between the resident's knees. If the resident has a weak knee, brace it against your knee.
9. *With transfer (gait) belt*: Place belt around resident's waist. Grasp the belt while helping the resident to stand.

   Without transfer belt: Place arms around resident's torso under resident's armpits. Help resident to stand.
10. *With transfer belt*: Walk slightly behind and to one side of resident for the full distance, while holding onto the transfer belt (Fig. 21-5).

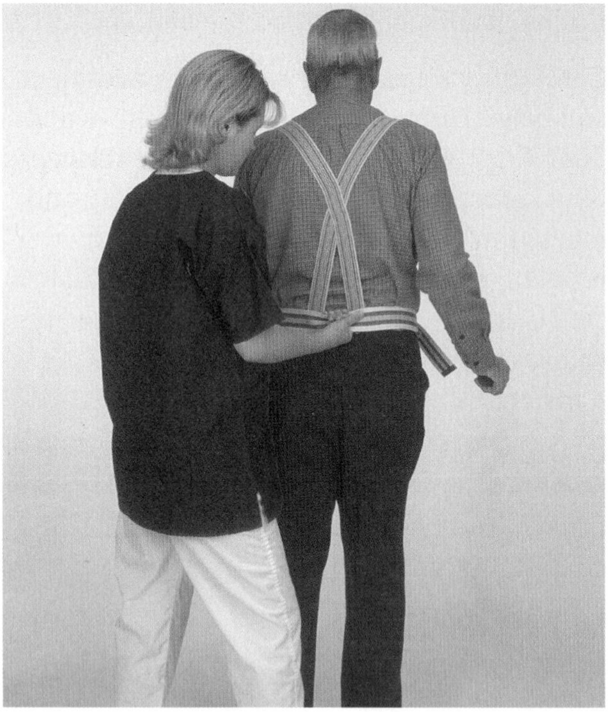

Fig. 21-5.

   Without transfer belt: Walk slightly behind and to one side of resident for the full distance. Support resident's back with your arm.
11. After ambulation, remove transfer belt if used. Help resident to a position of comfort and safety.
12. Return bed to appropriate position. Remove privacy measures.
13. Before leaving, place call light within resident's reach.
14. Wash your hands.
15. Report any changes in resident to nurse.
16. Document procedure using facility guidelines.

When a resident uses a walker or cane, follow these guidelines. They will help keep the resident safe.

GUIDELINES
Cane or Walker Use

- Be sure the walker or cane is in good condition. It must have rubber tips on bottom. Walker may have wheels. If the walker has wheels, check them for safety.
- Be sure the resident is wearing non-skid shoes.
- Have the resident use the cane on his or her strong side.
- Have the resident use both hands on the walker. The walker should not be over-extended. It should be placed no more than 12 inches in front of the resident.
- Stay near the person. Stay on the weak side.
- Purses or clothing cannot hang on the walker.
- If the height of the cane or walker does not fit a resident, tell the nurse or physical therapist.

Assisting with ambulation for a resident using a cane, walker, or crutches

Equipment: transfer belt, non-skid shoes for resident, cane, walker, or crutches

1. Wash your hands.
2. Identify yourself by name. Identify resident by name.

3. Explain procedure to resident. Speak clearly, slowly, and directly. Maintain face-to-face contact whenever possible.
4. Provide for resident's privacy with curtain, screen, or door.
5. Before ambulating, put and properly fasten non-skid footwear on the resident.
6. Adjust bed to a safe level, usually waist high. Lock bed wheels.
7. Stand in front of and face the resident.
8. Brace the resident's lower extremities. Bend your knees. Place one foot between the resident's knees. If the resident has a weak knee, brace it against your knee.
9. Place transfer belt around resident's waist. Grasp the belt while helping the resident to stand.
10. Help as needed with ambulation.
    a. *Cane.* Resident places cane about 12 inches in front of his stronger leg. He brings weaker leg even with cane. He then brings stronger leg forward slightly ahead of cane. Repeat (Fig. 21-6).

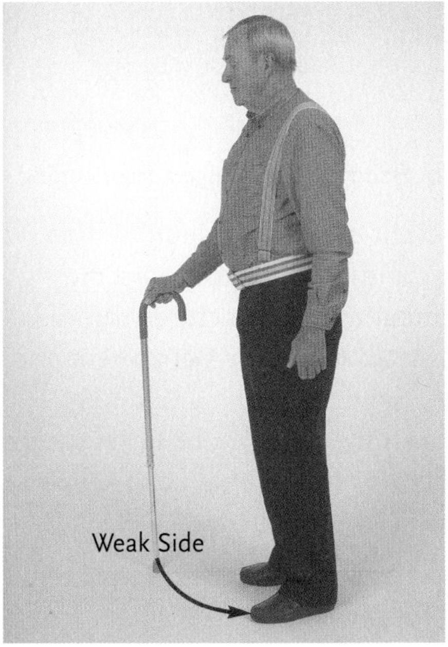

Fig. 21-6.

    b. *Walker.* Resident picks up or rolls the walker. He places it about 12 inches in front of him. All four feet or wheels of the walker should be on the ground before resident steps forward to the walker. The walker should not be moved again until the resident has moved both feet forward and is steady (Fig. 21-7). The resident should never put his feet ahead of the walker.

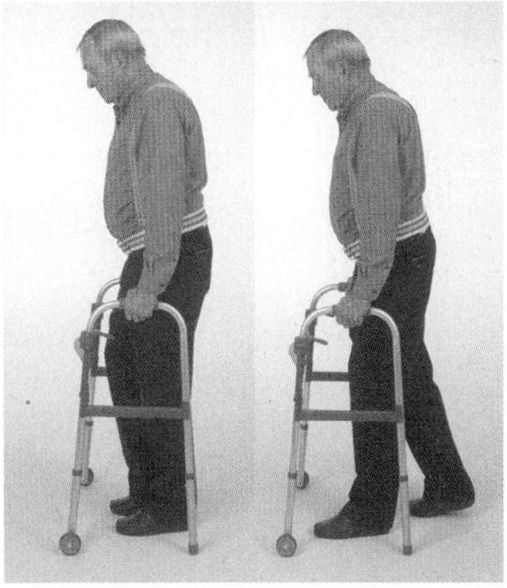

Fig. 21-7.

    c. *Crutches.* Resident should be fitted for crutches and taught to use them correctly by a physical therapist or nurse. The resident may use the crutches several different ways. It depends on what his weakness is. No matter how they are used, weight should be on the resident's hands and arms. Weight should not be on the underarm area (Fig. 21-8).

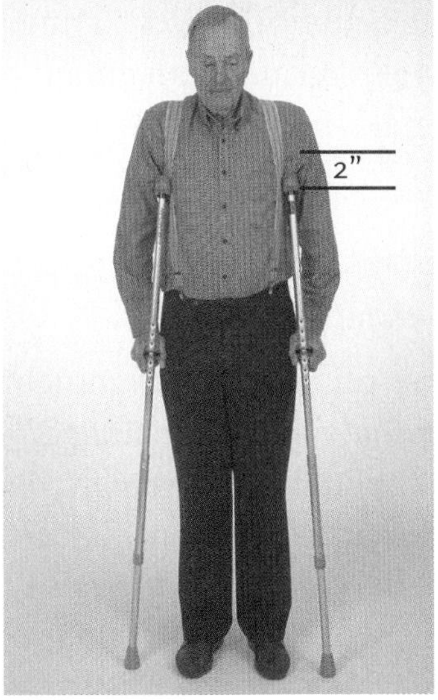

Fig. 21-8.

11. Walk slightly behind and to one side of resident. Hold the transfer belt if one is used.
12. Watch for obstacles in the resident's path. Ask the resident to look ahead, not down at his feet.
13. Encourage the resident to rest if he is tired. When a resident is tired, it increases the chance of a fall. Let the resident set the pace. Discuss how far he plans to go based on the care plan.
14. After ambulation, remove transfer belt. Help resident to a position of comfort and safety.
15. Return bed to appropriate position. Remove privacy measures.
16. Before leaving, place call light within resident's reach.
17. Wash your hands.
18. Report any changes in resident to nurse.
19. Document procedure using facility guidelines.

4. Explain guidelines for maintaining proper body alignment

Residents who are bedbound need good body alignment. This aids recovery and prevents injury to muscles and joints. Chapter 10 gives specific instructions for positioning. These guidelines help residents maintain good alignment and make progress when they can get out of bed.

GUIDELINES
Alignment and Positioning

- Observe principles of alignment. Proper alignment is based on straight lines. The spine should be in a straight line. Pillows or rolled or folded blankets can support the small of the back and raise the knees or head in the supine position. They can support the head and one leg in the lateral position (Fig. 21-9).

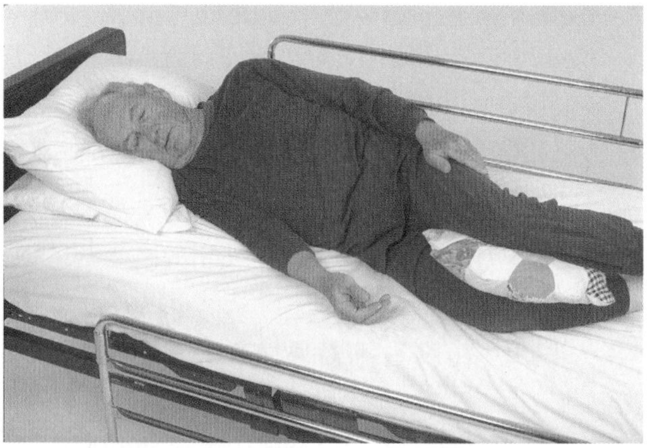

Fig. 21-9. **Pillows or rolled or folded blankets give extra support.**

- Keep body parts in natural positions. In a natural hand position, the fingers are slightly curled. Use a rolled washcloth, gauze bandage, or rubber ball inside the palm to support the fingers in this position (Fig. 21-10). Use footboards to keep covers from resting on feet in the supine position.

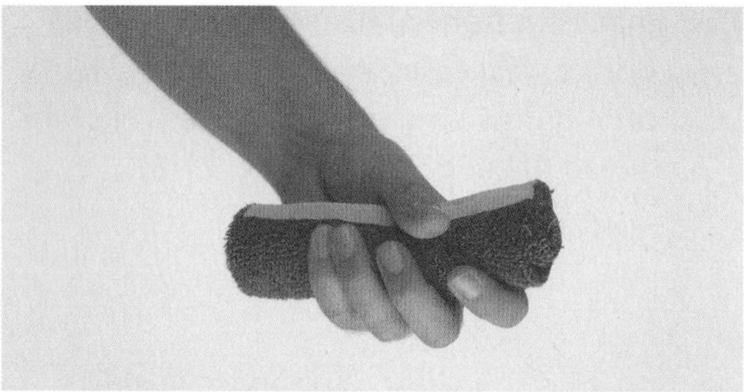

Fig. 21-10. **Handrolls keep fingers from curling tightly.**

- Prevent external rotation of hips. When legs and hips turn outward during bedrest, hip contractures can result. A **contracture** is the permanent and often very painful stiffening of a joint and muscle. A rolled blanket or towel tucked alongside the hip and thigh can keep the leg from turning outward.
- Change positions often to prevent muscle stiffness and pressure sores. This should be done at least every two hours. The position used will depend on the resident's condition and preference. Check the skin every time you reposition the resident.

5. Describe how to assist with range of motion exercises

Exercise helps people regain strength and mobility. It helps to prevent disabilities. People who are in bed for long periods are more likely to develop contractures. Contractures are often caused by immobility. They can result in the loss of ability.

Range of motion (ROM) exercises put a joint through its full arc of motion. The goal of ROM exercises is to decrease or prevent contractures, improve strength, and increase circulation. **Passive range of motion** (PROM) exercises are used when residents cannot move on their own. When helping with PROM exercises, support the resident's joints. Move them through the range of motion. **Active range of motion** (AROM) exercises are done by a resident himself. Your role in AROM exercises is to encourage the resident. **Active assisted range of motion** (AAROM) exercises are done by the resident with some help and support from you.

You will not do ROM exercises without an order from a doctor, nurse, or physical therapist. Follow the care plan. You will repeat each exercise two to five times, once or twice a day. You will work on both sides of the body. During ROM exercises, begin at the resident's head. Work down the body. Exercise the upper extremities (arms) before the lower extremities (legs). Give support above and below the joint. Stop the motion if the resident reports pain. Report pain to the nurse. These exercises are specific for each body area. They include the movements below (Fig. 21-11).

- **Abduction**: moving a body part away from the body
- **Adduction**: moving a body part toward the body
- **Dorsiflexion**: bending backward
- **Rotation**: turning a joint
- **Extension**: straightening a body part
- **Flexion**: bending a body part
- **Pronation**: turning downward
- **Supination**: turning upward

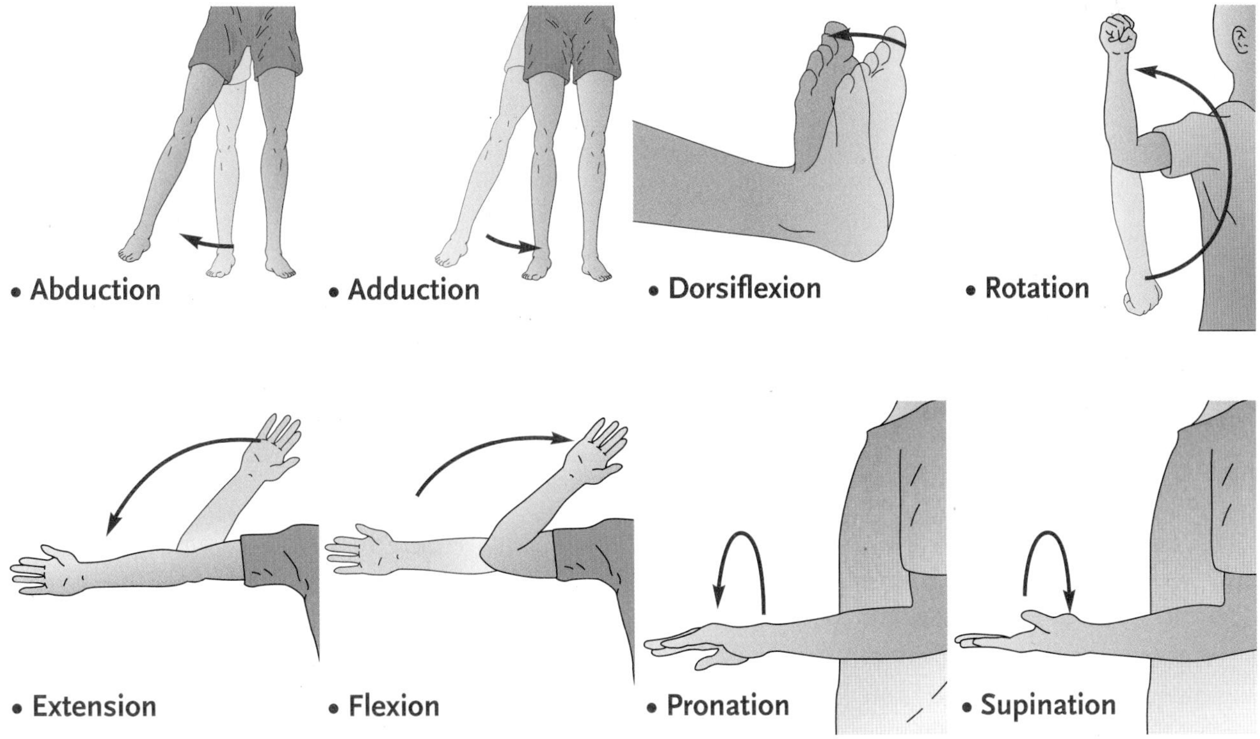

Fig. 21-11. **The different range of motion body movements.**

Assisting with passive range of motion exercises

1. Wash your hands.
2. Identify yourself by name. Identify the resident by name.
3. Explain procedure to resident. Speak clearly, slowly, and directly. Maintain face-to-face contact whenever possible.
4. Provide for resident's privacy with curtain, screen, or door.
5. Adjust bed to a safe level, usually waist high. Lock bed wheels.
6. Position the resident lying supine—flat on his or her back—on the bed. Use good alignment.
7. **Shoulder**. Support the resident's arm at the elbow and wrist during ROM for the shoulder. Place one hand above the elbow. Place the other hand around the wrist. Move the arm up so that the upper arm is aligned with the side of the head (forward flexion) (Fig. 21-12).

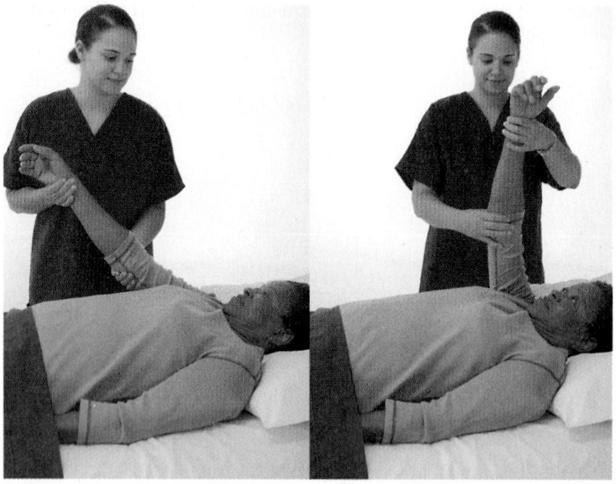

Fig. 21-12.

Move the arm downward to the side (extension) (Fig. 21-13). Return arm to side.

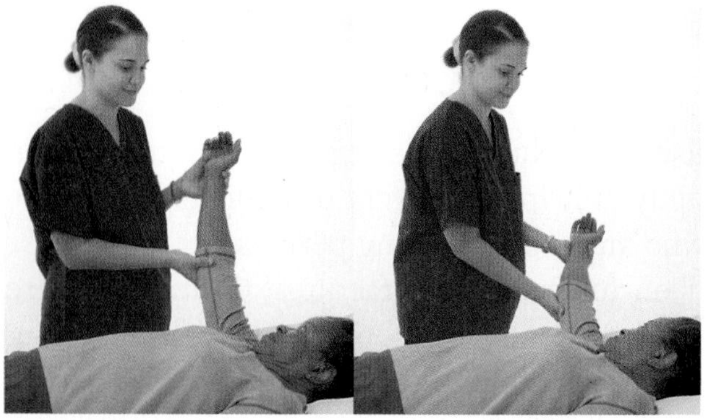

Fig. 21-13.

Bring the arm sideways away from the body to above the head (abduction) and back down to midline (adduction) (Fig. 21-14).

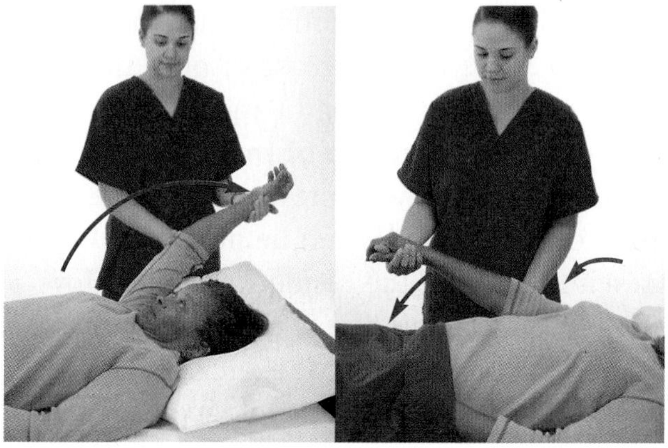

Fig. 21-14.

Bend the elbow. Position it at the same level as the shoulder. Move the forearm down toward the midline of the body (internal rotation). Now move the forearm toward the head (external rotation) (Fig. 21-15).

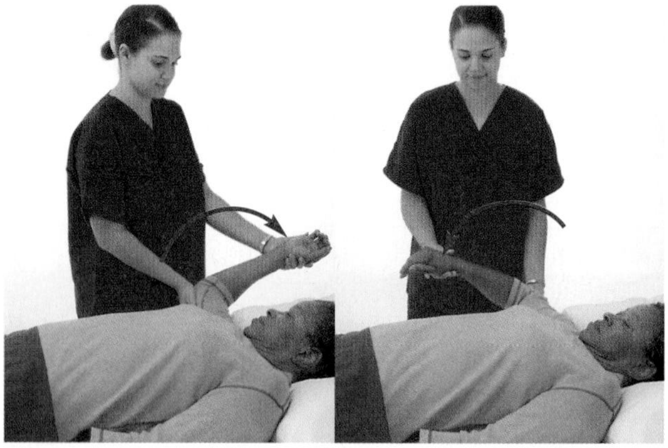

Fig. 21-15.

8. **Elbow**. Hold the resident's wrist with one hand. Hold the elbow with the other hand. Bend the elbow so that the hand touches the shoulder on that same side (flexion). Straighten the arm (extension) (Fig. 21-16).

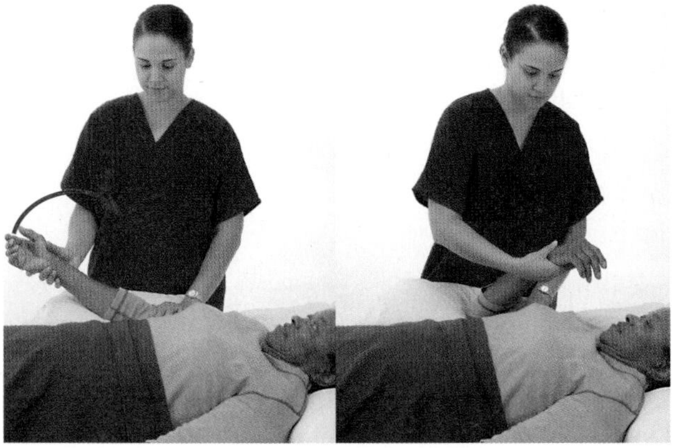

Fig. 21-16.

Exercise the forearm by moving it so the palm is facing downward (pronation) and then upward (supination) (Fig. 21-17).

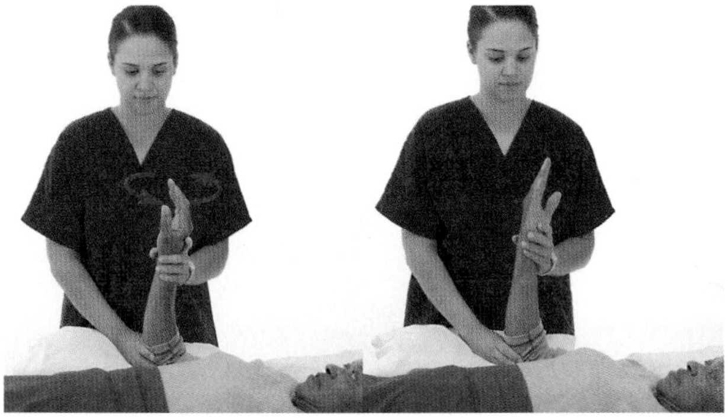

Fig. 21-17.

9. **Wrist**. Hold the wrist with one hand. Use the fingers of the other hand to help the joint through the motions. Bend the hand down (flexion). Bend the hand backwards (extension) (Fig. 21-18).

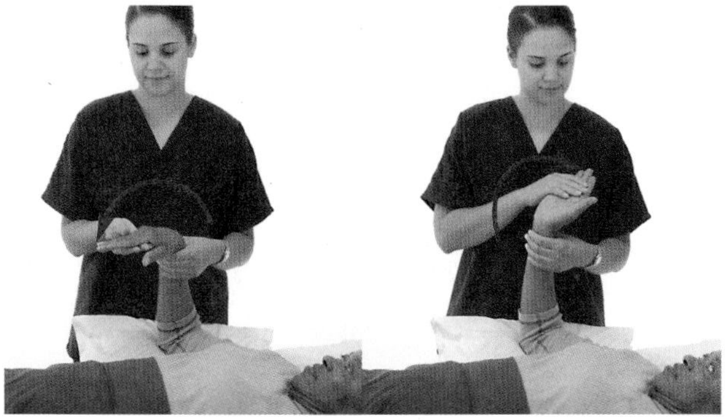

Fig. 21-18.

Turn the hand in the direction of the thumb (radial flexion). Then turn it in the direction of the little finger (ulnar flexion) (Fig. 21-19).

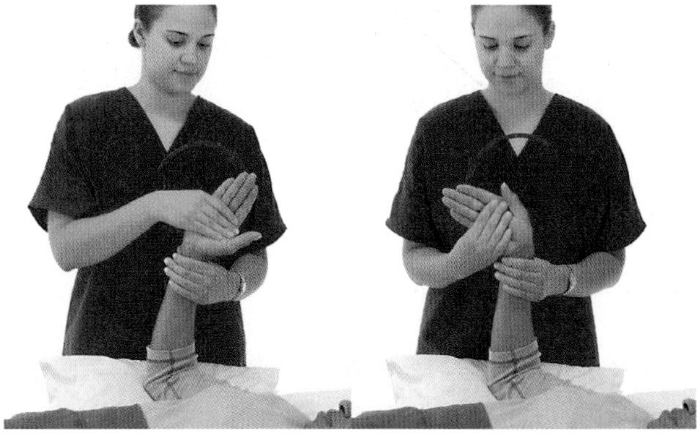

Fig. 21-19.

10. **Thumb**. Move the thumb away from the index finger (abduction). Move the thumb back next to the index finger (adduction) (Fig. 21-20).

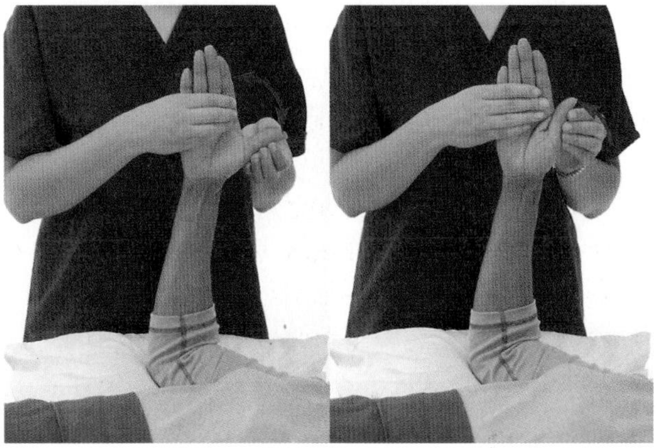

Fig. 21-20.

Touch each fingertip with the thumb (opposition) (Fig. 21-21).

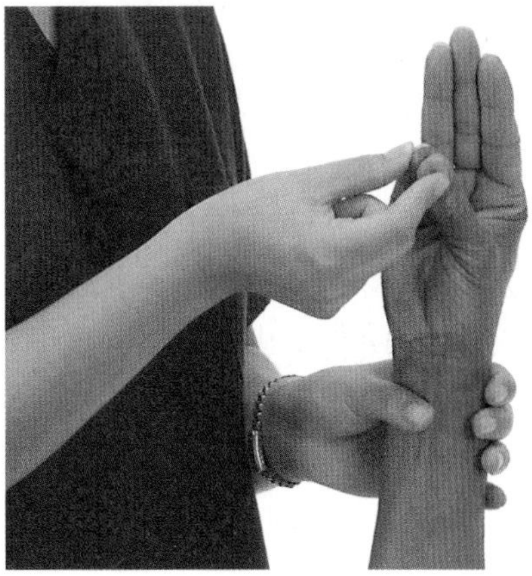

Fig. 21-21.

Bend thumb into the palm (flexion). Bend it out to the side (extension) (Fig. 21-22).

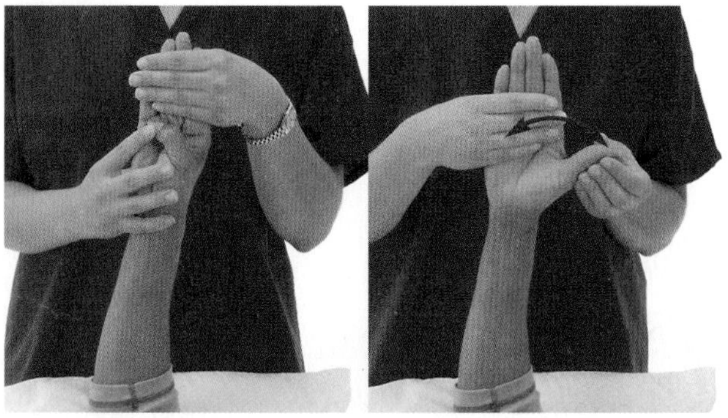

Fig. 21-22.

11. **Fingers**. Make the hand into a fist (flexion). Gently straighten out the fist (extension) (Fig. 21-23).

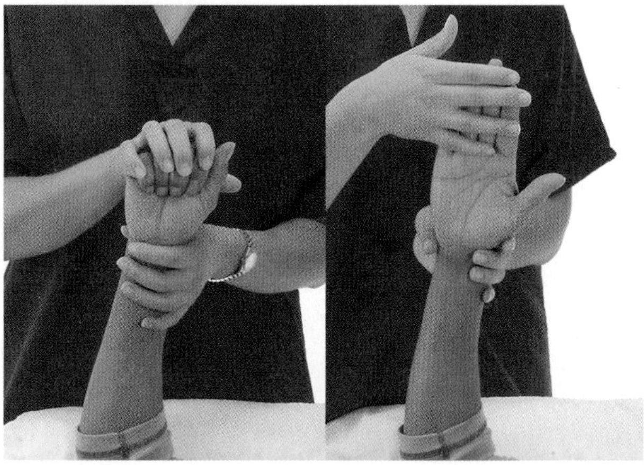

Fig. 21-23.

Spread the fingers and the thumb far apart from each other (abduction). Bring the fingers back next to each other (adduction) (Fig. 21-24).

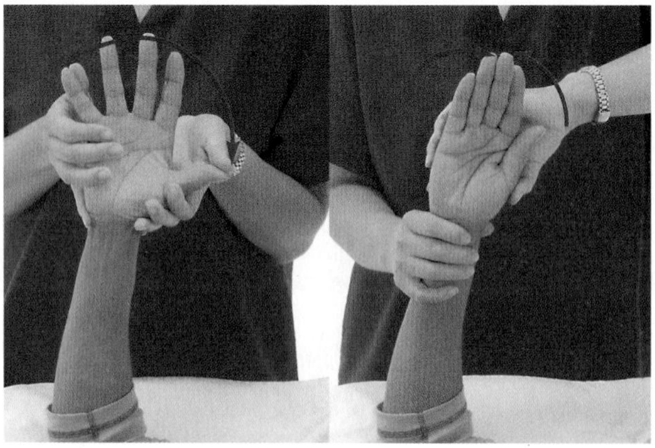

Fig. 21-24.

12. **Hip**. Support the leg by placing one hand under the knee and one under the ankle. Straighten the leg. Raise it gently upward. Move the leg away from the other leg (abduction). Move the leg toward the other leg (adduction) (Fig. 21-25).

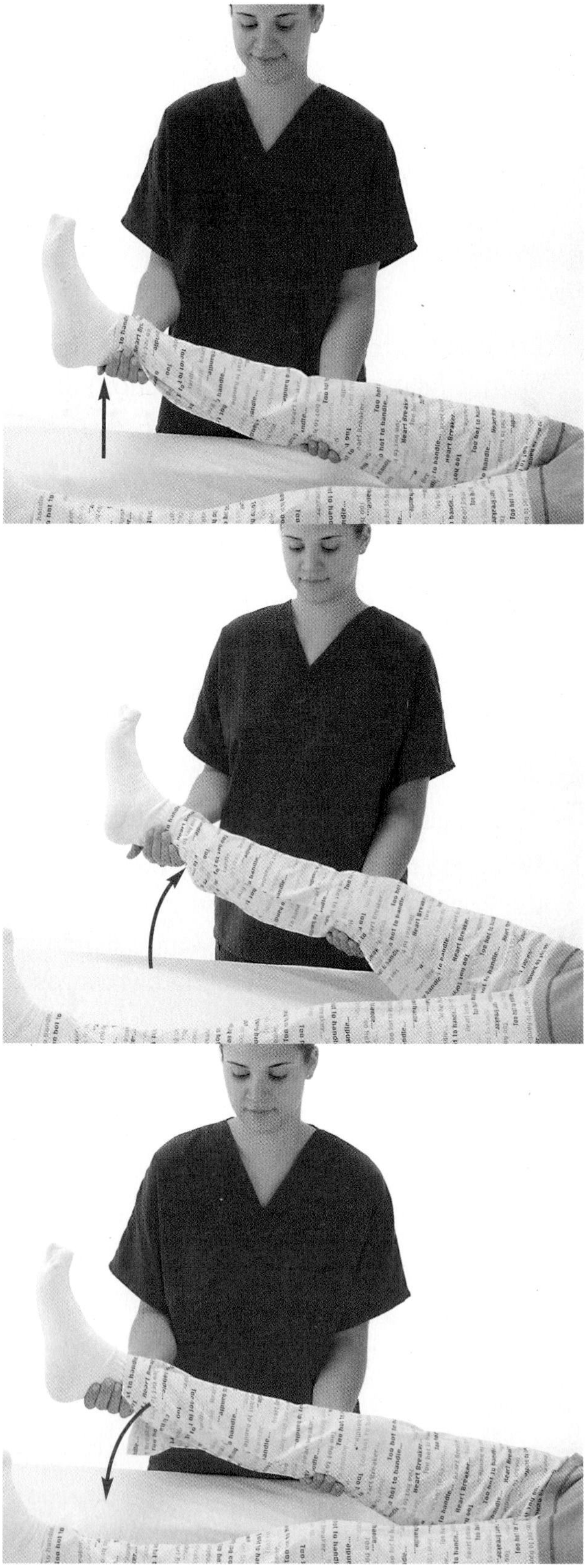

Fig. 21-25.

Gently turn the leg inward (internal rotation). Turn the leg outward (external rotation) (Fig. 21-26).

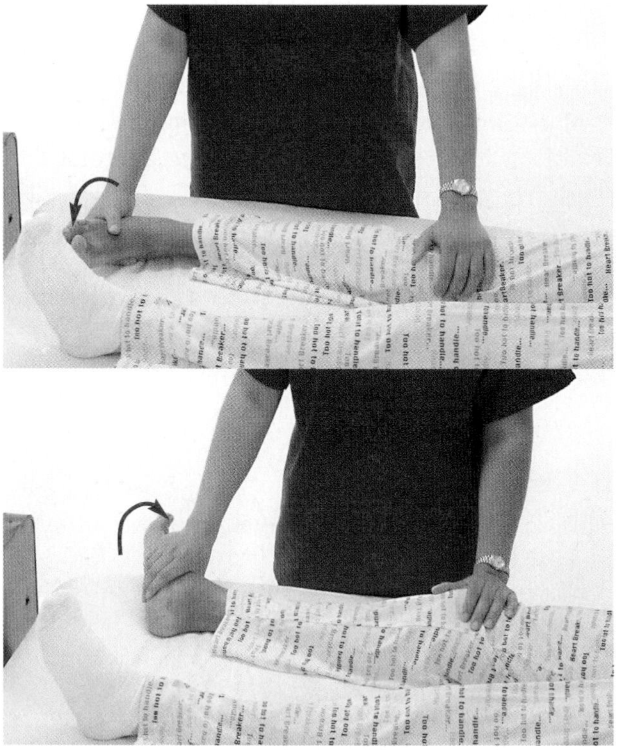

Fig. 21-26.

13. **Knees**. Bend the leg at the knee (flexion). Straighten the leg (extension) (Fig. 21-27).

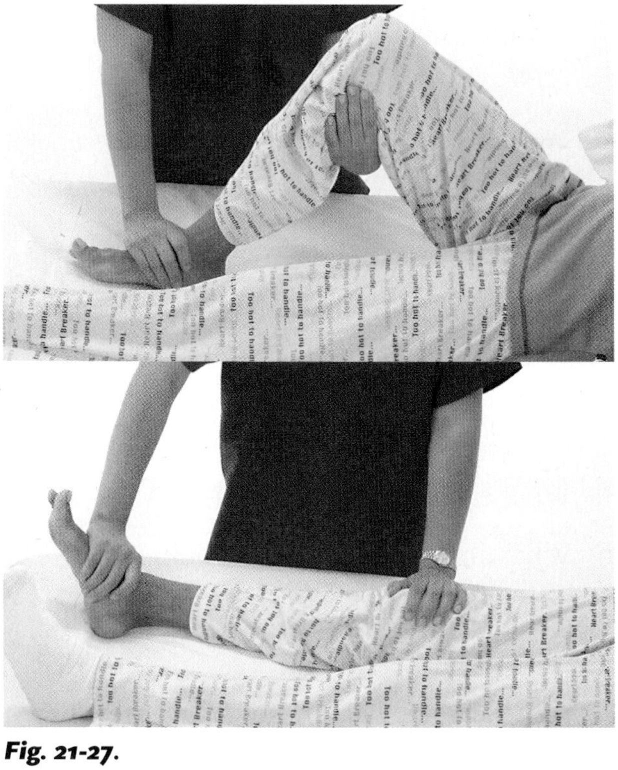

Fig. 21-27.

14. **Ankles**. Bend the foot up toward the leg (dorsiflexion). Turn the foot down away from the leg (plantar flexion) (Fig. 21-28).

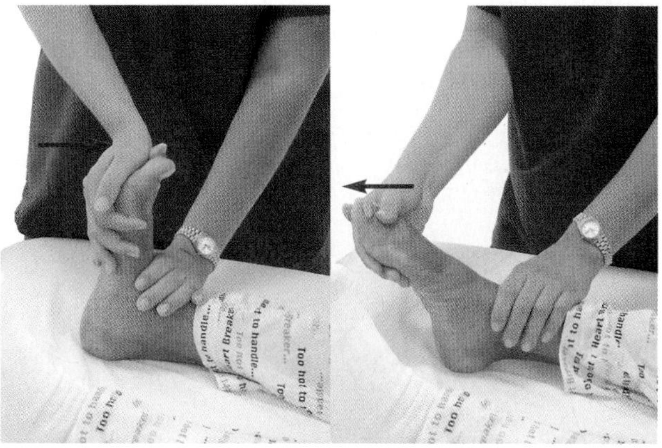

Fig. 21-28.

Turn the inside of the foot inward toward the body (supination). Bend the sole of the foot away from the body (pronation) (Fig. 21-29).

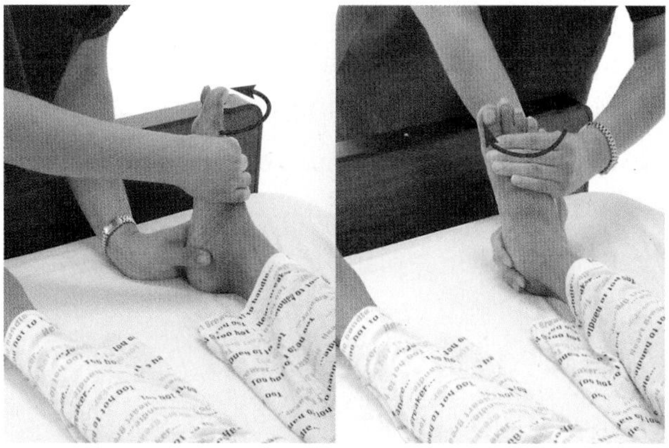

Fig. 21-29.

15. **Toes**. Curl and straighten the toes (flexion and extension) (Fig. 21-30).

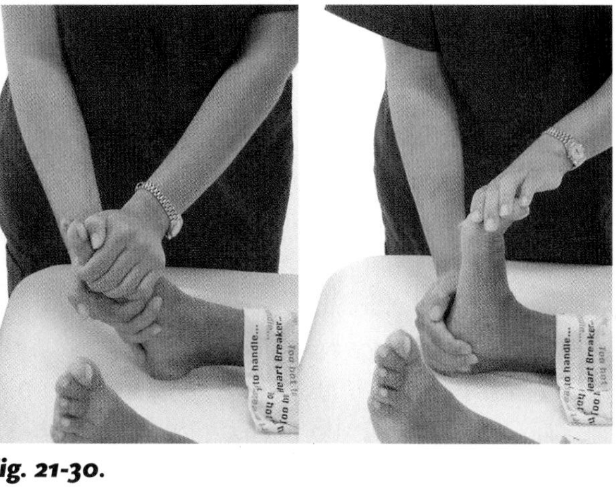

Fig. 21-30.

Gently spread the toes apart (abduction) Fig. 21-31).

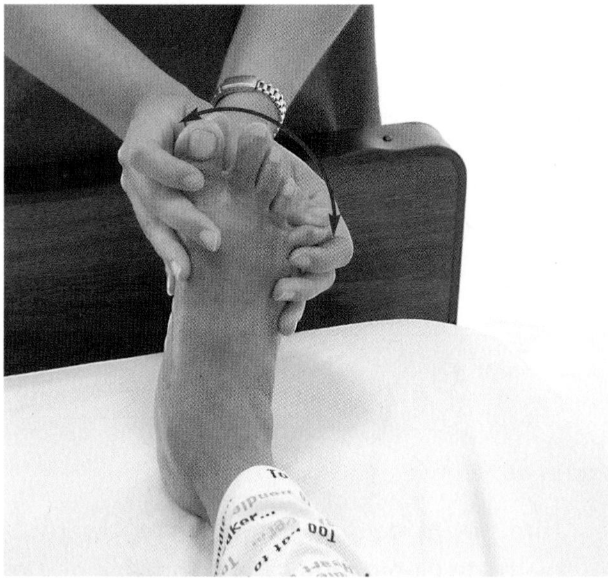

Fig. 21-31.

16. While supporting the limbs, move all joints gently, slowly, and smoothly through the range of motion to the point of resistance. Stop if any pain occurs.
17. Return bed to appropriate position. Remove privacy measures.
18. Before leaving, place call light within resident's reach.
19. Wash your hands.
20. Report any changes in resident to nurse.
21. Document procedure using facility guidelines.

"No pain, no gain" does not apply to residents.

Range of motion exercises are important. They keep muscles strong and healthy. Make sure you know how to help with these exercises. Doing ROM exercises in an overly-aggressive way may cause pain and injury. Causing unnecessary pain during these exercises is abuse. If residents report pain during ROM exercises, stop immediately. Tell the nurse.

6. Describe the benefits of deep breathing exercises

Deep breathing exercises help expand the lungs, clearing them of mucus and preventing infections (such as pneumonia). Residents who are paralyzed or who have had surgery are often told to do deep breathing exercises regularly to expand the lungs.

The care plan may include using a deep breathing device called an **incentive spirometer** (Fig. 21-32). Do not assist with these exercises if you have not been trained. Ask the nurse for instructions.

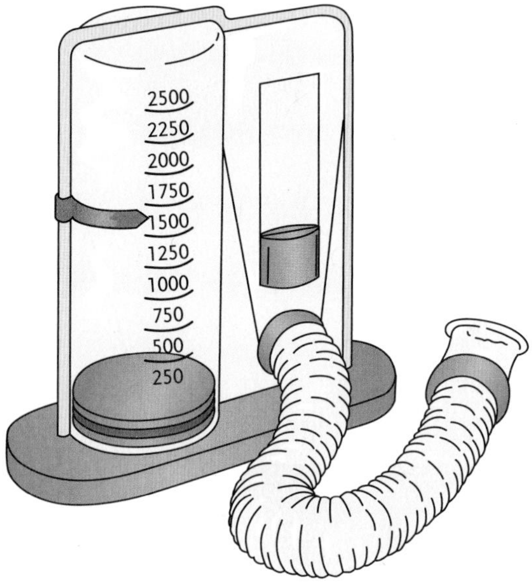

Fig. 21-32. **Incentive spirometers are used for deep breathing exercises.**

Chapter Review

1. What does restorative care or rehabilitation involve?
2. What attitudes can you adopt to help with restorative care? Give an example of each.
3. What can a lack of mobility cause?
4. What does regular exercise help improve?
5. What is one difference between a straight cane and a quad cane?
6. To which side should you stay close when a resident is using adaptive equipment?

7. Look at the adaptive devices in Figure 21-2. Choose one. Describe how it might help a resident recovering from or adapting to a physical condition.
8. List guidelines to follow to help residents maintain good alignment.
9. Why should you change a resident's position often?
10. What is the purpose of ROM exercises?
11. Describe the difference between passive, active, and active assisted range of motion exercises.
12. What do deep breathing exercises help?

Chapter 22
Subacute Care

1. Understand the types of residents who are in a subacute setting

A subacute setting is a special unit or facility. It is for people who need more care than most long-term care facilities can give. Hospitals and nursing homes can provide subacute care. Residents in subacute settings need a higher level of care than other residents. They will need more direct care and close observation by staff. The cost is usually less than a hospital but more than long-term care.

Recent surgery and chronic illnesses, such as AIDS or cancer, may call for subacute care. Other conditions that need subacute care are serious burns and dialysis. Dialysis cleanses the body of waste that the kidneys cannot remove due to kidney failure. Residents in subacute units may also be on a **mechanical ventilator**. This is a machine that literally breathes for a person.

2. List care guidelines for pulse oximetry

When residents are on oxygen, going to or coming from surgery, or bleeding or having another problem, a pulse oximeter may be used. A **pulse oximeter** measures a person's blood oxygen level and the pulse rate (Fig. 22-1). Blood oxygen is the oxygen level inside the arteries. It is also called oxygen saturation.

A sensor is clipped on a finger, ear lobe, or toe. It warns of a low blood oxygen level before any observable signs or symptoms develop. It works by moving red and infrared light through the skin. It then measures the amount of each type of light absorbed by the hemoglobin in the blood. Blood with oxygen absorbs more of the infrared light. Blood without oxygen absorbs more red light.

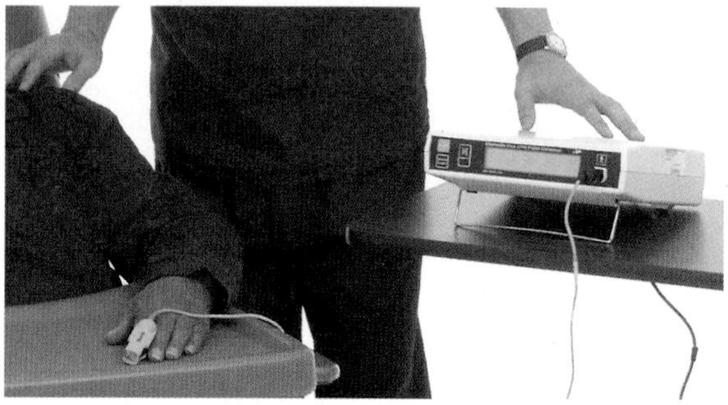

Fig. 22-1. **A pulse oximeter.**

A normal blood oxygen level is usually measured between 95% and 100%. However, what is normal for one person may be different from the normal range for another person. Report to the nurse if the alarm on the pulse oximeter sounds or if you notice that the level is increasing or decreasing.

GUIDELINES
Pulse Oximeter

- If the alarm on the pulse oximeter sounds, tell the nurse right away.

- Be careful when moving and positioning residents. Do not cause the oximeter to come off or move.
- Report pale or cyanotic (bluish) skin.
- Report difficulty breathing (**dyspnea**).
- Observe and report any signs of skin breakdown from the device. Report any cracks, breaks, rashes, or sores on the skin around and under the oximeter.
- Check vital signs as ordered. Report changes to the nurse.

3. Describe telemetry and list care guidelines

Telemetry is the application of a device that sends information about the heart rhythm and rate. A skilled staff member can then assess it. The data is sent to an area within a facility. Monitoring screens are watched constantly by trained specialists.

The unit attaches to a resident's chest. It is carried in a pack that allows for movement. There are different ways to connect the device to a person's chest. One type uses sponge-like adhesive pads or patches (also called leads or electrodes) that stick to different parts of the chest. The pad attaches to a wire connected to the telemetry pack.

GUIDELINES

Telemetry

- Do not get the unit, wires, pads/patches, or electrodes/leads wet during bathing. Report if they become wet.
- If an alarm sounds, notify the nurse. The alarm may sound with movement, a disconnected lead, or a low battery.
- Check vital signs as ordered. Report changes to the nurse.
- Check the skin for signs of irritation under or around the leads.
- Report if leads become loose.
- Report resident complaints of chest pain, discomfort, and dizziness. Report if the resident is sweating or seems short of breath.

4. Explain artificial airways and list care guidelines

An **artificial airway** is any plastic, metal, or rubber device inserted into the respiratory tract to promote breathing. Artificial airways keep the airway open. This is needed when the airway is obstructed from illness, injury, secretions, or aspiration. Some residents who are unconscious will need an artificial airway.

Intubation is the method used to insert an artificial airway. It involves passing a plastic tube through the mouth or nose and into the trachea or windpipe. There are different types of artificial airways (Fig. 22-2):

- An oropharyngeal airway is inserted into the mouth. It goes behind the tongue and into the pharynx.
- A nasopharyngeal airway is lubricated and then gently passed up a nostril and down into the pharynx.
- An endotracheal tube is put in the mouth or nose and then into the trachea.
- A tracheostomy is an opening surgically created through the neck into the trachea. A tracheostomy tube is placed through this opening. It is also called a "trach tube."

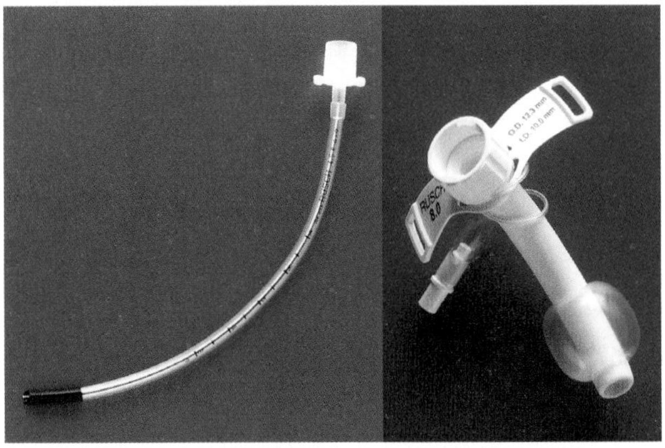

Fig. 22-2. An endotracheal tube and a tracheostomy tube. (Photos courtesy of Rusch - A Teleflex Company.)

GUIDELINES
Artificial Airways

- Observe resident closely. If the tubing falls out, tell the nurse immediately.
- Check vital signs as ordered. Report changes to the nurse.
- Perform oral care as ordered.
- Watch for biting and tugging on tube. If a resident is doing this, tell the nurse.
- Use other methods of communication if the person cannot speak. Try writing notes, drawing pictures, and using communication boards. Watch for hand and eye signals.
- Be supportive and reassuring. It can be frightening and uncomfortable to have an artificial airway. Some residents may choke or gag. Be empathetic. Imagine how it might feel to have a tube in your nose, mouth, or throat.

More information on tracheostomies is in the next learning objective.

5. Discuss care for a resident with a tracheostomy

A tracheostomy is a common type of artificial airway seen in nursing homes. This procedure is usually temporary, but it can be permanent. It is easier to suction and attach respiratory equipment with a tracheostomy than with other artificial airways.

Some reasons why tracheostomies are necessary are:

- tumors/cancer
- infection
- severe neck or mouth injuries
- facial surgery and facial burns
- long-term unconsciousness or coma
- obstruction in the airway
- paralysis of muscles relating to breathing
- aspiration related to muscle or sensory problems in the throat
- severe allergic reaction
- gunshot wound

While the tracheostomy is in place, the resident may be unable to speak. Being unable to speak can cause fear. Be supportive and responsive. Use other methods of communication. Try notepads, communication boards, or hand signals. Answer call lights promptly.

General tracheostomy care includes keeping the skin around the opening, or stoma, clean, helping with dressing changes, and helping with the cleansing of the inner part of the device. Suctioning may be needed often. Gurgling sounds during breathing may be one sign that suctioning is needed. Generally, NAs do not do tracheostomy care or suctioning. However, careful observing and reporting is vital. Report shortness of breath, trouble breathing, and gurgling to the nurse right away.

Do oral care as directed. Observe and report mouth sores or discomfort.

6. List care guidelines for a resident requiring mechanical ventilation

Residents in a subacute unit may be on a ventilator (Fig. 22-3). A ventilator performs the process of breathing for a person who cannot breathe on his own. Many problems cause a person to need a mechanical ventilator. Injuries that affect breathing or diseases, such as cancer, are examples.

Residents on a ventilator will not be able to speak. This is because air will no longer reach the larynx (vocal cords). This may increase anxiety. The resident may think that no one will know if he or she is having trouble breathing. Being on a ventilator has been compared to breathing through a straw. Residents will need a lot of support while being connected to the ventilator. Enter the room (so the resident can see you) often. This reassures residents that they are being carefully observed. Clipboards, pads, and communication boards will help with communication.

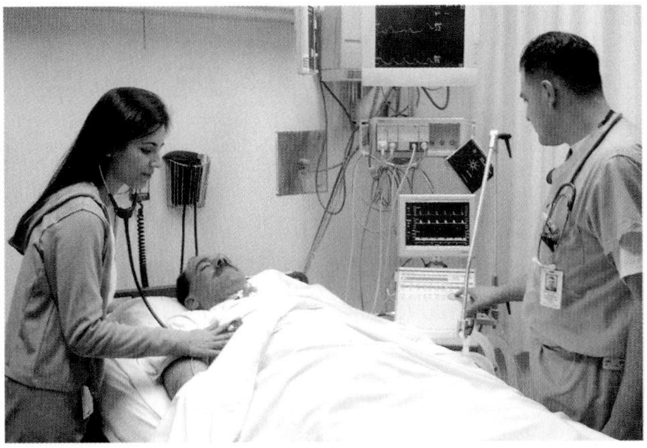

Fig. 22-3. **A mechanical ventilator. (Photo courtesy of Pulmonetic Systems.)**

Residents on a ventilator are often heavily sedated. This prevents them from feeling discomfort. Some residents may be alert. If the resident is unconscious, act and speak appropriately. Assume that he or she is able to understand everything that is happening.

GUIDELINES

Mechanical Ventilator

- Report to the nurse right away if the alarm sounds.
- Watch for kinks or disconnected tubing. Report them immediately.
- Answer the call light promptly.
- Give oral care as directed. Observe and report mouth sores or discomfort.
- Reposition at least every two hours. Follow instructions carefully when moving and positioning. Always get enough help. Have the nurse check the resident after repositioning.
- Give regular skin care to prevent pressure sores. Observe for cracks, breaks, or sores on the skin, especially at the intubation site.
- Watch for biting on the tube. If a resident is doing this, tell the nurse.
- Be patient during communication.
- Allow time for rest.
- Give support during difficult times. Being dependent can cause feelings of despair.

7. Describe suctioning and list signs of respiratory distress

Residents in subacute care may need frequent suctioning by the nurses. Suctioning is needed when a person has collected secretions in the upper respiratory system. A resident may need suctioning with or without a tracheostomy.

Suction comes from a wall hook-up or a portable pump. A bottle collects the suctioned material from the airway. The nurse or the respiratory therapist will suction the resident (Fig 22-4). Sterile water is normally used to rinse the suction catheter after suctioning.

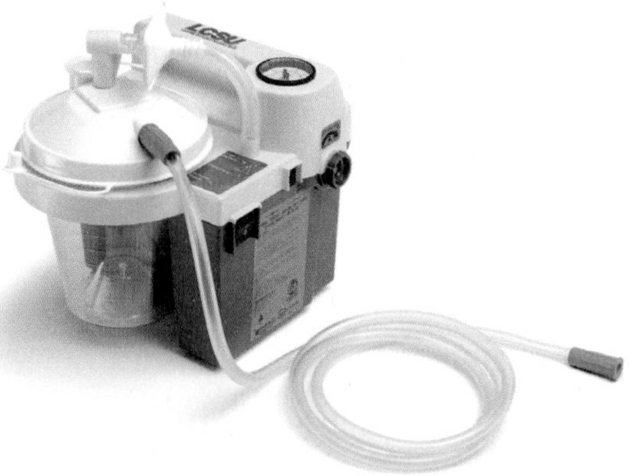

Fig. 22-4. **NAs do not perform suctioning. They can help by telling the nurse immediately if there is any sign of respiratory distress. (Photo courtesy of Laerdal Medical Corporation.)**

A resident who has frequent suctioning may show signs of respiratory distress. Signs of respiratory distress are:

- gurgling
- high respiratory rate
- shortness of breath
- trouble breathing

- pale skin
- bluish skin

GUIDELINES
Suctioning

- If you note any signs of respiratory distress, report them immediately. An inability to breathe freely causes great anxiety. Staying in respiratory distress for any period of time is dangerous.
- Answer call lights promptly.
- Observe skin color carefully. Report if skin is bluish or very pale.
- Monitor vital signs closely, especially respiratory rate. Report changes.
- Follow Standard Precautions. Put on gloves, gown, mask, or goggles as directed.
- Place resident in position as directed by nurse, normally semi-Fowler's or lateral.
- Place pad or towel under the chin before suctioning. Have wet washcloth ready.
- Give oral care after suctioning as directed.
- Give support during periods of difficult breathing. Use touch if appropriate.

8. Describe chest tubes and explain related care

Chest tubes are hollow drainage tubes that are inserted into the chest during a sterile procedure. They can be inserted at the bedside or during surgery. Chest tubes drain air, blood, or fluid that has collected inside the pleural space or cavity. This is the space surrounding the lungs. Chest tubes are also inserted to allow a full expansion of the lungs. Some conditions that require chest tube insertion include:

- pneumothorax: air or gas in the pleural space
- hemothorax: blood in the pleural space
- empyema: pus in the pleural space
- certain types of surgery
- injuries

A doctor normally inserts chest tubes at the hospital. The chest tube is connected to a bottle of sterile water. Suction is sometimes attached to the system sometimes to encourage drainage. This system must be sealed so that air cannot enter the pleural space. The system must be airtight.

When X-rays show that the air, blood, or fluid has been drained, the tube is removed. Medications may prevent or treat infection.

GUIDELINES
Chest Tubes

- Be aware of the number and location of chest tubes. Tubes may be in the front, back, or side of the body.
- Check vital signs as directed. Report any changes immediately to the nurse.
- Report signs of respiratory distress to the nurse immediately. Report complaints of pain.
- Keep the drainage system below the level of the resident's chest.
- Make sure drainage containers remain upright and level at all times.
- Make sure that tubing is not kinked. If tubing becomes kinked, report to the nurse right away.
- Watch for disconnected tubing. If this happens, report it immediately.
- Certain equipment is kept nearby in case tubes are pulled out. Do not remove these items from the area.
- Observe chest drainage for amount and color. If the amount or color changes, report it immediately.
- Report if there is an increase or decrease in bubbling in the drainage system. Report if there are clots in the tubing.

- Follow the repositioning schedule. Be very gentle with turning and repositioning. You must move the resident and the tubes at the same time to prevent tubes from coming out. Always get enough help.
- Report odor in the chest tube area.
- Provide rest periods as needed.
- Follow fluid intake orders. Measure intake and output carefully as ordered.
- If asked to help with coughing and deep breathing exercises, be encouraging and patient.

Other residents who require more direct care and close observation by staff include residents with IVs (chapter 17) and residents with tube feedings (chapter 16).

Chapter Review

1. What is different about the type of care in provided in a subacute setting?
2. List two reasons why a resident may need a pulse oximeter.
3. What is telemetry?
4. What are alternate methods of communication you can use with residents who have an artificial airway?
5. What does general tracheostomy care include?
6. Why do you think a resident might be anxious while on a ventilator?
7. List five signs of respiratory distress.
8. What types of fluids are drained by chest tubes?
9. List four conditions that should be reported to the nurse immediately regarding chest tubes.

Chapter 23
Death and Dying

1. Discuss the stages of dying

Death can occur suddenly without warning, or it can be expected. Older people, or those with terminal illnesses, may have time to prepare for death. A **terminal illness** is a disease or condition that will eventually cause death. Preparing for death is a process. It affects the dying person's emotions and behavior.

Dr. Elisabeth Kubler-Ross studied and wrote about the process of dying. Her book, *On Death and Dying*, describes five stages that dying people and their loved ones may reach before death. These five stages are listed below. Not all residents go through all the stages. Some may stay in one stage until death. Residents may move back and forth between stages during the process.

Denial. People in this stage may refuse to believe they are dying. They may think a mistake has been made. They may demand lab work be repeated. They may talk about the future and avoid discussion about their illnesses. They may simply act like it is not happening. This is the "No, not me" stage.

Anger. Once they start to face the possibility of death, people become angry. They may be angry because they think they are too young or that they have always taken care of themselves. Anger may be directed at staff, visitors, roommates, family, or friends. Anger is a normal, healthy reaction. The caregiver must not take it personally. This is the "Why me?" stage.

Bargaining. Once people have begun to believe they really are dying, they may make promises to God. They may somehow try to bargain for recovery. This is the "Yes me, but..." stage.

Depression. As dying people get weaker and symptoms get worse, they may be deeply sad or depressed (Fig. 23-1). They may cry or withdraw. They may be unable to do even simple things. They need physical and emotional support. Listen and be understanding.

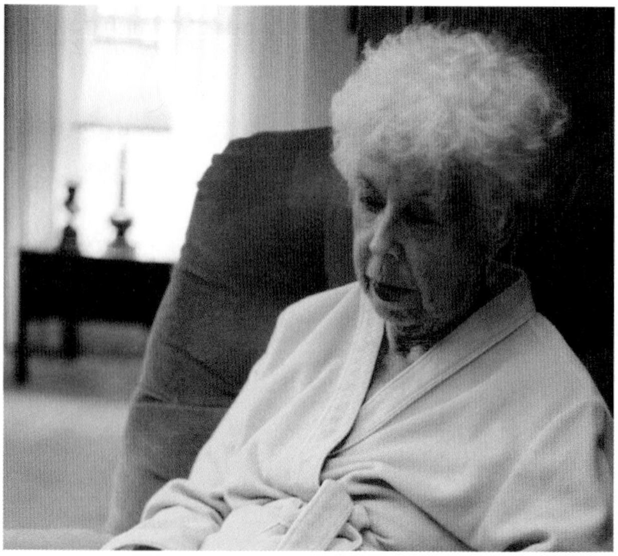

Fig. 23-1. **A person who is dying may become depressed.**

Acceptance. Most people who are dying are eventually able to accept death and prepare for it. They may ask to see an attorney or accountant. They may arrange with loved ones for the care of important people or things. They may plan for their last days or for the ceremonies to follow. At this stage, people who are dying may seem detached.

These stages of dying may not be possible for someone who dies suddenly, unexpectedly, or quickly. You cannot force anyone to move from stage to stage. You can only listen, and be ready to offer your help.

2. Describe the grief process

Dealing with grief after the death of a loved one is a process as well. Grieving is individual. No two people will grieve in exactly the same way. Clergy, counselors, or social workers can help people who are grieving. Family members or friends will have different reactions to the death of a loved one. These reactions are called coping mechanisms. **Coping mechanisms** are responses to stress. They include:

Shock. Even when death was expected, family members and friends may still be shocked after it occurs. Many of us do not know what to expect after the death of a loved one. We may be surprised by our feelings.

Denial. Sometimes we want to think that everything will quickly return to normal. Denying or refusing to believe we are grieving can help people deal with the hours or days after a death. But eventually we must face our feelings. Grief can be overwhelming. Some people may take years to face their feelings. Professional help can be very valuable.

Anger. Although it is hard to admit it, many of us feel angry after a death. We may be angry with ourselves, at God, at the doctors, or even at the person who died. There is nothing wrong with feeling anger as a part of grief.

Guilt. It is very common for families, friends, and caregivers to feel guilty after a death. We may wish we had done more for the person. We may simply feel that he or she did not deserve to die. We may feel guilty that we are still living.

Regret. Often we regret what we did or did not do for the dying person. We may regret things we said or did not say. Many people carry regrets with them for years.

Sadness. Feeling depressed is very common after a death. We may cry or feel emotionally unstable. We may have headaches or insomnia when we cannot express our grief.

Loneliness. Missing someone who has died is very normal. It can bring up other feelings, such as sadness or regret. Many things may remind us of the person. The memories may be painful at first. With time, we usually feel less lonely. Memories are less painful.

Grieving

You and other staff and residents may be upset by a resident's death. It is important to understand the grief you may experience. Do not underestimate your feelings. Do not be ashamed because you feel grief about a resident's death. This grief is a testament to the kind of person you are and the kind of person your resident was. Grieve at your own pace. Allow other staff and residents to grieve at their own pace. Listen and provide emotional support when needed. Many facilities allow staff and residents to participate in memorial or religious services following a death. Some services are held in the facility.

3. Discuss how feelings and attitudes about death differ

Death is a very sensitive topic. Many people find it hard to discuss. Feelings and attitudes about death can be formed by many factors.

Experience with death. Someone who has been through other deaths may have a different understanding of death than someone who has not.

Personality type. Open, expressive people may have an easier time talking about and coping with death than those who are very reserved or quiet. Sharing feelings is a way of working through fears and concerns.

Religious beliefs. Religious practices and beliefs affect the experience with death (Fig. 23-2). This includes the dying process, rituals at the time of death, burial or cremation, services after death, and mourning. For example, some Catholics do not believe in cremation. Orthodox Jews may not believe in viewing the body after death. Beliefs about what happens after death can also influence grieving. Those who believe in an afterlife, such as heaven, may be comforted by this.

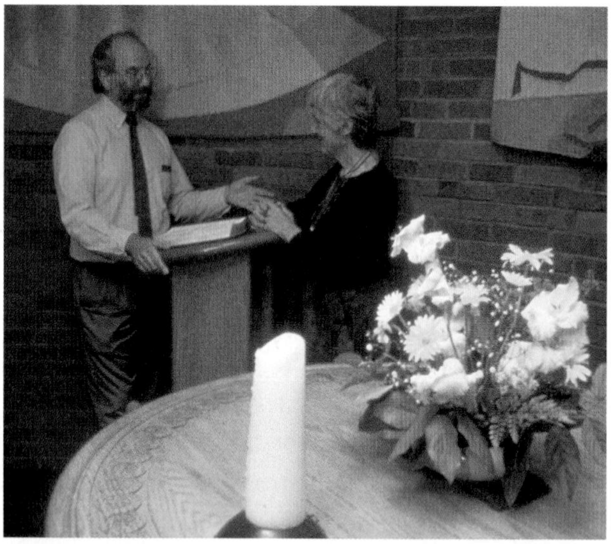

Fig. 23-2. **Religious beliefs influence a person's feelings about death.**

Cultural background. The customs we grow up with will affect how we deal with death. Cultural groups may have different practices to deal with death and grieving. Some have meals and other services but say very little about death. In other groups, talking about and remembering the person may be a comfort to family and friends (Fig. 23-3).

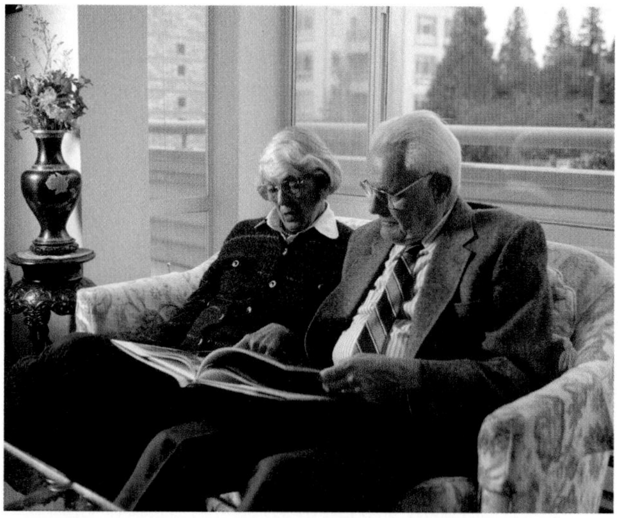

Fig. 23-3. **Cultural practices affect the way a family grieves.**

4. Explain common signs of approaching death

Death can be sudden or gradual. Physical changes occur that can be signs of approaching death. Vital signs and skin color are often affected. Disorientation, confusion, and reduced responses may occur. Vision, taste, and touch usually lessen. However, hearing is often present until death occurs.

Signs of approaching death include:

- blurred and failing vision
- unfocused eyes
- impaired speech
- diminished sense of touch
- loss of movement, muscle tone, and feeling
- a rising or below-normal body temperature
- decreasing blood pressure
- weak pulse that is abnormally slow or rapid
- slow, irregular respirations or rapid, shallow respirations, called **Cheyne-Stokes** respirations
- a "rattling" or "gurgling" sound as the person breathes
- cold, pale skin

- mottling (looks like bruises), spotting, or blotching of the skin caused by poor circulation
- perspiration
- incontinence (both urine and stool)
- disorientation or confusion

5. Discuss how to care for a dying resident

Follow the care plan when caring for a dying resident. Keep these guidelines in mind to help you make the resident as comfortable as possible:

GUIDELINES

Dying Resident

- **Diminished Senses**. Reduce glare and keep room lighting low (Fig. 23-4). Hearing is usually the last sense to leave the body. Speak in a normal tone. Tell them about any procedures that are being done. Describe what is happening in the room. Do not expect an answer. Ask few questions. Encourage family to speak to the resident, but to avoid subjects that are disturbing. Observe body language to anticipate a resident's needs.

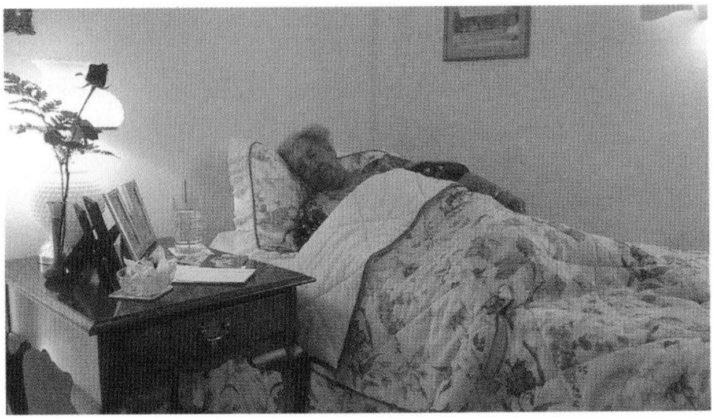

Fig. 23-4. **Keep a dying resident's room softly lit without glare.**

- **Care of the Mouth and Nose**. Give mouth care often. If the resident is unconscious, give mouth care every two hours. The lips and nostrils may be dry and cracked. Apply lubricant, such as lip balm, to lips and nose.
- **Skin Care**. Give bed baths and incontinence care as needed. Bathe perspiring residents often. Skin should be kept clean and dry. Change sheets and clothes for comfort. Keep sheets wrinkle-free. Skin care to prevent pressure sores is important.
- **Comfort**. Pain relief is critical. Residents may not be able to tell you that they are in pain. Observe for signs of pain. Report them. Frequent changes of position, back massage, skin care, mouth care, and proper body alignment may help. Body temperature usually rises. Many residents are more comfortable with light covers. However, fever may cause chills. Use extra blankets if residents need more warmth.
- To control pain, residents may be connected to patient-controlled analgesia (PCA) (Fig. 23-5). Residents control PCA by themselves. They press a button to give themselves a dose of pain medication.

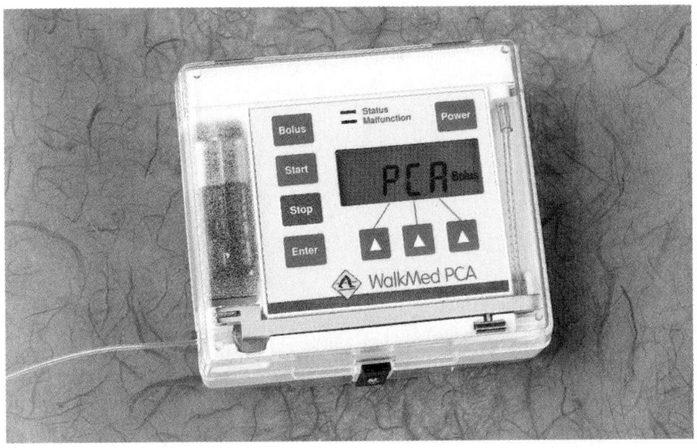

Fig. 23-5. **A patient-controlled analgesia (PCA) (Photo courtesy of McKinley Medical www.mckinleymed.com.)**

- **Environment**. Put favorite objects and photographs where the resident can easily see them. They may give comfort. Make sure the room is comfortable, appropriately lit, and well ventilated.
- **Emotional and Spiritual Support**. Listening may be one of the most important things you can do for a dying resident. They may also need the quiet, reassuring, and loving presence of another person. Touch can be

very important. Holding your resident's hand can be very soothing.

- Some dying residents may seek spiritual comfort from clergy. Tell the nurse immediately if resident requests a clergy person. Give privacy for visits from clergy, family, and friends.
- If talking to residents and their families, do not discuss your religious beliefs. Do not judge anything a resident tells you about his or her past.

Remember that hearing is the last sense to disappear.

Do not say anything inappropriate around dying residents. The sense of hearing is usually the last sense to leave a person. Be professional. Treat this person as you would any resident. Explain procedures and talk to the person normally. Never act like the resident is not there or cannot understand you.

6. Describe ways to treat dying residents and their families with dignity

Working in a nursing home with older and ill residents will probably expose you to death more often than other people. You can treat residents with dignity when they are approaching death by respecting their rights and their preferences.

Some legal rights to remember when caring for the terminally ill include:

1. **The right to refuse treatment.**

Remember that whether you agree or disagree with a resident's decisions, the choice is not yours. It belongs to the person involved. Sometimes, when a resident is not able to make a decision, he has told family members how he wishes things to be done. Be supportive of family members. Do not judge them. They are most likely following the resident's wishes.

2. **The right to have visitors.**

It may be inconvenient to have visitors coming and going at odd hours. When death is close, it is an emotional time for all those involved. Saying goodbye can be a very important part of dealing with a loved one's death. It may also be very reassuring to the dying person to have someone in the room, even if they do not seem to be aware of their surroundings.

3. **The right to privacy.**

Privacy is a basic right, but privacy for visiting, or even when the person is alone, may be even more important now.

Other rights of a dying person are listed in Figure 23-6.

Legal Rights

Residents may have advance directives or DNR orders. You learned about these legal rights in chapter 3. Advance directives allow people to choose what medical care they wish to have if they cannot make those decisions themselves. Advance directives can also name someone to make decisions for a person if that person becomes ill or disabled. A DNR order tells medical professionals not to perform CPR. By law, advance directives and DNR orders must be honored.

Ways to treat dying residents and their families with dignity include:

- Respect their wishes in all possible ways. Communication between staff is extremely important at this time so that everyone understands what the resident's wishes are.
- Listen carefully for ideas on how to provide simple gestures that may be special and appreciated.
- Be careful not to make promises that cannot or should not be kept.
- Listen if a dying resident wants to talk.

I have the right to:

be treated as a living human being until I die.

maintain a sense of hopefulness, however changing its focus may be.

be cared for by those who can maintain a sense of hopefulness, however changing this might be.

express my feelings and emotions about my approaching death in my own way.

participate in decisions concerning my care.

expect continuing medical and nursing attention even though "cure" goals must be changed to "comfort" goals.

not die alone.

be free from pain.

have my questions answered honestly.

not be deceived.

have help from and for my family in accepting my death.

die in peace and dignity.

retain my individuality and not be judged for my decisions, which may be contrary to beliefs of others.

discuss and enlarge my religious and/or spiritual experiences, whatever these may mean to others.

expect that the sanctity of the human body will be respected after death.

be cared for by caring, sensitive, knowledgeable people who will attempt to understand my needs and will be able to gain some satisfaction in helping me face my death.

Fig. 23-6. **The Dying Person's Bill of Rights. (This was created at a workshop on "The Terminally Ill Patient and the Helping Person," sponsored by Southwestern Michigan In-service Education Council, and appeared in the *American Journal of Nursing*, Vol. 75, January, 1975, p. 99.)**

- Do not babble or be especially cheerful or sad. Sometimes you may be nervous when you know that a resident is dying. That nervousness may lead to giggling or talking too much. Or, if you let your emotions get out of hand, you may be so sad and upset that you cannot be any help to the resident who needs you.
- Keep the resident as comfortable as possible. The nurse needs to know immediately if pain medication is requested. Keep the resident clean and dry.
- Do not isolate or avoid residents who are dying.
- Assure privacy when it is desired.
- Respect the privacy of the family and other visitors. They may be upset and not want to be bothered with others now. They may welcome a friendly smile, however, and should not be isolated, either.

7. List changes that may occur in the human body after death

When death occurs, the body will not have heartbeat, pulse, respiration, or blood pressure. Other signs you may see are:

- the jaw drops, causing the mouth to stay open
- eyelids partially open with eyes in a fixed stare
- incontinence of both urine and stool
- pupils are fixed and dilated (this means there is no blood flow inside the brain)

Though these things are a normal part of death, they can be frightening. Tell the nurse immediately to help confirm the death.

8. Describe postmortem care

Postmortem care is care of the body after death. Be sensitive to the needs of the family and friends after death. They may wish to sit by the bed to say goodbye. They may wish to stay with the body for a while. Allow them to do so. Be aware of religious and cultural practices of the family. Facilities will have different policies on postmortem care. A shroud kit containing a large white piece of material for covering the body may be used. It may include special pads and ID tags. Always follow your facility's policies and procedures. Do only assigned tasks.

GUIDELINES

Postmortem Care

Follow your facility's guidelines. They may include:

- Bathe the body. Be very gentle to avoid bruising.
- Place drainage pads where needed. This is most often under the head and/or under the perineum. Follow Standard Precautions.
- Do not remove any tubes or other equipment. A nurse or the funeral home will do this.
- Put dentures back in the mouth if instructed by the nurse. Close the mouth. You may need to place a rolled towel under the chin to support the closed-mouth position. If this is not possible, place dentures in cup near the head.
- Close the eyes carefully.
- Position the body on the back with legs straight. Fold arms across the abdomen.
- Put a small pillow under the head.
- Follow facility policy on personal items. Check to see if you should remove jewelry. Always have a witness if personal items are removed or given to a family member. Document what was given and to whom.
- Document using your facility's policy.
- Strip the bed after the body has been removed.
- Open windows to air the room, as needed. Straighten up.
- Respect the wishes of family and friends. Be sensitive to their needs. Only perform assigned tasks.

9. Define the goals of a hospice program

Hospice is the term for the special care that a dying person needs. It is a compassionate way to care for dying people and their families. Hospice care uses a holistic approach. It treats the person's physical, emotional, spiritual, and social needs. Hospice care can be given seven days a week, 24 hours a day. There is always a nurse on call to answer questions, make a visit, or solve a problem. Hospice care may be given in a hospital, at a care facility, or in the home. Hospice care is available with a doctor's order.

Any caregiver may give hospice care. Often specially-trained nurses, social workers, and volunteers provide hospice care. The hospice team may include doctors, nurses, social workers, counselors, nursing assistants, therapists, clergy, dietitians, and volunteers.

Hospice care helps meet all needs of the dying resident. Family and friends, as well as the resident, are directly involved in care decisions. The resident is encouraged to participate in family life and decision-making as long as possible.

In long-term care, goals focus on recovery, or on the resident's ability to care for him- or herself as much as possible. However, in hospice care, the goals are the comfort and dignity of the resident. This type of care is called **palliative** care. This is an important difference. You will need to change your mind-set when caring for hospice residents. Focus on pain relief and comfort, rather than on teaching them to care for themselves. Report complaints or signs of pain to the nurse immediately. Residents who are dying need to feel independent for as long as possible. Caregivers should allow residents to have as much control over their lives as possible. Eventually, caregivers may have to meet all basic needs.

Other attitudes and skills useful in hospice care are:

Be a good listener. It is hard to know what to say to someone who is dying or to his or her loved ones. Most often, people need someone to listen to them (Fig. 23-7). Review the listening skills in chapter 4. A good listener can be a great comfort. Some people will not want to confide in you. Never push someone to talk.

Respect privacy and independence. Relatives, friends, clergy, or others may visit a dying resident. Make it easy for these difficult visits to take place. Stay out of the way when you can. Do not join in the conversation unless you are asked to do so. Dying residents can have some independence even when they need total care. Let the resident make choices, such as when to bathe. Understand that some people wish to be alone with their dying loved ones.

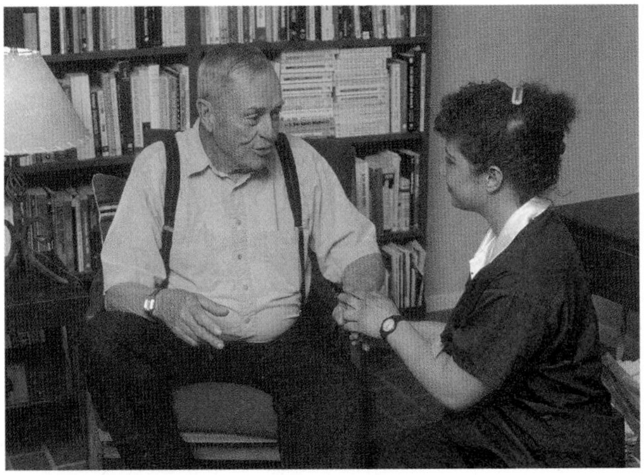

Fig. 23-7. **Being a good listener can be a great help to a dying resident and his or her family.**

Be sensitive to individual needs. Different residents and families will have different needs. The more you know what is needed, the more you can help. Some residents need a quiet and calm atmosphere. Others like a cheery presence. They might like you to talk or stay close by. Ask family members or friends how you can help.

Be aware of your own feelings. Caring for people who are dying can be draining. Know your limits. Respect them. Discuss your feelings of frustration or grief with another care team member.

Recognize the stress. Just realizing how stressful it is to work with people who are dying is a first step toward caring for yourself. Talking with a counselor about your experiences at work can help you understand and work through your feelings. Remember, however, you must keep specific information confidential. Your supervisor may be able to refer you to a counselor or support group.

Take good care of yourself. Eating right, exercising, and getting enough rest are ways of taking care of yourself. Remember to care for your emotional and spiritual health, too. Talk about and acknowledge your feelings. Take time out to do things for yourself, such as reading a book, taking a bubble bath, or whatever you enjoy. Spiritual needs may be met by attending religious services, reading, praying, meditating, or just taking a quiet walk. Meeting your needs allows you to best meet other people's needs.

Take a break when you need to. Find ten minutes to sit down and relax or stand up and stretch. These ideas may be enough of a break in some situations.

Hospice cares.

According to the National Hospice and Palliative Care Organization, there are now more than 3,200 hospices across the country. They gave care to more than 775,000 people in 2001. About 200,000 hospice volunteers give more than 10 million hours each year to help people who are dying. Hospice volunteers go through a training program for hospice work. The volunteers provide a variety of services. These include caring for the home or family of a dying person, driving or doing errands, and emotional support.

Chapter Review

1. Describe one behavior you might see at each stage of dying.
2. Describe five possible feelings/emotions in the grief process.
3. What helps you work through difficult feelings like those associated with grief?
4. Which sense is often present until death occurs?
5. What are some of the ways to give emotional and spiritual support for a dying resident?
6. What measures may help a dying resident who is in pain?
7. List three legal rights to remember when caring for the terminally ill.
8. List five changes you may see in the body after death occurs.
9. Define "postmortem."
10. Where are drainage pads most often needed during postmortem care?
11. What is the focus in dealing with hospice residents? How does it differ from the usual care you provide?
12. What needs does hospice care treat?

Chapter 24
Caring for Your Career and Yourself

1. Explain how to find a job and how to write a résumé

If you are in school, you may soon be looking for a job. To find a job, you must first find potential employers. Then you must contact them to find out about job opportunities. To find employers, use the newspaper, the telephone book, the Internet, or personal contacts (Fig. 24-1). Ask your instructor about potential employers. Some schools keep a list of employers seeking nursing assistants.

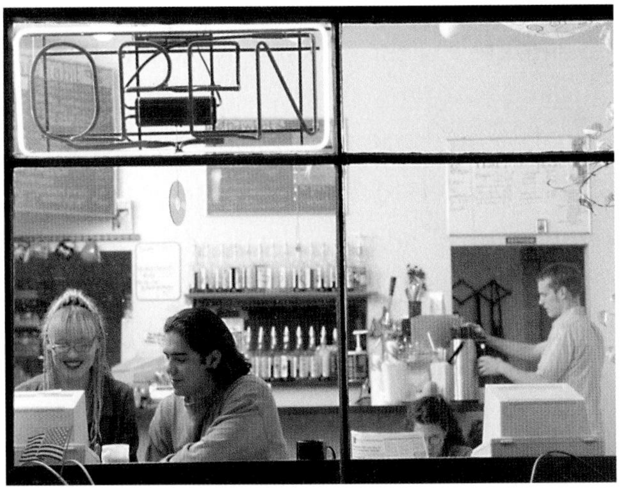

***Fig. 24-1.* Searching the Internet is one good way to find a job.**

Once you have a good list of potential employers, you need to contact them. Phoning first is a good way to learn what jobs are available and how to apply.

When making an appointment, ask what information to bring with you. Make sure you have it when you go. Some documents you may need to show a potential employer are:

- Identification: driver's license, social security card, birth certificate, passport, or other official form of identification
- Proof of your legal status in this country and proof that you are legally able to work, even if you are a U.S.-born citizen. Employers must have files showing that employees are legally allowed to work in this country. Do not be upset by this request.
- High school diploma or equivalency, school transcripts, and diploma or certificate from your nursing assistant training course. It is a good idea to have your instructor's name and phone number, too.
- References are people who can be called to recommend you as an employee. They can include former employers, former teachers, or your minister. Do not use relatives or friends. You can ask them beforehand to write letters for you, addressed "To whom it may concern," explaining how they know you and describing your skills, qualities, and habits. Take copies of these with you.

Some potential employers will ask you for a résumé and a cover letter. A **résumé** is a summary of your education and experience. You will need to include these topics when preparing a résumé:

- An objective states your main goals in the field in which you wish to work.
- Your education lists schools or G.E.D. courses completed, from high school through college.
- Your work experience includes jobs you have held to this point, from the most current moving backwards. A general rule is to list jobs you have held for more than six months.
- Describe all of your volunteer work. Emphasize work in the healthcare field.
- List all of your special skills. Include things like typing, computer skills, and speaking other languages.
- State that your references are available upon request.

Here are some rules for writing a résumé:

- Limit your résumé to one page. Use short sentences.
- Do not add borders or color. Use quality, white paper.
- Use a basic, size-12, plain font. Boldface your name and address at the top of the page and center it.
- If using a computer, do not rely only on a spell-check program. Use it first, then check spelling yourself. Have a friend check the spelling. Read the résumé out loud to make sure you have not made any errors.
- Do not staple anything to your résumé.

A well-written NA résumé is shown in Fig. 24-2. Pay attention to your résumé. Make it the best it can be.

The cover letter is a letter included with your résumé. A sample cover letter is shown in Fig. 24-3. This letter should be brief. It serves as your introduction to the interviewer. It explains why you seek the job and why you are qualified for it. Emphasize skills you have that would be a good match.

2. Identify information that may be required when filling out a job application

Completing a job application can be stressful. Being prepared will help you present yourself well. On one sheet of paper, write down the information you will need. Take it with you, along with your résumé, if you have one. This will save time and avoid mistakes.

Include the following general information:

- your address and phone number
- your birth date
- your social security number
- the name and address of the school or program where you were trained and the date you completed it, as well as certification numbers and expiration dates from a nursing assistant certification card, if you have one
- the names, titles, addresses, and phone numbers of former employers, and the dates you worked there
- salary information from your former jobs
- why you left each of your former jobs
- the names, addresses, and phone numbers of your references
- the days and hours you can work (facilities usually have shifts on days, nights, and weekends)
- a brief statement of why you are changing jobs or why you want to work as a nursing assistant

Fill out the application carefully and neatly (Fig. 24-4). Never lie. Before you write anything, read it all the way through. If you do not understand what is being asked, find out

Sarah Harris

1234 Sandia Court • Albuquerque, NM 87126 • 505-555-4211

Objective

To secure an entry-level nursing assistant job in a long-term care facility.

Education

Hobbs High School, Hobbs, NM, Diploma 1996
Hartman Medical Institute, Albuquerque, NM 2000
Certified Nursing Assistant

Experience

Sunnyvale Nursing Home 2000 - present
Albuquerque, NM
Nursing Assistant

- Perform personal care duties and assisted with ADLs.
- Work mostly with residents with dementia.
- Help plan activities for residents.

Happy Home Nursing Center 1998-2000
Austin, Texas
Receptionist

- Managed multi-line phone system.
- Made appointments for staff.
- Visited residents and read to them.
- Made arrangements for resident activities out of the facility.

Skills

Microsoft Word, Microsoft Excel, Adobe Acrobat, and ACT database on a PC.

Volunteer Work

National Diabetes Foundation, Hospice Foundation

References

Available upon request.

Fig. 24-2. A sample résumé.

Sarah Louise Harris
1234 Sandia Court
Albuquerque, NM 87126
505-555-4211

January 10, 2005
Mr. David Pomazal
Human Resources Manager
Nursing Assistant Finders
PO Box 555
Albuquerque, NM 87102

Dear Mr. Pomazal:

Please consider this letter and the enclosed resume and application for the NA position advertised in last Sunday's edition of the *Albuquerque Journal.*

I am an energetic, detail-oriented person who has strong organizational skills, experience, and the ability to work well with people from all walks of life. In addition, I have held positions of responsibility in four community organizations over the last eight years and was chosen as the "2004 National Diabetes Foundation Volunteer of the Year."

As you can see from my résumé, I thrive in a busy atmosphere that involves many different tasks, the opportunity to work with residents, and the chance to excel. I would appreciate an interview to discuss the possibility of my joining your staff. I will call you next week to request an appointment, or you may call me at your convenience at (505) 555-4211.

Thank you for your consideration of my application. I look forward to meeting you soon.

Sincerely,

Sarah Louise Harris

Fig. 24-3. **A sample cover letter.**

Employment Application

Personal Information	
Name: Rosie Ferguson	Date: 1/15/05
Social Security Number: 555-99-9999	
Home Address: 8529-A Indian School Rd. NE	
City, state, Zip: Albuquerque, NM 87112	
Home Phone: 505-291-1274	Business Phone: N/A
US Citizen? Yes	If Not Give Visa No. & expiration:

Position Applying For	
Title: Nursing Assistant	Salary Desired: $8.50/hr
Referred By: Ms. McClain Instructor, NA Training Center	Date Available: 1/15/05

Education	
High School (Name, City, State): Laguna High School Albuquerque, NM	
Graduation Date: December 2004	
Technical or Undergraduate School: NA Training Center Albuquerque, NM	
Dates Attended: July – Dec. 2004	Degree Major:

References
Mr. Robert Castro, Instructor, NA Training Center, 505-291-1284
Ms. Scott, Health Occupations, Laguna HS, 505-555-6255
Kate Crawford, Instructor, NA Training Center, 505-291-1294

Fig. 24-4. A sample job application.

before filling in that space. Do not leave anything blank. You may write N/A (not applicable) if the question does not apply to you.

Before going to the facility, think about any potential problems in your job application. If you have a time when you did not work at all, an interviewer may ask you about it. Be prepared to give that answer.

By law, your employer must do a criminal background check. You may be asked to sign a form granting permission to do this. Do not take it personally. It is a law to protect residents.

3. Discuss proper job interview techniques

Use these tips to make the best impression at a job interview:

- Dress neatly and appropriately.
- Shower or bathe. Use deodorant.
- Wash your hands. Clean and file your nails. Nails should be medium length or shorter.
- Men should shave right before the interview.
- Brush your teeth.
- Do not smoke. You will smell like smoke during the interview.
- Do not wear perfume or cologne. Many people dislike or are allergic to scents.
- Wear simple makeup and jewelry or none at all.
- Wear your hair in a simple style.
- Wear a nice pair of pants, a skirt, or a dress. Make sure your clothes are not wrinkled. A skirt or a dress should be no shorter than knee-length. Do not wear jeans or shorts.
- Make sure your shoes are polished. Do not wear sneakers or open-toed sandals.
- Arrive ten or 15 minutes early.
- Introduce yourself. Smile and shake hands (Fig. 24-5). Your handshake should be firm and confident.

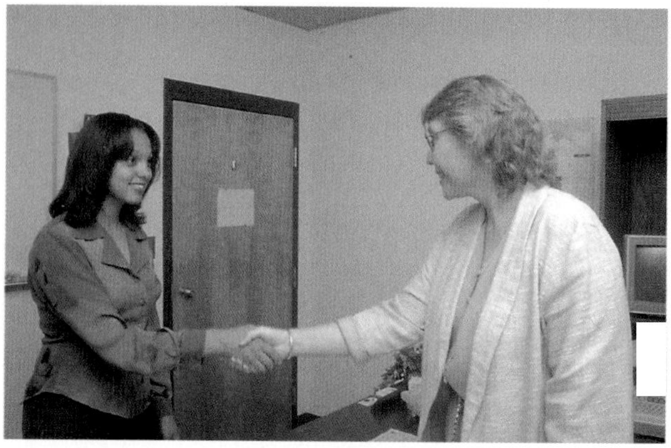

Fig. 24-5. **Smile and shake hands when you arrive at a job interview.**

- Answer questions clearly and completely.
- Make eye contact to show you are sincere (Fig. 24-6).

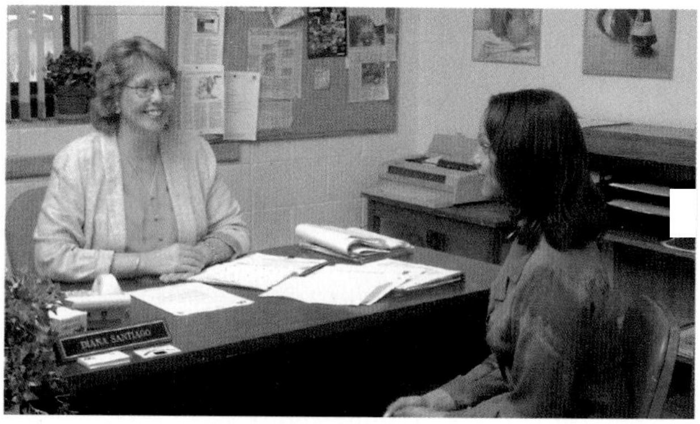

Fig. 24-6. **Be polite. Make eye contact during an interview.**

- Avoid slang words or expressions.
- Never eat, drink, chew gum, or smoke in an interview.
- Sit up or stand up straight. Look happy to be there.
- Do not bring friends or children with you.
- Relax. You have worked hard to get this far. You understand the work and what is expected of you. Be confident!

Be positive when answering questions. Emphasize what you enjoy or think you will enjoy about being a nursing assistant. Do not complain about previous jobs. Make it clear that you are hardworking and willing to work with all kinds of residents.

Some questions you may be asked include:

- Why did you become an NA?
- What do you like about working as an NA?
- What do you not like? (If this is your first job, you may be asked what you expect to like or dislike.)
- What are your best qualities? What are your weaknesses?
- Why did you leave your last job?

Usually interviewers will ask if you have any questions. Have some prepared. Write them down so you do not forget things you really want to know. Questions you may want to ask include:

- What hours would I work?
- What benefits does the job include? Is health insurance available? Would I get paid sick days or holidays?
- What orientation or training will be provided?
- Will my supervisor be available when needed?
- How soon will you be making a decision about this position?

Later in the interview, you may want to ask about salary or wages if you have not already been told what it would be.

Listen carefully to the answers to your questions. Take notes if needed. You will probably be told when you can expect to hear from the employer. Do not expect to be offered a job at the interview. When the interview is over, stand up and shake hands again. Say something like, "Thank you for taking the time to meet with me today. I look forward to hearing from you."

Send a thank-you letter after every job interview. This states your continued interest in a job (Fig. 24-7). If you have not heard from the employer within the time frame you discussed with your interviewer, call and ask if the job was filled.

April 22, 2005
Nancy Proust, Personnel Manager
Nursing Care Providers
332 S. Main
Rio Grande, TX 74568

Dear Ms. Proust:

Thank you for taking the time to interview me last week for a nursing assistant position with Nursing Care Providers. It was a pleasure to talk to you and to learn more about your facility. I look forward to hearing from you soon regarding the nursing assistant openings listed in the newspaper.

Sincerely,

Marilyn Michaels
4356 12th St.
Rio Grande, TX 74568
505-291-1274

Fig. 24-7. **After a job interview send a professional thank-you letter.**

4. Describe a standard job description and list steps for following the scope of practice

A **job description** is an outline of what will be expected of you in your job. It can be a long, complex form. Read it before you sign it. Ask questions if you do not understand something.

You learned about scope of practice in chapter 2. A scope of practice defines the things you are allowed to do and how to do them. Follow these tips when deciding whether or not to do something:

1. Do not do a procedure if it is not listed in your job description. Doing things that are beyond your scope of practice could harm a resident, you, or another staff member. If a

resident asks you to do a task outside your scope of practice, explain why you cannot do it. Tell the nurse about the request.

2. Do not perform a procedure you have not been trained to do.
3. Do not perform a procedure if you have forgotten how to do it. Ask the nurse to remind you how to perform the procedure before you do it.
4. If you have been trained to perform a procedure within your scope of practice, but you think it may not be appropriate for a certain resident, ask the nurse.

5. Explain an employer's responsibilities regarding TB and hepatitis

Each year facilities must test all employees for exposure to diseases like tuberculosis. You will get a notice when it is time to have an annual TB skin test. It is your responsibility to get the test. Once this is done, you will be asked to return within a certain time, usually 48 to 72 hours, for the test results.

As you learned in chapter 5, hepatitis B and C are bloodborne diseases that can cause death. Many people have hepatitis B (HBV). It is a serious threat to healthcare workers. Your employer must offer you a free vaccine to protect you from hepatitis B. You will usually get the vaccine when you begin your new job. There is no vaccine for hepatitis C.

6. List guidelines for managing time and assignments

When you take care of residents, it is important to manage your time well every day. You will have a variety of tasks to do during your shift. Managing time properly will help you to complete these tasks. Many of the ideas for managing time on the job can be used to manage your personal time as well. The following are basic ways to manage time:

1. **Plan ahead**. Planning is the single best way to help you manage your time better. Sometimes you may feel you do not even have the time to plan. Take the time to sit down and list everything you have to do. Take time to check to see if you all the supplies needed for a procedure. Often just making the list and taking the time to recheck will help you feel better. This will get you focused.

   The nurse will make your work assignments. He or she bases this on needs of residents and availability of staff. The assignments will allow staff to work as team. Your responsibilities in completing assignments include:
   - helping others when needed
   - never ignoring a resident who needs help
   - answering all call lights even if you are not assigned to a particular resident
   - notifying your supervisor if you cannot complete an assignment
2. **Prioritize**. Identify the most important things to get done. Do these first.
3. **Make a schedule**. Write out the hours of the day and fill in when you will do what. This will help you be realistic.
4. **Combine activities**. Can you visit with residents while providing care? Can you prepare tomorrow's dinner while the laundry is in the dryer? Work more efficiently when you can.
5. **Get help**. It is not reasonable for you to do everything. Sometimes you will need help to ensure a resident's safety. Do not be afraid to ask for help.

7. Describe employee evaluations and discuss appropriate responses to criticism

Handling criticism is hard for most people.

Being able to accept and learn from criticism is important in all relationships, including employment. From time to time you will get evaluations from your employer. They contain ideas to help you improve your job performance. Here are some tips for handling criticism and using it to your benefit:

- Listen to the message that is being sent. Do not get so upset that you cannot understand the message.
- Hostile criticism and constructive criticism are not the same. Hostile criticism is angry and negative. Examples are, "You are useless!" or "You are lazy and slow." Hostile criticism should not come from your employer or supervisor. You may hear hostile criticism from residents, family members, or others. The best response is something like, "I'm sorry you are so disappointed," and nothing more. Give the person a chance to calm down before trying to discuss their comments.
- Constructive criticism may come from your employer, supervisor, or others. Constructive criticism is meant to help you improve. Examples are, "You really need to be more accurate in your charting," or "You are late too often. You'll have to make more of an effort to be on time." Listening and acting on constructive criticism can help you be more successful in your job. Pay attention to it (Fig. 24-8).
- If you are not sure how to avoid a mistake you have made, always ask for suggestions. Avoiding making mistakes will help you improve your performance.
- Apologize and move on. If you have made a mistake, apologize as needed (Fig. 24-9). This may be to your supervisor, a resident, or others. Learn from the incident and put it behind you. Do not dwell on it or hold a grudge. Responding professionally to criticism is important for success in any job.

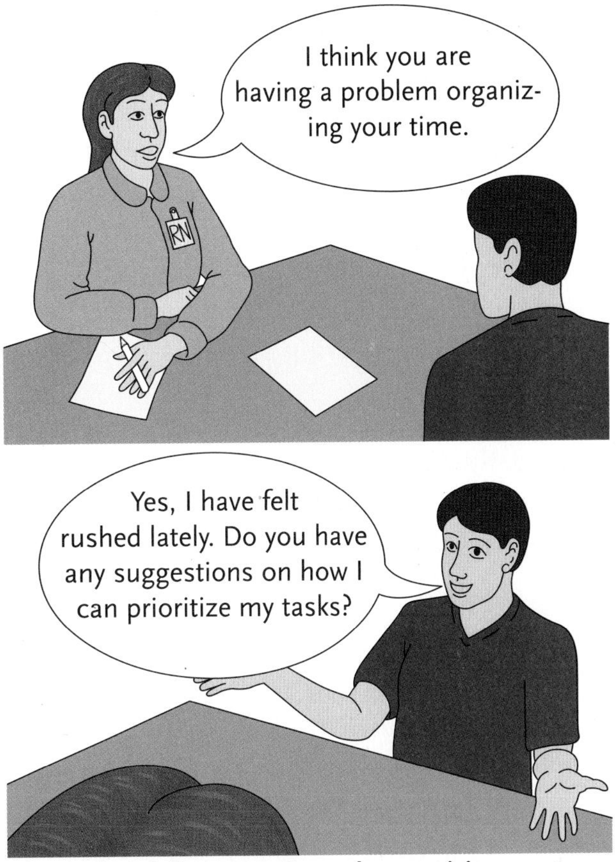
I think you are having a problem organizing your time.
RN
Yes, I have felt rushed lately. Do you have any suggestions on how I can prioritize my tasks?

Fig. 24-8. **Ask for suggestions when receiving constructive criticism.**

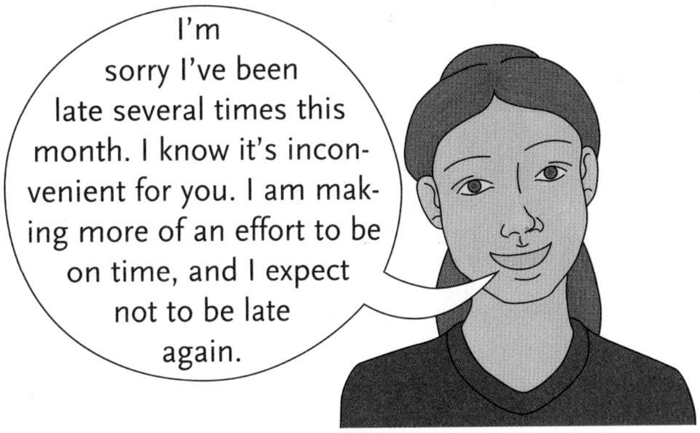
I'm sorry I've been late several times this month. I know it's inconvenient for you. I am making more of an effort to be on time, and I expect not to be late again.

Fig. 24-9. **Be willing to apologize if you have made a mistake.**

Your evaluation will also cover overall knowledge, conflict resolution, and team effort. Flexibility, friendliness, trustworthiness, and customer service are other things considered. Evaluations are often the basis for salary increases. A good evaluation can help you advance within the facility. Being open to criticism and suggestions for improvement will help you be more successful.

8. Explain how to make job changes

If you decide to change jobs, be responsible. Always give your employer at least two weeks' written notice that you will be leaving. Otherwise, your facility may be understaffed. Both the residents and other staff will suffer. Future employers may talk with past supervisors. People who change jobs too often or who do not give notice before leaving are less likely to be hired.

9. Identify guidelines for maintaining certification and explain the state's registry

To meet OBRA's requirements, several organizations, including the National Council of State Boards of Nursing, created competency evaluation programs. These programs are a guide for each state for developing NA testing programs. OBRA requires that NAs complete at least 75 hours of training before being employed. Many states' requirements exceed the minimum 75 hours.

After completing a state's required hours of training, NAs may then take the test in that state. A fee may be charged. Once a nursing assistant has passed both the written and manual skills test, a certificate is mailed.

Each state has different requirements for maintaining certification. Learn your state's requirements. Follow them exactly or you will not be able to keep working. General guidelines on obtaining and keeping certification are:

1. You will have a certain amount of time from the date you are employed to take the state test. Your employer will give you that information when you are hired. Pay attention to the time frame. If you do not take the test during the time given, you will not be able to work as a nursing assistant until you have passed the test.
2. Usually you must take the state test within 24 months of training or you will have to take a new training course and state examination.
3. You must work for pay during a 24-month period. If you do not, you will have to take a new training program and examination.
4. In most states, you will have three chances to pass the state test.
5. You must keep your certification current if the state requires certification. File a change-of-address with your state agency if you move to make sure you get your certification renewal.

Your employer may require that you show proof of renewal of your certificate each time it expires. Do not let your certificate expire. Respond immediately to your state's request to renew your certification. There may be a fee.

In the United States, each state keeps a registry for certified nursing assistants (CNAs). This registry keeps track of each nursing assistant working in that state. Information kept in the registry includes:

- a nursing assistant's full name and any other names the person may have used
- a nursing assistant's home address and other information, such as date of birth and social security number
- the date that a nursing assistant was placed in the registry and the results from the state test
- expiration dates of nursing assistants' certificates
- information about investigations and hearings regarding abuse, neglect, or theft, which becomes a part of a nursing assistant's permanent record

NAs can ask for a written statement to be added to the file. This includes information explaining events in the nursing assistants' own words. NAs have the right to correct any errors in a registry file.

10. Describe continuing education for nursing assistants

The federal government requires nursing assistants to have 12 hours of continuing education each year. Some states may require more. In-service continuing education courses help you keep your knowledge and skills fresh. Classes also give new information about conditions, challenges in working with residents, or regulation changes. Your facility must provide and document this continuing education. It is sometimes called an in-service.

Your employer is responsible for offering in-service courses. You are responsible for successfully attending and completing them. It is your responsibility to meet education requirements:

- Sign up for the course or find out where it is offered.
- Attend all class sessions.
- Pay attention and complete all the class requirements.
- Make the most of your in-service programs. Participate! (Fig. 24-10)

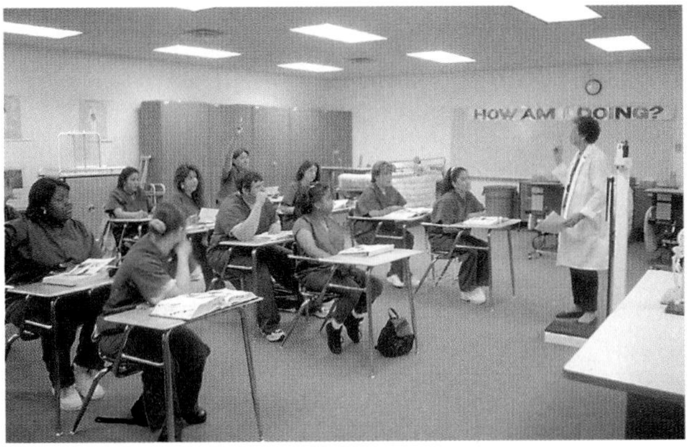

Fig. 24-10. **Pay attention and participate during in-service courses.**

- Keep original copies of all certificates and records of your successful attendance so you can prove you took the class.

11. Define "stress" and "stressors"

Stress is the state of being frightened, excited, confused, in danger, or irritated. We may think only bad things cause stress. However, positive situations cause stress, too. For example, getting married or having a baby are usually positive situations. But both can bring enormous stress from the changes they bring to our lives (Fig. 24-11).

You may be thrilled when you get a new job as a nursing assistant. Starting work may also cause you stress. You may be afraid of making mistakes, excited about earning money or helping people, or confused about your new duties. Learning how to recognize stress and its causes is helpful. Then you can master a few simple methods for relaxing and learn to manage stress.

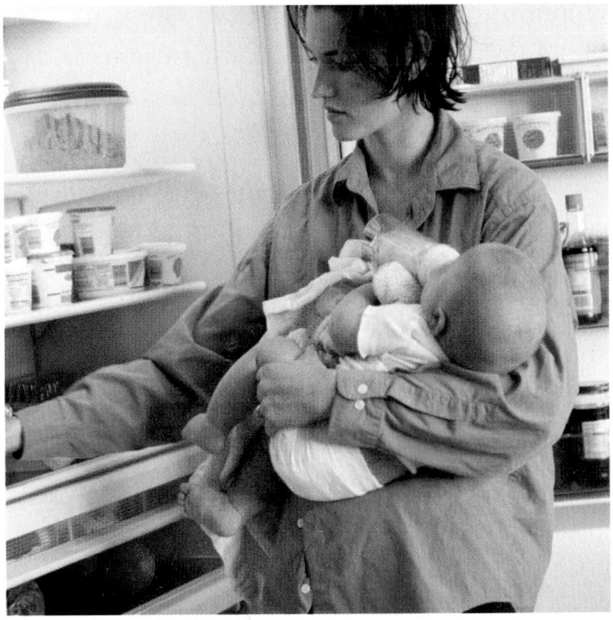

Fig. 24-11. **Although having a new baby is usually a happy time, it can also cause stress.**

A **stressor** is something that causes stress. Anything can be a stressor. Some examples are:

- divorce
- marriage
- a new baby
- children leaving home

- feeling unprepared for a task
- starting a new job
- losing a job
- new responsibilities at work
- problems at work
- supervisors
- co-workers
- residents
- illness
- finances

12. Explain ways to manage stress

Stress is not only an emotional response. It is also a physical response. When we have stress, changes occur in our bodies. The endocrine system may make more of the hormone adrenaline. This can increase nervous system response, heart rate, respiratory rate, and blood pressure. This is why, in stressful situations, your heart beats fast, you breathe hard, and you feel warm or perspire.

Each of us has a different tolerance level for stress. What one person would find overwhelming may not bother another person. Your tolerance for stress depends on your personality, life experiences, and physical health.

GUIDELINES
Managing Stress

- Develop healthy habits of diet, exercise, and lifestyle.
- Eat nutritious foods.
- Exercise regularly (Fig. 24-12). You can exercise alone or with a partner.
- Get enough sleep.
- Drink only in moderation.
- Do not smoke.
- Find time at least a few times a week to do something relaxing, such as taking a walk, reading a book, or sewing.

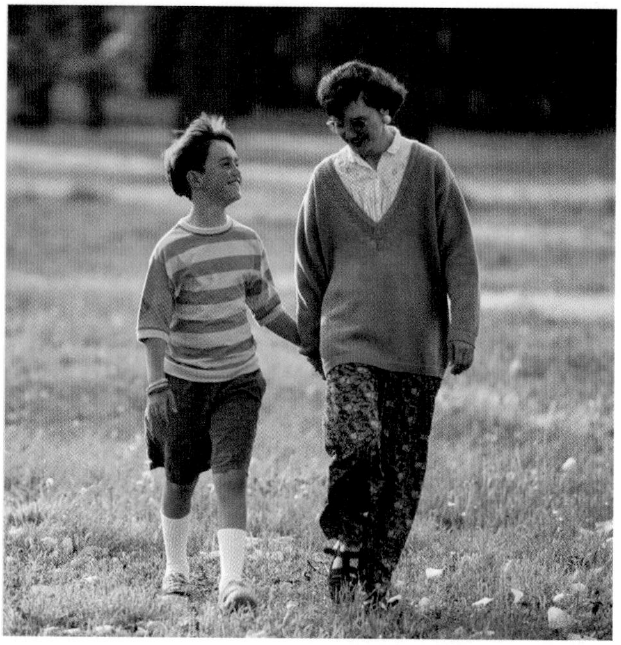

Fig. 24-12. **Exercising regularly is one healthy way to decrease stress.**

Not managing stress can cause many problems. Some of these will affect how well you do your job. Signs that you are not managing stress are:

- showing anger or being abusive to residents
- arguing with your supervisor about assignments
- poor relationships with co-workers and residents
- complaining about your job and your responsibilities
- feeling work-related burn-out
- feeling tired even when you are rested
- trouble focusing on residents and procedures

Stress can seem overwhelming when you try to handle it yourself. Often talking about stress or stressors can help you manage it better. Sometimes another person can offer helpful suggestions. You may think of new ways to handle stress just by talking it through. Get help from one or more of these when managing stress (Fig. 24-13):

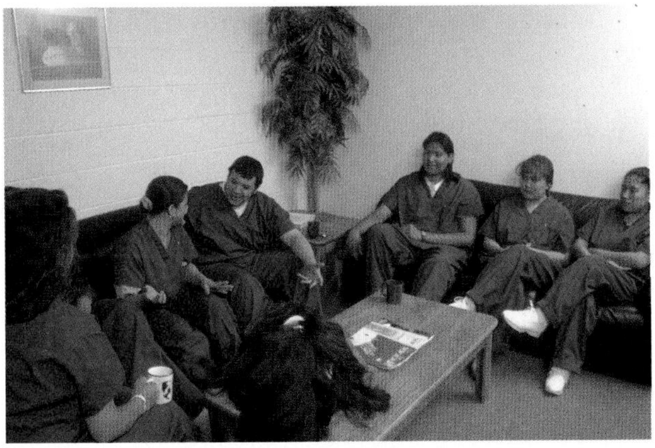

Fig. 24-13. **Support groups can help you deal with different types of stress.**

- your supervisor or another member of the care team for work-related stress
- your family
- your friends
- your church, synagogue, mosque, or temple
- your doctor
- a local mental health agency
- any phone hotline that deals with related problems (check your local yellow pages)

It is not appropriate to talk to your residents or their family members about your personal or job-related stress.

One of the best ways of managing stress is to develop a plan. The plan can include nice things you will do for yourself every day and things to do in stressful situations. When you think about a plan, you first need to answer these questions:

- What are the sources of stress in my life?
- When do I most often feel stress?
- What effects of stress do I see in my life?
- What can I change to decrease the stress I feel?
- What things must I learn to cope with because I cannot change them?

When you have answered these questions, you will have a clearer picture of the challenges you face. Then you can come up with strategies for managing stress.

13. Describe a relaxation technique

Sometimes a relaxation exercise can help you feel refreshed and relaxed in a short time. Below is a simple relaxation exercise. Try it out. See if it helps you feel more relaxed.

The body scan. Close your eyes. Focus on your breathing and posture. Be sure you are comfortable. Start at the balls of your feet. Concentrate on your feet. Find any tension hidden in the feet. Try to relax and release the tension. Continue very slowly. Take a breath between each body part. Move up from the feet. Focus on and relax the legs, knees, thighs, hips, stomach, back, shoulders, neck, jaw, eyes, forehead, and scalp. Take a few very deep breaths. Open your eyes.

This exercise takes only about two minutes. If it is helpful for you, try it the next time you need a break, at work or at home.

Look back over all you have learned. Your work as a nursing assistant is very important. Every day may be different and challenging. In a hundred ways every week you will offer help that only a caring person like you can give.

14. List ways to remind yourself of the importance of the work you have chosen to do

Value the work you have chosen to do. It is important. Your work can mean the difference between living with independence and dignity and living without. The difference you make is sometimes life versus death. Look in the face of each of your residents. Know that you are doing important work. Look in a mirror when you get home. Be proud of how you make your living (Fig. 24-14).

An important life skill is reflecting on how you spend your time. Learn ways to fully appreciate that what you do has great meaning. Few jobs have the challenges and rewards of working as a nursing assistant. Congratulate yourself for choosing a path that includes helping others along the way.

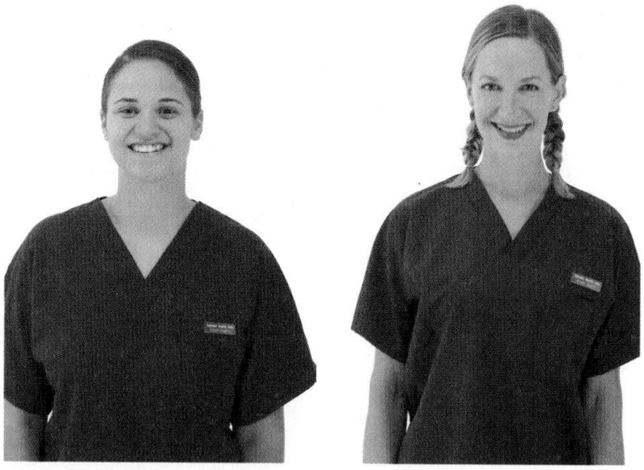

Fig. 24-14. **Be proud of the work you have chosen to do. It is important.**

Chapter Review

1. What is a good way to find out about job opportunities with a potential employer?
2. List three documents you may need to take when applying for a job.
3. What is a résumé? Ideally, how many pages should it be?
4. What should you do before writing anything on a job application?
5. Why do you think employers are required to do criminal background checks on nursing assistants?
6. How can you follow up on a job interview?
7. List three things you can do to show a potential employer your professionalism during an interview.
8. Why do you think it is important to be positive during a job interview?
9. List three ways you can comply with your scope of practice.
10. What must your employer do with regards to the hepatitis B vaccine?
11. List five guidelines for managing time.
12. What is the difference between hostile and constructive criticism?
13. Why might an employer not hire a person who has changed jobs often?
14. What information does a registry for certified nursing assistants keep?
15. How many hours of continuing education does the federal government say that nursing assistants must have each year?
16. What can you do to get the most out of continuing education?
17. Give three examples of stressors you've experienced in the last year. How did you respond to them?
18. What steps can you take to manage stress in your life?
19. What do you think you will like best about being a nursing assistant?

Common Abbreviations

The Joint Commission on Accreditation of Healthcare Organizations (JCAHO) evaluates and accredits different types of healthcare facilities. JCAHO is an independent, not-for-profit organization. JCAHO's standards focus on improving the quality and safety of care provided by healthcare facilities.

In 2003, JCAHO approved the 2004 National Patient Safety Goals. These goals include information on standardizing abbreviations, acronyms and symbols used in facilities. They also include a list of abbreviations, acronyms and symbols not to use. The list below does not include abbreviations that JCAHO does not want facilities to use.

abd.	abdomen
ABR	absolute bedrest
ac	before meals
ad lib	as desired
adm.	admission
ADL	activities of daily living
AFB	acid-fast bacillus (TB)
AIDS	acquired immune deficiency syndrome
AKA	above-knee amputation
AL	assisted living
am, AM	morning
amb	ambulatory
amt	amount
ap	apical
approx.	approximately
AROM	active range of motion
ASAP	as soon as possible
as tol	as tolerated
ax	axillary (armpit)
BID, b.i.d.	two times a day
BKA	below-knee amputation
bld	blood
BM	bowel movement
BP, B/P	blood pressure
BR	bedrest
BRP	bathroom privileges
BS	blood sugar
BSC	bedside commode
$\bar{c}$	with
C	centigrade
CA	cancer
cath	catheter
CBC	complete blood count
CBR	complete bedrest
cc	cubic centimeter
CCU	coronary care unit
CDC	Centers for Disease Control
CHF	congestive heart failure
cl liq	clear liquid
CMS	circulation, motion, sensation
CNA	certified nursing assistant
CNS	central nervous system
c/o	complains of, in care of
COPD	chronic obstructive pulmonary disorder
CPR	cardiopulmonary resuscitation
CVA	cerebrovascular accident, stroke
CVS	cardiovascular system
DAT	diet as tolerated
DM	diabetes mellitus
DNR	do not resuscitate

DOA	dead on arrival
DOB	date of birth
DON	director of nursing
Dr.	doctor
drsg	dressing
DVT	deep vein thrombosis
dx	diagnosis
ECG, EKG	electrocardiogram
EEG	electroencephalogram
ER	emergency room
ETOH	alcohol
exam	examination
F	fahrenheit
FBS	fasting blood sugar
FF	force fluids
fl, fld	fluid
FSBS	fingerstick blood sugar
ft	foot
FWB	full weight-bearing
FYI	for your information
F/U, f/u	follow-up
fx	fracture
gal	gallon
geri chair	geriatric chair
GI	gastrointestinal
h, hr	hour
H_2O	water
H/A	headache
HBV	hepatitis B virus
HIV	human immunodeficiency virus
HOB	head of bed
HOH	hard of hearing
ht	height
HTN	hypertension
hyper	above normal, too fast, rapid
hypo	low, less than normal
I&O	intake and output
ICU	intensive care unit
inc	incontinent
irr., irrig	irrigation
isol	isolation
IV	intravenous
kg	kilogram
l	liter
L, lt.	left
lab	laboratory
lb	pound
LLE	left lower extremity
lg	large
liq	liquid
LLQ	left lower quadrant
LOC	level of consciousness
LPN	Licensed Practical Nurse
LTC	long-term care
LUQ	left upper quadrant
LVN	Licensed Vocational Nurse
M.D.	medical doctor
meds	medications
MI	myocardial infarction
min	minute
ml	milliliter
mm Hg	millimeters of mercury
mod	moderate
MRSA	methicillin-resistant *Staphylococcus aureus*
N/A	not applicable
NA	nursing assistant
N/C	no call
neg	negative
NF	nursing facility
NKA	no known allergies
NPO	nothing by mouth
NWB	non-weight-bearing

O_2	oxygen
OBRA	Omnibus Budget Reconciliation Act
occ	occasionally
OOB	out of bed
OPD	outpatient department
OR	operating room
os	mouth
OSHA	Occupational Safety and Health Administration
OT	occupational therapy
oz	ounce
p	after
pc, p.c.	after meals
PCA	patient-controlled analgesia
PEG	percutaneous enteral gastrostomy
per os	by mouth
peri care	perineal care
pm, PM	afternoon
PNS	peripheral nervous system
p.o.	by mouth
post op	after surgery
PPE	personal protective equipment
pos.	positive
pre op	before surgery
prep	preparation
p.r.n., prn	when necessary
PROM	passive range of motion
Pt.	patient
PT	physical therapy
PVD	peripheral vascular disease
PWB	partial weight-bearing
$\bar{q}$	every
qh, qhr	every hour
qhs	every night at bedtime
q2h, q3h, q4h	every two hours, every three hours, every four hours
q.i.d., qid	four times a day
Q.S.	every shift or once a shift
quad	four, quadriplegic
R	respirations, right
R/A	rheumatoid arthritis
RBC	red blood cell/count
reg.	regular
rehab	rehabilitation
req.	requisition
res.	resident
resp.	respiration
R.I.C.E.	Rest, Ice, Compression, Elevation (acronym)
RLE	right lower extremity
RLQ	right lower quadrant
RN	Registered Nurse
R/O	rule out
ROM	range of motion
RR	respiratory rate
rt.	right
RUE	right upper extremity
RUQ	right upper quadrant
$\bar{s}$	without
ss	one-half
sm.	small
SNAFU	situation normal, all fouled up (slang)
SNF	skilled nursing facility
spec.	specimen
SOB	shortness of breath
S&S, S/S	signs and symptoms
SSE	soapsuds enema

staph	staphylococcus
stat	immediately
STD	sexually transmitted diseases
std. prec.	standard precautions
strep	streptococcus
T.	temperature
TB	tuberculosis
T, C, DB	turn, cough and deep breathe
temp	temperature
TIA	transient ischemic attack
t.i.d., tid	three times a day
TLC	tender loving care
TPN	total parenteral nutrition
TPR	temperature, pulse, and respirations
TWE	tap water enema
Tx	traction, treatment
U/A, u/a	urinalysis
UGI	upper gastrointestinal
unk	unknown
URI	upper respiratory infection
UTI	urinary tract infection
vag.	vaginal
VRE	vancomycin-resistant enterococcus
vs, VS	vital signs
WBC	white blood cell/count
w/c	wheelchair
WNL	within normal limits
wt.	weight

Glossary

24-hour urine specimen: specimen consisting of all urine voided in a 24-hour period.

abuse: purposely causing physical, mental, or emotional pain or injury to someone.

acquired immune deficiency syndrome (AIDS): disease caused by the human immunodeficiency virus (HIV) in which the body's immune system is weakened and unable to fight infection.

active assisted range of motion: exercises done by a person with some help and support from the caregiver.

active range of motion: exercises done by a person alone, without help.

activities director: person who plans activities at a facility to help residents socialize and stay physically and mentally active.

activities of daily living (ADLs): the personal care tasks a person does every day to care for him- or herself; ADLs include bathing or showering, dressing, caring for teeth and hair, toileting, eating and drinking, and moving from place to place.

activity therapy: therapy for people with Alzheimer's disease that uses activities to prevent boredom and frustration.

acute illness: an illness that has severe symptoms.

acute care: care given in hospitals and ambulatory surgical centers.

adaptive devices: special equipment that helps a person who is ill or disabled to perform ADLs; also called assistive devices.

additive: a substance added to another substance changing its effect.

adult daycare: care given at a facility during daytime hours; generally for people who need some help but are not seriously ill or disabled.

advance directives: documents that allow people to choose what medical care they wish to have if they cannot make those decisions themselves; they can also name someone to make decisions for a person if that person becomes ill or disabled.

affected side: a weakened side from a stroke or injury; also called the weaker or involved side.

ageism: prejudice toward, stereotyping of, and/or discrimination against older persons or the elderly.

agitated: the state of being excited, restless, or troubled.

AIDS dementia complex: condition in the late stages of AIDS in which damage to the central nervous system causes memory loss, poor coordination, paralysis, and confusion.

Airborne Precautions: special measures used for diseases that can be transmitted through the air after being expelled.

Alzheimer's disease (AD): a progressive, degenerative, and irreversible disease that causes dementia; there is no cure.

ambulation: walking.

amputation: the removal of some or all of a body part.

angina pectoris: chest pain.

antimicrobial: an agent destroys or resists pathogens.

anxiety: uneasiness or fear, often about a situation or condition.

apathy: a lack of interest.

aphasia: the inability to speak or to speak clearly.

apical pulse: the pulse on the left side of the chest, just below the nipple.

arthritis: a general term that refers to inflammation of the joints.

artificial airway: any plastic, metal or rubber device inserted into the respiratory tract to promote breathing.

asepsis: a state in which no pathogens are present.

aspiration: : the inhalation of food or drink into the lungs; can cause pneumonia or death.

assisted living: facilities where residents live who need some assistance, but do not usually require skilled care.

assistive devices: special equipment that helps a person who is ill or disabled to perform ADLs; also called adaptive devices.

asthma: a chronic inflammatory disease that makes it difficult to breathe and causes coughing and wheezing.

atrophy: the wasting away, decreasing in size, and weakening of muscles.

barrier: a block or obstacle.

baseline: initial values that can be compared to future measurements.

bed sore: a serious wound resulting from skin breakdown; also known as pressure sore or decubitus ulcer.

benign: non-cancerous.

benign prostatic hypertrophy: a disorder in which the prostate becomes enlarged, causing problems with urination and/or emptying the bladder.

bias: prejudice.

bipolar disorder: a type of depression that causes a person to swing from deep depression to extreme activity; also called manic depression.

bloodborne pathogens: microorganisms found in human blood; can cause infection and disease in humans.

body mechanics: the way the parts of the body work together whenever a person moves.

bony prominences: areas of the body where the bone lies close to the skin.

bowel elimination: the process of emptying the colon of stool or feces.

brachial pulse: the pulse inside of the elbow.

bronchiectasis: a condition in which the bronchi are opened out too wide; causes coughing and shortness of breath.

bronchitis: an irritation and inflammation of the lining of the bronchi.

calculi: kidney stones.

cancer: a general term used to describe many types of malignant tumors.

cardiopulmonary resuscitation (CPR): medical procedures used when a person's heart or lungs have stopped working.

care plan: a plan developed for each resident to achieve certain goals; it outlines the steps and tasks the care team must perform.

care team: people with different kinds of education and experience who help care for residents.

cataract: a condition in which the lens of the eye becomes cloudy, causing vision loss.

catastrophic reaction: overreacting to something in an unreasonable way.

catheter: a tube used to drain urine from the bladder.

cells: building blocks of the body; they divide, grow, and die, renewing tissues and organs.

Centers for Disease Control and Prevention (CDC): a federal government agency that issues guidelines to protect and improve health.

cerebral palsy: a disorder resulting from brain damage while a person is in the uterus or during birth; can cause physical and mental disabilities.

cerebral vascular accident (CVA): a condition caused when the blood supply to the brain is cut off suddenly by a clot or a ruptured blood vessel; also called stroke.

chain of command: term to describe the line of authority in a facility.

chain of infection: a way to describe how disease is transmitted from one living being to another.

charting: writing down information.

chemical restraints: medications given to control a person's behavior.

chest tubes: hollow drainage tubes inserted into the chest; they drain air, blood, or fluid that has collected inside the pleural space.

Cheyne-Stokes: slow, irregular respirations or rapid, shallow respirations that usually occur when a person is dying.

chlamydia: an infection is caused by organisms in the mucous membranes of the reproductive tract; can cause pelvic inflammatory disease (PID) and sterility.

chronic illness: an illness or condition that is long-term or long-lasting.

chronic kidney failure: condition in which the kidneys cannot eliminate certain waste products; becomes worse over time.

chronic obstructive pulmonary disease: a chronic lung disease that causes trouble breathing.

circadian rhythm: the 24-hour day-night cycle.

cite: to find a problem through a survey.

claustrophobia: the fear of being in a confined space.

clean: a condition in which an object has not been contaminated with pathogens.

clean catch specimen: specimen that does not include the first and last urine; also called mid-stream.

closed bed: a bed completely made with the bedspread and blankets in place.

cognition: the act of thinking logically and quickly.

colostomy: removal of part of the intestine; causes stool to be semi-solid.

combative: violent or hostile.

combustion: the process of burning.

communication: the process of exchanging information with others.

compassionate: being caring, concerned, considerate, empathetic, and understanding.

condom catheter: a catheter that has an attachment on the end that fits onto the penis; also called an external or Texas catheter.

confusion: an inability to think clearly.

congestive heart failure: a condition in which the heart muscle is damaged and cannot pump effectively; blood backs up into the heart instead of circulating.

conscientious: always trying to do one's best.

conscious: the state of being mentally alert and having awareness of surroundings, sensations, and thoughts.

constipation: the inability to have a bowel movement.

constrict: to narrow.

Contact Precautions: special measures used when a person is at risk of transmitting or contracting a microorganism from touching an infected object or person.

contracture: the permanent and painful stiffening of a joint and muscle.

coping mechanisms: reactions used to cope with stress.

coronary artery disease: a condition in which blood vessels in the coronary arteries narrow, lowering blood supply to the heart and depriving it of oxygen and nutrients.

crutches: adaptive devices used for people who can bear no weight or limited weight on one leg.

cultural diversity: the variety of people living and working together in the world.

culture: a system of behaviors people learn from the people they grow up and live with.

cyanotic: skin that is pale or blue.

cystitis: inflammation of the bladder; may be caused by bacterial infection.

dandruff: excessive shedding of dead skin cells from the scalp.

dangle: to sit up with the feet over the side of the bed to regain balance.

decubitus ulcer: a serious wound resulting from skin breakdown; also known as pressure sore or bed sore.

defense mechanisms: unconscious behaviors used to release tension or cope with stress.

degenerative: something that continually gets worse.

dehydration: a serious condition in which there is not enough fluid in the body.

delegation: transferring authority to a person for a specific task.

delirium: a state of severe confusion.

delusion: a belief in something that is not true, or is out of touch with reality.

dementia: a serious loss of mental abilities such as thinking, remembering, reasoning, and communicating.

dentures: artificial teeth.

depression: an illness that causes withdrawal, lack of energy, and loss of interest in activities, as well as other symptoms.

developmental disabilities: a chronic condition that restricts physical or mental abilities.

diabetes: a condition in which the pancreas does not produce enough insulin; causes problems with circulation and can damage vital organs.

diabetic coma: a life-threatening complication of diabetes that can result from undiagnosed diabetes, not enough insulin, eating too much, not getting enough exercise, and stress; also known as acidosis or hyperglycemia.

diagnoses: medical conditions.

dialysis: a process that cleanses the body of waste that the kidneys cannot remove due to kidney failure.

diarrhea: frequent elimination of liquid or semi-liquid feces.

diastolic: second measurement of blood pressure; phase when the heart relaxes.

diet cards: cards that list residents' names and information about special diets, allergies, likes and dislikes, and any other instructions.

digestion: the process of breaking down food so that it can be absorbed into the cells.

dilate: to widen.

direct contact: way to transmit pathogens through touching the infected person or his or her secretions.

dirty: a condition in which an object has been contaminated with pathogens.

disinfection: a measure used to decrease the spread of pathogens and disease by destroying pathogens.

disorientation: confusion about person, place, or time.

disposable: equipment designed to be thrown away after one use.

disruptive: any behavior that disturbs others.

diuretics: drugs that reduce fluid in the body.

DNR: an order tells medical professionals not to perform CPR.

domestic violence: abuse by spouses, intimate partners, or family members.

dorsal recumbent: a position in which the person is flat on his or her back with the knees flexed and the feet flat on the bed.

double-bagging: putting waste in a trash bag, closing it, and putting the first bag in a second, clean trash bag and closing it.

Down syndrome: a type of developmental disability in which people have different degrees of mental retardation, along with physical symptoms.

drainage: fluid from a wound or a cavity.

draw sheet: an extra sheet placed on top of a bottom sheet; it allows repositioning of a person without causing shearing.

Droplet Precautions: special measures used when the disease-causing microorganism does not stay suspended in the air and usually travels only short distances after being expelled.

Durable Power of Attorney for Health Care: a signed, dated, and witnessed paper that appoints someone else to make the medical decisions for a person in the event he or she becomes unable to do so

dysphagia: trouble swallowing.

dyspnea: difficulty breathing; shortness of breath.

edema: swelling caused by excess fluid in body tissues.

elimination: the process of expelling wastes.

emotional lability: laughing or crying without any reason, or when it is inappropriate.

empathy: being able to enter into the feelings of others.

emphysema: a chronic lung disease; usually results from chronic bronchitis and smoking.

enema: a specific amount of water flowed into the colon to eliminate stool.

epilepsy: an illness of the brain that causes seizures.

epistaxis: the medical term for a nosebleed.

ergonomics: the practice of designing equipment and work tasks to suit a worker's abilities.

ethics: the knowledge of right and wrong.

expiration: exhaling air out of the lungs.

expressive aphasia: an inability to express needs through speech or written words.

fallacy: a false belief.

farsightedness: the ability to see distant objects better than objects nearby.

fecal impaction: a hard stool stuck in the rectum that cannot be expelled.

fecal incontinence: the inability to control the bowels.

feces: solid waste products eliminated by the colon; also called stool.

financial abuse: stealing, taking advantage of, or improperly using the money, property, or other assets of another.

first aid: care given in an emergency before trained medical professionals can take over.

flammable: easily ignited and capable of burning quickly.

flatus: air in the intestine that is passed through the rectum; also called gas.

fluid balance: taking in and eliminating equal amounts of fluid.

fluid overload: a condition in which the body cannot handle the fluid consumed.

Food Guide Pyramid: A guide for healthy eating developed by the U.S. Department of Agriculture.

force fluids: a medical order for a person to drink more fluids.

fracture pan: a bedpan that is flatter than the regular bedpan; used for people who cannot assist with raising their hips onto a regular bedpan.

fractures: broken bones.

gait belt: a belt made of canvas or other heavy material used to assist people who are able to walk but are weak, unsteady, or uncoordinated; also called a transfer belt.

gait: manner of walking.

gastroesophageal reflux disease (GERD): a chronic condition in which the liquid contents of the stomach back up into the esophagus; causes bleeding or ulcers and difficulty swallowing.

gastrostomy: an opening in the stomach and abdomen.

geriatrics: the study of health, wellness, and disease later in life.

gerontology: the study of the aging process in people from mid-life through old age.

gingivitis: an inflammation of the gums.

glands: structures that secrete hormones.

glaucoma: a condition in which the pressure in the eye increases, damaging the optic nerve and causing blindness.

glucose: natural sugar.

gonorrhea: a sexually transmitted diesase that can cause sterility if not treated.

graduate: a measuring container.

groin: the area from the pubis (area around the penis and scrotum) to the upper thighs.

grooming: practices to care for oneself, such as caring for fingernails and hair.

halitosis: bad breath.

hallucinations: seeing or hearing things that are not really there.

hand hygiene: handwashing with either plain or antiseptic soap and water and using alcohol-based hand rubs.

health: a state of complete physical, mental, and social well-being, and not merely the absence of disease.

hearing aid: a battery-operated device that amplifies sound.

heart attack: a condition in which blood flow to the heart is completely blocked and muscle cells die; also called a myocardial infarction.

heartburn: a condition that results from a weakening of the sphincter muscle which joins the esophagus and the stomach.

Heimlich maneuver: a procedure that uses abdominal thrusts to move a blockage upward, out of the throat, when a person is choking.

hemiparesis: weakness on one side of the body.

hemiplegia: paralysis on one side of the body.

hemorrhoids: enlarged veins in the rectum that can cause itching, burning, pain, and bleeding.

hepatitis: inflammation of the liver caused by infection; can cause damaged liver function and other chronic, life-long illnesses.

herpes simplex II: a sexually transmitted disease caused by a virus; repeated outbreaks of the disease occur for the rest of the person's life and it cannot be cured.

hoarding: collecting and putting things away in a guarded way.

holistic: care that involves the whole person, including physical and psychosocial needs.

home health care: care that takes place in a person's home.

homeostasis: the condition in which all of the body's systems are working their best.

hormones: chemical substances created by the body that control numerous body functions.

hospice: special care for a dying person needs; uses a holistic, compassionate approach and involves the dying person and his or her family.

human immunodeficiency virus (HIV): a virus that attacks the body's immune system and gradually disables it; eventually causes AIDS.

hygiene: ways to keep bodies clean and healthy.

hypertension: high blood pressure.

hypotension: low blood pressure.

ileostomy: removal of part of the intestine; causes liquid stool.

impairment: a loss of function or ability.

incident: an accident or unexpected event during the course of care.

incontinence: the inability to control the bladder or bowels.

indirect contact: way to transmit pathogens from touching something contaminated by the infected person.

indwelling catheter: a catheter that stays inside the bladder for a period of time; urine drains into a bag.

infection: the state resulting from pathogens invading and growing within the human body.

infection control: set of methods used to control and prevent the spread of disease.

infectious: contagious.

inflammation: swelling.

informed consent: the process in which a person, with the help of a doctor, makes informed decisions about his or her health care.

input: the fluid a person consumes; also called intake.

inspiration: the process of breathing air into the lungs.

insulin shock: a life-threatening complication of diabetes that can result from either too much insulin or too little food; also known as hypoglycemia.

intake: the fluid a person consumes; also called input.

integument: natural protective covering.

intervention: a way to change an action or development.

intravenous (IV): into a vein.

intubation: the method used to insert an artificial airway; involves passing a plastic tube through the mouth or nose and into the trachea or windpipe.

involuntary seclusion: confinement or separation from others in a certain area; done without consent or against one's will.

involved: a weakened side from a stroke or injury; also called the affected or weaker side.

irreversible: a disease or condition that cannot be cured.

irritable bowel syndrome: a chronic form of stomach upset that gets worse from stress.

isolate: to keep something separate or by itself.

job description: an outline of what will be expected in a job.

knee-chest: a position in which a person is lying on his or her abdomen with the knees pulled towards the abdomen and legs separated; arms are pulled up and flexed, and the head is turned to one side.

kosher: prepared according to Jewish dietary laws.

lactose intolerance: the inability to digest lactose, a type of sugar found in milk and other dairy products.

laws: rules set by the government to protect people and help them live peacefully together.

length of stay: the number of days a person stays in a healthcare facility.

lever: something that moves an object by resting on a base of support.

liability: a legal term that means someone can be held responsible for harming someone else.

licensed practical nurse or licensed vocational nurse: a licensed professional who has completed one to two years of education; LPN/LVN passes medications, gives treatments, and supervises daily care of residents.

lithotomy: position in which a person lies on his or her back with hips at the edge of the exam table, legs flexed, and feet in stirrups.

Living Will: document that states the medical care a person wants, or does not want, in case he or she becomes unable to make those decisions him- or herself.

localized infection: an infection limited to a specific part of the body; has local symptoms.

logrolling: method of moving a person as a unit, without disturbing the alignment of the body.

long-term care: care for people who require 24-hour care and assistance for conditions that are long-term.

major depression: a type of depression that may cause a person to lose interest in everything he or she once cared about.

malabsorption: a condition in which a body cannot absorb or digest a particular nutrient properly.

malignant: cancerous.

malnutrition: a serious condition in which a person is not getting proper nutrition.

manic depression: a type of depression that causes a person to swing from deep depression to extreme activity; also called bipolar disorder.

masturbation: to touch or rub sexual organs in order to give oneself or another person sexual pleasure.

Material Safety Data Sheet: a sheet detailing chemical ingredients, chemical dangers, emergency response actions to be taken, and safety handling procedures for dangerous chemicals.

mechanical ventilator: a machine that literally breathes for a person.

medical social worker: person who helps with social needs at a facility.

menopause: the stopping of menstrual periods.

mental abuse: emotionally harming a person by threatening, scaring, humiliating, intimidating, isolating, insulting, or treating him or her as a child; includes verbal abuse.

mental health: the normal function of emotional and intellectual abilities.

mental illness: a disease that disrupts a person's ability to function at a normal level in the family, home, or community.

mental retardation: a developmental disorder that causes people to develop at a below-average rate and to have below-average mental functioning; difficulty in learning and problems adjusting socially may be present.

metabolism: physical and chemical processes.

microorganism: a tiny living thing always present in the environment; not visible to the eye without a microscope.

Minimum Data Set (MDS): a detailed form with guidelines for assessing residents in nursing homes; also details what to do if resident problems are identified.

modified diet: a special diet for people who have certain illnesses; also called therapeutic diet.

MRSA: an infectious disease caused by bacteria that are resistant to many antibiotics; can develop when people do not take all of the medication prescribed to them.

mucous membranes: the linings of the mouth, nose, eyes, rectum, or genitals.

multi-drug resistant TB: disease that occurs when the full course of medication is not taken for tuberculosis (TB); the "strongest" bacilli are left and are less likely to be killed by medication.

multi-drug-resistant organisms: microorganisms, mostly bacteria, that are resistant to one or more antimicrobial agents.

multiple sclerosis: a progressive disease of the nervous system in which the protective covering for the nerves, spinal cord, and white matter of the brain breaks down over time; without this covering, nerves cannot send messages to and from the brain in a normal way.

myocardial infarction: a condition in which blood flow to the heart is completely blocked and muscle cells die; also called a heart attack.

NPO: medical abbreviation that stands for "nothing by mouth."

nasogastric tube: a special feeding tube that is inserted into the nose going to the stomach.

nearsightedness: the ability to see things near but not far.

neglect: harming a person physically, mentally, or emotionally by failing to give needed care.

nitroglycerin: medication that relaxes the walls of the coronary arteries.

nonverbal communication: communication without using words.

non-weight bearing (NWB): the inability to support any weight on one or both legs.

nosocomial infection: an infection acquired in a hospital or other healthcare facility; also known as hospital-acquired infection (HAI).

nursing assistant: person at a facility who does assigned tasks and gives personal care.

nursing process: an organized method used by nurses to determine the nursing care for residents.

nutrition: how the body uses food to maintain health.

nutritionist: person at a facility who creates diets for residents with special needs; also called a registered dietitian.

objective information: information collected by using the senses.

obsessive compulsive disorder: disorder in which a person uses obsessive behavior to cope with anxiety.

obstructed airway: a condition in which a person has something blocking the tube through which air enters the lungs.

occult: hidden.

occupational therapist: person at a facility who helps residents learn to compensate for disabilities.

occupied bed: a bed made while a person is in the bed.

ombudsman: person assigned by law as the legal advocate for residents; this person visits the facility, listens to residents, and decides what course of action to take if there is a problem.

Omnibus Budget Reconciliation Act (OBRA): law passed by the federal government; includes minimum standards for nursing assistant training, staffing requirements, resident assessment instructions, and information on rights for residents.

onset: the time the signs and symptoms of a disease begin.

open bed: bed made with linen folded down to the foot of the bed.

organ: a structural unit in the human body that performs a specific function.

OSHA: a federal government agency that makes rules to protect workers from hazards on the job.

osteoarthritis: a type of arthritis that usually affects hips and knees and joints of the fingers, thumbs, and spine.

osteoporosis: a condition in which the bones become brittle and weak; may be due to age, lack of hormones, not enough calcium in bones, alcohol, or lack of exercise.

ostomy: an operation to create an opening from an area inside the body to the outside.

outpatient care: care usually given for less than 24 hours; for people who need short-term skilled care.

output: eliminated fluid in urine, feces, and vomitus; also includes perspiration and moisture in the air that is exhaled.

oxygen concentrator: a device that changes air in the room into air with more oxygen.

pacing: walking back and forth in the same area.

palliative: care that focuses on the comfort and dignity of the person, rather than on curing him or her.

panic disorder: a disorder in which a person is terrified for no known reason.

paranoid schizophrenia: a brain disorder that centers mainly on hallucinations and delusions.

paraplegia: a loss of function of lower body and legs.

paresis: paralysis, or loss of ability, of only part of the body.

Parkinson's disease: a progressive disease that causes the brain to degenerate; causes stooped posture, shuffling gait, pill-rolling, and tremors.

partial bath: a bath that includes washing the face, underarms, and hands, and performing perineal care.

partial weight bearing (PWB): the ability to support some weight on one of both legs.

passive range of motion: exercises that are used when people cannot move on their own.

pathogen: disease-causing microorganism.

pediculosis: an infestation of lice.

PEG tube: a tube placed through the skin directly into the stomach to assist with eating.

peptic ulcers: raw sores in the stomach or the small intestine; can cause pain, vomiting and bleeding.

perineum: the genitals and anus and the area between them.

peripheral vascular disease: a condition in which the legs, feet, arms or hands do not have enough blood circulation.

perseveration: the repetition of words, phrases, questions, or actions.

personal: refers to life outside one's job, such as family, friends, and home life.

personal protective equipment (PPE): a barrier between a person and disease.

phantom sensation: pain or feeling from a body part that has been amputated; caused by remaining nerve endings.

phlegm: thick mucus from the respiratory passages.

phobia: an intense form of anxiety.

physical abuse: any treatment, intentional or not, that causes harm to a person's body; includes slapping, bruising, cutting, burning, physically restraining, pushing, shoving, or rough handling.

physical therapist: person at a facility who gives therapy in the form of heat, cold, massage, ultrasound, electricity, and exercise to people with muscle, bone, and joint problems.

pillaging: taking things that belong to someone else.

plaque: a substance that forms in a brief period of time if oral care is not done regularly.

pneumonia: acute inflammation in the lung tissue caused by a bacterial, viral, or fungal infection; causes high fever, chills, cough, chest pains, and rapid pulse.

policy: a course of action to be followed.

portable commode: a chair with a toilet seat and a removable container under it.

positioning: helping people into positions that will be comfortable and healthy for them.

post-traumatic stress disorder: anxiety-related disorder caused by a traumatic experience.

postmortem care: care of the body after death.

pre-diabetes: condition in which a person's blood glucose levels are above normal but not high enough for a diagnosis of type 2 diabetes.

prehypertension: condition in which a person does not have high blood pressure now but is likely to develop it in the future.

pressure points: areas of the body that bear much of its weight.

pressure sore: a serious wound resulting from skin breakdown; also known as decubitus ulcer or bed sore.

procedure: a method, or way, of doing something.

professional: having to do with work or a job.

professionalism: how a person behaves when he or she is on the job.

progressive: something that continually gets worse.

prosthesis: an artificial body part.

protected health information (PHI): health information must be kept private by law; includes name, address, telephone number, social security number, e-mail address, and medical record number.

psychological abuse: emotionally harming a person by threatening, scaring, humiliating, intimidating, isolating, insulting, or treating him or her as a child; also includes verbal abuse.

psychosocial needs: needs which involve social interaction, emotions, intellect, and spirituality.

pulse oximeter: device that measures a person's blood oxygen level and pulse rate.

puree: to chop, blend, or grind food into a thick paste of baby food consistency.

quad cane: a cane with four rubber-tipped feet; used for people can bear a little weight.

quadriplegia: loss of function of legs, trunk, and arms.

radial pulse: the pulse on the inside of the wrist, where the radial artery runs just beneath the skin.

range of motion: exercises that put a joint through its full arc of motion.

Reality Orientation: uses calendars, clocks, signs, and lists to help people with Alzheimer's disease remember who and where they are.

registered dietitian: person at a facility who creates diets for residents with special needs; also called a nutritionist.

registered nurse (RN): a licensed professional who has completed two to four years of education; RNs assess residents' status, monitor progress, provide skilled nursing care, give treatments, and supervise nursing assistants' daily care of residents.

rehabilitation: managed by professionals to restore a person to the highest possible level of functioning after an illness or injury.

Reminiscence Therapy: encouraging people with Alzheimer's disease to remember and talk about the past.

repetitive phrasing: repeating a word or phrase over and over.

residents: the people who live in nursing homes.

Residents' Rights: numerous rights identified by the OBRA law for residents in nursing homes; purpose is to inform residents and others of their rights within these facilities and to provide an ethical code of conduct for healthcare workers.

resistant: condition in which drugs no longer work to kill specific germs.

respiration: the process of breathing air into the lungs and exhaling air out of the lungs.

restorative services: services used to keep a person at the level achieved by the rehabilitation team.

restraint: a physical or chemical way to restrict voluntary movement or behavior.

restraint alternatives: any intervention used in place of a restraint or that reduces the need for a restraint.

restraint-free: an environment in which restraints are not used for any reason.

restrict fluids: a medical order that limits the amount of fluids a person takes in.

résumé: a summary of education and experience.

rheumatoid arthritis: a type of arthritis in which joints become red, swollen, and very painful and movement is restricted.

routine urine specimen: a specimen collected any time a person voids.

scalds: burns caused by hot liquids.

schizophrenia: a brain disorder that affects a person's ability to think and communicate clearly, as well as manage emotions, make decisions, and understand reality.

scope of practice: defines the things a nursing assistant is allowed to do and how to do them correctly.

sexual abuse: forcing a person to perform or participate in sexual acts.

sexual harassment: any unwelcome sexual advance or behavior that creates an intimidating, hostile or offensive working environment.

sexually transmitted diseases: diseases passed through sexual contact; includes sexual intercourse, contact of the mouth with the genitals or anus, and contact of the hands to the genitals.

sharps: needles or other sharp objects.

shearing: friction and pressure on the skin from rubbing or dragging it across surfaces.

situation response: a temporary condition caused by a crisis, temporary physical changes in the brain, side effects or interactions from medications, and severe change in the environment.

sitz bath: a warm soak of the perineal area to clean perineal wounds, and reduce inflammation and pain.

skilled care: medically necessary care given by a skilled nurse or therapist.

slip knot: a quick-release knot used to tie restraints so that they can be removed quickly when needed.

special diet: a diet for people who have certain illnesses; also called therapeutic or modified diet.

specimen: a sample.

speech language pathologist or speech therapist: a person at a facility who helps with speech and swallowing problems.

sphincter: a ring-like muscle that opens and closes an opening in the body.

sphygmomanometer: device that measures blood pressure.

spina bifida: a condition in which part of the backbone is not well-developed at birth; can cause the spinal cord to bulge out of the back; can cause a range of disabilities.

sputum: mucus coughed up from the lungs.

Standard Precautions: a method of infection control in which all blood, body fluids, non-intact skin (like abrasions, pimples, or open sores), and mucous membranes (lining of mouth, nose, eyes, rectum, or genitals) are treated as if they were infected with a disease.

sterilization: a measure used to decrease the spread of pathogens and disease by destroying all microorganisms, not just pathogens.

stethoscope: an instrument for listening to sounds within the body.

stoma: an artificial opening in the body.

stool: solid waste products eliminated by the colon; also called feces.

straight cane: a cane that helps with balance; it is not designed to bear weight.

straight catheter: a catheter that does not stay inside the person; it is removed immediately after urine is drained.

stress: the state of being frightened, excited, confused, in danger, or irritated.

stressor: something that causes stress.

stroke: a condition caused when the blood supply to the brain is cut off suddenly by a clot or a ruptured blood vessel; also called CVA.

subacute care: care given in a hospital or in a nursing home; used for people who need more care and observation than some long-term care facilities can give.

subjective information: information that cannot be or was not observed; it is based on something reported that may or may not be true.

substance abuse: the use of legal or illegal drugs, cigarettes, or alcohol in a way that is harmful to oneself or others.

sundowning: a condition in which a person gets restless and agitated in the late afternoon, evening, or night.

suppository: a medication given rectally to cause a bowel movement.

surgical bed: a bed made to easily accept residents who must return to bed on stretchers.

surveys: inspections done every nine to 15 months by the state agency that licenses facilities.

sympathy: sharing in the feelings and difficulties of others.

syphilis: a sexually transmitted disease, that if left untreated, can cause brain damage, mental illness, and death.

systemic infection: an infection that occurs when pathogens enter the bloodstream and move throughout the body; causes general symptoms.

systolic: first measurement of blood pressure; phase where the heart is at work, contracting and pushing blood out of the left ventricle.

tact: the ability to understand what is proper and appropriate when dealing with others.

tartar: hard deposits on the teeth that are filled with bacteria; may cause gum disease and loose teeth if it is not removed by a dentist.

TB disease: a type of tuberculosis in which a person who shows symptoms of tuberculosis and can spread it to others; also called active TB.

TB infection: a type of tuberculosis in which a person who carries tuberculosis but does not show symptoms and cannot infect others; also called latent TB.

telemetry: the application of a device that collects information about the heart rhythm and rate.

terminal illness: a disease or condition that will eventually cause death.

therapeutic diet: a special diet for people who have certain illnesses; also called special or modified diet.

tissues: groups of cells that perform similar tasks.

total parenteral nutrition (TPN): a special type of feeding that bypasses the digestive system; the person receives nutrients directly into the bloodstream.

transfer belt: a belt made of canvas or other heavy material used to assist people who are able to walk but are weak, unsteady, or uncoordinated; also called a gait belt.

transient ischemic attack (TIA): a warning sign of a CVA, or stroke.

trigger: a situation that leads to agitation.

tuberculosis (TB): a bacterial infection that affects the lungs; it is transmitted through the air and causes coughing, difficulty breathing, fever, and fatigue.

tumor: a group of abnormally growing cells.

ulcerative colitis: a chronic inflammatory disease of the large intestine; causes cramping, diarrhea, pain, rectal bleeding, and loss of appetite.

unoccupied bed: a bed made while no person is in the bed.

ureterostomy: a condition in which an ureter is opened to abdomen for urine to be eliminated.

urinary tract infection: a disorder that causes inflammation of the bladder and the ureters; causes burning during urination and a frequent feeling of needing to urinate.

urination: the process of emptying the bladder of urine.

vaginitis: an infection of the vagina; may be caused by a bacteria, protozoa (one-celled animals), or fungus (yeast).

validating: giving value to or approving.

Validation Therapy: lets people with Alzheimer's disease believe they live in the past or in imaginary circumstances.

vegans: vegetarians who do not eat or use any animal products, including milk, cheese, other dairy items, eggs, wool, silk, and leather.

vegetarians: people who do not eat meat, fish, and poultry for religious, moral, or health reasons; they may or may not eat eggs and dairy products.

verbal abuse: oral or written words, pictures, or gestures that threaten, embarrass, or insult a person.

verbal communication: communication using words or sounds, spoken or written.

violent: actions that include attacking, hitting, or threatening someone.

vital signs: measurements that show how well the vital organs of the body are working.

voiding: emptying the bladder of urine.

VRE: a mutant strain of the bacterium enterococcus; it is a resistance caused by a person not taking all of a powerful antibiotic Vancomycin.

walker: adaptive equipment that is used when the resident can bear some weight on the legs; gives stability for people who are unsteady or lack balance.

wandering: walking aimlessly around the facility.

weaker: a weakened side from a stroke or injury; also called the affected or involved side.

wellness: successfully balancing things that happen in everyday lives; includes five different types: physical, social, emotional, intellectual, and spiritual.

will: a legal declaration of how a person wishes his or her possessions to be disposed of after death

workplace violence: abuse of staff by staff or a resident; can be verbal, physical, or sexual.

Index

A

B

C

D

E

F

G

Index

P

Q

R

S

T

Index

U

V

W